MEDICINE FOR
EXAMINATIONS

R. J. Epstein trained in medicine at the University of Sydney, University of Cambridge, and at Harvard Medical School. He is currently Reader at the University of London.

MEDICINE FOR EXAMINATIONS

Third edition

R. J. Epstein MD PhD FRACP

Senior Lecturer
University of London

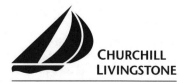

CHURCHILL LIVINGSTONE

EDINBURGH LONDON MADRID MELBOURNE NEW YORK SAN FRANCISCO AND TOKYO 1996

CHURCHILL LIVINGSTONE
Medical Division of Pearson Professional Limited

Distributed in the United States of America by
Churchill Livingstone Inc., 650 Avenue of the Americas,
New York, 10011 and by associated companies,
branches and representatives throughout the world.

First edition 1985
Second edition 1990
Third edition 1996

ISBN 0 443 05377 4

British Library Cataloguing in Publication Data
A catalogue record for this book is available from the
British Library.

Library of Congress Cataloging in Publication Data
A catalog record for this book is available from the
Library of Congress.

Medical knowledge is constantly changing. As new
information becomes available, changes in treatment,
procedures, equipment and the use of drugs become
necessary. The author and the publishers have, as far as
it is possible, taken care to ensure that the information
given in this text is accurate and up to date. However,
readers are strongly advised to confirm the information,
especially with regard to drug usage, complies with
current legislation and standards of practice.

The
publisher's
policy is to use
**paper manufactured
from sustainable forests**

Produced by Longman Singapore Publishers (Pte) Ltd.
Printed in Singapore

Contents

Preface to the Third Edition

FIRST, PASS YOUR EXAM . . .

Many medical trainees approach examinations as deadly serious affairs, but this is a mistake. Medical exams are a game and, as with all games, you get the most out of them by first learning the rules. The catch is that the 'rules' of medical exams are unwritten; as a result, all too many candidates end up learning these rules only by going from one exam to the next (a painful and costly approach). This third edition of *Medicine for Examinations* aims to transform the exam experience from one of academic 'musical chairs' to one which reflects the candidate's knowledge and ability.

Despite the claims of medical educators to be cutting back on boring old 'facts', in truth not even the most esoteric pearl of wisdom can be assumed unexaminable. If you flip through any well-thumbed textbook in your medical library, you'll observe an interesting phenomenon: namely, that readers have succeeded in emphasizing certain snippets of information using a variety of graphic techniques. That so much is left unemphasized suggests that the important information is camouflaged within a morass of verbiage.

The exam candidate can overcome this handicap by realizing that certain subsets of information lend themselves to the exam format. You are more likely to be asked something which has a specific and topical answer, for instance, than something which is equivocal or passé. *Medicine for Examinations* has been structured to take advantage of this bias. By presenting important clinical topics as discrete *packets of information,* this book aims to optimize study efficiency.

Since the last edition, the text has been completely revised, expanded and updated, with new sections concerning:

- updates on disease entities related to *Helicobater pylori*; Kawasaki syndrome; significance of Δ_{508} mutation in cystic fibrosis; alpha-1-antitrypsin deficiency; Lyme disease, catscratch disease; diseases mediated by prion particles or trinucleotide repeats; hepatitis C and E; factor V Leiden (protein C resistance); food-dependent Cushing's syndrome; myocardial reperfusion injury; in situ breast cancer; hormonal 'flare' reactions; colorectal carcinogenesis; HHV-8; and MALT
- new investigations such as high-resolution chest CT; ANCA; transesophageal echocardiography; and ^{99m}Tc-HIDA biliary scintigraphy
- new treatments such as colony-stimulating factors and erythropoietin; anti(retro)virals; proton pump inhibitors, misoprostol, sucralfate; mifepristone (RU486); atypical neuroleptics such as clozapine, risperidone; SSRIs such as fluoxetine (Prozac™); infertility treatments; somatostatin analogs; magnesium therapy; opioid receptors; new macrolides (clarithromycin, azithromycin) and fluoroquinolones (ciprofloxacin, norfloxacin); sumatriptan; new GABA agonists; and the therapeutic use of botulinum toxin

Serendipity plays a key role in clinical examinations. In the overall scheme of things, however, good candidates make their own luck. Discrepancies arise between the results of comparable candidates in any exam, but in the long run things even out. So don't be too downhearted if events fail to go as well as you had hoped; on the other hand, don't make the mistake of blaming Lady Luck when a little more preparation would have made the difference.

Instead, think positive — and pass.

London, 1996   R.J.E.

Acknowledgements

Many of the improvements to this third edition of *Medicine for Examinations* have been contributed by readers and colleagues. I would like particularly to thank Steve Cannistra, Mark Nidorf and Ian Turner for their very helpful suggestions; Laszlo Kondor for typing assistance; and Anne for support.

Any errors or oversimplifications, on the other hand, are my own responsibility, and I would be grateful to any person who takes the trouble to bring such matters to my attention.

All efforts have been made to check the accuracy of drug dosages and other therapeutic recommendations in this book. It is advised, however, that physicians consult other sources prior to prescribing any course of therapy mentioned in the book.

The Short Case

Q *Should I take beta-blockers before my viva?*

A Some people will regard even the mention of beta-blockers as a tacit advocation of pill-popping, analogous to drug abuse by Olympic athletes and racehorses. Hence, let it be clearly stated from the outset that most prospective clinical exam candidates will find the best remedy for disabling exam nerves to be plain hard work — practice, practice, and more practice.

Beta-blockers *are* used, however, by an increasing number of people who suffer from stage fright. Indeed, many irrepressibly 'adrenergic' exam candidates have come to regard beta-blockers as a godsend. After all, if you find that every time you present a case your voice dries up, palpitations set the walls shaking, and puddles (of perspiration) appear on the floor, then you really can't be blamed for at least *thinking* about using a beta-blocker.

If the decision is made to seek pharmacologic assistance for exam nerves, a number of caveats apply:

1 Beta-blockers should be prescribed in the ordinary way by your own physician — not yourself — in accordance with all the usual precautions.

2 You should try them (in the same dosage you plan to use) in a comparable situation *before* your exam — and preferably on several occasions. The horror stories you have heard about the candidate who became so hypotensive that she had to lie down on the floor during the viva or the one who had his first experience of asthma in the middle of the oral are probably true.

3 Do not, whatever you do, use benzodiazepines, alcohol or cannabis to calm your nerves; apart from anything else, remember that such drugs induce amnesia and obtundation (some say this is also true to some extent of beta-blockers).

Q *What instruments should I carry into the exam?*

A You should carry the same instruments you've carried into all your previous practice cases. If there's one situation where your well-practised routines are going to break down, it will be under the duress of an exam and especially if your attention is distracted by an unfamiliar instrument, causing you to bungle something which would otherwise have won you brownie points. You must carry a watch with a second hand while other items advisable to sequester within your white coat include:

Stethoscope
Pen-light torch (with fresh batteries)
Tongue depressors
Red-topped hat pin
Disposable pins (for testing sensation; one per patient; discard safely), cotton wool
Short ruler (6", 15 cm) or tape measure (though width of fingers or hand can be used
Pocket visual acuity chart (read at 24"/60 cm)
Pen(s) and paper; tendon reflex hammer
Ophthalmoscope (with fresh batteries)
Tuning forks magnifying glass (for skin)

There is no need to get carried away with your armamentarium, since no amount of instruments will compensate for lack of skill in using them. It is not necessary to invest in a massive stethoscope, for example, if you can hear the low-pitched rumbling diastolic murmur of mitral stenosis with your current model — proper positioning of the patient and knowing what to listen for are more important than the acoustics of your tubes. Nor is it mandatory to carry a white-topped pin for testing peripheral vision or separate tuning forks for vibration and auditory testing (128 cps and 256/512 cps respectively). You won't be penalized if you can't afford your own ophthalmoscope, but it doesn't hurt if you do have one — the big advantage is that you're used to using it.

Don't bother carrying your own auriscope, thermometer or blood pressure cuff; even in a long case, any diagnostic items not present can be requested from an attendant. Inevitably, some obsessional long-case candidates will feel more secure in bringing additional diagnostic aids such as mydriatic drops, urinalysis strips (plus an MSU container), Hemoccult kits (together with glove, gauze, lubricant) and/or Schirmer's test papers — but this is probably going over the top.

In the event of a neurologic examination (speech or higher centres), you could impress by coming with a 'test kit' including such items as: (1) written orders, e.g. 'Stick out your tongue', 'Point to a chair'; (2) a card to read aloud, e.g. 'The war broke out last December'; (3) illustrations, e.g. the Queen, Donald Duck, map of England; (4) paper and pen for writing words, drawing clockfaces, five-pointed stars, houses and other items of neurologic interest.

Irrespective of whether or not you carry your own instruments, be sure to mention that you would like to take the temperature and blood pressure, look at the fundi, test sensation, do a pelvic examination, urinalysis and all those little things necessary for persuading the examiner that you are the real clinical McCoy and not just an exam day tripper.

Q *How do I impress the examiners on the day?*

A Most of the books written about medical exams tell you to keep your fingernails clean, do not wear a low-cut dress (particularly if you are male), etc. More constructive advice, however, will depend on what sort of qualification you are seeking. If you are sitting for medical school finals, the examiners will be (or at least should be) trying their hardest to pass you. They will expect only that your performance confirms that:

1 Your knowledge is sound;
2 Your demeanor is sensible;
3 Your approach is safe.

That is, they want to see that you have bothered to spend at least *some* time in the wards and that you are not a Martian or some sort of lunatic. In this context the examiners are definitely on your side: set your standards to what you are, not to what you imagine they might want you to be.

If, on the other hand, you are sniffing around for a postgraduate qualification, your examiners will be more discerning — it's not only Martians and lunatics who find themselves poorly regarded in this setting. The successful candidate will appear knowledgeable and sensible, but will also exude an aura of sufficient experience and maturity that their examiners would sleep happily at night if that candidate was looking after their patients. If you find this point difficult to grasp, try getting somebody to videotape you presenting a case; it may prove a salient exercise in self-criticism.

Alternatively, practise your presentation style on your partner or even into a mirror. Ask yourself the question: am I convincing? Don't just dream it, be it. Treat the exam (and your rehearsals for it) not as some sort of audition but rather as a discussion between peers. If you can't persuade yourself that you're ready to take on this role, then perhaps you're not yet ready to sit your exam.

Apart from these considerations, the best advice is still to be found in the old chestnuts which have been trotted out to prospective examinees for decades:

1 **More is missed by not looking than not knowing** (Riordan's corollary: *if you don't put your finger in it, you put your foot in it*). The reassurance you can draw from this is that motivation and hard work are more important than talent, flair or genius — in medical exams, that is, albeit not necessarily in life. Fortune, as Pasteur once mumbled, favors the prepared mind. If you are given an ambiguous introduction to a short case (such as, 'Examine this man's chest'), err on the side of being too thorough — that is, go for the *systematic* approach wherever possible. At worst you'll get a growling reprimand

EXAMINER: *'I told you to examine his **chest**, didn't I, not his frigging hands!'*

which will make the instruction immediately clear.

Having said this, you should also try to get to the 'guts' of any case in reasonable time, minimizing the time spent on parts of the examination likely to be non-contributory. For example, if a patient's legs reveal gross fasciculations, wasting, brisk reflexes and extensor plantar responses, you are not automatically obliged to proceed to pin-sticking and cotton wool dabbing.

Instead, don't be afraid to suggest to your examiners that you would now like to tap out the reflexes in the upper limbs and jaw and to examine the bulbar musculature. After all, even if you are directed to persevere with the sensory examination, you will have at least given notice that you're capable of thinking on your feet.

2 **Common things are common** — even, it must be said, in medical exams. Don't speculate that the fundal hemorrhages might be due to hyperviscosity unless you have actively excluded diabetes and hypertension. Of course, the real fun of short case vivas lies in the paradox that *certain* (chronic) uncommon things appear relatively commonly, e.g. Argyll-Robertson pupils, pretibial myxedema, Eisenmenger's syndrome, etc. Everyone admits that such conditions are rare in day-to-day clinical practice — but, oh boy, if there's one in the vicinity at the time of the exam, you can rest assured it'll be trotted out.

3 **Take your time,** especially at the beginning of each case. Show concern for the patient — this needs to be done as theatrically as any other aspect of the physical examination. Introduce yourself by name, shake hands, ask permission to examine them, help them get undressed and in position. Do not, whatever you do, treat the patient like a piece of meat. When exposing the area to be examined, at least pay lip service to their modesty by enquiring whether they are warm. Don't poke, flick or bash and take care when examining plantar reflexes, breasts, testicles and other sensitive areas. If you inadvertently distress the patient during the performance (sorry, examination), display enough remorse to ensure you can't be accused of wanton inhumanity. Private anguish may win you a place in heaven, but it won't help you through a short case viva.

When you have finished your examination and have been asked for your findings, *think before you speak*. A candidate who thinks before speaking (and, just as importantly, is seen to do so) will be regarded as safe; whereas one who speaks without thinking will seem immature and foolhardy. If you are questioned by the examiner, listen closely and then answer — sounds simple, doesn't it? It becomes a lot simpler if you get into the habit of consciously thinking while you are examining. To do this well requires lots of practice; if you start describing your findings without any idea of how they fit together, you'll be unlikely to impress. Don't underestimate the value of information gleaned from the end of the bed — if you can see immediately that you're being asked to examine a patient with ascites or exophthalmos or hemiparesis or a mastectomy, it makes life a lot easier. The 'Diagnostic Pathways' in this book are intended to illustrate how recognition of an obvious physical sign such as this may be the seed around which a diagnostic pattern can be crystallized. If you leave the patient without a 'bottom line' diagnosis, always ask to go back if given the chance; it's worth being a bit pushy if it saves having to do the exam again.

4 **Only state 'barn-door' clinical signs in the first instance** — at all costs avoid indecisive references to 'early clubbing', 'slight papilledema', etc. If the patient really does have cerebral metastases from a lung carcinoma, the examiners will generally redirect your attention to the equivocal signs, e.g.:

EXAMINER: *Did you . . . ah . . . think he was clubbed?*

CANDIDATE: *Sir, to be honest I did at first glance — but on closer inspection the nailfold angle seemed relatively normal, and there was rather less nailbed fluctuation than expected . . .*

EXAMINER: *I see. And, er, the fundi, you thought they were . . .*

CANDIDATE: *Well, sir, I couldn't see any venous pulsations and the disc margins were somewhat indistinct – so I'd like to . . . er . . . examine for enlargement of the blind spot since this would . . . ah . . . be consistent with papilledema.*

EXAMINER (sighing): *Mmmm, well . . . yes, why don't you go ahead and do that . . .*

If you can justify your uncertainty, it is difficult for an examiner to penalize you too severely; whereas if you claim abnormalities which aren't there, you could easily talk yourself into a corner from which there is no escape. In the event that you realize you've made an error, be decisive in admitting it — if you can rechannel the conversation quickly enough, the damage may be minimal.

Avoid mix-and-matching signs and 'cliché' jargon. If for some reason you think a patient with all the signs of pure aortic stenosis has a somewhat 'tapping' quality to his apex beat — irrespective of how beautifully the term may seem to describe this particular patient's sign — don't say so. Similarly, don't refer to the malar flush of a patient with a valvotomy scar as a 'butterfly rash', the high-stepping gait of a patient with footdrop as 'stamping' or the rusty sputum of a patient with pneumonia as 'anchovy sauce'. By the same token, of course, not all patients with hypopituitarism have 'alabaster' skin, just as not all acromegalics have bitemporal hemianopia — so don't get too tendentious. You should also eschew the use of sloppy language, such as brand names (e.g. Lasix for frusemide, Zantac for ranitidine) or abbreviations:

EXAMINER: *All right then, how could your findings help explain his symptoms?*

CANDIDATE: *Sir, I believe this man's neurological symptoms are due to MS, his lethargy to MF, his indigestion to his HSV, and his backache to PID.*

The examiner may be less than impressed if he misinterprets your 'multiple sclerosis' acronym as 'mitral stenosis', your 'myelofibrosis' as 'mycosis fungoides', your 'highly selective vagotomy' as 'herpes simplex virus' and your 'prolapsed intervertebral disc' as 'pelvic inflammatory disease'. . . Unless you say what you mean, you'll never mean what you say.

5 The greatest fool may ask questions which the wisest man can't answer. While it's best to avoid quoting this particular rule of thumb during the exam, don't get all defensive if you happen to hit a bare patch of hippocampus — just admit it and get on to something else, keeping in mind that there are plenty of things your examiners don't know either. Indeed, some are notorious for saying things like, 'No, I don't know that either' after asking you something weird. Don't waffle; instead, disarm them with candour. If the examiner persists in asking 'difficult' questions, it could mean:

1 You are doing brilliantly and they are simply trying to stretch your obviously considerable talents to the limit;

2 You have completely misunderstood the line of questioning and they are desperately trying to redirect you; or

3 You are stuck with a rotten examiner who wants to play the 'guess-what-I'm-thinking-of' game (they do exist) and who justifies such torture by alluding to the stresses of clinical practice.

A reasonable ploy if you are in this fix is to ask for the question to be rephrased (rather than risking irritation by demanding that it be 'repeated'), thus giving you a few more seconds to think and putting the onus on them to clarify what they're getting at. Don't cave in and moan, 'I don't understand', or they'll be sure to take you for a ninny. Put the ball back in their court by obliging them to guide your thoughts.

On no account betray any sign of agitation throughout the ordeal. Rather, concentrate on impressing the examiners with your professionalism and imperturbability — as distinct from aloofness or overconfidence, which are politically fatal. Never give up, no matter how badly you feel things are going; exams are too traumatic to be used simply as a tutorial for a repeat performance.

6 It's all show biz. Clinical examinations are not a showcase for shrinking violets or wallflowers, but a chance to be the centre of attention (if not quite famous) for 15 minutes. And that's a chance you need to grasp with both hands. Exaggerate things a little bit, don't be shy. You are not there just to elicit physical signs, but also to *be seen* eliciting them — not unlike a magician is seen to pull a rabbit from a hat. If the liver is enlarged or the jugular venous pulse elevated, don't just leave it at that: take out your ruler and (hey presto) measure the abnormality. If you are demonstrating a straightforward neurological deficit, do so with as much flair as you can muster, just short of declaring *'Voilà!'*. If, after completing the examination requested, you are asked if there is anything else you would like to look at, this is your cue to spring into action:

CANDIDATE: *Sir, I would also like to examine the lungfields for basal crepitations, feel for sacral and peripheral edema, check for ascites and hepatic distension, look for calf tenderness, take the temperature and blood pressure, examine the fundi, and perform a urinalysis.*

When asked to present your findings, don't be coy if you are fairly sure you have twigged to the diagnosis: instead, try bowling them over at the outset with something solid like:

CANDIDATE: *Sir, this patient has physical signs consistent with aortic stenosis of moderate severity. On general inspection . . .*

If you are unsure of the diagnosis, on the other hand, limit yourself to describing the signs; volunteer a differential diagnosis (with all the attendant pros and cons of each one) only when asked. Use non-eponymous signs to describe your findings in the first instance, rather than insisting on baffling your examiners with biographical irrelevancies.

In summary:

1 Be calm, but not blasé
2 Be well-prepared, but not stale
3 Be thorough, but not mechanical
4 Be decisive, but not foolhardy
5 Be confident, but not arrogant

The Long Case

APPROACH TO THE LONG CASE

1 **Your priority in the long case is to keep the examiners entertained.** This requirement does not feature on the scorecard and may come as a surprise to the candidate who believes the examiners are hell-bent on finding an excuse to fail him or her. No, one of the better-kept secrets of the clinical examination system is that more often than not the main concern of the examiner is to resist nodding off during the case presentation. This is understandable when you realize that the examiner may be worried about mortgage debt, behind schedule with research, due to deliver a lecture on an unrehearsed topic in two hours' time, and — most critically — all but mesmerized from having just sat through two presentations of the same case.

How, then, does one go about entertaining one's examiners? The prerequisite is to make sure that the examiner does the minimal amount of *work*. In practice this means that *you* do the talking, that *you* ensure there are no embarrassing gaps in the monologue during which they must compose a question for you, and that *you* refrain from exasperating them by talking stuff and nonsense.

Like nature itself, long-case examiners abhor vacuums. The most ominous sign of a long case spiralling into oblivion is the protracted silence. Don't let things degenerate into a monosyllabic question-and-answer session. Show off your knowledge. Express concern for all possible aspects of your patient's plight — don't just mumble abstractly as if discussing a crossword puzzle. Explore every nuance of every problem. Prove to the examiners that you have experience, sensitivity, integrity, judgement; in short, *sell yourself*. By the time you've finished talking, the case should be all but over and the examiners too overwhelmed to fight back — and, with luck, you may find before you know it that you have done your last-ever long case presentation (and just when it was starting to be fun too, right?).

2 **Success in the long case requires a successful encounter with the patient.** People will volunteer all sorts of advice about how long to spend on the various sections of the case, but it clearly must be about 20 minutes each for history, examination and writing up alike. Don't be concerned if you find yourself prompted to ask more historical details by the results of physical examination or if, when writing up, you suddenly remember to examine something extra: real-life medicine is an organic process, not a stereotyped protocol. On the other hand, if you find yourself in the lion's den (i.e. being examined) and realize that you have

missed doing something critical to the case, it may be best to make a clean breast of it rather than hoping to get off scot free — if it is your lucky day, you may get to re-examine the patient.

Always clarify two key points from the history:

1 What is your main problem?
2 How is your life affected by it?

Don't forget to ask the patient the time-honoured 'long case' questions at the end (yes, the end) of the interview. After all, many of your less scrupulous colleagues will do exactly this and it is not in the public interest for you to concede a survival advantage to such degenerates. So, since you are morally obliged to do so, ask:

1 What do the doctors say is wrong with you?
2 What part of your anatomy were the examiners most interested to examine when they visited you this morning?
3 What investigations or treatments are planned for you in the immediate future?
4 Is there anything else you think I should know? Mmmnh? [Bat eyelashes]

If the patient is under the misapprehension that they are not meant to give you such information, simply clarify for them that such precautions only apply to the candidates who come *after* you!

3 **It is essential to show off in the correct manner.** One must, it seems, show off confidently but humbly. This means managing to communicate knowledge and clinical skill while at the same time avoiding any hint of smugness or complacency. If you have personally managed to see 23 cases similar to the one you are presenting, let your experience show. If you are familiar with the clinical research background relevant to the problem under discussion, use that knowledge to add authority and pizzazz to your conclusions. Keep in mind that what you are really seeking is *approval* to be admitted into the exclusive club currently patronized by your examiners. Provided that you have got the case itself sorted out, don't be afraid to add a pinch of charm to your presentation — suitably peppered as it will need to be with deference and tact.

4 The eruption of an all-out no-holds-barred argument with any examiner is obviously a dire prognostic indicator, but **a mature degree of self-assertion is a plus**. If challenged over some finding (or lack thereof) simply be honest: if you were a little dubious about it, say so, while if you were solidly convinced then stand your ground. Don't, in your paranoia, assume that the examiner will try to mislead

you, but be prepared to have the strength of your conviction tested. If you have just claimed that a cardiac valve lesion is hemodynamically severe, be prepared to argue this from clinical facts rather than gut feeling. The biggest mistake is to assert something which you cannot substantiate — particularly if it is wrong. Most examiners will try to lead you back to the correct diagnosis, so consider very carefully what they say to you.

5 **Don't be put off if the diagnosis doesn't appear clear-cut.** After all, even the consultant managing the case may not have worked it out and the last thing he wants to hear is some young whippersnapper saying it's a cut-and-dried example of (say) mulibrey nanism or Tourette's syndrome. Real-life medicine tends to be shades of grey rather than black and white; your only problem will be if they've dragged in an 'exam classic' (in which context you'll often be alerted by the uneasy feeling that you're 'missing something') but these are far commoner in short cases. If the diagnosis is obscure, begin by giving a 'first-phase' diagnosis ('lower motor neurone lesion'), advancing then to the second-phase ('involving lumbosacral nerve roots') and finally to a third-phase differential diagnosis ('polio', 'motor neurone disease', etc.) which may be clarified by relevant investigations. Rest assured that numerous clues, inadvertent or otherwise, can be given away by the examiners' subsequent questions. You should never be stuck for a differential diagnosis; have a mental list of generic causes ('tumor, trauma, infection, infarction . . .') which you can conjure up even when the cerebral computer has gone down in the heat of battle.

Never underestimate your ability to answer a question in the absence of specific knowledge. You may find yourself asked, for instance:

EXAMINER (smiling): *Tell me then, what proportion of patients with this condition would you expect to have an elevated serum rhubarb?*

to which you could answer,

CANDIDATE: *I . . . I . . . (gulp) . . . don't know, sir . . .*

[which would prompt the following reply:

EXAMINER (licking his lips): *Ah. I see.]*

or, alternatively, you could answer:

CANDIDATE: *Er, I believe it's around 10%, sir, if I recall correctly.*

[which might in turn prompt the reply:

EXAMINER (scowling): *Hmm, I think you might find it's actually 19% ... All right then, what about . . .]*

Similarly, you could be asked about a drug you have never actually prescribed yourself, and your memory regarding its effects may need jogging:

EXAMINER: *So what do you know of the toxicity of amiodarone, then?*

CANDIDATE: *Ah yes, amiodarone. Well, sir, it can cause skin rashes in some individuals, nausea in others, at times vomiting, occasional diarrhea . . .*

EXAMINER: *Yes, yes . . . what about . . . do you know of any . . . ah . . . endocrinological side-effects?*

Remember that even if one of the examiners insists on proving he knows more than you do about Binswanger's disease, say, or congenital hepatic fibrosis, there should be at least one other examiner available to prevent undue emphasis being placed on such fringe knowledge. Don't let yourself be floored — by anything.

Have the justification for any recommended investigation at the ready, including those that you know are often ordered 'routinely' (i.e. without thinking) in everyday hospital practice. Furthermore, when presenting (say) a jaundiced patient, start by recommending the most conservative, non-invasive and inexpensive investigations (e.g. urinalysis, liver function tests) rather than the more definitive (ERCP, percutaneous biopsy). Simply imagine what you would do in real life, why you would do it and the order in which you would do it. Wisdom born of experience is undoubtedly the most impressive persona to create in a clinical viva.

In summary:

KEEP TALKING
SOUND AUTHORITATIVE
SELL YOURSELF
THINK POSITIVE
BE A PHYSICIAN

PRESENTING THE LONG CASE: A FORMAT FOR EXAM CANDIDATES

The most time-honored way to fritter away precious minutes during preparation of a long case is to enter the patient's room armed only with blank sheets of paper. This means that you have automatically lost several minutes in having to write headings all the way through, such as 'Allergies', 'Pulse rate', 'Main problems', 'Investigations' or whatever. Moreover, you are constantly having to fret about whether you are doing everything in the conventional order and whether you might inadvertently omit a key finding — something you would *never* do under normal circumstances.

This is not the way you would run things if you were trying to develop, say, an efficient private practice. In that situation it would make far more sense to have your own 'new case' format already formulated and printed, leaving you with the relatively simple task of filling in the gaps. This has the additional advantage of systematizing your approach to the case despite the pressures of the moment. Since there is no reason why such an approach shouldn't be used in day-to-day clinical practice, there seems little theoretical objection to its use in a long case examination viva.

In the next few pages you will find an example of such a long case format. You may find that your own particular style is better suited to a custom-made version — in which case, write it up!

LONG CASE PROTOCOL: I HISTORY

EXAMINER: Hello there, I'm Professor Smith and this is Dr Jones—would you like to tell us about the patient you've just seen?

CANDIDATE: Certainly, sir. I saw _____

NAME

who is a _____

AGE   SEX   NATIONALITY   OCCUPATION

admitted to hospital _____ because of/for investigation of

WHEN?

_____ . (S)he had been completely

PRESENTING SYMPTOM(S)

well until _____ when (s)he developed

WHEN WERE THE VERY FIRST SYMPTOMS?

_____ . (S)he then/since that

INITIAL SUSPICIOUS SYMPTOMS

time _____ (now go into ENORMOUS DETAIL)

_____

EXACT SEQUENCE OF EVENTS;   DURATION AND PERIODICITY OF SYMPTOMS;

_____

NATURE AND SEVERITY;   LOCATION AND RADIATION OF PAIN;

_____

EXACERBATING AND RELIEVING FACTORS;   RESPONSE TO PREVIOUS TREATMENT;

_____

RESULTS OF PREVIOUS INVESTIGATIONS;   HOW HAS THE DISEASE BEEN MONITORED?

_____

ASSOCIATED FEATURES

Her/his main problem(s) in coping with this disease is/are _____

PAIN;

_____

DAY-TO-DAY INCAPACITY;   INABILITY TO WORK;

_____

SOCIAL HANDICAP;   SEXUAL PROBLEMS;

_____

EFFECT ON FAMILY;   SUFFERING AND DEMORALIZATION

Her/his doctors have recently told her/him that (s)he has _____

DIAGNOSIS IF KNOWN

and that the outlook is _____

PROGNOSIS IF KNOWN

Currently (s)he remains in hospital because of _____

ONGOING MANAGEMENT;

_____

PLANNED INVESTIGATIONS   DISEASE COMPLICATIONS

Checklist:
short of breath chest pain palpitations dizziness orthopnea nocturnal dyspnea claudication syncope fatigue
wheeze stridor cough sputum hemoptysis pleurisy sweats
dysphagia nausea vomiting diarrhea constipation weight loss heartburn abdominal pain jaundice hematemesis melena rectal bleeding
headache photophobia blurred vision loss of vision vertigo deafness funny turns unconsciousness paresthesiae numbness weakness paralysis difficulty walking dysarthria dysphasia
hematuria nocturia dysuria oliguria polyuria polydipsia loin pain pruritus incontinence
skin rash joint pain/swelling

DIRECT QUESTIONS RELATING TO SYSTEM(S) INVOLVED IN PRESENT ILLNESS
(positives and significant negatives only)

DIRECT QUESTIONS RELATING TO OTHER SYSTEMS
(significant positives and negatives only)

PAST MEDICAL HISTORY

PREVIOUS OPERATIONS AND BLOOD TRANSFUSIONS

DAILY LIFESTYLE
Past smoking
Current smoking
Past alcohol
Current alcohol
Analgesics
Laxatives
Oral contraceptives
Illicit drug use

OCCUPATIONAL HISTORY

ACTIVITIES OF DAILY LIVING
Functional capacity
Handicaps
Aids

MISCELLANEOUS
Allergies
Pet; animal contact
Recent travel
Diet
Menstrual/sexual
history (if relevant)

CURRENT MEDICATIONS AND OTHER TREATMENT
Vitamins
Radiotherapy
Physiotherapy

FAMILY HISTORY

SOCIAL HISTORY

II PHYSICAL EXAMINATION   OTHER SYSTEMS:

GENERAL APPEARANCE

young/old

well/distressed

cachectic/obese

jaundiced/pale/
pigmented

plethoric/cyanosed

deformity/paralysis

alopecia/hirsutism

MENTAL STATE

oriented/disoriented

lucid/confused

hostile/co-operative

SPECIFIC STIGMATA

surgical scars

IV therapy

fan/oxygen

inhaler/nebulizer

fistula/shunt

VITAL SIGNS

temperature

pulse

rate/rhythm/quality

blood pressure

respiratory rate

hydration status

MAJOR SYSTEM(S)

GENERAL

POSITIVE SIGNS

SIGNIFICANT NEGATIVES

EQUIVOCAL/DIFFICULT SIGNS

MANEUVRES

FUNCTIONAL ASSESSMENT

DISEASE EXTENT

DISEASE ACTIVITY/SEVERITY

CARDIAC

JVP? PULSATIONS? HEAVE?

THRILL? APEX? HEART

SOUNDS? EXTRA SOUNDS?

MURMURS?

LUNG CREPITATIONS?

EDEMA? PULSES?

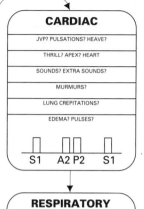

S1   A2 P2   S1

RESPIRATORY

CLUBBING? ADENOPATHY?

TRACHEA? EXPANSION?

FREMITUS? PERCUSSION?

RESONANCE?

BREATH SOUNDS?

GASTROINTESTINAL

PALMAR ERYTHEMA?

DUPUYTREN'S? FLAP?

SPIDERS? NODES? MOUTH?

FETOR? GYNECOMASTIA?

JAUNDICE? ASCITES?

LIVER? SPLEEN? KIDNEYS?

HERNIAE? TESTICLES? PR?

NEUROLOGICAL

WASTING?

FASCICULATION? TONE?

CLONUS? WEAKNESS?

REFLEXES? PLANTARS?

CEREBELLAR? SENSORY?

FUNDI? CRANIAL NERVES?

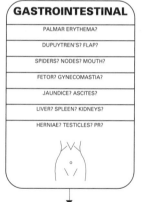

Checklist:

hands

nails

hair

skin

scalp

eyes: acuity/fundi

visual fields

dental hygiene

tongue

speech

parietal lobe
  function

neck; bruits

parotids

goiter

lymph nodes

back

breasts

bladder distension

abdominal reflexes

renal/femoral bruit

genitalia

perineum

pelvic examination

sacroiliac joints

bony tenderness

peripheral joints

gait

tendon reflexes

plantar reflexes

pigmentation

urinalysis

III LONG CASE SUMMARY

CANDIDATE: In summary, then, Mrs/Mr _____
                                                                                NAME
is a very interesting patient with a _____
                                                                 DURATION OF SYMPTOMS
history of _____ who now presents with
                                           SYMPTOMS
_____ . (S)he presents several
                               MAJOR SYMPTOMS AND SIGNS
challenging diagnostic/management problems. I believe that her/his MAIN PROBLEM is

_____ .
            SYMPTOM(S)?   PROVISIONAL DIAGNOSIS?   DIFFERENTIAL DIAGNOSIS?
However, her/his case does present some unusual aspects: _____

_____
                            PROS AND CONS OF POSSIBLE DIAGNOSIS

_____

_____
                              STRATEGIES FOR CLARIFYING DIAGNOSIS

_____

There are also a number of other problems related to this patient's _____
                                                                                                    MAIN PROBLEM
_____ and these include _____
                                                                         RELATED PROBLEMS
MY APPROACH to these problems is to begin by _____
                                                                       APPROACH TO MAIN PROBLEM;

_____

_____
                  INVESTIGATIONAL SEQUENCE (NON-INVASIVE FIRST) AND JUSTIFICATION;

_____
                       MANAGEMENT STRATEGY (CONSERVATIVE MEASURES FIRST)

_____

I'd also like to discuss _____
                                               APPROACH TO RELATED PROBLEMS

_____

_____
                     INVESTIGATION AND MANAGEMENT OF RELATED PROBLEMS

_____

So let me now give you some details about exactly what I'd like to do for this patient

_____

_____

IV LONG CASE DISCUSSION

REVIEW DIAGNOSIS
(if indicated)

↓

EXCLUSION OF POTENTIALLY REVERSIBLE FACTORS

↓

ELIMINATION OF RISK FACTORS FOR FURTHER COMPLICATIONS

↓

INVESTIGATIONS IMPINGING ON FURTHER MANAGEMENT
(see over)

↓

SYMPTOMATIC MEASURES

DEFINITIVE TREATMENT

Drug therapy:

Surgery:

Radiotherapy:

Hormones/vitamins:

Plasma exchange:

↓

PHYSIOTHERAPY

Mobilization:
Splints:
Braces:
Exercise:

↓

OCCUPATIONAL THERAPY

Home appliances:

Domestic help:

↓

DIETARY SUPERVISION

Ideal body weight:
Special diet:
Fluid/salt restriction:

FOLLOW-UP

Disease monitors:

Compliance monitors:
— drug levels
—

Anticipation/exclusion of drug toxicity:
Vaccinations:
Contraception:
Sperm banking:
Genetic counselling:
Care of shunt/stoma/catheter:
Involvement of local doctor/nurse/social worker:

↓

SOCIAL

Change of occupation:

Change of climate:

Identification locket (on steroids, insulin, etc.):

Social placement:

V LONG CASE INVESTIGATIONS

HEMATOLOGY	
Hb	
film	
WCC	
differential	
platelets	
MCV/MCHC	
reticulocytes	
ESR	
PT/INR	
APTT/PTTK	
fibrinogen	
FDPs, D-dimer	
folate/B$_{12}$	
Schilling test	
Fe/TIBC/ferritin	
Coombs' test	
haptoglobin	
NAP score	
lysozyme	
cold agglutinins	
marrow aspiration	
marrow trephine	

RADIOLOGY	
CXR	
AXR	
SXR	
XR (specify)	
skeletal survey	
IVP	
myelogram	
CT scan:	
( )	
ultrasound:	
( )	
nuclear scan:	
( )	
angiogram:	
( )	
MRI	

PATHOLOGY	
review sections	
biopsy:	
( )	
cytology:	
( )	
immunofluorescen	
electron microscopy	

CARDIOLOGY	
ECG	
echocardiography	
stress test	
ejection fraction	
cardiac catheter	
nuclear scan:	
( )	

NEUROLOGY	
EMG/nerve conduction	
muscle/nerve biopsy	
CSF studies	
EEG/evoked responses	
porphyrins	
lead level	

ENDOCRINOLOGY	
GTT	
fT$_4$/fT$_3$/TSH	
ACTH/urinary cortisol	
pituitary function tests:	
-TRH/GnRH/Arg/Synacthen	
Hypothalamic function tests	

URINE STUDIES	
urinalysis	
microscopy	
culture sensitivity	
osmolality	
24-h calcium	
24-h urate	
serum iPTH	

BIOCHEMISTRY	
Na$^+$	
K$^+$	
HCO$_3$	
BUN, S.Cr.	
Ca^{2+}	
Mg^{2+}	
albumin	
bilirubin	
AST/ALT	
alk.phos.	
GGT	
glucose	
uric acid	
cholesterol	
triglycerides	
CPK (-MB)	
amylase	
LDH	

MICROBIOLOGY	
MSU	
blood culture	
sputum culture	
AFB	
Mantoux	
viral titers	
VDRL, FTA	
HIV Ab	
HBsAg	
ASO titer	
thick/thin film	
darkfield examination	
Indian ink	
stool examination	
CSF examination	

IMMUNOLOGY	
ANA, dsDNA Ab	
rheumatoid factor	
lupus anticoagulant	
C$_3$ C$_4$	
EPG/IEPG	
Ig levels	
urinary BJP	
smooth muscle Ab	
antimitochondrial Ab	
cryoglobulins	
tissue typing	

GASTROENTEROLOGY	
endoscopy	
colonoscopy	
ERCP	
liver biopsy	
hepatitis serology	
oral cholecystogram	
IV cholangiogram	
fasting serum gastrin	
breath test(s)	

RESPIRATORY	
FEV$_1$/VC	
PEFR	
DL$_{CO}$	
blood gases	
bronchoscopy	
diagnostic lavage	
lung biopsy	

TUMOR MARKERS	
AFP; βHCG	
paraprotein level	
CEA	
acid phosphatase	
thyroglobulin	
5HIAA, catecholamines	

EYE	
slit lamp examination	
fluorescein angiography	

VI SHORT CASE/LONG CASE SCORESHEET

SHORT CASE	unsatisfactory	borderline	good
APPROACH TO THE PATIENT			
WAS THE EXAMINATION TECHNICALLY SMOOTH?			
WAS THE EXAMINATION SYSTEMATIC AND THOROUGH?			
ACCURACY OF FINDINGS			
INTERPRETATION OF FINDINGS			

LONG CASE	unsatisfactory	borderline	good
HISTORY			
PHYSICAL FINDINGS			
INVESTIGATIONS			
MANAGEMENT			
CONCLUSIONS			

OVERALL ASSESSMENT: medical school finals (e.g. final MB)   { This candidate is clinically safe to work under supervision }   TRUE (pass) ☐   FALSE (fail) ☐

OVERALL ASSESSMENT: postgraduate internal medicine diploma (e.g. MRCP)   { This candidate is clinically safe to work without supervision }   TRUE (pass) ☐   FALSE (fail) ☐

Medicine for Examinations

CHAPTER 1

Cancer medicine

Physical examination protocol 1.1   You are asked to assess the current clinical status of a patient who has been receiving treatment for malignant disease

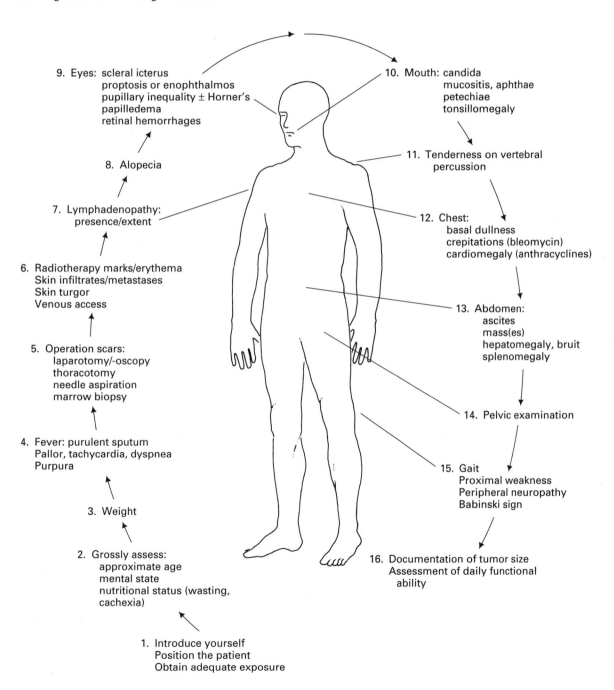

9. Eyes: scleral icterus
    proptosis or enophthalmos
    pupillary inequality ± Horner's
    papilledema
    retinal hemorrhages

8. Alopecia

7. Lymphadenopathy:
   presence/extent

6. Radiotherapy marks/erythema
   Skin infiltrates/metastases
   Skin turgor
   Venous access

5. Operation scars:
   laparotomy/-oscopy
   thoracotomy
   needle aspiration
   marrow biopsy

4. Fever: purulent sputum
   Pallor, tachycardia, dyspnea
   Purpura

3. Weight

2. Grossly assess:
   approximate age
   mental state
   nutritional status (wasting,
   cachexia)

1. Introduce yourself
   Position the patient
   Obtain adequate exposure

10. Mouth: candida
    mucositis, aphthae
    petechiae
    tonsillomegaly

11. Tenderness on vertebral
    percussion

12. Chest:
    basal dullness
    crepitations (bleomycin)
    cardiomegaly (anthracyclines)

13. Abdomen:
    ascites
    mass(es)
    hepatomegaly, bruit
    splenomegaly

14. Pelvic examination

15. Gait
    Proximal weakness
    Peripheral neuropathy
    Babinski sign

16. Documentation of tumor size
    Assessment of daily functional
    ability

Physical examination protocol 1.2   You are asked to examine a patient who has recently presented with metastatic disease of unknown primary etiology

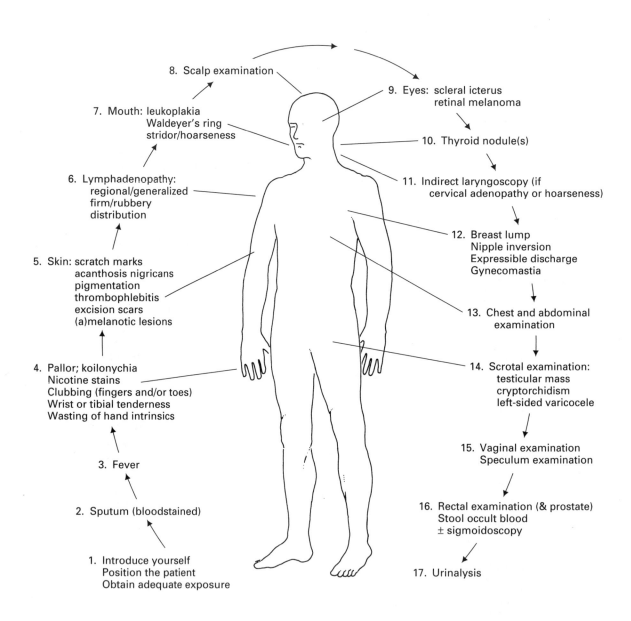

8. Scalp examination

9. Eyes: scleral icterus
   retinal melanoma

7. Mouth: leukoplakia
   Waldeyer's ring
   stridor/hoarseness

10. Thyroid nodule(s)

6. Lymphadenopathy:
   regional/generalized
   firm/rubbery
   distribution

11. Indirect laryngoscopy (if
    cervical adenopathy or hoarseness)

12. Breast lump
    Nipple inversion
    Expressible discharge
    Gynecomastia

5. Skin: scratch marks
   acanthosis nigricans
   pigmentation
   thrombophlebitis
   excision scars
   (a)melanotic lesions

13. Chest and abdominal
    examination

4. Pallor; koilonychia
   Nicotine stains
   Clubbing (fingers and/or toes)
   Wrist or tibial tenderness
   Wasting of hand intrinsics

14. Scrotal examination:
    testicular mass
    cryptorchidism
    left-sided varicocele

3. Fever

15. Vaginal examination
    Speculum examination

2. Sputum (bloodstained)

16. Rectal examination (& prostate)
    Stool occult blood
    ± sigmoidoscopy

1. Introduce yourself
   Position the patient
   Obtain adequate exposure

17. Urinalysis

Diagnostic pathway 1.1   This patient has ascites. What is the most likely cause?

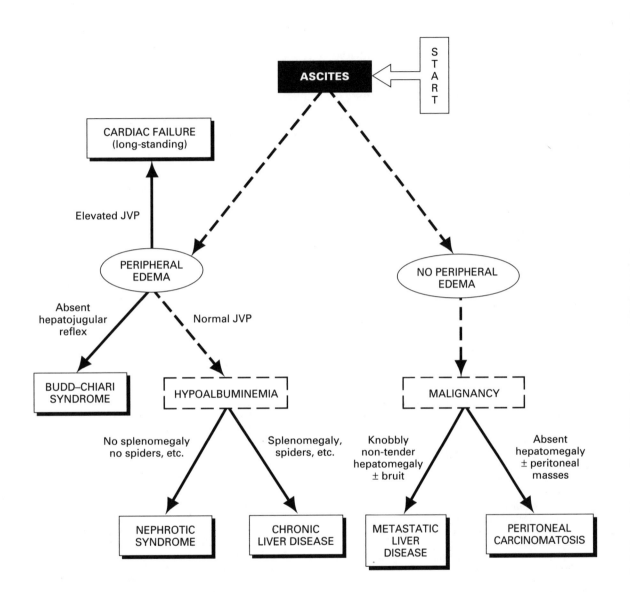

CLINICAL ASPECTS OF MALIGNANT DISEASE

Commonest oncology short cases
1 Lung cancer
2 Metastatic liver disease

Patient performance status*: modified ECOG criteria
1 Grade 0 — asymptomatic
2 Grade 1 — symptomatic, fully ambulant
3 Grade 2 — symptomatic, ambulant > 50% waking hours
4 Grade 3 — symptomatic, in bed > 50% waking hours
5 Grade 4 — symptomatic, confined to bed

* 'Performance status' = assessment of patient well-being

The palpable lump: how to describe it
1 **S:** **s**ite, **s**ize, **s**hape
2 **F:** **f**irmness, **f**ixation, **f**luctuation
3 **T:** **t**exture, **t**emperature, **t**enderness

Differential diagnosis of fever in the cancer patient
1 Infective
   — Septicemia, esp. if neutropenic (< 0.5 x 10⁹/L)
   — Intermittent bacteremias, e.g. from central line
   — Occult localized infections, e.g. cryptococcal meningitis
   — Viremia, esp. CMV (e.g. following marrow transplant)
2 Iatrogenic
   — Drug-induced: e.g. L-asparaginase, interferon
   — Transfusion-associated
3 Intrinsic (i.e. disease manifestation; a diagnosis of exclusion)
   — Lymphoma (esp. Hodgkin's); leukemia (esp. CML)
   — Retroperitoneal tumors, e.g. renal cell carcinoma
   — Metastatic liver disease

Differential diagnosis of confusion in the cancer patient
1 Metabolic
   — Hypercalcemia
      • With bone metastases (e.g. Ca breast, myeloma)
      • Humorally mediated (e.g. in SCC lung)
   — Hyponatremia (SIADH; e.g. in small-cell lung cancer)
   — Hyperviscosity (esp. in IgM dysproteinemias)
2 Septic, esp.
   — Pneumonia
   — Cryptococcal meningitis
   — Progressive multifocal leukoencephalopathy (p. 23)
3 Hypoxic, esp.
   — Pulmonary emboli
4 Iatrogenic
   — Opiates
   — Steroids (may be fatal)
   — Procarbazine, L-asparaginase
   — Ifosfamide encephalopathy
5 Tumor-related
   — Paraneoplastic encephalopathy/dementia
   — Cerebral metastases

Differential diagnosis of vomiting in the cancer patient
1 Iatrogenic
   — Chemotherapy and/or anticipatory
   — Other drugs (e.g. opiates)
2 Gastrointestinal obstruction
   — Primary gastrointestinal tumors (e.g. linitis plastica)
   — Peritoneal seedlings (e.g. Ca ovary, lobular Ca breast)
3 Raised intracranial pressure due to intracranial metastases
   — Cerebral edema
   — Ventricular obstruction
4 Hypercalcemia

Differential diagnosis of alopecia in the cancer patient
1 Wispy alopecia
   — Chemotherapy
2 Asymmetric alopecia
   — Post-craniotomy (for brain tumor)
3 Total alopecia*
   — Cranial irradiation

* NB: Some drugs (e.g. taxol, high-dose anthracyclines) may cause total alopecia; or patients may elect to shave head

CLINICAL PRESENTATIONS OF TUMOR SUBTYPES

Clinical presentations of lung tumors
1 Local endobronchial symptoms
   — Hemoptysis
   — Stridor ± dyspnea
2 Local extrabronchial obstructive presentations
   — Superior vena caval obstruction (esp. SCC, small-cell)
   — Chylous pleural effusion (rare)
3 Syndromes due to nerve palsies
   — *Hoarseness* due to recurrent laryngeal nerve compression, esp. with left-sided tumors
   — *Hemidiaphragmatic paralysis* (phrenic nerve palsy)
   — *Pancoast's syndrome* (p. 23) due to T1 nerve root compression (esp. by upper lobe apical tumors)
   — *Horner's syndrome* (ptosis, miosis, ipsilateral facial dryness) due to interruption of ascending cervical sympathetic supply (esp. by Pancoast tumors)
4 Metastatic presentations
   — Serosal spread: pleural effusion, pericardial tamponade
   — Other: jaundice, convulsions, weight loss
5 Paraneoplastic syndromes (see below)

Common presentations of pathologic lung tumor subtypes
1 Non-small-cell lung cancer (→ 80%: SCC, adenoCa, large-cell)
   — Hypertrophic pulmonary osteoarthropathy (HPO)
   — Non-metastatic hypercalcemia (esp. SCC); due to PTHrP
2 Small-cell lung cancer (20%; SCLC)
   — Metastases at presentation

— Leukoerythroblastic anemia
— Cerebral metastases, meningeal carcinomatosis
— SIADH* (due to 1° tumor *or* intracranial spread)
— Ectopic ACTH syndrome
— Eaton-Lambert ('myasthenic') syndrome
— Extensive mediastinal involvement‡
— SVC obstruction (→ 50% of all cases)
— Rapid, transient response to chemotherapy
3 Bronchioloalveolar cell carcinoma
— Copious clear sputum (often in a non-smoker)
— Respiratory insufficiency ± pulmonary infiltrate
4 Bronchial adenoma (usually a carcinoid tumor)
— Hemoptysis with normal CXR (tumor usually central)
— Recurrent chest infections, e.g. abscess, pneumonia¶
— Left-sided cardiac valve lesions (*very* rare)
— Incidental CXR finding in a non-smoker
— Brisk hemorrhage if biopsied (highly vascular)

* DD$_x$ = Syndrome of increased atrial natriuretic peptide (ANP)
‡ DDx = Lymphoma, germ-cell tumor
¶ Due to bronchial obstruction

Predominant localization of lung tumor subtypes
1 Central
— Small-cell lung cancer
— Squamous cell carcinoma
— Bronchial adenoma
2 Peripheral
— Adenocarcinoma*
— Large cell carcinoma

* Metastasis from other primary site may require exclusion if no luminal lesion visualized at bronchoscopy

Clinical presentations of colorectal cancer
1 Distal (left-sided) colon tumors
— Changed bowel habit
— Rectal bleeding
2 Transverse colon tumors
— Obstruction
3 Proximal (right) colon tumors
— Iron-deficiency anemia
4 Other (rare) presentations
— *Strep. bovis* endocarditis
— *Clostridium septicum* myonecrosis
— Perforation

Clinical presentations of pancreatic cancer
1 'Head' tumors
— Common:
• Progressive jaundice
• Back pain (due to invasion of celiac plexus)
— Classical:
• Palpable non-tender gallbladder (Courvoisier's sign)
2 'Tail' tumors
— Common:
• Weight loss
— Classical:
• Endogenous depression, *angor animi*
• Migratory thrombophlebitis (Trousseau's syndrome)

Clinical presentations of gastric cancer
1 Common
— Weight loss
— Epigastric discomfort
2 Classical
— Troisier's sign (enlargement of Virchow's node)
— Sister Mary Joseph nodule (umbilical mass)
— Blumer's (prerectal) shelf on digital examination
— Krukenberg tumors (ovarian metastases) at laparotomy
— Acanthosis nigricans (symmetric pigmented warty skin lesions → axillae, pubis, neck and umbilicus)

Clinical presentations of primary liver tumors
1 Hepatoma (often associated with HBsAg and ↑ AFP)
— Common:
• Onset of ascites in a previously stable cirrhotic
• Unexplained weight loss in an alcoholic
• Tender hepar with bruit (DDx: alcoholic hepatitis)
— Uncommon:
• Polycythemia
• Dysproteinemia
• Porphyria
— Investigations:
• HBsAg, HCV serology
• AFP (positive in 50%)
• Lipiodol CT
2 Hepatic adenoma (→ young women)
— Intraperitoneal rupture in a previously well woman taking oral contraceptives for at least 5 years
3 Hepatoblastoma (→ infants only)
— Clubbing; precocious puberty

SYMPTOMS AND SIGNS OF SPECIFIC TUMORS

Symptoms and signs of renal cell carcinoma
1 Common
— Hematuria
— Flank pain)
— Flank mass) in 25% each
— Anemia)
2 Uncommon
— Polycythemia (5%)
— Fever; thromboembolism
— Left-sided varicocele
— Non-metastatic hypercalcemia
— Non-metastatic liver dysfunction (Stauffer's syndrome)

Symptoms and signs of choriocarcinoma
1 Hyperemesis gravidarum
2 Metastatic presentation usual (cf. seminoma)
3 Hemorrhagic metastases → hemoptysis, stroke
4 Painful gynecomastia (in males)
5 Rare: mild hyperthyroidism (HCG shares TSH β-subunit)

Symptoms and signs of cervical carcinoma
1 Majority detected by routine pelvic examination and Pap smear of *asymptomatic* patients

2 Symptomatic presentations
   — Vaginal discharge
   — Pelvic pain (advanced disease)
   — Fistulas (e.g. rectovaginal → pneumaturia)*
   — Obstructive uropathy (frequently terminal)

* Often iatrogenic, e.g. post-radiotherapy

Symptoms and signs of ovarian tumors
1 Adenocarcinoma
   — Abdominal fullness and/or dyspepsia due to ascites
   — Bowel obstruction
   — Peritoneal carcinomatosis at laparotomy
2 Stromal tumors (rare)
   — Fibroma, thecoma   → Meigs' syndrome
   — *Struma ovarii*   → thyrotoxicosis
   — Granulosa cell tumor   → vaginal bleeding
   — Sertoli–Leydig tumor*   → virilization

* Formerly termed arrhenoblastoma

Symptoms and signs of melanoma
1 Common
   — Primary skin lesion: suspicious if A,B,C,D:
     • <u>A</u>symmetric shape
     • <u>B</u>order irregularity
     • <u>C</u>olor variegated (incl. black)
     • <u>D</u>iameter > 6 mm
   — Spread to regional lymph nodes
   — Cerebral metastases, meningeal carcinomatosis
   — Pulmonary metastases
   — Skin metastases (may be indolent)
2 Classical
   — Hepatomegaly and unilateral scleral icterus (i.e. liver metastases from retinal primary; glass eye)

Symptoms and signs of brain tumors
1 Local neurologic effects
   — Focal motor seizures
   — Hemiparesis ± hemisensory deficit
   — Aphasia
   — Homonymous/bitemporal hemianopia
   — Cranial nerve palsies
2 Raised intracranial pressure
   — Headache, malaise, vomiting
   — Visual blurring, papilledema, diplopia
   — CN VI (abducens) palsy, Parinaud's syndrome
   — Personality change, amnesia, dementia

The solitary thyroid nodule: factors favoring malignancy
1 Positive family history of medullary thyroid cancer
2 Past history of low-dose neck irradiation, esp. in childhood
3 Clinical features: hard nodule, lymphadenopathy
4 Elevated serum thyroglobulin (papillary/follicular cancer)
   Elevated serum calcitonin (medullary carcinoma)
5 'Cold' nodule on scintigraphy
6 Solid lesion on ultrasound

Medullary thyroid carcinoma (MTC): features
1 80% are sporadic (no family history of MEN2; p. 115–116)
2 *Familial* MTC may be either:
   — Isolated familial MTC (least aggressive type)

   — MTC with type IIa MEN
     • + Pheochromocytoma, parathyroid adenoma
   — MTC with type IIb MEN (rarest and most aggressive)
     • 'Mucosal neuroma' syndrome (± pheo-, etc.)
3 Familial transmission is autosomal dominant
   — 90% get MTC by age 60
   — 50% develop hyperparathyroidism
4 Clinical presentation*
   — Lumps in neck
   — Watery diarrhea
   — Flushing (less marked than in carcinoid syndrome)
5 Screen family members (i.e. of *all* index cases) using:
   — DNA analysis (if MEN suspected)
     • Mutations affecting the *RET* protooncogene; *or*
   — Biochemical screening tests
     • Pentagastrin-stimulated calcitonin, *or*
     • Calcium-stimulated calcitonin, *or*
     • Alcohol-stimulated calcitonin
6 Prognosis
   — Calcitonin < 1000 pg/mL: 95% cure
   — Calcitonin > 10,000 pg/mL: 5% cure

* Note that calcium remains *normal* despite gross elevation of calcitonin

PATTERNS OF NEUROLOGIC DEFICIT IN CANCER

Common presentations of intracranial neoplasms
1 Headaches
   — Morning esp.; ± diplopia, projectile vomiting
2 Convulsions
   — May be focal
3 Cranial nerve deficit
   — May be mixed or 'false localizing'
4 Personality change
   — Dementia included

Cerebrovascular manifestations of malignant disease
1 Intracranial hemorrhage
   — Leukemia (e.g. DIC in acute promyelocytic leukemia)
   — Bleeding metastases (melanoma, choriocarcinoma)
2 TIAs/cerebral infarction
   — Leukemia (DIC or leukostasis: WCC > 100,000)
   — Waldenström's macroglobulinemia (hyperviscosity)
   — Non-bacterial endocarditis
3 Sagittal sinus thrombosis
   — DIC (e.g. in Ca breast/prostate, APL)

Clinical features of meningeal carcinomatosis
1 Commonest causes
   — Small-cell lung cancer
   — Breast cancer
   — Melanoma, lymphoma
2 Presentation
   — Cranial nerve deficits
   — Disseminated or mixed deficits (e.g. upper and lower motor neuron lesions)
   — Bizarre sensory disturbances (e.g. jaw numbness)

3 Diagnosis
— CSF cytology (positive for malignant cells*)
— ↑ CSF protein ± ↓ CSF glucose
— MRI may confirm nodules within spinal canal

*NB: CSF examination may need to be repeated several times for diagnosis

Clinical features of progressive multifocal leukoencephalopathy
1 Commonest cause
— Leukemias (esp. CLL), lymphomas
2 Pathology
— Deep corticocerebellar demyelination
3 Presentation
— Progressive cortical (visual, speech, higher centres) deficits, weakness; normal intracranial pressure
4 Diagnosis
— CSF exam typically normal
— Antibodies to JC virus (a papovavirus)
— CT or NMR scanning may show discrete lesions
— Brain biopsy for viral studies (definitive)
5 Course
— Survival averages 3 months from diagnosis

Clinical features of Pancoast's syndrome
1 Commonest cause
— Lung cancer, esp. SCC
2 Symptoms
— Shoulder pain, radicular pain (due to plexus invasion)
3 Signs
— Interossei wasting; T1 sensory loss; Horner's
4 CXR
— May show erosion of first and second ribs

Clinical features of myasthenic (Eaton-Lambert) syndrome
1 Commonest cause
— Small-cell lung cancer
2 Symptoms
— Weakness; myalgias, paresthesiae
— Impotence; dry mouth
3 Signs
— Minimal wasting; hyporeflexia
— Ocular/bulbar sparing
4 Diagnosis
— Negative edrophonium (Tensilon) test
— Post-tetanic facilitation on EMG
5 Treatment
— Ablation of underlying malignancy
— Corticosteroids, plasmapheresis
— Diaminopyridine; guanidine HCl*

* Both enhance acetylcholine release at neuromuscular junction

Back pain: clinical features suggesting malignant etiology
1 Insidious onset, progressive course, general ill health
2 Often worse at night
3 Pain in thoracic or upper lumbar nerve root distribution

4 Disseminated sites of vertebral tenderness
5 Signs of multiple and/or bilateral nerve root lesions
6 Coexisting upper motor neuron signs
7 Sphincter dysfunction, perianal anesthesia, leg weakness

NB: Back pain due to spinal cord compression of malignant origin is a medical emergency which may require rapid treatment to prevent permanent neurologic sequelae (p. 32)

INVESTIGATING MALIGNANT DISEASE

RADIOGRAPHIC ABNORMALITIES IN NEOPLASTIC DISEASE

Pulmonary infiltrates in the cancer patient
1 Infiltration (by tumor)
— Lymphangitis carcinomatosa (esp. in breast cancer)
— Lymphoma, bronchioloalveolar cell carcinoma
2 Infection (opportunistic)
— Neutropenic: esp. Gram-negative pneumonia
— Immunosuppressed: CMV, *Pneumocystis,* fungi
3 Infarction (pulmonary)
— Thromboembolism
4 Collapse/consolidation (hypostatic)
— Obstructing primary tumor
5 Aspiration
— Intrinsic/extrinsic esophageal obstruction by tumor
— Cytotoxic-induced emesis in a sedated patient (rare)
6 Iatrogenic
— Radiation pneumonitis or fibrosis
— Cytotoxic-induced lung disease (e.g. bleomycin)

Osteolytic lesions in the cancer patient
1 Focal lesions
— Myeloma
— Metastatic renal cell carcinoma
— Other metastatic carcinoma, esp.
• Ca breast
• Ca lung
• Ca thyroid
— Primary bone tumors
2 Generalized osteopenia
— Myeloma
— Old age ± immobilization
— Prolonged steroid therapy

Osteosclerotic lesions in the cancer patient*
1 Metastatic prostate cancer
2 Metastatic breast cancer
— De novo mixed lytic/blastic
— Treatment → lytic healing → sclerosis
3 'Ivory vertebrae' or patchy sclerosis
— Hodgkin's disease
— Myelofibrosis
— Coincidental Paget's disease

* *Rarely* associated with hypercalcemia; cf. osteolytic lesions

Factors distinguishing osteosarcoma from Ewing's sarcoma
1 Osteosarcoma
  — Usually affects metaphysis
  — cf. Ewing's → diaphysis
2 Osteosarcoma
  — Usually affects long bones
  — cf. Ewing's → flat bones
3 Osteosarcoma X-ray
  — 'Sunburst', Codman's triangle*
  — cf. Ewing's → 'onionskinning'
4 Osteosarcoma
  — Usually radioresistant
  — cf. Ewing's: usually radiosensitive

* cf. osteoid osteoma: dense sclerotic lesion surrounded by radiolucent zone

TUMOR MARKERS*

Diagnostic significance of tumor markers in serum
1 AFP
  — Non-seminomatous germ-cell tumors (80%)
  — Hepatoma (50%; too insensitive for screening)
2 β-HCG
  — Choriocarcinoma (100%)
  — Non-seminomatous germ-cell tumors (50%)
  — Seminoma (10% *only*; elevation is typically mild)
3 CEA
  — Colorectal cancer, esp. with liver metastases‡
  — Useless for *screening*
  — May be useful for *follow-up* (e.g. for monitoring efficacy of palliative chemotherapy for metastases
  — May help in *diagnosis* of undifferentiated carcinoma (if +) from poorly differentiated lymphoma or amelanotic melanoma (−)
4 Prostate-specific antigen (PSA)
  — Elevated in 95% primary prostate cancers
  — Levels reflect degree of extraprostatic extension
  — Elevation in asymptomatic patients may indicate need for transrectal ultrasound and/or needle biopsy
  Prostatic acid phosphatase (PAP)
  — Prostatic carcinoma, esp. bony secondaries (85% +ve)
  — Poor sensitivity for early-stage disease (50% false −ve)
  — Less sensitive monitor of tumor activity than PSA¶
5 Alkaline phosphatase
  — Elevations may signify metastasis to bone *or* liver; in bone disease the enzyme is *heat-labile* ('bone burns') and there is no elevation of GGT
  — Bone-derived enzyme is marker of osteoblastic activity; correlates with ^{99m}Tc bone scan
  — *Placental* isoenzyme (PLAP) is elevated in 50% of seminomas and dysgerminomas, and is a sensitive marker for (rare) *extragonadal* germ-cell tumors
6 Calcitonin
  — Medullary carcinoma of the thyroid
  — Invaluable in screening, diagnosis and follow-up

7 Thyroglobulin
  — Papillary/follicular thyroid cancer
  — Useful in follow-up
8 Paraprotein
  — B-cell neoplasm, esp. myeloma
  — Useful in initial diagnosis and follow-up
  β₂-Microglobulin
  — Myeloma (in follow-up)
9 ESR
  — Hodgkin's, myeloma
  — Useful in follow-up (and diagnosis of myeloma)
10 Urinary 5-HIAA
  — Carcinoid syndrome
  — Useful in diagnosis and follow-up
11 Urinary/plasma catecholamines
  — Pheochromocytoma
  — Useful in initial diagnosis, less so in follow-up
12 Ca 125
  — Ovarian cancer (esp. non-mucinous; cf. inhibin)
  — Positive in 80% cases; predicts recurrence in 75%
  — Not specific for ovarian; e.g. also → endometrial Ca, peritoneal seedlings
13 Ca 15-3
  — Breast cancer
  — Positive in 75% metastatic cases (cf. CEA ~ 50%)
14 Ca 19-9
  — Gastrointestinal Ca, esp. pancreas, bile ducts (± colon)
15 Inhibin
  — Ovarian tumors, esp.:
    • Granulosa-cell tumors (also have ↑ E₂)
    • Mucinous ovarian adenocarcinomas

* = Serum assays which correlate with presence/progression of a tumor type
‡ *Poor* sensitivity for early-stage disease; often also elevated in advanced-stage gastric, breast and lung cancer
¶ NB: Borderline elevations of PAP or PSA often occur in benign hypertrophy

DETERMINING THE ORIGIN OF METASTATIC CANCER

Metastases from unknown primary*: investigative rationâle
1 Diagnosis of treatable disease, esp.
  — Hormone-responsive disease
  — Chemosensitive disease
2 Avoidance of iatrogenic morbidity in resistant disease
3 Prevention of complications related to occult primary, e.g. bowel obstruction, pathologic fracture
4 Prognostic clarification

* i.e. no clue to organ of origin from history, examination or CXR

Unknown primary diagnoses requiring active exclusion
1 Chemosensitive tumors, esp.
  — Non-Hodgkin's lymphoma
  — Germ-cell tumors
  — Neuroendocrine tumors (incl. SCLC)
  — Ovarian cancer

2 Hormone-sensitive tumors
— Breast cancer
— Prostate cancer
— Endometrial cancer
— Thyroid cancer

Approach to evaluation of metastatic disease
1 Squamous cell carcinoma in cervical nodes
— Meticulous inspection of scalp and skin
— ENT exam: indirect laryngoscopy ± examination under anesthesia (EUA) with blind biopsies from nasopharynx, base of tongue
— CXR (± barium swallow)
2 Anaplastic carcinoma in cervical nodes
— CXR; sputum cytology (most reliable in SCLC)
— Thyroid scan + needle biopsy
— Nasopharyngeal assessment
— Consider diagnosis of undifferentiated lymphoma; exclude with monoclonal light chain staining
3 Squamous cell carcinoma in inguinal nodes
— Careful examination of legs, vulva, penis, perineum
— Pelvic examination (exclude vaginal/cervix cancer)
— Proctoscopy/colposcopy (exclude anal/cervix cancer)
4 Metastatic adenocarcinoma
— Hormone receptor (ER/PR) expression in females
— Serum PSA/acid phosphatase in males
— Serum AFP/HCG (if positive, histology needs review)
— Consider diagnosis of poorly differentiated lymphoma
5 Axillary node adenocarcinoma in a female
— ER/PR immunocytochemistry
— Bilateral mammography (irrespective of ER result)
6 Retroperitoneal/mediastinal mass, or multiple pulmonary metastases, in a young male*
— AFP, β-HCG; ± testicular ultrasound
— Blood count, differential, film, marrow examination (exclude lymphoma, T cell leukemia)

* Presence of *gynecomastia* in this context is virtually diagnostic of germ-cell tumor (primary may be extragonadal, e.g. in sympathetic ganglia)

Histopathologic characterization of tumor tissue
1 Light microscopy
— Signet ring cells (favor gastric primary)
— Melanin (melanoma)
— Mucin
• *Common* in gut/lung/breast/endometrial cancer
• Less common in ovarian cancer
• *Rare* in renal cell or thyroid cancer
— Psammoma bodies
• Ovarian cancer (mucin +)
• Thyroid cancer (mucin –)
2 Immunoperoxidase
— AFP, β-HCG, ± PLAP (p. 24)
— PSA, PAP (p. 24)

— CEA, cytokeratin, EMA (carcinomas)
— Leukocyte common antigen (lymphomas)
— Neuron-specific enolase (neuroblastoma, SCLC)
— Thyroglobulin (follicular thyroid carcinoma)
— Calcitonin (medullary thyroid carcinoma)
— S-100, vimentin (melanoma)
— Vimentin (sarcomas)
— Desmin, muscle-specific actin (rhabdomyosarcoma)
— Factor VIII antigen (angiosarcoma)
3 Surface immunoglobulin
— Anti-light chain monoclonal antibodies
— Phenotypic T cell markers (e.g. CD4)
4 Hormone receptor immunocytochemistry (Ca breast)
5 Electron microscopy
— Distinguishes
• Adenocarcinoma and mesothelioma
• Spindle-cell tumors (sarcomas, melanoma, SCC)
• Small round-cell tumors (see below)
— May identify
• Amelanotic melanoma (melanosomes)
• Carcinoids (neurosecretory granules)
• Undifferentiated lymphomas, histiocytosis X

Differential diagnosis of small round-cell tumors
'LEMON':
1 **L**ymphoma
2 **E**wing's tumor; rhabdomyosarcoma
3 **M**edulloblastoma
4 **O**at-cell (small-cell) carcinoma
5 **N**euroblastoma, primitive neuroectodermal tumor (PNET)

SCREENING FOR MALIGNANT DISEASE

General principles of cancer screening
1 *Effectiveness* of a screening test depends on
— The availability of *effective treatment*
— The ability to identify (and test) *high-risk groups*
2 The most effective screening test in current use is the *Papanicolaou (cervical) smear*
3 *Mammography* of women aged 50–70 reduces breast cancer-specific mortality by 20–30%

Sources of bias in evaluating cancer screening tests
1 *Lead time bias*
— By detecting disease at an earlier (presymptomatic) stage, subsequent survival is spuriously prolonged when compared with a symptomatic cohort
2 *Length time bias*
— By instituting mass screening programs, a relative excess of patients with *indolent* disease will be detected initially (since at any one time the *prevalence* of slowly growing tumors will tend to be greater, even if the *incidence* of aggressive tumors is similar), leading to an illusory survival improvement in the screened cohort

Colorectal cancer: recommendations for high-risk screening and follow-up

1 Ulcerative colitis (pancolitis > 10 years duration *or* left-sided colitis > 20 years duration)
   — 6-monthly sigmoidoscopy + annual colonoscopy with multiple biopsies
   — Proctocolectomy is indicated if high-grade dysplasia
2 Familial adenomatous polyposis (FAP): first-degree relative
   — Children have 50% chance of inheriting disease
   — Annual flexible sigmoidoscopy after age 15
   — Extend to 3-yearly sigmoidoscopy if clear at age 35
   — Genetic screening (5q- mutation) may be useful
   — Prophylactic surgery if polyps develop
3 Hereditary non-polyposis colorectal cancer (HNPCC)
   — Lynch syndrome I (site-specific Ca colon)
   — Lynch syndrome II (cancer family syndrome, with additional cancers of endometrium, ovary, etc.)
   — Annual fecal occult blood testing from age 25
   — 2-yearly colonoscopy from age 30
4 Patients with previous adenoma(s) or carcinoma
   — Colonoscopy every 3–5 years; occult blood testing has a purely supplementary role in follow-up here
5 First-degree relative of patient with colorectal cancer
   — Annual fecal occult blood testing from age 40
   — ± Flexible sigmoidoscopy every 5 years
   — Positive occult blood? Colonoscopy

Fecal occult blood testing in standard-risk patients

1 2–5% of tests performed in standard-risk subjects will be positive and of these, 75% will have no abnormality
   — i.e. False-positive rate for polyp/Ca detection is 75%
   — False-positive rate for Ca detection alone is ~ 95%
   — These rates translate into many unnecessary tests
2 20% of cancers appear never to bleed
   — i.e. False-negative rate for Ca detection is > 20%
   — False-negative rate for polyp detection is much higher
3 Less than 1% of screened standard-risk subjects will have a carcinoma. Tumors detected in this way are twice as likely to be Dukes' stage A or B than are symptomatic tumors
4 Annual screening of standard-risk subjects *may* reduce cancer-specific mortality (ref. 1.1). Hence, annual occult blood testing + digital rectal exam (?± 10-yearly sigmoidoscopy) *may* be justifiable after age 50
5 The *cost-effectiveness* of fecal occult blood screening remains unproven

False-positive and -negative fecal occult blood tests

1 *False-negatives* may arise due to
   — Sampling error or delay in test development
   — Proximal site of bleeding
   — Vitamin C ingestion
2 *False-positives* may arise due to
   — Red meat, iron tablets
   — Aspirin, other NSAIDs

Asymptomatic mammographic lesions meriting biopsy

1 Mass lesion
   — May be stellate ± spiculated margins
2 'Suspicious' microcalcifications*
   — Linear
   — Branching

* May indicate intraductal carcinoma (p. 36) accompanying invasive tumors

Common causes of false-positive mammograms

1 Fat necrosis (e.g. post-traumatic)
2 Fibrocystic disease
3 Scarring
   — Post-surgical (e.g. lumpectomy)
   — Post-irradiation

Investigation and management of the abnormal cervical smear

1 Mild-to-moderate dyskaryosis
   — Repeat smear in 6 months (± endocervical curettage)
2 Two further smears → mild dyskaryosis, *or*
   One further smear → moderate dyskaryosis, *or*
   Severe dyskaryosis (once)
   — Proceed to colposcopy and punch-directed biopsy
3 Minor cervical intraepithelial neoplasia (CIN grade I–II)
   — Cryocoagulation/cold coagulation
4 CIN III (localized or upper limits undefinable)
   — Cone biopsy (large loop excision of transformation zone) using diathermy loop CIN III involving most of cervix or → vaginal fornix
   — CO_2 laser photovaporization
5 Invasive SCC cervix
   — Hysterectomy or radiotherapy

Early detection of prostate cancer*

1 Elevated PSA (if > 4 ng/mL; but *esp.* if > 10 ng/mL)
2 Transrectal ultrasound ± needle biopsy
3 Digital rectal examination (less sensitive than PSA)

* Too non-specific and insensitive to justify routine screening; these measures only reliably detect tumors > 0.5 cm diameter. Annual rectal examination after age 50 (± PSA before) is reasonable, though *not* yet proven effective

INVESTIGATION OF THE SYMPTOMATIC PATIENT

Investigation of colorectal symptoms

1 Patients presenting de novo with rectal bleeding
   — Sigmoidoscopy and colonoscopy
2 Patients presenting with other colorectal symptoms
   — Digital rectal examination
   — Sigmoidoscopy
   — Assess the need for colonoscopy and/or barium studies on the basis of these results
3 The false-negative rate for fecal occult blood testing in patients with symptoms of colorectal cancer is > 20%
   — i.e. This is an *inappropriate* test in such patients

The symptomatic breast: triple assessment
1 Physical examination
2 Mammogram*
— Two views: mediolateral, craniocaudal
— Compression views of abnormality
— ± Ultrasound of ?cystic lesions
3 Tissue diagnosis
— Fine-needle aspiration cytology
— Percutaneous biopsy
— Excision biopsy

* NB: Mammography in the evaluation of symptomatic breast disease (lumps) is purely adjunctive, i.e. a negative examination is *unhelpful* and provides *no* reassurance (15–20% of palpable carcinomas are mammogram-negative)

STAGING OF SOLID TUMORS

Staging of testicular germ-cell tumors
1 Stage I — Involvement limited to testis
2 Stage II — Abdominal nodal involvement
3 Stage III — Mediastinal involvement, *and/or*
— Supraclavicular node involvement, *and/or*
— Lung parenchyma involvement
4 Stage IV — Extranodal, extrapulmonary disease

Adverse prognostic features in testicular germ-cell tumors
1 Bulky disease
— Infradiaphragmatic tumor mass > 10 cm diameter
— Supradiaphragmatic tumor mass > 5 cm diameter
2 Extragonadal primary tumor (esp. 1° mediastinal disease)
3 AFP > 1000 ng/L; β-HCG > 50 000 mIU/mL
4 Non-pulmonary visceral spread (esp. to liver, bone, CNS), *or*
Pulmonary metastases: > 20 tumors or > 3 cm diameter
5 Unfavorable histology (e.g. pure choriocarcinoma)

Histologic subtypes of testicular tumors
1 Seminoma (dysgerminoma) — 40%
2 Embryonal carcinoma — 20%
3 Teratoma — 10%
4 Mixed teratoma/embryonal — 25%
5 Choriocarcinoma — 1%

Staging of colorectal carcinoma
1 Dukes' A
— Confined to (sub)mucosa
— > 90% 5-year survival
2 Dukes' B
— Spread through muscularis layer
— 70–85% 5-year survival
3 Dukes' C
— Involvement of local nodes
— 30–60% 5-year survival
4 Dukes' D
— Distant metastases
— < 5% 5-year survival

Staging of cervical cancer
1 FIGO stage 0 — Carcinoma *in situ*
2 FIGO stage 1 — Confined to cervix
3 FIGO stage 2 — Extends to upper vagina or parametrium
4 FIGO stage 3 — Extends to lower vagina/pelvic sidewall
5 FIGO stage 4 — Extends beyond true pelvis

Staging of small-cell lung cancer
1 Limited disease
— Confined to hemithorax
— Includes ipsilateral supraclavicular nodes
2 Extensive disease
— Spread beyond hemithorax
— Includes ipsilateral pleural effusion

TNM staging: breast cancer as an example
1 **T** = tumor
— T1: tumor < 2 cm diameter
— T2: tumor ≥ 2 cm diameter
— T3: tumor fixed to pectoralis muscle/fascia
— T4: tumor involving chest wall or skin; includes
• Peau d'orange
• Dermal lymphatic invasion ('inflammatory' Ca)
2 **N** = nodes
— N0 = impalpable nodes (± negative histology)
— N1 = mobile axillary adenopathy (positive histology)
— N2 = matted/fixed axillary nodes
— N3 = supraclavicular or internal mammary adenopathy
3 **M** = metastases
— M0 = no evidence of metastases
— M1 = distant metastases

Staging and management of malignant melanoma
1 Breslow thickness (depth of invasion) ≤ 1 mm
— i.e. Confined to superficial dermis
— Good prognosis (90% cure)
— Excise with 1 cm margin
2 Breslow thickness 1–2 mm
— Moderate prognosis
— (Re)excise with 2 cm margin
3 Breslow thickness > 2 mm
— i.e. Invading subcutaneous fat
— Poor prognosis (20% cure only)
— Reexcise with 3 cm margin
4 Clinically suspicious regional nodes *or* > 3 mm thick 1°
— Check CXR and LFTs
— Proceed to en bloc dissection if negative

MANAGING MALIGNANT DISEASE

Extent of disease: influence on treatment
1 Local treatments
— Surgery
— Radiotherapy

2 Systemic treatments
 — Hormone therapy
 — Cytotoxic chemotherapy

Therapeutic approaches in oncology
1 Adjuvant
 — Prophylactic treatment of presumed
   micrometastases
2 Neoadjuvant
 — Initial systemic therapy of locally advanced
   disease aimed at 'downstaging', thus permitting
   local treatment
3 Radical
 — Maximal treatment, usually with curative intent
4 Palliative
 — Specific antitumor treatment administered
   without anticipated survival prolongation, but
   with hope of improved quality of life
5 Symptomatic
 — Non-specific measures only; no anticancer
   treatment

Malignancies curable with chemotherapy
1 70–90% cure rate
 — Testicular teratoma or seminoma
 — Choriocarcinoma (in women)
 — Hodgkin's disease
 — Wilms' tumor
2 40–60% cure rate
 — Acute lymphoblastic leukemia (in childhood)
 — Burkitt's lymphoma (endemic variety)
 — Ewing's sarcoma, osteosarcoma
 — Non-Hodgkin's lymphoma (diffuse large-cell)
3 20–30% cure rate
 — Acute lymphoblastic leukemia (in adults)
 — Acute myeloblastic leukemia

Malignancies responsive to palliative chemotherapy
1 Low-grade lymphomas
   Chronic leukemias
   Myeloma
2 Breast cancer
3 Ovarian cancer
4 Small-cell lung cancer

Malignancies responsive to adjuvant chemotherapy
1 Premenopausal breast cancer*
2 Wilms' tumor
3 Osteogenic sarcoma, embryonal
   rhabdomyosarcoma

* cf. postmenopausal breast cancer: adjuvant
tamoxifen

Malignancies curable with radical radiotherapy
1 Non-melanomatous skin cancer
2 Seminoma, dysgerminoma (non-bulky)
3 Hodgkin's disease stages IA and IIA (unless bulky
   disease)
4 Non-Hodgkin's lymphoma pathologic stage I and II
5 Early-stage head/neck tumors (incl. laryngeal or
   lingual SCC)
6 Early-stage carcinoma of the cervix or bladder

Malignant complications responsive to palliative radiotherapy
1 Painful bone metastases (local or hemibody
   irradiation)
2 Refractory lymphomas (e.g. whole-body irradiation)
3 Neoplastic skin ulceration/fungation
4 Obstructed hollow viscus (esp. trachea, esophagus,
   vena cava)
5 Neural compression (cerebral, spinal cord, nerve)
6 Uncontrolled tumor bleeding (e.g. hemoptysis,
   hematuria)

Malignancies responsive to hormonal manipulation
1 Breast cancer (p. 36)
2 Prostate cancer (p. 38)
3 Endometrial cancer (progestogens)
4 Papillary/follicular thyroid cancer ($T_4 \rightarrow$ TSH
   suppression)

Malignancies resistant to treatment
1 Gastrointestinal adenocarcinomas, esp. pancreas
2 Renal cell carcinoma
3 Melanoma
4 Mesothelioma
5 Hepatoma

NB: 'Radioresistance' of many tumors is technical
in origin, i.e. the tumor cells may be 'sensitive' but toxicity to
adjacent normal tissue precludes effective treatment

Malignancies which may undergo spontaneous regression
1 Neuroblastoma (esp. stage IV S)
2 Kaposi's sarcoma (endemic variety)
3 Rarely – melanoma, renal cell carcinoma

Common fallacies in cancer management
1 A dire prognosis justifies toxic treatment even if
   therapeutic benefit is unproven
2 Tumor responsiveness (i.e. shrinkage) to a given
   therapy justifies treatment even if quality-of-life
   benefit unproven
3 Lack of toxicity justifies presumptive treatment even
   if cost-effectiveness is unproven

MECHANISMS OF CYTOTOXIC DRUG ACTION

Classification of common chemotherapeutic agents
1 Alkylators
 — Chlorambucil, cyclophosphamide
 — Nitrogen mustard (mustine in MOPP)
 — Melphalan (phenylalanine mustard), busulphan
 — Platinum derivatives (cisplatin, carboplatin)
2 Intercalators
 — Anthracyclines (doxorubicin, daunorubicin)
 — Anthraquinones (mitoxantrone); m-AMSA
3 Nitrosoureas (alkylate and crosslink DNA)
 — BCNU, CCNU, streptozotocin
4 Antitumor antibiotics (variable mechanisms of
   action)
 — Bleomycin, mithramycin, mitomycin C

5 Spindle toxins
   — Vinca alkaloids: vincristine, vinblastine
   — Yew bark derivatives: taxol (paclitaxel)
6 Topoisomerase II inhibitors
   — Podophyllotoxin derivatives: e.g. VP-16
     (etoposide)
7 Protein synthesis inhibitors
   — L-asparaginase
8 Antimetabolites
   — Purine analogues
     • Azathioprine, 6MP, 6TG
   — Enzyme inhibitors
     • Methotrexate (→ dihydrofolate reductase)
     • Hydroxyurea (→ ribonucleotide reductase)
     • 5FU (→ thymidylate synthetase)
     • Ara-C (→ DNA polymerase)
     • Deoxycoformycin (→ cytosine deaminase)

Relationships of cytotoxic action to cell cycle kinetics
1 Cycle-specific drugs (preferentially toxic to
   proliferating cells)
   — Alkylating agents
   — Anthracyclines
   — Topoisomerase II inhibitors
2 Phase-specific drugs (preferentially act in cell cycle
   phases)*
   — S-phase (DNA **s**ynthesis) drugs: antimetabolites
   — M-phase (**m**itosis) drugs: vinca alkaloids

* Phase-specific drugs are also cycle-specific

Indications for corticosteroids in malignant disease
1 Intracranial tumor with edema + raised intracranial
   pressure
2 Nerve (incl. spinal cord) compression, esp.
   preradiotherapy
3 Acute inflammation following radiotherapy, e.g.
   radiation proctitis (steroid enemas), non-candidal
   esophagitis
4 Dyspnea due to lymphangitis carcinomatosa
5 Hypercalcemia (in myeloma)
6 Antiemetic prophylaxis
7 Appetite stimulation
8 Antitumor effect (e.g. in B cell malignancies)

Mechanisms of tumor resistance to anticancer drugs
1 General
   — Tumor heterogeneity: genetic instability of
     primary tumor → clonal loss of sensitive drug
     targets
   — Small growth fraction: many tumors replicate no
     faster than normal tissues and are therefore no
     more sensitive to cycle-specific chemotherapeutic
     drugs
2 Specific
   — Reduced drug uptake
   — Increased drug inactivation or efflux
   — Enhanced lesion repair (e.g. induction of DNA
     alkyltransferase activity during alkylator therapy)
   — Gene amplification (e.g. of the dihydrofolate
     reductase gene during prolonged methotrexate
     therapy)
   — Reduced requirement for metabolic product (e.g.
     acquired L-asparaginase resistance)

   — Loss of drug target (e.g. ER loss → tamoxifen
     resistance)

MORBIDITY OF CYTOTOXIC THERAPY

Common problems limiting use of cytotoxic therapy
1 Myelosuppression
   — Alkylators, nitrosoureas
   — Anthracyclines; ara-C; vinblastine
2 Severe nausea
   — Cisplatin
   — Anthracyclines; IV alkylating agents
3 Total alopecia
   — Anthracyclines, cranial irradiation
   — Cyclophosphamide; VP-16, ara-C; taxol
4 Mucositis, stomatitis
   — Methotrexate
   — Anthracyclines, bleomycin, 5FU
5 Pulmonary fibrosis
   — Bleomycin, busulphan (dose-related)
   — Methotrexate, etc. (idiosyncratic)
6 'Radiation recall' reactions
   — Actinomycin D, anthracyclines
   — Methotrexate
7 Extravasation necrosis
   — Anthracyclines, actinomycin D
   — Nitrogen mustard
8 Expense
   — New drugs, e.g. taxol
   — Chronic therapy, esp. hormones (e.g. megestrol,
     flutamide, LHRH agonists)

Drug interactions with cytotoxic therapy
1 Azathioprine, oral 6MP
   — 4-fold potentiation by allopurinol
     (inhibits drug catabolism by xanthine oxidase)
2 Methotrexate
   — Potentiated by aspirin, NSAIDs (see below)
3 Procarbazine
   — Hypertension on tyramine ingestion (MAO
     inhibitor)
4 Cyclophosphamide
   — Activated in liver (hence, potentiated) by enzyme
     inducers, e.g. barbiturates

Genitourinary morbidity of cyclophosphamide/ifosfamide
1 Hemorrhagic cystitis (preventable by hydration and
   MESNA)
2 Bladder telangiectasia and/or fibrosis
3 Azoospermia, amenorrhea
4 Inappropriate ADH secretion
5 Transitional cell carcinoma of the bladder

Methotrexate toxicity: precipitants, potentiation and prevention
1 Precipitants (drugs competing for renal tubular
   secretion)
   — Aspirin: displaces drug from plasma protein
     binding
   — Probenecid, phenylbutazone, trimethoprim

2 Potentiation
  — Concurrent radiotherapy
3 Prevention (esp. in high-dose regimens)
  — Forced diuresis (intravenous prehydration)
  — Urinary alkalinization
  — Oral folinic acid (leukovorin) 'rescue'

Relative contraindications to anthracycline therapy
1 Frail and/or elderly patient
2 Left ventricular dysfunction or arrhythmia
3 Obstructive jaundice
4 History of mediastinal irradiation and/or
   cyclophosphamide

Relatively non-myelosuppressive cytotoxics
1 Bleomycin
2 L-Asparaginase
3 Vincristine (cf. vinblastine)
4 Cisplatin (cf. carboplatin)
5 Methotrexate with leukovorin 'rescue'

TOXICITY OF RADIATION THERAPY

Modes of radiotherapy administration
1 External beam
  — Superficial (25–150 kV)
    • Limited penetration
    • Used for skin cancers (BCC, SCC)
  — Orthovoltage (250–350 kV)
    • Moderate penetration
    • Used to palliate painful bone metastases
    • Skin toxicity may be a problem
  — Megavoltage (> 1 MV; usually 4–10 MV)
    • Produced by cobalt machines or linear
      accelerators
    • Excellent penetration ('skin-sparing' radiation)
2 Brachytherapy
  — Unsealed sources
    • ^{32}P (polycythemia vera)
    • ^{131}I (Graves' disease, thyroid cancer)
    • ^{137}Cs (cesium: Ca cervix)
  — Sealed sources
    • ^{192}Ir (iridium e.g. head & neck tumors)

Determinants of radiation-induced toxicity
1 Volume irradiated
2 Tissue/organ irradiated
3 Fraction size (i.e. dose per treatment session)
4 Total dose

Normal tissue tolerance: radiation dose thresholds*
1 Brain   — 50 Gy
2 Heart, small intestine   — 30 Gy
3 Liver, lung, kidney   — 20 Gy
4 Whole body   — 3–5 Gy

* (= the 5% injury risk for an 'average' treatment volume and
fractionation)

Common problems following therapeutic irradiation
1 Acute local toxicity
  — Skin erythema, desquamation, photosensitivity
  — Hair loss (usually transient)
  — Mucositis; inflammation of any organ
2 Acute systemic toxicity (radiation sickness)
  — Fatigue and malaise
  — Nausea, anorexia
3 Late toxicity caused by endarteritis obliterans, e.g.
  — Radiation nephritis
  — Radiation pneumonitis
  — Radiation myelopathy (cord ischemia)
  — ↓ Hemopoietic reserve (compromising
    chemotherapy)
4 Following mantle irradiation (Hodgkin's)
  — Hypothyroidism (30% within 20 years)
  — Graves' disease, thyroiditis, carcinoma
5 Following cranial irradiation
  — Intellectual deterioration, somnolence (esp.
    children)
  — Hypopituitarism due to hypothalamic damage:
    • Low GH, high prolactin, low FSH/LH
    • Low free T4 without ↑ TSH
6 Mutagenicity
  — Leukemia (esp.) after megavoltage therapy or ^{32}P
  — CNS tumors after neuraxis irradiation for ALL

NB: *Late* toxicity (e.g. stricture, second malignancy) is a major
concern in *radical* treatment, but less so (or not at all) in
palliative treatment

Problems following abdominal or pelvic irradiation
1 Nausea, esp. following abdominal irradiation
   (e.g. for ovarian cancer, seminoma, lymphoma)
  — Management: antiemetics (p. 31)
2 Diarrhea, esp. following radical pelvic irradiation
   (for gynecological or genitourinary malignancies)
  — Management: loperamide, codeine, low-residue
    diet
3 Tenesmus, rectal bleeding (radiation proctitis)
  — Management: prednisolone suppositories
4 Urinary frequency/dysuria
  — Management: exclude infection; anticholinergics;
    alkalinizers, analgesics; repeat cystoscopy
5 Vaginal discharge ± cervicitis
  — Management: exclude *Candida, Trichomonas*
  Vaginal adhesions
  — Management: treat with dilators
6 Nephrotoxicity (dose-related)
  — Management: prevent by shielding

THERAPEUTIC USE OF CYTOTOXIC DRUGS

Points to discuss with patients prior to commencing treatment
1 Prognosis with and without treatment
2 Probability of therapeutic benefit (cure, complete or
   partial remission, disease-free interval, symptoms)
3 Risks of infertility/teratogenicity/premature
   menopause; availability of sperm banking
4 Likely severity of alopecia; availability of wig-making
5 Likely severity and duration of nausea; prophylactic
   drugs
6 Need for allopurinol (in hematologic malignancies)
7 Requirement for regular blood tests
8 Urgent significance of fever or bruising/bleeding

9 Rationâle of clinical trials and informed consent
10 Long-term risk of second malignancy, esp. in good-prognosis disease treated with alkylating agents ± radiotherapy

Clinical assessment of the patient commencing treatment

1 Assessment and documentation of disease extent
 — Measurement (and/or photography) of visible lesions
 — Radiographic corroboration
 — Measurement of tumor markers
 — Invasive staging *if* stage-specific therapy exists
2 Assessment of vital organ function
 — Left ventricular function (pre-doxorubicin)
 — Lung function (pre-bleomycin)
 — Renal function (pre-platinum)
3 Assessment of immune status (in leukemia, transplantation)
 — CXR, tuberculin test
 — Viral (CMV, HSV, hepatitis B) and toxoplasma serology
4 Assessment of venous access
 — Consideration of an implantable infusion port/catheter
5 Assessment of psychological adjustment to disease and to disease- and treatment-related disability

Chemotherapeutic agents commonly used for solid tumors

1 Germ-cell tumors
 — Cisplatin, bleomycin, VP-16 (BEP)
2 Small-cell lung cancer
 — Etoposide (incl. oral)
 — Doxorubicin, cyclophosphamide, vincristine
3 Breast cancer
 — Cyclophosphamide, methotrexate, 5FU (CMF)
 — Doxorubicin/epirubicin
4 Ovarian cancer
 — Cisplatin or carboplatin (see below)
 — Chlorambucil or cyclophosphamide
 — Taxol
5 Choriocarcinoma
 — Methotrexate, actinomycin D
6 Osteosarcoma
 — Methotrexate, doxorubicin, platinum
7 Colorectal cancer
 — 5FU + leukovorin
8 Adrenocortical carcinoma
 — Mitotane
9 Langerhans cell histiocytosis (histiocytosis X)
 — Etoposide

Cisplatin or carboplatin for cancer chemotherapy?

1 Testicular germ-cell tumors
 — Cisplatin (more effective)
2 Ovarian cancer
 — Carboplatin (more convenient)
3 Poor bone marrow reserve
 — Cisplatin
4 Pre-existing renal failure or hearing impairment
 — Carboplatin

PRE-TREATMENT CONSIDERATIONS

Antiemetic drugs in cancer chemotherapy

1 $5HT_3$ (serotonin) receptor antagonists
 — Ondansetron, granisetron
2 D_2 (dopamine) receptor antagonists
 — Metoclopramide*, metopimazone
3 Dexamethasone (IV or oral)
 — esp. Effective for late nausea
4 Lorazepam (oral)
 — esp. Effective for anticipatory nausea
5 Cyclizine (± via pump); phenothiazines, butyrophenones

* Causes $5HT_3$ receptor blockade at high dosage

Indications for hematopoietic colony-stimulating factors (p. 167)

1 After febrile neutropenia in a previous chemotherapy cycle (if dose needs to be maintained for anticancer efficacy)
2 To reduce likelihood of febrile neutropenia in high-risk scenarios, e.g. high-dose regimens
3 After high-dose chemotherapy and autologous stem-cell transplantation

NB: Use of hemopoietic growth factors for hypoplastic and metastatic cytopenias is generally *not* effective

Infertility following cancer chemotherapy

1 MOPP chemotherapy for Hodgkin's disease
 — 80% menstruating women → premature menopause
 — 90% men → infertile (i.e. without sperm banking)
 — Males may be rendered infertile by only 1–2 treatments
 — Younger adults have better prospects for fertility; prepubertal children are least likely to be sterilized
2 Chemotherapy for testicular germ-cell tumors
 — Patients may be oligospermic pretreatment
 — Virtually *all* become infertile during chemotherapy*
 — 80% show partial recovery within 18 months
3 Leukemias and lymphomas
 — High-dose *intermittent* treatment causes less sterility
 — Long-term maintenance therapy (incl. oral alkylating agents) is associated with high incidence of sterility

* cf. gestational trophoblastic tumors: patients *rarely* sterilized by therapy

SECOND PRIMARY NEOPLASMS AFTER CANCER THERAPY

Common antecedents of cytotoxic-induced malignancy

1 Treatment of hematological malignancy
 — Hodgkin's disease, non-Hodgkin's lymphoma
 — Multiple myeloma (melphalan)
 — Polycythemia vera (chlorambucil, ^{32}P)

2 Treatment of 'solid' tumors
— Ovarian cancer (chlorambucil) esp.

Cytotoxic agents predisposing to second malignancies
1 Alkylating agents (e.g. chlorambucil, melphalan)
— Associated with 5q- and 7q- deletions
2 Etoposide (VP-16)
— Cause 11q23 and 21q22 translocations
3 Nitrosoureas; procarbazine
4 Azathioprine*

* Via *immunosuppression* (e.g. → EBV-linked lymphomas), not mutagenicity

Cytotoxic agents not implicated in second malignancies
1 Antimetabolites (except azathioprine; see above)
2 Vinca alkaloids
3 Tumor antibiotics*

* NB: Doxorubicin may potentiate carcinogenicity of radiotherapy

Cytotoxic-induced malignancies
1 Acute non-lymphocytic leukemia*
— esp. Myelomonocytic
2 Non-Hodgkin's lymphoma
— Post-transplant/-Hodgkin's
3 SCC (skin, cervix)
— Post-transplant
4 TCC (bladder)
— Post-cyclophosphamide
5 Miscellaneous adenocarcinomas and soft-tissue sarcomas
— Colon, lung, bone, thyroid

* Up to 5% incidence within 10 years, esp. if also treated with radiotherapy

Radiation-induced malignancies
1 Thyroid tumors
— After low-dose external radiation, *not* ^{131}I
2 Myeloma, non-lymphocytic leukemias
— AML, CML; *not* CLL
3 Breast cancer
— e.g. following multiple fluoroscopies for TB
4 Lung cancer, esp. SCLC
— e.g. in Hiroshima survivors
5 Osteo-/soft tissue sarcoma
— Including hepatic angiosarcoma (post-Thorotrast)
6 Skin tumors
— e.g. after scalp irradiation for ringworm
7 CNS tumors (meningiomas, other neural tumors)
— after low-dose (1–2 Gy) scalp irradiation for tinea capitis

Hormone-induced neoplasms

1 Hepatocellular carcinoma	— Androgenic anabolic steroids
2 Hepatic adenoma	— Combined oral contraceptive
3 Endometrial carcinoma	— Exogenous estrogens
4 Breast cancer	— Estrogens
Prostate cancer	— Endogenous androgens
5 Clear-cell vagina carcinoma	— Maternal diethylstilbestrol

Familial syndromes predisposing to multiple malignancies
1 Multiple endocrine neoplasia type 1 (MEN-1)
— Pituitary/parathyroid/pancreatic islet cell tumors
2 Multiple endocrine neoplasia type 2 (MEN-2)
— Medullary thyroid Ca, bilateral pheochromocytoma
3 Familial retinoblastoma
— Bilateral retinoblastoma ± osteosarcoma
4 Intestinal polyposis syndromes (see also p. 40)
— Familial polyposis
• Colorectal carcinomas
— Gardner's syndrome
• Small and large intestinal Ca
• Mesodermal tumors
— Turcot's syndrome
• Colonic adenomatosis
• Brain tumors
5 Gorlin's (basal cell nevus) syndrome
— Multiple BCCs
— Medulloblastoma, intestinal polyps
6 Familial breast cancer
— Pre-menopausal breast cancer, esp. bilateral
— Sometimes associated with ovarian cancer
7 Li-Fraumeni (mutant p53) syndrome
— Breast/ovary/endometrium/gliomas/sarcomas
— Colorectal carcinoma, esp. right-sided; no polyps
8 Dysplastic nevus syndrome
— Skin tumors (esp. melanoma)
9 Von Hippel–Lindau syndrome
— Retinal, cerebellar hemangioblastomas
— Pheochromocytomas, islet cell tumors
— Renal cell carcinomas

Inherited syndromes predisposing to non-melanoma skin cancer
1 Xeroderma pigmentosum
2 Basal cell nevus syndrome
3 Epidermodysplasia verruciformis
4 Albinism

ONCOLOGIC EMERGENCIES

Management of suspected spinal cord compression
1 Have a high index of suspicion prior to onset of paraparesis or urinary symptoms. Confirm the diagnosis with urgent myelography or (if available) MRI scanning. If compressive lesions at *multiple* levels are demonstrated, surgical management is generally *not* appropriate
2 Refer for immediate surgical decompression if
— Paraplegia or incontinence have not supervened, *and*
— Prognosis following surgery is reasonable, *and*
— The primary pathology is unknown, *or*
— Tumor is probably radioresistant (e.g. melanoma) *or*
— The tumor has recurred following cord irradiation
3 Refer for immediate radiotherapy if
— The tumor is at least moderately radiosensitive, *and*
— Corticosteroids have been commenced

4 Refer for initial cytotoxic therapy (rarely) if
   — The tumor is exquisitely chemosensitive, *and*
   — The neurologic deficit is not serious nor
     fulminant, *or*
   — Both surgery and radiotherapy are
     contraindicated

Management of superior vena caval obstruction
1 Confirm the diagnosis with CXR showing
   mediastinal widening (or, if necessary, contrast
   venography or CT)
2 If the primary histological diagnosis is not known,
   this should be sought by either bronchoscopy with
   biopsy (safe) or by mediastinotomy; careful
   evaluation for peripheral adenopathy may spare
   invasive diagnostic procedure. A small proportion
   (5%) of cases arise due to benign lesions (e.g.
   retrosternal goiter, aortic aneurysm)
3 If a tissue diagnosis cannot be obtained,
   symptomatic relief may be achieved using
   mediastinal irradiation + steroids
4 Obstruction due to SCLC or lymphoma may be best
   treated with systemic chemotherapy in the first
   instance
5 Although often described as an emergency, SVC
   obstructions present subacutely and can be
   managed non-urgently
6 Intravenous lines (esp. if used for administration of
   vesicant cytotoxic therapy) should not be sited in the
   arms

Management of cancer-associated hypercalcemia
1 Evaluate prospects for survival before embarking
   upon definitive intervention
2 The mainstay of management is *intravenous saline*,
   1 litre every 3–4 hours. Frusemide also promotes
   calcium excretion and may be indicated in cardiac or
   renal failure
3 Initial management should also include
   — Treatment of the underlying malignancy
   — Mobilization if feasible (ensuring adequate
     analgesia)
   — Cessation of possible iatrogenic precipitants, e.g.
     tamoxifen (p. 36), thiazides, vitamins A or D
4 Specific hypocalcemic drugs
   — Biphosphonates (osteoclast inhibitors)*
     • Pamidronate infusion (repeat after ~ 3 weeks)
     • Clodronate infusion (repeat after ~ 2 weeks)
   — Plicamycin (mithramycin; osteoclast inhibitor)
     • Daily x 2, then weekly @ 15–25 mg/kg
     • Toxic: nausea, coagulopathy, ↓ platelets
     • Highly effective but needs close monitoring
   — Prednisone 40 mg/day
     • For myeloma or lymphoma *only*
   — Calcitonin (100 U subcut. t.d.s.)
     • For myeloma with renal impairment
   — Gallium nitrate (binds hydroxyapatite)
     • Nephrotoxic
   — IV sodium phosphate
     • Only indicated in life-threatening hyper-
       calcemia

* Now the drug treatment of choice for hypercalcemia

Management of bleeding
1 Iatrogenic (cytotoxic-induced) thrombocytopenia
   — Platelet transfusion
2 Leukoerythroblastic thrombocytopenia (e.g. in
   lymphoma)
   — Cytotoxic therapy with transfusion cover
3 Autoimmune thrombocytopenia (e.g. in CLL)
   — Steroids
4 Hypersplenic thrombocytopenia (e.g. in hairy cell
   leukemia)
   — Splenectomy, splenic irradiation
5 Hyperviscosity
   — Plasmapheresis
6 Obstructive jaundice
   — Parenteral vitamin K
7 Uncontrolled neoplastic hemorrhage
   — Radiotherapy
8 Disseminated intravascular coagulation
   — Fresh frozen plasma ($\geq$ 6 units; no heparin)
   — Platelet transfusion if count < 80 x 10^9/L
   — Cytotoxic therapy of underlying malignancy

Management of urological emergencies
1 Hemorrhagic cystitis
   — Alum irrigation
2 Ureteric obstruction
   — Stent(s) or percutaneous nephrostomy*
3 Priapism
   — Control of underlying disease (e.g. CML)
4 Acute retention
   — Catheterization

* i.e. *if* prognosis warrants active intervention

PAIN IN MALIGNANT DISEASE

**Principles of treating refractory pain in malignant
disease**
1 Adequate (large) doses
2 Regular rather than 'p.r.n.' administration
3 Oral route if possible
4 Single rather than multiple drugs
5 Hospital admission for severe pain control
6 Narcotic infusions via pump for relief of refractory
   pain

Indications for parenteral*/rectal analgesia
1 Rapid effect desired
2 Inability to swallow (dysphagia, cachexia)
3 Persistent vomiting *or* bowel obstruction
4 Intractable pain despite optimal regular oral dosing
5 In the last few hours of life

* e.g. subcutaneous diamorphine infusion via pump

Suboptimal narcotic analgesics for malignant pain
1 Propoxyphene, pentazocine, oral pethidine
   — Weak agonists which may precipitate dysphoria
     (i.e. simulate withdrawal) in opiate-dependent
     patients
2 Dextromoramide (Palfium)
   — Short (2-hour) duration of action
   — Rapid development of *tolerance*

3 Methadone (Physeptone)
— Long (18–36 h) half-life → ↑ risk of toxicity

Clinical guidelines for use of narcotic analgesics
1 Approximate oral equivalents for 30 mg oral morphine
— 300 mg dextropropoxyphene
— 200 mg codeine phosphate
— 150 mg pethidine
— 30 mg methadone (less frequent dosing)
— 30 mg diamorphine (heroin)
— 15 mg dextromoramide (peak effect)
2 Oxycodone suppositories
— 30 mg every 6 hours is equipotent to 20 mg oral morphine every 4 hours
3 Morphine
— Oral–parenteral bioavailability ratio is about 1:3, though patient dosage requirements vary markedly
— No advantage from using oral diamorphine (heroin)
4 Nausea, if it occurs, usually settles after 72 hours of opiate use; constipation, on the other hand, is invariable and should be prevented by *routine* laxative administration
5 Addiction (cf. tolerance) is *rarely* a problem in malignant pain (nor is respiratory depression)

Opioid receptors mediating opiate function and toxicity
1 μ (mu) receptors
— Mediate analgesia and respiratory depression
— Also mediate euphoria and dependence
— Best agonists: morphine, diamorphine
— Partial agonist: buprenorphine
— Weak affinity: dextropropoxyphene
— Partial antagonist: pentazocine
— Full antagonist: naloxone
2 κ (kappa) receptors
— Mediate spinal analgesia
— Also mediate miosis and sedation
— Partial agonists: pentazocine, nalbuphine
3 δ (delta) receptors
— Responsible for constipation, nausea
— Also → respiratory depression, euphoria
— (Dihydro)codeine activates these receptors; some is metabolized to morphine → μ receptors (analgesia)

Oral analgesic regimens for cancer-associated pain
1 Mild
— Paracetamol (acetaminophen) 1 g q 4 h
— Aspirin 600 mg q 4 h (or other NSAID)
2 Moderate
— Dextropropoxyphene 65 mg q 4 h, or
— Dihydrocodeine 30–60 mg q 4 h (constipating), or
— Buprenorphine 0.2–0.4 mg q 6–8 h sublingually (emetic)
3 Severe
— Morphine 5–200 mg q 3–4 h

Specific indications for adjuvant non-narcotic drug therapy
1 Bone pain — NSAIDs, e.g. ketorolac
— Biphosphonates

2 Nerve compression — Steroids (dexamethasone)
— Tricyclics
3 Neuralgias — Carbamazepine, valproate, phenytoin, clonazepam
— Tricyclics; flecanide
4 Muscle spasm — Baclofen, diazepam
5 Neoplastic ulcer — Metronidazole (etc.)
6 Insomnia/depression — Tricyclics, hydroxyzine
7 Opiate constipation — Lactulose
8 Opiate augmentation — Phenothiazines
9 Opiate antiemesis — Haloperidol
10 Opiate sedation — Amphetamines

Neurosurgical approaches to intractable pain in cancer patients
1 Phenol nerve block
— e.g. Celiac axis (Ca pancreas)
2 Dorsal rhizotomy
— For pain in trunk, neck, perineum
3 Percutaneous cordotomy
— For unilateral pain below C_5 dermatome
4 Thalamotomy
— For 'central' pain
5 Epidural anesthesia

Management of bony metastases
1 Bilateral cortical erosion on X-ray of long bone (esp. femur)
— Pin prophylactically
— Irradiate following surgical fixation
2 Bone pain without gross cortical erosion
— Systemic treatment, esp. if hormone-responsive disease
— Palliative irradiation
3 Intractable pain in resistant, terminal disease
— Hemibody irradiation

SURGICAL MANAGEMENT OF MALIGNANT DISEASE

Potential indications for surgery in premalignant conditions
1 Orchiopexy in children with testicular maldescent
Orchidectomy in adolescents or adults with cryptorchidism
Bilateral orchidectomy in testicular feminization
2 Oophorectomy in Turner's syndrome (incl. mosaics)
3 Colectomy in hereditary polyposis *or* in long-standing ulcerative colitis with severe dysplasia on biopsy

Potential indications for cytoreductive (debulking) surgery
1 Pre-chemotherapy
— Ovarian cancer
— Burkitt's lymphoma
2 Post-chemotherapy
— Germ-cell tumors
— Osteosarcoma
— Breast cancer*
3 Post-radiotherapy
— Germ-cell tumors
— Head and neck tumors

* Salvage mastectomy following neoadjuvant chemotherapy for locally advanced tumors

Opportunities for surgical palliation in malignant disorders

1 Colostomy, gastrojejunostomy or feeding gastrostomy for neoplastic gastrointestinal obstruction
2 Placement of intraluminal silastic (e.g. Celestin) or infant feeding tube in esophageal obstruction
3 Percutaneous insertion of biliary drainage catheter following transhepatic cholangiography for extrahepatic obstruction
4 Nephrostomy drainage, or passage of ureteric stent(s), for malignant ureteric obstruction
5 Creation of tracheostomy for obstructing laryngeal carcinoma
6 Insertion of Hickman's catheter or implantable infusion port
7 Le Veen shunt for intractable malignant ascites
8 Prophylactic pinning of impending pathological fracture
9 Ventriculoatrial or peritoneal shunt for hydrocephalus
10 Resection of (apparently) solitary metastasis, e.g. in germ-cell tumors, osteosarcoma, hepatic spread of bowel cancer

Approach to intestinal obstruction in the cancer patient

1 Commence nasogastric suction and intravenous fluids
2 If obstruction does not resolve following supportive measures, surgical palliation should be considered
3 Plain abdominal films may help establish the obstructive site
4 Small bowel intubation may resolve incomplete obstructions
5 Right transverse colostomy relieves large bowel obstruction and can be done under local anesthesia if necessary

Sexual morbidity of cancer treatment

1 Hysterectomy
   — Infertility
2 Radical prostatectomy
   — Impotence; infertility
3 Mastectomy, intestinal stoma
   — Disturbed sexual self-image
   — Impaired libido
4 Pelvic interstitial radiation
   — Vaginal fibrosis, dyspareunia
5 Abdominoperineal resection, cystectomy
   — Impotence (exclude depression)
6 Paraaortic lymphadenectomy
   — Retrograde ejaculation
7 Oophorectomy, menopausal induction
   — Loss of libido, lubrication difficulties
8 Drugs inhibiting libido or sexual responsiveness
   — Hormonal agents
   — Cytotoxic drugs
   — Narcotics, hypnotics, antidepressants

MANAGEMENT OF LUNG CANCER

Contraindications to thoracotomy for lung cancer*

1 Small-cell histology on biopsy or sputum cytology

2 Evidence of local extrapulmonary invasion
   — Hoarseness, bovine cough (laryngeal nerve palsy)
   — Superior vena caval obstruction; dysphagia
   — Horner's (± Pancoast's) syndrome
   — Basal dullness due to pleural effusion (unless chylous) *or* phrenic nerve palsy
3 Evidence of mediastinal involvement
   — Carinal widening on chest X-ray
   — Tumor < 2 cm from carina on bronchoscopy
   — Positive node biopsy on mediastinoscopy
4 Evidence of distant spread
   — Positive liver/bone/brain scan
   — Malignant cells in marrow or CSF
5 Inability to tolerate surgery
   — Age: > 65 (for pneumonectomy), > 70 (for lobectomy)
   — FEV_1 < 1.5 L (pneumonectomy) or < 1.0 L (lobectomy)
   — $PaCO_2$ > 45 mmHg *unless* due to distal collapse
   — Pulmonary hypertension ± cor pulmonale
   — Anesthetic risk factors, e.g. ischemic heart disease

* Note that only 10% of patients are found to be suitable for surgery on initial assessment, and of these only a minority prove resectable; note also that *paraneoplastic syndromes* (p. 20–21) per se are *not* contraindications

Favorable prognostic features in non-small-cell lung cancer

1 Age < 60 with no lung disease or recent smoking history
2 Symptoms minimal, no weight loss
3 Right-sided tumor with no demonstrable spread
4 Well-differentiated squamous cell histology
5 Small primary removable by single lobectomy

Therapeutic modalities in non-small-cell lung cancer

1 Surgery if no contraindications
2 Observation only for minimally symptomatic patients with extrapulmonary (metastatic or locally invasive) disease
3 Palliative irradiation for unresectable symptomatic disease
4 Radical irradiation for patients with small-volume localized disease and contraindications to thoracotomy

Adverse prognostic features in small-cell lung cancer

1 Symptoms, esp. weight loss
2 Extensive disease (p. 27), esp. CNS/liver/marrow spread
3 Cytopenia, esp. thrombocytopenia
4 Mixed (small- and large-cell) histology
5 Failure to achieve complete remission with chemotherapy

Therapeutic modalities in small-cell lung ancer

1 Combination chemotherapy: radical in patients with limited-stage disease (p. 27), palliative if adverse prognosis
2 Prophylactic cranial irradiation for patients achieving complete remission following cytotoxic treatment

3 Palliative cranial irradiation for known cerebral metastases
4 Palliative intrathecal methotrexate ± neuraxis irradiation for meningeal carcinomatosis
5 Palliative irradiation for symptomatic chemoresistant disease

MANAGEMENT OF BREAST CANCER

Biologic and prognostic considerations in breast cancer
1 Long-term follow-up of breast cancer patients suggests that there is no disease-free plateau
2 Axillary dissection is a valuable prognostic, but not therapeutic, measure (i.e. nodes do not 'limit' spread)
3 The post-surgical (mastectomy, lumpectomy) *disease-free survival* is best predicted by axillary node status
4 The *post-relapse survival* is best predicted by the response to hormonal manipulation

Precursor lesions in breast cancer: in situ carcinoma
1 Ductal carcinoma in situ (DCIS; 'intraductal carcinoma')
   — Different histologic subtypes (e.g. comedo-DCIS)
   — Directly gives rise to invasive cancer (infiltrating ductal carcinoma) in 30–50% of cases
   — Prominently associated with 'suspicious' mammographic microcalcifications (p. 26)
   — Microcalcifications may be localized by needle insertion under radiographic guidance, then biopsied/excised
   — Extensive DCIS may necessitate mastectomy
2 Lobular carcinoma in situ (LCIS)
   — Not a precancerous lesion per se; rather, a marker of increased cancer risk in *both* breasts
   — Incidence of subsequent invasive cancer ~ 1%/year
   — Subsequent tumors may be ductal in origin (i.e. *not* usually lobular carcinomas)
   — Subsequent tumors may *not* arise from LCIS region
   — Best managed by close mammographic follow-up

Management of locally recurrent breast cancer
1 Intramammary (post-lumpectomy) recurrence
   — Mastectomy
2 Chest wall recurrence* (e.g. post-mastectomy)
   — Palliative systemic therapy
3 Nodal recurrence
   — Isolated axillary relapse
     • Dissection and/or irradiation
   — Supraclavicular/internal mammary nodes
     • Palliative systemic therapy

* Same prognostic significance as distant metastases

Risk factors for intramammary recurrence post-excision and therapeutic implications
1 Indications for post-lumpectomy irradiation
   — Heavy involvement of axillary lymph nodes (esp. > 3)

   — Histopathologic criteria
     • Lymphatic or vascular invasion (LVI)
     • Disease reaches resection lines ('dirty margins')*
2 Indications for mastectomy
   — Diffuse multifocal carcinoma
   — Extensive intraductal carcinoma
   — Unacceptable cosmetic result from breast conservation‡

* Reexcision (± radiotherapy) is also an option if technically feasible
‡ i.e. relatively large tumor; better cosmesis (if desired) achieved with immediate reconstruction

Estrogen receptor (ER) status and hormone responsiveness
1 About 50% of primary breast tumors are ER+
2 About 50% of ER+ tumors respond to hormonal treatment*
3 About 50% of ER+ tumors have progesterone receptors (PR)
4 About 50% more responses are seen in tumors which are both ER+ and PR+ (i.e. 75% will respond)
5 About 50% of tumors responding to tamoxifen will respond to a second-line hormonal manipulation on relapse

* cf. < 5% for ER- tumors

Factors favoring response to hormonal manipulation
1 ER (PR) +
2 High absolute level of ER (e.g. > 100 fmol/mg protein)
3 Response to previous hormonal manipulation
4 Long disease-free interval following resection of primary
5 Metastatic disease confined to bone/soft tissue/pleura
6 Post-menopausal status; increasing age

Varieties of hormonal manipulation in breast cancer
1 Tamoxifen
   — An antiestrogen; binds ER
2 Progestogens (medroxyprogesterone, megestrol acetate)
   — Bind PR; mechanism of action unclear
3 Aromatase inhibitors (e.g. 4-hydroxyandrostenedione)
   — Inhibit peripheral aromatization of androstenedione to estrone
   — Effective for painful bone metastases esp.
   — Used in *postmenopausal* patients only
4 LHRH analogs (pp. 38, 112)
   — Used in *premenopausal* patients only
5 Oophorectomy (in premenopausal patients)
   — May be performed by laparoscopy

Choice of adjuvant systemic therapy in breast cancer
1 Premenopausal*, esp. if node-positive
   — Adjuvant cytotoxic therapy (esp. if ER/PR-negative)
   — Ovarian ablation (esp. if ER/PR-positive)
2 Post-menopausal women‡
   — Adjuvant tamoxifen (all may benefit)

* In practice, includes patients menstruating normally *or* plasma FSH < 20 *or* age < 50 years (unless iatrogenically rendered menopausal)
‡ Includes *all* patients > 60 years; 50–60 year olds may also benefit from chemo

Clinical features of 'flare' reactions to hormonal interventions

1 Most commonly seen now with tamoxifen (the commonest hormonal intervention) but formerly reported most often after androgens or estrogens; affects about 1% of patients
2 Usually presents 3 days to 3 weeks after initiating treatment; typically occurs in setting of widespread bone metastases
3 Manifests with
  — Subacute worsening of bone pain (may be severe)
  — Hypercalcemia
4 Alkaline phosphatase may rise and bone scan 'worsen', indicating osteoblast activation
5 Treatment consists of analgesia, reversing hypercalcemia and continuing hormonal medication where possible
6 Occurrence predicts neither failure nor efficacy of treatment

Indications for palliative chemotherapy in breast cancer

1 Symptomatic ER– metastatic disease
2 Symptomatic ER+ metastatic disease with no response to an adequate (6-week) trial of hormonal therapy
3 Metastatic liver disease
4 Lymphangitic pulmonary spread
5 Mastitis carcinomatosa ('inflammatory' primary carcinoma)

Surgical and radiotherapeutic aspects of primary breast cancer

1 Chest wall irradiation reduces local disease recurrence (25% → 5%) but does *not* improve overall survival
2 Tumors < 4 cm diameter may be treated with lumpectomy + radiotherapy with no major loss of local control
3 Combining axillary node dissection and axillary nodal irradiation results in high morbidity from arm lymphedema and is thus contraindicated

Breast cancer in pregnancy: management considerations

1 Stage-specific prognosis may be little different from other premenopausal breast cancers
2 No role has been proven for therapeutic abortion in modifying the natural history of the disease
3 Surgery appears to be tolerated by mother and fetus at any stage of pregnancy
4 Chemotherapy is contraindicated in the first trimester and best postponed if possible until after delivery
5 Ionizing radiation should be avoided throughout pregnancy
6 Subsequent pregnancies are not contraindicated, but mothers should realize that their life expectancy remains reduced

MANAGEMENT OF TESTICULAR GERM-CELL NEOPLASMS

Surgical considerations in testis tumors

1 Exploration of *any* undiagnosed testicular mass should be undertaken via a transinguinal (not scrotal) approach, thus reducing tumor spread to inguinal nodes; testicular ultrasound may be helpful
2 Tumor markers (AFP, β-HCG) should be sent prior to surgery for *any* undiagnosed testicular mass
3 Retrograde ejaculation and sterility may result from paraaortic lymphadenectomy for suspected stage II disease, esp. if *bilateral* lymphadenectomy is performed
4 Surgical debulking of residual (post-chemotherapy) tumor may be of value diagnostically and therapeutically, since
  — Non-malignant masses may persist after therapy
  — Chemotherapy may be more effective after debulking
5 Resection of pulmonary metastases may be of value in selected patients

Diagnostic considerations in testis tumors

1 Computed tomographic (CT) scanning of abdomen and chest is the staging procedure of choice; > 50% of teratoma patients have metastases at presentation (cf. seminoma)
2 Residual abdominal lymph node enlargement on CT scanning following chemotherapy may signify benign differentiated teratoma rather than tumor persistence. If tumor markers have returned to normal, surgical exploration is indicated to exclude residual disease
3 Persistent elevation of markers (even in the absence of radiographic disease recurrence) is an indication for recommencement of radical cytotoxic therapy
4 The plasma half-life of AFP is 5 days while that of β-HCG is 30 hours; the *rate of decline* of these markers can therefore be used to *predict* the success or otherwise of therapy administered with curative intent. If β-HCG level on day 22 is > 0.5% pre-treatment, response will be incomplete
5 Elevated serum AFP is inconsistent with a diagnosis of pure seminoma. However, 5–10% of seminomas have elevated β-HCG (i.e. indicating choriocarcinomatous elements)

Therapeutic considerations in testis tumors

1 Frequent serial tumor markers should be assayed after any therapeutic intervention (if elevated pre-treatment) to assess response and need for further treatment
2 Sperm banking should be offered prior to initiation of cytotoxic therapy, though patients may already be too azoospermic for preservation of fertility
3 There is an increased incidence of neoplasia in the remaining testicle; clinical/ultrasound monitoring may be of value
4 Radiotherapy may be curative in stage I and II seminomas

5 Platinum-based chemotherapy (cisplatin or carboplatin) is the most effective modality in teratoma (> stage I) and in seminoma (> bulky stage II); combination bleomycin, etoposide (VP-16) and cisplatin (BEP) is standard

6 Grossly elevated tumor markers (AFP > 500 ku/L, β-HCG > 1000 IU/L, high LDH) indicate a lower probability of complete remission, especially with bulky disease

7 Surveillance studies of stage I teratoma suggest that deferral of consolidation treatment ('adjuvant' paraaortic irradiation or cytotoxics) is appropriate in early disease

MANAGEMENT OF MISCELLANEOUS MALIGNANCIES

Prostatic carcinoma: available endocrine therapies
1 *Testicular* (LH-dependent) androgen ablation
   — Long-acting LHRH analogues, incl.
      • Buserelin, goserelin, leuprolide
      • Induce *continuous* LH release leading to LH receptor *downregulation*, with suppression of testosterone secretion after 3–4 weeks
   — Not thrombogenic (no ↓ AT-III; cf. estrogens) but may cause disease *flare* (p. 37)
2 Antiandrogens
   — Non-steroidal antiandrogens
      • Flutamide, nilutamide, casodex
         → Block androgen receptors (AR), thus *preventing* LHRH-induced flare if used beforehand
         → Hence, block peripheral effects of *adrenal* (LH-independent) androgens
         → Compensatory ↑ plasma LH/testosterone
   — Progestational antiandrogens
      • Cyproterone acetate: LH-reducing (progestational) *and* AR-blocking (antiandrogen) effects
      • Hence, opposes testicular *and* adrenal androgens
3 'Complete androgen blockade'
   — Due to combined LHRH agonist + 'pure' antiandrogen
   — Testicular and adrenal androgens effectively blocked
4 Estrogens
   — Stilbestrol (DES)
      • Acts by reflexly inhibiting LHRH secretion
      • Plasma testosterone declines to castrate levels
      • Cardiovascular side-effects limit popularity
5 Bilateral orchidectomy
   — Efficacy and cost-effectiveness remain unsurpassed
      • Popularity limited by psychological factors

Efficacy of endocrine treatment for prostate cancer
1 Benefits
   — Pain relief (in 75%)*
   — Lower incidence of ureteric obstruction
   — Fewer neurologic complications

2 Limitations
   — *No* significant survival prolongation

* Note, however, that only 30% respond to second-line hormonal intervention

Bladder carcinoma
1 Superficial tumors
   — Cystoscopic fulguration and monitoring
   — Intravesical agents (prophylactic or therapeutic)
      • BCG (→ antitumor T cell response; best R_x)
      • Mitomycin C; doxorubicin
2 Invasive tumors (± nodal involvement)
   — Radical cystectomy + ileal bladder
   — Partial cystectomy + radical irradiation
3 Extensive disease
   — Palliative irradiation (i.e. for symptoms)
   — Cytotoxic therapy, e.g. MVAC

Ovarian cancer
1 Surgical staging and debulking
2 Systemic cytotoxic therapy
   — Oral chlorambucil, cyclophosphamide or melphalan
      • For minor disease or frail patients
   — Single-agent IV cisplatin or carboplatin
      • For major disease in fit patients

Papillary/follicular thyroid carcinoma
1 Subtotal thyroidectomy (*if* tumor < 1 cm diam.; else total)
2 Ablation of metastases with high-dose (50–150 mCi) ^{131}I
   (= *therapeutic* scan)
3 Long-term TSH suppression using thyroxine (~ 200 µg/day)
4 Monitoring of disease with serum thyroglobulin and/or whole-body iodine uptake scanning (= *diagnostic* scan)

Medullary carcinoma of the thyroid
1 Total thyroidectomy (i.e. as for anaplastic carcinoma)
2 Exclusion of pheochromocytoma, parathyroid tumor (p. 115)
3 Family screening: plasma calcitonin levels following stimulation by pentagastrin, alcohol or calcium infusion
4 Octreotide

UNDERSTANDING MALIGNANT DISEASE

CLINICAL TRIALS OF CANCER TREATMENT

Types of clinical drug trials
1 *Phase 1 study*
   — Toxicologic 'dose-finding' study which determines maximum tolerated dose (i.e. side-effects) in heavily pre-treated, poor prognosis patients

2 *Phase 2 study*
   — Using doses found 'safe' in the phase 1 study, patients with various tumor types are treated to determine the drug's anticancer activity when used alone
3 *Phase 3 study*
   — Sensitive tumor types identified by the phase 2 study are treated with the new drug in a prospective randomized comparison with standard treatment

Factors commonly confounding interpretation of clinical trials
1 Small numbers
2 Inadequate controls
3 Lack of endpoint definition
4 Insufficient long-term follow-up
5 Publication bias towards positive studies
6 Unstated criteria for patient exclusion/attrition

Strengths and weaknesses of epidemiological studies
1 *Case-control* studies
   — Advantages
     • Cheap and quick
     • Relatively few participants required
     • Suitable for rare diseases
   — Disadvantages
     • Difficult to select control group
2 *Cohort* studies
   — Advantages
     • Minimal bias
     • Measures incidence as well as relative risk
   — Disadvantages
     • Large number of participants needed
     • Long follow-up required
     • High attrition rate usual
     • Expensive and slow

PATHOGENESIS OF MALIGNANCY

Cell kinetics in tumor evolution
1 Tumor too small to be detected by sensitive screening tests:
   — 1 mm tumor diameter
   — Roughly equivalent to 10^6 tumor cells
   — Represents approximately 20 tumor cell doublings
2 Tumor too small to be symptomatic; detectable by screening
   — 1 cm tumor diameter (~ 1 g tumor burden)
   — Roughly equivalent to 10^9 tumor cells
   — Represents approximately 30 tumor cell doublings
3 Tumor clinically evident; advanced disease, usually incurable
   — 1 kg total tumor burden
   — Roughly equivalent to 10^{12} tumor cells
   — Represents approximately 40 tumor cell doublings

Premalignant syndromes of chromosomal instability (DNA repair defects)
1 Xeroderma pigmentosum
   — Ultraviolet light sensitivity
   — Prone to skin SCCs
2 Ataxia telangiectasia
   — X-radiation sensitivity
   — Prone to leukemias and lymphomas esp.
3 Fanconi's anemia
   — DNA crosslinking drug sensitivity
   — Prone to leukemias
4 Bloom's syndrome
   — Oncogenic virus sensitivity
   — Prone to leukemias

Cytogenetic aspects of tumor evolution
1 Hereditary retinoblastoma/osteosarcoma
   — 13q deletion leading to loss of Rb gene heterozygosity
2 Wilms' tumor
   — 11p deletion
   — Associated aniridia/hemihypertrophy (WAGR syndrome) due to adjacent gene deletions
3 Ewing's tumor
   — t(11q;22q) in 90% cases
4 Burkitt's lymphoma
   — 8:14 translocation affecting c-*myc*
5 Chronic myeloid leukemia
   — 9:22 translocation affecting c-*abl*
6 Low-grade non-Hodgkin's lymphoma
   — t(14:18) *bcl*-2 translocation in > 80%
7 Small-cell lung cancer
   — 3p14-23 deletion* (> 90%)

* Also seen in almost 100% bronchial carcinoids

ONCOGENES AND TUMOR SUPPRESSORS

Critical genes in cancer development
1 Cellular 'oncogenes' (protooncogenes, c-*onc*) are normal regulatory genes homologous to retroviral oncogenes
2 Putative mechanisms of oncogene action include
   — Cellular 'immortalization', e.g. *myc*
   — Transformation of immortalized cells, e.g. *ras, src*
   — Growth factor (autocrine) agonism, e.g. *sis* (PDGF)
   — Growth factor receptor production, e.g. EGFR, c-*erb*B-2
3 Disease associations of oncogene activation include
   — *abl/bcr* gene fusion in chronic myeloid leukemia
   — *sis* overexpression in myelofibrosis
   — N-*myc* amplification in neuroblastoma, retinoblastoma
   — L-*myc* amplification in small-cell lung cancer
   — *erb*B-2 overexpression in breast/ovarian cancer
4 *Tumor suppressor genes* ('recessive oncogenes' which, if even one allele is present, prevent neoplastic transformation) have been implicated in the development of many tumors, e.g.
   — Retinoblastoma (Rb)
   — Familial cancer (Li-Fraumeni) syndrome (p53)

— Breast–ovary cancer syndrome (BRCA1, BRCA2)
— Neurofibromatosis (NF-1)
— Wilms' tumor (WT-1)

Genetic changes in colorectal cancer evolution
1 Hereditary genetic defects*
   — Familial adenomatous polyposis (FAP)
     • APC (adenomatous polyposis coli) mutations
   — Hereditary non-polyposis colorectal cancer (HNPCC)
     • DNA mismatch repair genes (e.g. hMSH2)
2 Defects seen in hyperplastic epithelium
   — DNA hypermethylation (leads to gene activation)
3 Defects seen in adenomas and/or carcinomas
   — K-*ras* mutation
   — DCC deletion
   — p53 mutations

* i.e. present in morphologically normal colorectal mucosa.
Mutations of these genes also seen in *Turcot's syndrome* of
colorectal adenomas and brain tumors

EXOGENOUS CARCINOGENESIS

Malignancies associated with cigarette smoking
1 Lung cancer
   — SCC > SCLC > large-cell > adenoCa > alveolar cell*
2 Squamous cell carcinoma of mouth, larynx and esophagus‡¶
3 Transitional cell carcinoma of bladder and renal pelvis
4 Pancreatic adenocarcinoma
5 SCC cervix

* cf. mesothelioma: *not* associated with smoking
‡ cf. nasopharyngeal carcinoma: *not* associated with either
smoking or alcohol ingestion
¶ NB: 'Smokeless' tobacco is also a potent cause of oral cancer

Malignancies associated with alcohol ingestion
1 Mouth, pharynx
2 Larynx
3 Esophagus
4 Liver
5 ?Breast ?rectum (beer)

Viruses implicated in tumorigenesis
1 Epstein–Barr virus
   — Endemic Burkitt's lymphoma
   — Nasopharyngeal carcinoma
   — Primary cerebral lymphoma (if immunosuppressed)
   — Hodgkin's disease (implicated)
   — Lethal midline granuloma (T cell NHL)
2 Hepatitis B and C
   — Hepatocellular carcinoma
3 Papillomavirus (HPV) serotypes 16 and 18
   — Squamous cell carcinoma (SCC) of the cervix
   — Penile, vulvar and anal carcinomas (SCC)
4 HPV serotypes 5/8
   — Skin SCCs in renal transplant patients
   — Epidermodysplasia verruciformis

5 HTLV-I and II
   — T cell leukemia/lymphoma
6 HHV-8
   — Kaposi's sarcoma

OCCURRENCE AND PREVENTION OF CANCER

Incidence of malignant disease: the commonest cancers*
1 Western-world males
   — Lung cancer (25% all cancers, 40% cancer mortality)
   — Colorectal cancer (10–15% cancers, similar mortality)
   — Prostate cancer (10% cancers, similar mortality)
2 Western-world females
   — Breast cancer (25% cancers, 15% mortality)
   — Colorectal cancer (10–15% cancers, similar mortality)
   — Lung cancer (10% cancers and rising: 15% mortality)
3 Commonest malignancies in third-world populations
   — Gastric cancer (commonest malignancy worldwide)
   — Esophageal and oral cancer
   — Hepatoma
   — SCC cervix

* Excluding non-melanomatous skin cancer

Prognosis of treated malignancies (all stages)
1 Breast cancer
  Bladder cancer } 50–60% 5-year survival
  SCC cervix
2 Colorectal cancer
  Prostate cancer } 30–40% 5-year survival
3 Ovarian cancer } 25% 5-year survival
4 Pancreatic cancer
  Gastric cancer
  Esophageal cancer } 1–9% 5-year survival
  Lung cancer

Malignancies changing in incidence
1 Cancers increasing in frequency
   — Lung cancer (in third world and in women)
   — Mesothelioma
   — Melanoma
   — Hepatoma
   — Early-onset (< 35 years old) SCC cervix
   — Kaposi's sarcoma
   — Testicular tumors
   — Lymphoma (esp. 1° cerebral)
2 Cancers declining in frequency
   — Gastric cancer
   — Lung cancer (in Western middle-class males)

Geographical clustering of various cancers
1 Hepatoma — Mozambique, South-East Asia
2 Gastric cancer — Japan, Chile, China, USSR
3 Oral cancer — India, South-East Asia
4 Esophageal cancer — Iran, Turkey, Afghanistan, China
5 Nasopharynx cancer — South China, Eskimos

6   Skin cancer   — Australia
7   SCC cervix   — Chile, Latin America, Asia
8   Penile cancer   — Uganda

How to prevent cancer

1   Lung cancer and other cigarette-induced neoplasms
    — Stop smoking
2   Skin cancer, esp. non-melanomatous
    — ↓ UV exposure
3   Hepatoma
    — Hepatitis B vaccination
4   SCC cervix
    — Cytology screening, condom usage
5   Oral cancer
    — Vitamin A, cessation of betel-nut ingestion
6   Penile cancer
    — Circumcision

Dietary factors implicated in carcinogenesis

1   Betel-nut and tobacco chewing ⎫ — Oral
    Alcohol, incl. mouthwashes   ⎭   cancer
2   Alcohol and tobacco   ⎫
    Opium; dietary deficiencies   ⎬ — Esophageal
    Bracken fern (in Japanese)   ⎭   cancer
3   Salted fish — Nasopharyngeal Ca
4   Aflatoxin — Hepatoma
5   Overnutrition (obesity) — Endometrial/gallbladder
    Ca

Major risk factors for various cancers

1   Breast
    — Affected first-degree relative(s), esp.
      premenopausal
    — Loss of heterozygosity for BRCA1 (or 2) gene
    — Late age of first full-term pregnancy
2   Endometrial
    — Prolonged exogenous estrogen administration
    — Obesity, nulliparity, high social class
3   Cervix
    — Early and/or promiscuous sexual activity (HPV)
    — Smoking
    — HLA DQw3
4   Hepatoma
    — Macronodular cirrhosis
      • HBV, HCV¶
      • Hemochromatosis
      • α_1-antitrypsin deficiency
    — Alcohol, aflatoxin, anabolic steroids
    Hepatic adenoma
    — Estrogens
    Angiosarcoma
    — Thorotrast, arsenic, vinyl chloride monomer
5   Gallbladder
    — Gallstones (chronic cholecystitis); obesity
    — 'Porcelain' (calcified) gallbladder
6   Bile ducts
    — Inflammatory bowel disease
    — *Clonorchis sinensis* infestation

7   Colorectal
    — Familial polyposis; villous adenoma
    — Inflammatory bowel disease, esp. ulcerative colitis
    — Affected first-degree relative(s); Gardner's
      syndrome
8   Esophageal (SCC)
    — Cigarettes, alcohol; corrosive ingestion
    — Pickled vegetables
    — Achalasia, celiac disease, Plummer–Vinson
      syndrome
    — Tylosis (palmar–plantar hyperkeratosis: rare)
    Esophageal (adenocarcinoma)
    — Barrett's (columnar) esophagus (probably low-risk)
9   Lung
    — Cigarettes (incl. passive smoking)
    — Asbestos* (synergy with cigarettes)
    — Scars (predispose to adenocarcinoma)
    — Scleroderma (→ alveolar-cell carcinoma)
10 Mesothelioma
    — Asbestos*: 'blue' (crocidolite) > white (chrysotile)
      > brown (amosite)
11 Bladder (TCC)
    — Male sex; past history of bladder cancer
    — Aromatic dye/naphthalene exposure
    — Cigarettes, analgesics, cyclophosphamide
    Bladder (SCC)
    — *Schistosoma hematobium* infestation
12 Thyroid
    — Low-dose (< 2000 rad) external beam irradiation
    — Multinodular goiter
    — Gardner's/Cowden's/Verner's syndromes
13 Lymphoma
    — Radiotherapy, chemotherapy
    — Sjögren's syndrome (also → pseudolymphoma)
    Leukemia
    — Chemotherapy, radiation therapy
    — DNA repair deficiencies (p. 40)
    — Ionizing radiation, incl. ?radon exposure
    — Miscellaneous mutagens, e.g. benzene
14 Osteosarcoma
    — Paget's disease
    — Osteogenesis imperfecta
    — Familial retinoblastoma
15 Testicular tumors
    — Cryptorchidism
    — Testicular feminization syndrome
16 Melanoma
    — Dysplastic nevus syndrome
    — Repeated childhood sunburn‡
17 Ovarian tumors, esp. granulosa-cell
    — Clomiphene fertility stimulation
18 Gastric (MALT) lymphoma
    — *Helicobacter pylori*

¶ May also be associated with hepatoma in non-cirrhotics (see
ref. 1.1, 4.9)
* Asbestos-related *neoplasms* may occur at lower exposures
than asbestosis
‡ May reflect genetic UV sensitivity rather than a causal event;
no relationship with retinal melanoma

1.1 Mandel JS et al (1993) Reducing mortality from colorectal cancer by screening for fecal occult blood. N Engl J Med 328: 1365–1371

Randomized screening study of 46,551 standard-risk individuals aged 50–80 using guiaic testing of rehydrated stool. Results suggested a 33% reduction in colorectal cancer deaths in patients screened once-yearly, but little reduction in those screened every 2 years.

1.2 Sigurgeirsson B et al (1992) Risk of cancer in patients with dermatomyositis or polymyositis. N Engl J Med 326: 363–367

Swedish study of 788 patients with dermatomyositis or polymyositis over 20 years. Confirmed an approximate 3-fold increase in cancer incidence and death in dermatomyositis only; polymyositis was associated with a 1.75-fold increase in cancer incidence, but no change in cancer death rates.

1.3 Jankovic M et al (1994) Association of 1800 cGy cranial irradiation with intellectual function in children with acute lymphoblastic leukemia. Lancet 344: 224–227

Randomized comparison of 203 children over 6 years receiving 'low-dose' cranial irradiation for ALL or high-dose intrathecal methotrexate. The IQ of the irradiated group declined progressively compared with the methotrexate group, with the most marked declines in those commencing irradiation at the youngest age.

1.4 Thun MJ et al (1991) Aspirin use and reduced risk of fatal colon cancer. N Engl J Med 325: 1593–1596

Busch O et al (1993) Blood transfusions and prognosis in colorectal cancer. N Engl J Med 328: 1372–1376

Garau I et al (1994) Blood transfusion has no effect on colorectal cancer survival. Eur J Cancer 30A: 759–764

The first of these papers described an intriguing 40% reduction in the risk of regular aspirin users developing colorectal cancer. The next two addressed an association previously described between blood transfusion frequency and adverse prognosis in colorectal cancer patients. Busch et al carried out a comparison of autologous vs. allogeneic transfusion post-surgery and found no difference in outcome. Similarly, perioperative transfusion failed to affect outcomes in the study of Garau et al.

1.5 Ohno R et al (1990) Effect of granulocyte colony-stimulating factor after intensive induction therapy in relapsed or refractory acute leukemia. N Engl J Med 323: 871–877

Crawford J et al (1991) Reduction by granulocyte colony-stimulating factor of fever and neutropenia induced by chemotherapy in patients with small-cell lung cancer. N Engl J Med 325: 164–170

Two early studies of the use of G-CSF as a marrow recovery aid in chemotherapy patients.
The first study showed its effectiveness in increasing neutrophil counts and its safety in not accelerating leukemic cell growth, while the second suggested a role in reducing morbidity from septic episodes.

1.6 Hong WK et al (1990) Prevention of second primary tumors with isotretinoin in squamous cell carcinoma of the head and neck. N Engl J Med 323: 795-801

Lippman SM et al (1993) Comparison of low-dose isotretinoin with beta carotene to prevent oral carcinogenesis. N Engl J Med 328: 15–20

Two studies showing efficacy of one vitamin A derivative (isotretinoin) but not another (β-carotene) to treat leukoplakia, prevent progression to invasive cancer and prevent second primary tumors. However, no effect on recurrence or progression of established invasive tumors was apparent.

1.7 Friedman GD et al (1991) Case-control study of screening for prostatic cancer by digital rectal examinations. Lancet 337: 1526–1529

Chadwick DJ et al (1991) Pilot study of screening for prostate cancer in general practice. Lancet 338: 613–616

Catalona WJ et al (1991) Measurement of prostate-specific antigen in serum as a screening test for prostate cancer. N Engl J Med 324: 1156–1161

Three studies documenting the insensitivity of digital rectal examination in detecting early-stage prostate cancer, with the latter two demonstrating the superior potential of PSA measurements in this regard.

1.8 Kinlen LJ et al (1990) Evidence from population mixing in British New Towns 1946–1985 of an infective basis for childhood leukemia. Lancet 336: 577–582

Alexander FE et al (1990) Community lifestyle characteristics and risk of acute lymphoblastic leukaemia in children. Lancet 336: 1461–1465

Hill C, Laplanche A (1990) Overall mortality and cancer mortality around French nuclear sites. Nature 347: 755–757

The last of these three studies showed no increase in leukemia associated with proximity to nuclear sites per se. However, the 'Kinlen hypothesis' suggests that the influx of new settlers into centres (such as those formed near nuclear sites) creates a temporary loss of childhood immunity to viruses and that the increased incidence of leukemia in such locations may thus reflect involvement of an infectious agent in the etiology of leukemias.

1.9 Janerich DT et al (1990) Lung cancer and exposure to tobacco smoke in the household. N Engl J Med 323: 632–636

Morabia A, Wynder EL (1992) Relation of brochiolo-alveolar carcinoma to tobacco. Br Med J 304: 541–543

Doll R et al (1994) Mortality in relation to smoking: 40 years' observations on male British doctors. Br Med J 309: 901–911

Three studies documenting the ever-increasing morbidity of smoking. The first suggested that 17% of lung cancers in 'non-smokers' may be due to passive smoking in childhood, while the second confirmed a link (previously unrecognized) between smoking and the rare alveolar-cell lung cancer subtype. The follow-up of Doll et al establishes that about 50% of smokers will die from cigarette-induced disease.

1.10 Colombo M et al (1991) Hepatocellular carcinoma in Italian patients with cirrhosis. N Engl J Med 325: 675–680

Study of 447 patients with established cirrhosis, showing a 3% per year incidence of hepatoma. Screening for this complication using AFP did not increase the number of early-stage lesions treated.

CHAPTER 2

Cardiology

Physical examination protocol 2.1   You are asked to examine the patient's cardiovascular system

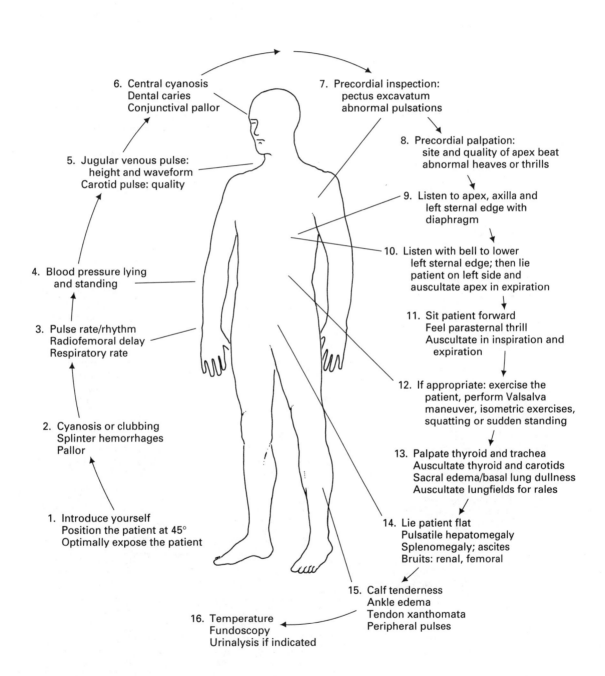

6. Central cyanosis
   Dental caries
   Conjunctival pallor

7. Precordial inspection:
   pectus excavatum
   abnormal pulsations

8. Precordial palpation:
   site and quality of apex beat
   abnormal heaves or thrills

5. Jugular venous pulse:
   height and waveform
   Carotid pulse: quality

9. Listen to apex, axilla and
   left sternal edge with
   diaphragm

10. Listen with bell to lower
    left sternal edge; then lie
    patient on left side and
    auscultate apex in expiration

4. Blood pressure lying
   and standing

11. Sit patient forward
    Feel parasternal thrill
    Auscultate in inspiration and
    expiration

3. Pulse rate/rhythm
   Radiofemoral delay
   Respiratory rate

12. If appropriate: exercise the
    patient, perform Valsalva
    maneuver, isometric exercises,
    squatting or sudden standing

2. Cyanosis or clubbing
   Splinter hemorrhages
   Pallor

13. Palpate thyroid and trachea
    Auscultate thyroid and carotids
    Sacral edema/basal lung dullness
    Auscultate lungfields for rales

1. Introduce yourself
   Position the patient at 45°
   Optimally expose the patient

14. Lie patient flat
    Pulsatile hepatomegaly
    Splenomegaly; ascites
    Bruits: renal, femoral

15. Calf tenderness
    Ankle edema
    Tendon xanthomata
    Peripheral pulses

16. Temperature
    Fundoscopy
    Urinalysis if indicated

Physical examination protocol 2.2   You are asked to examine a patient with refractory hypertension

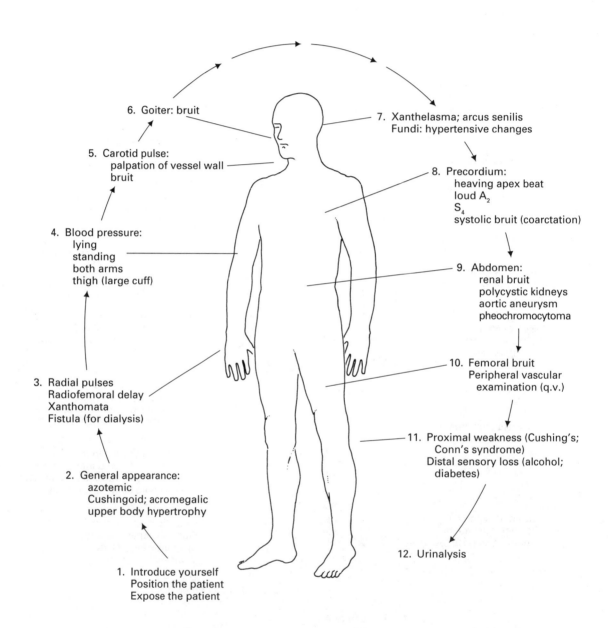

6. Goiter: bruit

7. Xanthelasma; arcus senilis
    Fundi: hypertensive changes

5. Carotid pulse:
    palpation of vessel wall
    bruit

8. Precordium:
    heaving apex beat
    loud A_2
    S_4
    systolic bruit (coarctation)

4. Blood pressure:
    lying
    standing
    both arms
    thigh (large cuff)

9. Abdomen:
    renal bruit
    polycystic kidneys
    aortic aneurysm
    pheochromocytoma

10. Femoral bruit
     Peripheral vascular
     examination (q.v.)

3. Radial pulses
    Radiofemoral delay
    Xanthomata
    Fistula (for dialysis)

11. Proximal weakness (Cushing's;
     Conn's syndrome)
     Distal sensory loss (alcohol;
     diabetes)

2. General appearance:
    azotemic
    Cushingoid; acromegalic
    upper body hypertrophy

12. Urinalysis

1. Introduce yourself
    Position the patient
    Expose the patient

Physical examination protocol 2.3   You are told that the patient is known to have aortic incompetence, and asked to examine him from that point of view

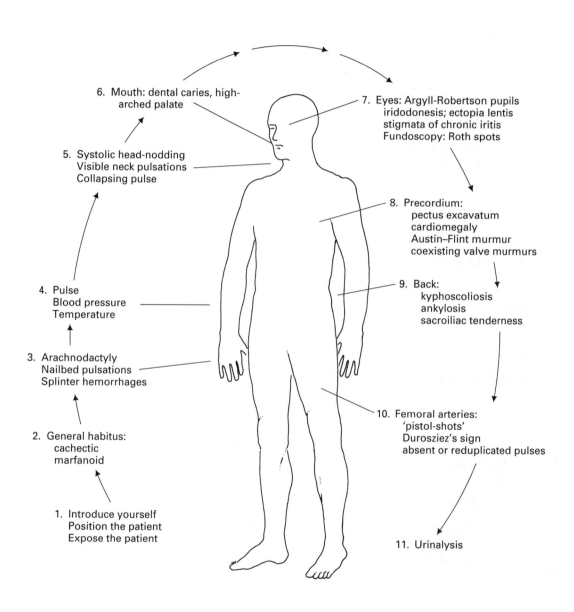

6. Mouth: dental caries, high-
   arched palate

5. Systolic head-nodding
   Visible neck pulsations
   Collapsing pulse

4. Pulse
   Blood pressure
   Temperature

3. Arachnodactyly
   Nailbed pulsations
   Splinter hemorrhages

2. General habitus:
   cachectic
   marfanoid

1. Introduce yourself
   Position the patient
   Expose the patient

7. Eyes: Argyll-Robertson pupils
   iridodonesis; ectopia lentis
   stigmata of chronic iritis
   Fundoscopy: Roth spots

8. Precordium:
   pectus excavatum
   cardiomegaly
   Austin–Flint murmur
   coexisting valve murmurs

9. Back:
   kyphoscoliosis
   ankylosis
   sacroiliac tenderness

10. Femoral arteries:
    'pistol-shots'
    Durosziez's sign
    absent or reduplicated pulses

11. Urinalysis

Physical examination protocol 2.4   You are asked to examine the patient looking specifically for signs of bacterial endocarditis

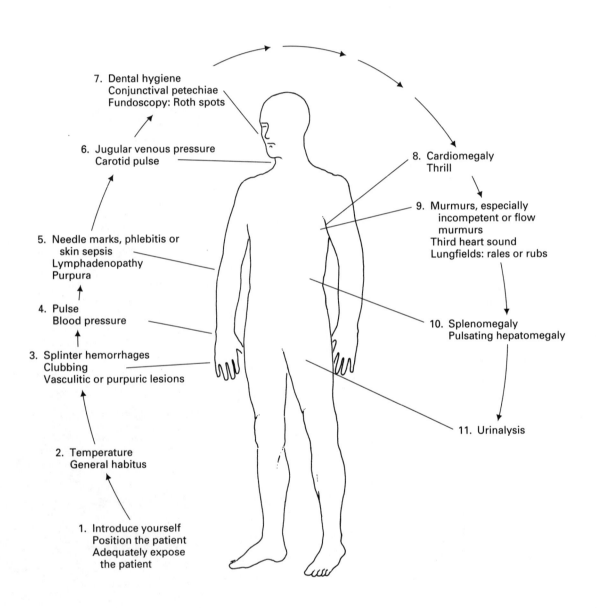

7. Dental hygiene
   Conjunctival petechiae
   Fundoscopy: Roth spots

6. Jugular venous pressure
   Carotid pulse

5. Needle marks, phlebitis or
      skin sepsis
   Lymphadenopathy
   Purpura

4. Pulse
   Blood pressure

3. Splinter hemorrhages
   Clubbing
   Vasculitic or purpuric lesions

2. Temperature
   General habitus

1. Introduce yourself
   Position the patient
   Adequately expose
      the patient

8. Cardiomegaly
   Thrill

9. Murmurs, especially
      incompetent or flow
      murmurs
   Third heart sound
   Lungfields: rales or rubs

10. Splenomegaly
    Pulsating hepatomegaly

11. Urinalysis

Physical examination protocol 2.5 You are asked to examine the patient's peripheral vascular system

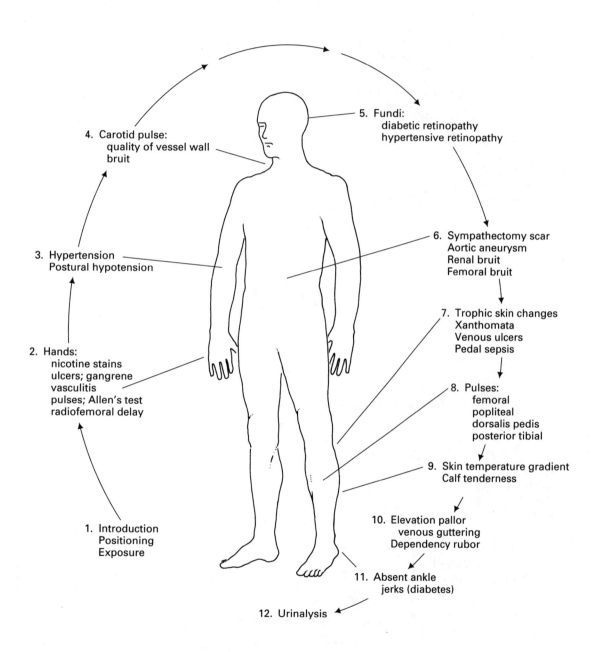

4. Carotid pulse:
   quality of vessel wall
   bruit

5. Fundi:
   diabetic retinopathy
   hypertensive retinopathy

3. Hypertension
   Postural hypotension

6. Sympathectomy scar
   Aortic aneurysm
   Renal bruit
   Femoral bruit

7. Trophic skin changes
   Xanthomata
   Venous ulcers
   Pedal sepsis

2. Hands:
   nicotine stains
   ulcers; gangrene
   vasculitis
   pulses; Allen's test
   radiofemoral delay

8. Pulses:
   femoral
   popliteal
   dorsalis pedis
   posterior tibial

9. Skin temperature gradient
   Calf tenderness

1. Introduction
   Positioning
   Exposure

10. Elevation pallor
    venous guttering
    Dependency rubor

11. Absent ankle
    jerks (diabetes)

12. Urinalysis

Diagnostic pathway 2.1 This patient has a fundoscopic abnormality. How would you characterize this?

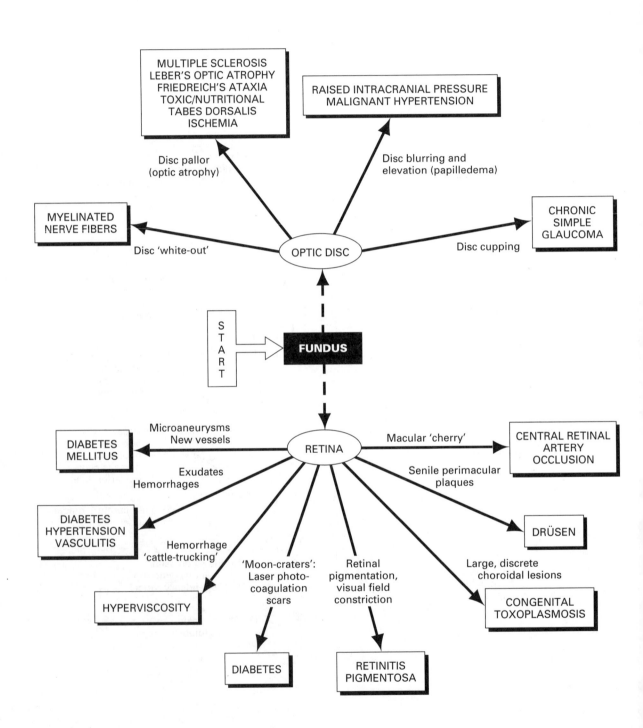

CLINICAL ASPECTS OF CARDIOVASCULAR DISEASE

Commonest cardiac short cases
1 Mitral and/or aortic valve disease
2 Cardiac failure/cardiomyopathy

THE CARDIOVASCULAR HISTORY

Assessment of cardiorespiratory capacity*
1 NYHA I — Dyspneic only on severe exertion
2 NYHA II — Dyspneic walking up hills or stairs
3 NYHA III — Dyspneic walking on a level surface
4 NYHA IV — Dyspneic at rest

* New York Heart Association — NYHA — criteria

Assessment of chest pain
(modified Canadian Cardiovascular Society criteria)
1 Grade I — Angina on strenuous/prolonged exertion
2 Grade II — Angina on climbing two flights of stairs
3 Grade III — Angina walking one block on the level
4 Grade IV — Angina at rest

Pain: how to describe it
1 When?
— First onset?
— Duration of individual episodes?
— Periodicity?
2 Where?
— Site of origin?
— Radiation?
— Effect of different postures?
3 How?
— Severity?
— Nature?
— Exacerbating and relieving factors?

THE PULSE

Describing pulse character
1 Volume
— Low/full
— Alternans
— Paradoxical (reduces on inspiration)
2 Upstroke
— Normal
— Slow/brisk

Clinical varieties of pulse character
1 Paradoxical
— Tamponade/constrictive pericarditis
— Severe asthma
Alternans
— Severe left ventricular failure
2 Collapsing
— Aortic incompetence

— Patent ductus arteriosus ('big' pulse)
Jerky
— Hypertrophic cardiomyopathy (HOCM)
3 Plateau
— Aortic valvular stenosis (diagnostic)
4 Bisferiens
— Mixed aortic valve disease

Differential diagnosis of unequal radial pulses
1 Atheroma
2 Proximal coarctation
3 Cervical rib
4 Takayasu's arteritis
5 Dissecting aneurysm

The irregularly irregular pulse: differential diagnosis
1 Atrial fibrillation
2 Sinus arrhythmia
3 Multiple atrial or ventricular premature beats
4 Atrial tachycardia or atrial flutter with varying block

Clinical signs of atrial fibrillation
1 Irregularly irregular pulse in time and amplitude
2 Absent 'a' waves in jugular venous pulse
3 Variation in intensity of first heart sound
4 Signs of mitral valve disease, cardiomyopathy, thyrotoxicosis

Analysing the jugular venous pulse (JVP)
1 Raised or not?
— Measure height above sternal angle
2 If raised, is it fixed?
— Stand the patient up
• Fixed: SVC obstruction (p. 33)
— Elicit hepatojugular reflux
• Absent: IVC obstruction, Budd–Chiari
3 Is the 'a' or 'v' wave dominant?
— Palpate contralateral carotid artery

Interpreting elevated 'a' and 'v' waves in the JVP
1 Normal
— 'a' wave: (right) atrial systole
— 'v' wave: venous filling
2 Abnormal 'a' wave
— Absent: atrial fibrillation
— Giant*: tricuspid/pulmonary stenosis
— Solitary: complete heart block
3 Cannon waves (= large 'a' waves)
— Atrial contraction against closed tricuspid valve
• Regular: nodal rhythm
• Irregular: complete heart block, ectopics
4 Systolic (ventricular) waves‡
— Tricuspid incompetence

* Associated with right atrial S_4
‡ *Not* 'v' waves; indicate 'ventricularization' of right atrium, and associated with pulsatile liver

Subclinical abnormalities of the JVP 'x' and 'y' descents
1 Definitions
— 'x' descent: systolic collapse (atrial relaxation)
— 'y' descent: diastolic collapse (tricuspid opening)
2 Rapid 'y' descent
— Tricuspid incompetence, constrictive pericarditis
3 Slow/absent 'y' descent
— Tricuspid stenosis, cardiac tamponade

4 Rapid 'x' descent
— Constrictive pericarditis, cardiac tamponade

THE PRECORDIUM

Cardiac significance of a left thoracotomy scar*
1 Mitral valvotomy
2 Repair of aortic coarctation or PDA
3 Pneumonectomy, splenectomy or gastrectomy

* cf. sternotomy scar

Reasons for failure to palpate the apex beat
1 Emphysema, obesity
2 Poor technique
3 Pericardial disease
— Effusion, constriction
4 Dextrocardia
— Any cause, incl. right pneumonectomy

Palpable heart sounds
1 Palpable S_1
— 'Tapping' apex beat (mitral stenosis)
2 Palpable S_4
— 'Double' apex beat (HOCM/severe aortic stenosis)
— Left ventricular aneurysm
3 Palpable P_2
— Pulmonary hypertension

Quality of the apex beat*
1 Heaving (sustained): LV pressure load
— Aortic stenosis, long-standing hypertension
2 Hyperdynamic, displaced: LV volume load
— Mitral/aortic incompetence, patent ductus arteriosus
3 Dyskinetic
— Left ventricular aneurysm
4 Displaced to right
— Dextrocardia, right pneumonectomy
5 Impalpable (see above)

* NB: *Location* of apex is more important than quality (as with real estate)

THE HEART SOUNDS

Conditions causing a soft first heart sound
1 Large pericardial effusion
2 Severe mitral regurgitation
3 Mitral stenosis with rigid valve
4 Cardiomyopathy, left ventricular failure
5 First degree heart block (intensity varies)

Conditions causing a loud first heart sound
1 Mitral stenosis with mobile valve
2 Sinus tachycardia (e.g. thyrotoxicosis)
3 Short PR interval
— Wolff–Parkinson–White syndrome
— Lown–Ganong–Levine syndrome

Splitting of the second heart sound
1 Physiological
— Single S_2 in expiration

— A_2 pre-P_2 appears on inspiration
2 Split, widens on inspiration
— RBBB
3 Split, paradoxical
— i.e. P_2 pre-A_2; widens on expiration
— LBBB
4 Widely split, fixed
— ASD
5 Narrow split with loud P_2 ($>>A_2$)
— Pulmonary hypertension
6 Wide split with soft P_2
— Pulmonary stenosis
7 Loud A_2
— Systemic hypertension
8 Single S_2 (inaudible A_2)
— Calcific aortic stenosis
Single S_2 (inaudible P_2)
— Obesity, emphysema

Differential diagnosis of the fixed split second heart sound
1 Atrial septal defect (ASD)
— Secundum (60%) or primum (30%)
2 Partial anomalous pulmonary venous drainage
— Associated with ASD (10%)
3 Misdiagnosis
— Opening snap (mitral stenosis) simulating P_2
— Midsystolic click (mitral valve prolapse) simulating A_2

Characterization of third heart sounds
1 Genuine S_3
— Low-pitched, localized
— Best heard with bell at apex, patient on left side
2 Other 'third sounds'
• Opening snap in mitral stenosis
• Fixed split second sound in atrial septal defect
• Mitral valve prolapse: systolic click simulating S_2
— High-pitched sounds heard all over precordium

MURMURS OF THE HEART

Features of an 'innocent' murmur
1 **S**ystolic ejection murmur
2 **S**hort (duration < 50% systole)
3 **S**oft, low-pitched and well-transmitted
4 **S**upine position best for auscultation
5 **S**ingle S_2 during expiration while standing
6 **S**atisfactory (normal) ECG and CXR

Characteristics of a venous hum*
1 Low-pitched sound best heard when sitting up
2 More common on right side, esp. in subclavian region
3 Increases during inspiration (often continuous)
4 Louder in diastole
5 Maximal with head turned away; abolished by finger pressure over internal jugular vein

* Usually in children

Differential diagnosis of continuous murmurs
1 Patent ductus arteriosus ('machinery' murmur)

2 Pulmonary flow murmur, cervical venous hum, AV fistula; ruptured sinus of Valsalva aneurysm; 'mammary souffle' (pregnancy)
3 Pseudocontinuous murmur (mixed aortic valve disease)

Causes of a late systolic murmur
1 Mitral (or tricuspid) valve prolapse
2 'Secondary' (ischemic) mitral prolapse
   — Papillary muscle dysfunction
   — Ruptured mitral chorda tendineae
3 Hypertrophic cardiomyopathy

Systolic sounds associated with myocardial infarction
1 Papillary muscle dysfunction or partial rupture (common)
   — Apical pansystolic murmur, no thrill; clinically stable
   Ruptured chorda tendineae (uncommon, serious)
   — Loud apical murmur (mitral regurgitation) + thrill
   Complete papillary muscle rupture (uncommon, often fatal)
   — Loud apical murmur, prominent thrill; usually fatal
2 Ruptured interventricular septum (common, often operable)
   — Loud medial murmur (VSD), thrill+++
3 Functional mitral incompetence due to cardiac dilatation
4 Pulmonary systolic murmur*
5 Pericardial rub
   — Transmural infarction
   — Dressler's syndrome
6 Aortic incompetence
   — Secondary to aortic dissection, esp. after inferior infarct

* Think of pulmonary embolism

MITRAL STENOSIS (MS)

Signs of valve mobility in mitral stenosis
1 Loud S_1
2 Opening snap*

* If S_2–OS gap easily audible, stenosis *not* severe; see below

Radiographic features of mitral stenosis
1 PA film
   — Straight (or convex) left heart border*
   — Double shadow of left atrium behind right atrium
   — Splaying of subcarinal angle greater than 90°
   — Dilated upper lobe veins
   — Prominent pulmonary conus
   — Pulmonary hemosiderosis
2 Lateral
   — Left atrial/right ventricular enlargement
   — Valvular calcification‡
   — McCallum's patch (left atrial calcification)
   — Esophageal indentation on barium swallow

* *Unless* auricle removed at valvotomy
‡ Calcification of the mitral annulus is associated with 2-fold ↑ stroke risk

M-mode echocardiography* in mitral stenosis
1 Thickened leaflets; calcification
2 Left atrial enlargement
3 Loss of 'A' point, if in atrial fibrillation
4 Excursion of anterior leaflet less than 20 mm
5 Anterior position of posterior leaflet throughout diastole
   — Most *specific* sign
6 Reduced EF slope
   — Semi-quantitative for *severity*

* M-mode little used now in most centers

Indicators of severity in mitral stenosis
1 Symptoms
2 Signs
   — Length of diastolic murmur
   — Proximity of opening snap to S_2
   — Signs of pulmonary hypertension/congestion
   — Functional pulmonary incompetence (Graham–Steell murmur) or tricuspid incompetence
3 CXR
   — Left atrial/right ventricular enlargement
   — Pulmonary hypertension and congestion
4 ECG
   — Atrial enlargement
   — Right ventricular strain pattern
5 Echo
   — M-mode: flattening of EF slope
   — Severity best quantitated by Doppler or 2-D echo
6 Catheter
   — Mitral valve gradient
   — Elevated right heart pressures
   — Decreased cardiac output during exercise

Severity of mitral stenosis assessed by 2-D echocardiography
1 Cross-sectional valve area > 2.5 cm²
   — Asymptomatic
2 Cross-sectional valve area 1.5–2.5 cm²
   — Symptoms on exercise only (mild)
3 Cross-sectional valve area 0.5–1.5 cm²
   — Symptoms at rest (think of valvuloplasty)
4 Cross-sectional valve area < 0.5 cm²
   — Severe stenosis (think of valve replacement)

Contraindications to valvotomy/valvuloplasty
1 Lack of symptoms
2 Significant mitral incompetence
3 Low chance of success*
   — Rigid valve
   — Heavily calcified leaflets (on echo, fluoroscopy)
4 Suspicion of left atrial thrombus

* esp. with balloon valvuloplasty

Indications for surgery in mitral stenosis
1 Progressive symptomatic deterioration due to pulmonary congestion in the absence of identifiable reversible factors
2 Recurrent embolic episodes

Mitral stenotic diastolic murmur: differential diagnosis
1 Flow murmur due to volume overload (like Austin–Flint)
   — Severe mitral regurgitation

— VSD, PDA
— Renal failure with fluid overload (functional AR)
2 Austin–Flint murmur
— Non-stenotic mitral flow murmur
— Due to severe aortic incompetence (p. 53)
3 Graham–Steell murmur
— Pulmonary incompetent murmur ($\uparrow$ on inspiration)
— Due to severe MS causing pulmonary hypertension
4 Carey–Coombs murmur
— Non-stenotic mitral flow murmur
— Occurs in rheumatic valvulitis
5 Tricuspid flow murmur with secundum ASD
6 Left atrial myxoma

Signs favoring an Austin–Flint murmur
1 Cardiomegaly* (apex *not* tapping)
2 Soft S_1
3 No opening snap ($\pm$ S_3)
4 ECG $\rightarrow$ left ventricular dominance
5 Echo $\rightarrow$ flutter on anterior mitral valve leaflet, posterior diastolic motion of posterior valve leaflet

* NB: Right ventricular dilatation (e.g. due to MS) can also cause apical displacement; may be tricky to distinguish clinically

MITRAL REGURGITATION (MR)

Signs of dominant MR in mixed mitral valve disease
1 Soft S_1
2 Left ventricular enlargement with thrusting apex
3 ECG $\rightarrow$ left ventricular hypertrophy + left axis deviation

Clinical assessment of severity in mitral regurgitation*
1 Degree of left ventricular enlargement
2 Mid-diastolic flow murmur
3 Thrill; murmur intensity; loud P_2; basal creps

* NB: Presence of S_3 does *not* correlate well with MR severity

Causes of mitral regurgitation
1 Rheumatic
2 Infective endocarditis
3 Mitral valve prolapse and/or Marfan's syndrome
4 Functional (left ventricular dilatation)
5 Ischemic
— Papillary muscle dysfunction
— Ruptured chorda tendineae
6 Rheumatoid arthritis, ankylosing spondylitis
7 Associations
— 1° ASD
— Hypertrophic cardiomyopathy
8 Congenital

Signs favoring acute rather than chronic mitral regurgitation
1 Acute onset of symptoms
2 Loud, short bruit (esp. in young male) radiating well to base
3 Other signs:
— Sinus tachycardia

— Large 'a' wave
— Minimally displaced apex beat
— Right ventricular heave with apical systolic thrill
— Normal intensity S_1, S_4; loud P_2

LEFT ATRIAL MYXOMA

Diagnostic clues to left atrial myxoma
1 Symptoms
— Constitutional
— Sudden onset; episodic
— Postural
2 Signs
— Pansystolic murmur; may be postural
— Mid-diastolic murmur
— Loud or soft S_1; $\pm$ 'tumor plop'
— Sinus rhythm
3 Investigations
— Normal CXR
— Left atrial mass on 2-D echocardiogram
— Positive embolus histology

Echocardiographic differential diagnosis of left atrial myxoma
1 Left atrial thrombus
2 Large mitral valve vegetation (e.g. staphylococcal, fungal)
3 Ruptured chorda tendineae; thick or redundant valve leaflets

MITRAL VALVE PROLAPSE (MVP)

Clinical associations of mitral valve prolapse
1 Marfan's syndrome; Ehlers–Danlos syndrome
2 Ostium secundum atrial septal defect
3 Wolff–Parkinson–White syndrome $\pm$ SLE

Maneuvers intensifying the murmur
1 Sudden standing
2 Valsalva (phases 2 and 3)

Maneuvers intensifying the click
1 Squatting
2 Isometric handgrip

Significance and timing of the midsystolic click
1 Caused by sudden tension on the chordae tendineae on stretching of the billowing valve
2 Sound occurs after beginning of carotid upstroke

ECG associations of mitral valve prolapse
1 Non-specific ST-T wave changes, esp. in inferior leads
2 Frequent atrial or ventricular ectopic beats
3 Prolonged Q-T$_c$; episodic ventricular tachycardia
4 Wolff–Parkinson–White syndrome (type A)
5 False-positive stress test*

* More likely *only* because this is a low-risk group

Approach to management of mitral valve prolapse
1 Incidental finding, asymptomatic patient
— Reassure, follow up

2 Atypical (non-anginal) chest pain, *or*
Exertional chest pain and/or dyspnea
— Stress test
3 'Funny turns', ECG ST-T wave changes, prolonged
$Q-T_c$
— Holter monitor
'Funny turns' with neurologic signs, normal ECG/
Holter
— Antiplatelet therapy
4 Significant degree of associated mitral regurgitation
— Antibiotic prophylaxis

AORTIC REGURGITATION (AR)

Eponymous signs associated with aortic regurgitation
1 Quincke's
— Capillary pulsation visible on nail compression
2 Corrigan's (pulse)
— Collapsing pulse
3 Corrigan's (sign)
— Visible carotid systolic pulsation
4 DeMusset's
— Systolic head nodding
5 Austin–Flint (murmur)
— Functional mitral diastolic flow murmur
6 Durosziez's
— To-and-fro bruit audible on lightly compressing
femoral arteries with diaphragm
7 Traube's
— Systolic 'pistol-shots' heard over femoral arteries
8 Marfan's (syndrome), Argyll-Robertson (pupils)
— Etiologic associations

Clinical indicators of severity in chronic aortic regurgitation
1 Presence of symptoms
2 Pulse character, pulse pressure
Absolute value of diastolic blood pressure
3 Degree of cardiomegaly
4 S_3; Austin–Flint murmur; length of diastolic murmur

Indicators of severity in acute aortic regurgitation*
1 Symptoms and signs of pulmonary venous congestion
2 Secondary mitral valve dysfunction
— Soft S_1
— Austin–Flint murmur; premature closure of mitral
valve on echo

* e.g. due to infective endocarditis, ruptured chorda
NB: Pulse pressure may *not* be wide despite severe (acute) aortic
regurgitation

Indications for valve replacement in aortic regurgitation
1 Symptoms
2 Declining exercise tolerance on stress testing
Fall in ejection fraction on exercise gated blood pool
scan
3 Increasing heart size on CXR
4 Development of left ventricular strain pattern on ECG
5 Echocardiogram showing left ventricular end-
diastolic diameter greater than 7 cm

Causes of aortic incompetence
1 Valvulitis
— Rheumatic

2 Infective endocarditis
— Rheumatoid arthritis
3 Aortitis
— Syphilis
— Ankylosing spondylitis
4 Annuloaortic ectasia
— Marfan's syndrome
— Atheroma
5 Hypertension
6 Bicuspid aortic valve
7 Aortic dissection; trauma
8 Fluid overload in renal failure

Predictors of heart failure following aortic valve surgery
1 Symptoms preoperatively
2 Echo
— Fractional shortening less than 25%
— Left ventricular end-systolic diameter > 55 mm
3 Gated blood pool scan
— Left ventricular dysfunction
— Fall in ejection fraction on exercise

AORTIC STENOSIS (AS)

Indicators of severity in aortic stenosis
1 Pulse character (slowly rising, 'plateau')*
Pulse pressure (narrow)
2 Signs of left ventricular failure, including S_3
3 Thrill
4 S_2: soft, single or paradoxically split
5 Presence of S_4; long, late-peaking murmur
6 Cardiac catheter
— Systolic transvalvular gradient > 50 mmHg (in
presence of normal left ventricular function‡)

* NB: Systolic hypertension does *not* exclude severe stenosis.
Pulse pressure width is unreliable in elderly patients, while
murmurs may become inaudible in patients with cardiac failure.
Accurate assessment may thus be *impossible* without
catheterization.
‡ The transvalvular gradient may decline in left ventricular
dysfunction

Prognosis: symptom-related actuarial outcome of aortic stenosis
1 Exertional angina
— Death within 3 years (if untreated)
2 Effort syncope
— Death within 2 years
3 Exertional dyspnea
— Death within 1 year
4 Overt cardiac failure
— Death within 6 months

Signs of dominant aortic stenosis in mixed aortic valve disease
1 Minimal cardiomegaly
2 Anacrotic pulse and narrow pulse pressure
3 S_4; no S_3

Causes and differential diagnosis of aortic stenosis
1 Valvular
— Rheumatic
— Calcific (degenerative)

— Congenital bicuspid valve
— Congenital aortic stenosis (with ejection click)
2 Subvalvar
— Hypertrophic cardiomyopathy
— Congenital subaortic membranous stenosis
3 Supravalvar
— Congenital aortic coarctation
— Congenital supravalvar aortic stenosis
with or without elfin facies and hypercalcemia

NB: Aortic stenotic murmurs may be simulated by pulmonary outflow bruits, esp. pulmonary stenosis

TRICUSPID VALVE DISEASE

Diagnostic clues to tricuspid stenosis*
1 History
— Unexplained spontaneous symptomatic improvement in patient with known mitral stenosis
2 Examination
— Giant 'a' waves but no parasternal heave or loud P$_2$
— Diastolic murmur increases on inspiration
— Hepatomegaly with presystolic pulsation
3 Investigations
— Clear CXR despite marked venous engorgement
— Isolated right atrial enlargement on CXR and ECG
4 Definitive diagnosis
— Echocardiography (makes the above redundant)

* Rare as hen's teeth, but anyhow . . .

Tricuspid incompetence: distinction from mitral incompetence
1 Murmur increases on inspiration
2 Murmur does not radiate well to axilla
3 Systolic waves and steep 'y' descents in jugular venous pulse
4 Pulsatile liver
5 Right (not left) ventricular enlargement *if* isolated lesion
6 Etiological stigmata
— Cyanosis and fixed split S$_2$: Ebstein's anomaly
— Nodular hepar, telangiectasia: carcinoid syndrome
— Needle marks: intravenous drug abuse

NB: Tricuspid valve lesions most commonly occur *with* other valvular lesions

INVESTIGATING CARDIOVASCULAR DISEASE

CHEST X-RAYS

Differential diagnosis of pulmonary plethora
1 Atrial septal defect
2 Ventricular septal defect
3 Patent ductus arteriosus (i.e. any left-to-right shunt)

Differential diagnosis of pulmonary oligemia
1 Pulmonic valvular stenosis
2 Pulmonary atresia
3 Primary pulmonary hypertension (peripheral oligemia)
4 Massive pulmonary embolism
5 Any right-to-left shunt
— Fallot's tetralogy, transposition
— Eisenmenger's syndrome

Differential diagnosis of enlarged cardiac silhouette
1 Cardiomyopathy
2 Multiple valvular defects
3 Ischemic heart disease with aneurysm
4 Complex congenital heart disease with RV enlargement
5 Pericardial effusion

The 'normal' chest X-ray: checklist
1 Patient's name; film date; correct siding
2 Adequate inspiration; optimal exposure; clavicles centered
3 Transradiancy of both lungfields (?mastectomy, Swyer–James)
4 *Actively* look for
— Retrocardiac mass
— Valvular calcification
— Rib resection/notching/erosions/fractures
— Small pneumothorax, effusion
— Gastric air bubble on right (*situs inversus*)
— Nipple shadow (absent on lateral)
5 Assess bones
— Osteoporosis (outer two-thirds of clavicle)
— Lytic lesions (e.g. myeloma, breast cancer)

Indications for additional X-ray views
1 Lateral
— Request routinely
2 Decubitus
— To confirm whether 'effusion' layers out (i.e. to exclude pleural thickening or loculation)
3 Expiratory
— To confirm or exclude pneumothorax
4 Erect
— To look for gas under diaphragm (suspected perforation of abdominal hollow viscus)
5 Apical lordotic
— Suspected TB

ECHOCARDIOGRAPHY

Echocardiographic features of left ventricular dysfunction
1 Left ventricular enlargement; wall thickness
2 Reduced fractional shortening
3 Paradoxical septal motion
4 'B' notch; reduced EF slope
5 Premature aortic valve closure or reduced valve opening

Differential diagnosis of paradoxical septal motion
1 Congestive cardiomyopathy

2 Ischemic heart disease, esp. septal infarction
3 Right ventricular volume overload (e.g. ASD)
4 Conduction disturbance
   — LBBB
   — WPW
   — Right ventricular pacing
5 Post-CABG

Asymmetric septal hypertrophy: differential diagnosis
1 Hypertrophic cardiomyopathy (incl. asymptomatic relatives*)
2 Infarction of left ventricular free wall
3 Rarely: LVH due to hypertension or valvular aortic stenosis‡

* i.e. these people have HOCM even if they don't think so
‡ i.e. probably HOCM in fact

Potential indications for transesophageal echocardiography
1 Diagnosis of thoracic aortic dissection
   — Investigation of choice (result in 15 mins)
2 Suspected left atrial thrombus or cardiogenic embolism
   — Commonest indication
3 Assessment of vegetations or abscesses in endocarditis
4 Evaluation of prosthetic valve dysfunction (esp. mitral)
5 Intraoperative assessment of LV function
6 Technically suboptimal transthoracic echocardiogram

Transthoracic better than transesophageal echocardiography?
1 Mitral or aortic stenosis
2 Mitral valve prolapse
3 Left ventricular thrombus

Valve surgery indicated by echo alone: prerequisites
1 Young patient (< 30 years)
2 Single valve involvement (esp. mitral)
3 Consistent clinical picture
4 Technically unequivocal echocardiogram

NUCLEAR CARDIOLOGY

Clinical utility of 'hot-spot' (^{99m}Tc pyrophosphate) scanning*
1 Suspected infarct with negative enzymes
   — e.g. Late presentation
2 Suspected infarct with equivocal enzymes
   — e.g. Post-surgery, intramuscular injection
3 Suspected infarct with non-diagnostic ECG
   — Previous infarction
   — Pacemaker in situ
   — Left bundle branch block, Wolff–Parkinson–White
4 Suspected right ventricular (or true posterior) infarct

*NB: Acute utility is limited, since may take 48 h to become positive

Indications for 'cold-spot' (thallium, ^{201}Tl) scanning*
1 Preangiographic evaluation of 'intermediate' chest pain

   — Non-diagnostic stress ECG
   — Male with atypical chest pain and positive stress ECG
   — Female with chest pains and positive stress ECG
2 Postangiography
   — To ascertain exact site of ischemia in patient with multivessel disease, some of which are ungraftable
   — To assess functional significance of stenoses seen at angiography and adequacy of collateral circulation
   — To assess the viability of myocardium apparently jeopardized by stenosis at angiography
3 Post-bypass assessment of chest pain
   — Graft occlusion vs post-(peri)cardiotomy syndrome
   — Graft occlusion vs chest wall pain
   — Graft occlusion vs ungrafted stenosis
4 Prior to thrombolytic therapy
   — To assess extent of jeopardized myocardium
   — MIBI has superseded thallium in this context

* Becomes positive within 4 h of infarct; cf. 'hot-spot'

Value of gated cardiac blood pool scanning
1 Assessment of left ventricular function prior to
   — Valve replacement
   — CABG
   — Heart transplant
2 Distinguishing global cardiomyopathy from segmental ventricular dysfunction*

* Rarely indicated; cardiomyopathy may also be segmental

CARDIAC CATHETERIZATION

Rationâle in valvular heart disease
1 To define the nature and severity of the suspected lesion
2 To detect coexisting valvular lesions
3 To assess left ventricular function
4 To determine the state of the coronary arteries
5 To assess pulmonary vascular resistance and/or pulmonary capillary wedge pressure

Other indications for cardiac catheterization
1 Detection and quantification of shunts
2 Electrophysiologic studies
3 Endomyocardial biopsy*
   — Cardiomyopathy/myocarditis
   — Intracardiac tumor
   — Post-transplant

* Precise role remains to be clarified

Indications for coronary angiography
1 Typical angina refractory to medical therapy
2 Typical angina and/or myocardial infarction in a patient younger than 40 years
3 Angina following myocardial infarction
4 Strongly positive exercise test
5 Atypical chest pain
   — In a male with a positive stress test
   — In a female with a positive exercise thallium scan

Morbidity of cardiac catheterization
1   Brachial or femoral arterial occlusion
2   Coronary dissection; aortic dissection; tamponade
3   Left ventricular perforation
4   Cerebral embolism
5   Complete heart block, esp. if pre-existing RBBB
6   Ventricular dysrhythmias*
7   Hypotension, pulmonary edema*
8   Death, esp. if left main disease (mortality 2/1000)

* Frequency reduced if low-osmolality contrast agents used (expensive)

EXERCISE STRESS (ECG) TESTING

Indications for exercise testing
1   Diagnosis of ischemic heart disease where the diagnosis cannot be made on clinical grounds (e.g. atypical pain)
2   Investigation of suspected exercise-induced arrhythmias
3   Objective evaluation of symptoms (and/or degree of incapacity) in patients with known coronary artery disease
4   Assessment of patients following myocardial infarction
    — Submaximal (symptom-limited) test prior to discharge
    — Maximal test 6 weeks later (prior to return to work)
5   Assessment of 'at-risk' individuals prior to exercise program

Exclusion criteria for exercise testing
1   Recent prolonged ischemic chest pain
2   Known severe left main coronary artery disease
3   Severe hypertension, cardiac failure or aortic stenosis
4   Debility
5   Relative
    — Recurrent ventricular tachyarrhythmias
    — Left bundle branch block
    — WPW; LV strain pattern on resting ECG
    — Digoxin R_x in previous week (→ false-positive)

Indicators of test positivity
1   Development of angina
2   Inability to achieve reasonable workload (> 5 Mets*)
3   ≥ 2 mm downward-sloping ST segment depression
    — Onset at heart rate < 120/min *or*
    — Post-test duration > 6 mins
    — Seen in multiple leads
4   Failure of blood pressure to rise (remains < 130 mmHg) despite increasing workload and pulse rate
5   Failure of heart rate to exceed 120/min (off β-blockers)

* A Met is a (metabolic) unit of work (O_2 utilization @ 3.5 mL/kg/min.)

Indicators for aborting test
1   Dizziness, leg pains, severe dyspnea and/or angina
2   Fall in systolic blood pressure of more than 10 mmHg
3   Sustained ventricular tachyarrhythmias

Associations of false-positive tests
1   Low-risk patient populations, e.g.
    — Female (general)
    — Mitral valve prolapse
2   Conditions which cause ischemia without vascular disease:
    — Anemia
    — Post-prandial
    — Valve stenosis, hypertension
    — Myxedema
3   Conditions causing ECG changes (see also Exclusions above)
    — Hypokalemia
    — Hyperventilation
    — Cardiomyopathy
    — Recent digoxin R_x (cf. β-blockers: false-negative)

ELECTROCARDIOGRAPHY (ECG)

Common cardiac rhythm anomalies in athletes
1   Sinus arrhythmia
2   Sinus bradycardia
3   First-degree heart block
4   Wenckebach phenomenon
5   Junctional rhythm

ECG effects of carotid sinus massage (CSM)
1   Left CSM → atrioventricular (AV) node
    Right CSM → Sinoatrial (SA) node
2   Sinus tachycardia
    — Transient slowing
3   Paroxysmal junctional (AV nodal reentry) tachycardia
    — Termination (sinus rhythm)
4   Atrial tachycardia/flutter/fibrillation
    — Slowing (AV block), may be abrupt
5   Wenckebach phenomenon
    — Slowing (AV nodal block) *if* intra-His block
6   Tachycardia-dependent bundle branch block
    — Disappearance of block
7   Bradycardia-dependent bundle branch block
    — Appearance of block
8   Demand pacemaker
    — Reinitiation of pacemaker rhythm
9   Ventricular tachycardia
    — No effect (*rarely* reverts)
10 WPW
    — Increased delta wave on ECG
    — Termination of tachycardia *or* no effect

Causes of a low-voltage ECG
1   Pulmonary emphysema
2   Cardiomyopathy ± ischemia, amyloid
3   Myxedema
4   Pericardial effusion (→ electrical alternans)
5   Incorrect calibration

Voltage criteria for left ventricular hypertrophy
1   None is absolute
2   $S(V_1) + R(V_6) > 35$ mm
3   Any R > 25 mm; any R + any S > 45 mm

4 R(lead 1) > 20 mm
R(aVl) > 13 mm if cardiac axis normal
R(aVl) > 16 mm if there is left axis deviation

Diagnostic criteria for right ventricular hypertrophy
1 Dominant R wave in V_1; $R(V_1)$ amplitude > 7 mm
2 Diagnosis supported by T-wave inversion in V_{1-4} ('strain')
3 Exclusion of other causes of tall $R(V_1)$
   — RBBB
   — WPW type A
   — Dextrocardia
   — Posterior infarction
   — Hypertrophic cardiomyopathy

Left anterior hemiblock: diagnosis and significance
1 Left axis deviation without other cause (LBBB, LVH)
2 Small 'q' in lead I, small 'r' in III
3 May mask inferior infarct

Left posterior hemiblock: diagnosis and significance
1 Axis to the right of +100° without other cause
2 Small 'r' in I, small 'q' in III
3 May mask anterior infarct

Complete heart block: important causes
1 Lenègre's disease: sclerodegeneration of conduction system
2 Lev's disease: fibrocalcareous encroachment onto the conduction system; often associated with calcific aortic stenosis and preceded by first-degree heart block
3 Ischemic heart disease; inferior infarct
4 Digoxin toxicity, esp. when associated with ischemia
5 Congenital (proximal block, narrow QRS)
6 Surgical, e.g. AVR or for congenital heart disease

Criteria for pathological Q wave in standard lead III
1 Duration of Q > 0.04 secs
2 Presence of Q (aVf) > 0.02 secs
3 Presence of Q in lead II
4 Q (III) > 2.5 mm amplitude*

* Unless R(III) > 5 mm and P(III) upright; does *not* disappear on inspiration

Pathological Q waves*
1 Transmural myocardial injury (indeterminate age)
   — Myocardial infarction
   — Myocarditis
   — Cardiac contusion
2 Cardiomyopathy
   — HOCM
   — Myocarditis
3 WPW
4 Recording artefact
   — Dextrocardia
   — Reversed limb leads
   — High lead placement

* Differential diagnosis = deep (not pathological) 'Q' waves

Causes of an elevated ST segment
1 Ischemia
   — Acute myocardial infarction
   — Coronary spasm

2 Pericarditis
3 Ventricular aneurysm
4 Early repolarization (normal variant)

Non-specific ST-T wave changes: some causes
1 Ischemic heart disease
2 Post-tachycardia
3 Hyperventilation; anxiety
4 Post-prandial; cold drinks
5 Mitral valve prolapse
6 Subarachnoid hemorrhage*
7 Smoking
8 Pheochromocytoma
9 Digoxin therapy and/or hypokalemia

* Causes deep 'T' waves in precordial leads

Causes of a prolonged Q-T$_c$*‡
1 Ischemic heart disease
2 Hypocalcemia
3 Rheumatic carditis
4 Heredofamilial long Q-T syndrome¶
5 Quinidine; tricyclics, phenothiazines, amiodarone

* In general, normal Q-T interval < 50% R-R interval. Non-specific causes of bradycardia (myxedema, hypothermia, raised intracranial pressure) may increase Q-T interval, but not when corrected for rate
‡ Sudden death in chronic CCF is commoner in patients with higher inter-lead Q-T variability ('Q-T dispersion')
¶ Left stellectomy (surgical denervation of left cardiac sympathetic supply) may help prevent arrhythmias in patients resistant to β-blockers

Absent 'p' waves: differential diagnosis
1 Atrial fibrillation
2 Nodal rhythm; sinoatrial block
3 Severe hyperkalemia

Inverted 'p' waves in standard lead I
1 Nodal rhythm
2 Dextrocardia
3 Reversed limb leads

ECG manifestations of digoxin therapy
1 Prolonged P-R interval
2 Shortened Q-T$_c$
3 S-T depression ('reverse-tick'); T wave flattening

ECG manifestations of quinidine therapy
1 Increased QRS width (25% increase may denote toxicity)
2 Prolonged Q-T$_c$; prolonged P-R interval; low wide T wave
3 *Torsade de pointes* *
   — Polymorphous VT with prolonged Q-T$_c$
   — Indicates toxicity

* May also complicate idiopathic long Q-T syndrome or perhexiline therapy

ECG manifestations of hyperkalemia
1 Peaked ('tent-shaped') T waves
2 P wave flattening
3 Broad QRS
4 Non-specific ST-T wave abnormalities
5 Asystole

ECG localization of acute myocardial infarction
1 Anterior
   — Q waves/ST elevation V_{2-4}
2 Extensive anterior
   — Q waves/ST elevation I, aVL, V_{1-6}
3 Anteroseptal
   — Q waves/ST elevation V_{1-3}
4 Anterolateral
   — Q waves/ST elevation V_{4-6}
5 Inferior
   — Q waves/ST elevation II, III, aVF
6 True posterior
   — Abnormalities in V_{1-2} (see below)
7 Right ventricular
   — ST elevation in V_{4R}

ECG in true posterior infarction
1 Dominant widened 'R' (V_{1-2}): no RBBB/RVH/WPW
2 Tall widened 'T' (V_{1-2})
3 Concave-up ST depression (V_{1-2})
4 Usually associated with signs of inferior infarction

ECG in cor pulmonale
1 Right axis deviation
2 P pulmonale
3 R:S > 1 in V_1 and aVR
   R:S < 1 in V_6
4 Right bundle branch block

ECG in rheumatic fever
1 Tachycardia: sinus or idionodal
2 Heart block: first degree (↑ PR)
3 Prolonged Q-T$_c$

ECG with reversed limb leads
1 Lead I appears to have reversed polarity
2 Leads II and III appear interchanged
3 aVr and aVl appear interchanged; aVf is normal

ECG in myotonic dystrophy
1 Sinus bradycardia
2 First-degree heart block (± higher-grade heart block)
3 Left axis deviation (± LAHB, LBBB)
4 Sporadic ventricular or reentrant arrhythmias

MANAGING CARDIOVASCULAR DISEASE

SURGERY AND THE HEART

Cardiovascular risk factors for general surgery
1 Poor left ventricular function
   — Myocardial infarction in last 6 months
   — Third heart sound
   — Elevated jugular venous pressure
   — Ejection fraction < 30% on echo
2 ECG
   — Not sinus rhythm, *or*
   — Sinus rhythm *plus* ≥ 5 VEB's/min
   — Ischemic S-T segment changes
3 General
   — Thoracic or upper abdominal surgery
   — *Severe* aortic stenosis or hypertension

Morbidity of open-heart surgery
1 LV dysfunction ± perioperative myocardial infarction
2 Cerebral sequelae
   — Stroke (mechanism unclear)
   — Personality change, confusion
   — Depression; sleep disturbance
3 Bleeding tendency
   — Post-pump syndrome (see below)
4 Exacerbation of peptic ulcer disease
5 Delayed complications
   — Post-cardiotomy syndrome
   — Endocarditis (after valve surgery)
   — CMV viremia; hepatitis
   — Wound infection

Coronary artery bypass grafting: rationâle
1 Operate for pain, not for dyspnea
2 Improved LV function *only* → hibernating myocardium

Coronary artery bypass grafting: survival benefit*
1 Accepted
   — Left main coronary artery disease
   — Triple-vessel disease
     • Symptomatic
     • Asymptomatic + poor LV function
2 Probable
   — Double-vessel disease + ↓ LV function
   — Double-vessel disease + high-grade proximal stenosis of ieft anterior descending branch of left coronary

* cf. low-risk patients: early CABG is associated with ↑ mortality

Factors influencing surgical evaluation of coronary disease
1 Severity of symptoms uncontrolled by medical therapy
   — i.e. Unstable angina
2 Size of left anterior descending branch of left coronary artery
   — Determines amount of myocardium jeopardized
3 Suitability for percutaneous angioplasty (PTCA; p. 60)
   — Age, prior surgery, other disease

Contraindications to coronary artery grafting
1 Absolute
   — Technically ungraftable vessels
2 Relative
   — Lack of symptoms*
   — Inadequate trial of medical therapy
   — Severe left ventricular dysfunction

* Exceptions: (1) left main disease, and (2) triple vessel disease with positive exercise test (silent ischemia) – though aspirin may have a role in the latter

Operability criteria in coronary artery grafting
1 Satisfactory general medical condition
2 Adequate left ventricular function
3 Discrete proximal stenoses with good distal run-off

The 'post-pump' (cardiopulmonary bypass) syndrome
1 Coagulopathy (may respond to dextran or dDAVP)
   — Heparin effect

— Thrombocytopenia
— Massive transfusion (see p. 166)
— Coagulation factor depletion
2 Anemia, leukopenia
— Mechanical intravascular hemolysis
3 Systemic inflammatory reactions
— e.g. 'Shock lung' (due to complement activation)
4 Pancreatitis
— Associated with perioperative $CaCl_2$ administration
5 Stroke
— e.g. Due to air embolism

Post-cardiotomy (Dressler's) syndrome: clinical features
1 Acute febrile illness within 6 months of heart surgery/infarct
2 Chest pain: pleuritic or pericarditic
3 CXR may show effusion(s), cardiomegaly; ECG often normal
4 Self-limiting; may need NSAIDs, aspirin, steroids, aspiration
5 Diagnosis of exclusion (DD$_x$: acute myocardial infarction)

PACEMAKING

Indications for permanent pacing
1 Major indication
— Symptomatic bradyarrhythmias
2 Relative indications
— Complete heart block (if symptomatic)
— 'At-risk' for complete heart block:
  • Intermittent Möbitz type II AV block (wide QRS)
  • Bi-/trifascicular block + ↑ H-V interval on EPS
  • Alternating RBBB and LBBB
— Drug-resistant tachyarrhythmias (incl. sick sinus)

Indications for transvenous pacing in anterior infarcts
1 Second- or third-degree AV block
2 Relative
— New RBBB with old 1° HB/LAHB/LPHB
— New LBBB with preexisting 1° HB
— Alternating RBBB and LBBB

Sources of interference
1 Arc welding
2 Intraoperative unipolar diathermy
3 Pectoralis overactivity (myoinhibition)
4 NMR scanners

Reasons for failure of pacemaker to prevent syncope
1 Failure of stimulus artefact
2 Failure of ventricular capture
3 Failure of demand function
— Oversensing (will not 'fire')
4 Symptoms not due to cardiac arrhythmia

Features of the pacemaker syndrome
1 Definition
— Retrograde ventriculoatrial conduction (despite blockade of anterograde conduction)

2 Mechanism
— Ventricular pacemaker induces atrial contraction, increasing atrial pressure + reducing cardiac output
3 Presentations
— Dizziness, episodic dyspnea

PROSTHETIC HEART VALVES

General considerations influencing valve selection
1 Topographic considerations
— Problems commoner in mitral/tricuspid position
  • Thromboembolism
  • Acute obstruction
— Problems commoner in aortic position
  • Intravascular hemolysis
  • Infection
  • Valve dysfunction
2 Mechanical valves (see below)
— Main advantage: durability
— Main disadvantage: anticoagulant requirement (hence, bleeding complications)
3 Tissue valves (e.g. Hancock, Carpentier–Edwards)
— Main advantage: no anticoagulant requirement*
— Main disadvantage: not durable‡, prone to calcify

* esp. in aortic position
‡ 50% need redoing by 8 years

Specific factors influencing mechanical valve selection
1 Ball-in-cage (Starr–Edwards)
— Disadvantage
  • Flow impediment (esp. with exercise)
— Advantage
  • Durability
2 Tilting disc (e.g. Björk–Shiley, St Jude)
— Disadvantages
  • Prone to massive valve thrombosis
  • Incidence of strut fracture
— Advantages
  • Excellent hemodynamics
  • Less peripheral thromboembolism

Features of valvar hemolysis
1 Diagnosis
— Normochromic (rarely, hypochromic) anemia
— Blood film: schistocytes, no spherocytes
— Haptoglobin with negative Coombs'/Ham's tests
— Hemosiderinuria (implies long-standing hemolysis)
2 Significance
— Suspect valve dysfunction (e.g. regurgitation)
— *Actively* exclude valve infection
3 Management
— Transfuse
— Treat infection
— Valve repair or replacement

Tissue valves: relative indications for use*
1 Elderly patient requiring aortic valve replacement
2 Elderly patient in sinus rhythm with normal size left atrium requiring mitral valve prosthesis

3 Young woman in sinus rhythm desiring pregnancy
4 Any absolute contraindication to anticoagulation

* NB: Durability is usually the most important consideration

Anticoagulant management of the pregnant patient
1 Use subcutaneous heparin prophylaxis
   (10 000 U b.d.) throughout first trimester to avoid
   warfarin embryopathy
2 Switch to warfarin at start of second trimester and
   maintain until halfway through third trimester
   (prolonged use of heparin prophylaxis may result in
   severe osteoporosis)
3 Change back to heparin (subcutaneous at home,
   infusion in hospital) and monitor closely using
   protamine sulfate neutralization and platelet count,
   esp. prior to delivery (neonatal intraventricular
   hemorrhage is a major risk)
4 Avoid epidural anesthesia throughout confinement.
   At delivery, reverse heparin with protamine sulfate
5 Recommence SC heparin immediately following
   delivery
6 Recommence warfarin 1 week after delivery (not
   contraindicated in lactation; cf. phenindione)

HEART TRANSPLANTS

Contraindications to transplantation
1 Satisfactory quality of life
2 Active infection (incl. HIV) or peptic ulcer
3 Severe pulmonary hypertension ($\geq$ 5 Wood units)
4 Past history of thromboembolism or CVA
5 Insulin-dependent diabetes
6 Renal or hepatic insufficiency
   Chronic hepatitis B/C
7 Major systemic/psychiatric illness, e.g. alcoholism
8 Positive cytotoxic crossmatch with donor organ
9 Prior thoracotomy
10 Advanced age

Signs of rejection
1 Fever (early sign)
2 CXR: cardiomegaly
3 ECG: conduction disturbances, reduced QRS voltage
4 Cardiac failure (late sign)

Indications for heart–lung transplantation
1 Pulmonary hypertension
   — Primary (advanced)
2 Pulmonary hypertension
   — Congenital heart disease (Eisenmenger's)
3 Pulmonary hypertension
   — Secondary to cystic fibrosis

CORONARY (BALLOON) ANGIOPLASTY

Percutaneous transluminal coronary angioplasty (PTCA)
1 All angiographic lesions are suitable for attempted
   PTCA
   Ischemia and angina commonly occur during PTCA
2 Commonest lesion (80%) is a proximal concentric
   non-calcified stenosis in a patient with single-vessel
   disease

3 80–90% of such lesions are successfully dilated 30%
   of dilated lesions reocclude within 6 months (stent
   placement may be more durable than PTCA)
4 2% require urgent thoracotomy post-PTCA (acute
   occlusion)
   2% incidence of non-Q wave myocardial infarction
   (p. 74)
   1% mortality from elective PTCA for single-vessel
   disease
5 Similar success (~ 80%) in restenosis and graft
   occlusion
   Efficacy approximates that of CABG (see ref. 2.7)

* i.e. 10–20% failure rate

Potential indications for PTCA
1 Angina
2 After thrombolysis for acute myocardial infarction

DRUG THERAPY

Elimination pathways of cardioactive drugs
1 Initial hepatic metabolism
   — Quinidine
   — Lignocaine
   — Antianginals
     • Nitrates
     • β-blockers (e.g. propranolol)
     • Verapamil
2 Initial renal excretion
   — Digoxin
   — Disopyramide
   — Procainamide

Popular drug combinations in cardiological practice
1 Nifedipine + aspirin
   — Coronary artery disease
2 ACE inhibitor + diuretic
   — Cardiac failure
3 Nitrates + dopamine/dobutamine
   — Acute LVF
4 β-blocker + isosorbide mononitrate*
   — Angina

* Note that further addition of calcium antagonists appears
unhelpful and most medically managed patients do well with β-
blocker monotherapy

Cardiovascular effects of tricyclic antidepressants
1 Tachycardia (anticholinergic effect)
2 Hypotension (esp. postural)
3 Prolonged Q-T_c (quinidine-like effect)
4 Prolonged P-R interval
5 Antagonism of guanethidine and methyldopa
6 Precipitation of ventricular arrhythmias (esp. in
   overdose)

CALCIUM ANTAGONISTS

Verapamil: absolute contraindications
1 High-degree AV block
2 Sick sinus syndrome*

3 Wolff–Parkinson–White syndrome with anterograde conduction causing recurrent atrial fibrillation/flutter
4 Digoxin toxicity
5 Heart failure, hypotension (incl. post-infarct)
6 Simultaneous IV use with β-blockers

* Unless manifests as atrial fibrillation

Calcium antagonists: which one?
1 Verapamil ($\rightarrow$ greatest AV nodal block)
   — Supraventricular tachycardia
   — Hypertrophic cardiomyopathy
   — Do not prescribe with β-blockers
2 Nifedipine ($\rightarrow$ greatest drop in peripheral resistance)
   — Angina (with β-blockers*)
   — Left ventricular dysfunction/cardiac failure
   — Hypertension*: systemic or pulmonary
   — Sinus bradycardia; impaired AV conduction
   — Coronary artery spasm
   — Peripheral vasospasm (Raynaud's)
   — Peripheral vascular disease
3 Diltiazem (intermediate in both respects)
   — Less negative ionotropy/chronotropy than verapamil; hence, least likely to precipitate heart failure‡
   — Permits increased heart rate with exercise
   — May be used for angina with (oral) β-blockers

* Short half-life of standard-preparation nifedipine makes monotherapy for hypertension/angina unsatisfactory
‡ New 2nd-generation agents (amlodipine, felodipine) may also be useful here

ANTIARRHYTHMIC THERAPY

Practical classification of antiarrhythmic drugs
1 'AV node' drugs
   — Digoxin
   — Verapamil
   — β-blockers
2 'Ventricle' drugs
   — Lignocaine
   — Mexiletine, tocainide
3 'Whole-heart' (incl. bundle of Kent) drugs
   — Amiodarone
   — Disopyramide
   — Quinidine, procainamide

Electrophysiological classification of antiarrhythmic drugs
1 #I
   — Block membrane Na^+ transport
   — $\downarrow$ Rate of action potential rise (phase O depolarization)
   — e.g. Quinidine, procainamide, disopyramide; lignocaine
2 #II
   — Sympathetic nervous system blockers
   — Reduce phase 4 depolarization
   — e.g. β-blockers
3 #III
   — Prolong duration of action potential/refractory period

— No effect on phase O depolarization
   — e.g. Amiodarone, bretylium
4 #IV
   — Calcium blockers
   — e.g. Verapamil (cf. nifedipine: *not* antiarrhythmic)

Drugs reducing ventricular rate in atrial fibrillation*
1 Digoxin
2 Adenosine
3 Verapamil
4 Amiodarone
5 β-blockers

* i.e. AV blockers

Quinidine: contraindications to use
1 Single agent use in atrial flutter/fibrillation
2 Prolonged Q-T$_c$
3 Hypotension
4 Sick sinus syndrome
5 Myasthenia gravis

Quinidine: toxicity
1 Diarrhea
2 Nausea, vomiting, abdominal pain, fever
3 Thrombocytopenia, agranulocytosis
4 Cinchonism
   — Tinnitus, deafness, vertigo, amblyopia
   — Sweats, flushing, urticaria
5 Potentiation of digoxin and warfarin toxicity

Disopyramide: toxicity
1 Anticholinergic, esp. urinary retention in males
2 Negative inotropy, esp. when given by IV bolus
3 Ventricular tachyarrhythmias (usually preceded by $\uparrow$Q-T$_c$)

Amiodarone: toxicity
1 Pneumonitis (10% incidence, 0.5% mortality)
2 Thyroid dysfunction*
   — Hypothyroidism (6–10% within 3 yrs)
   — Hyperthyroidism (< 3% within 3 yrs)
   — Euthyroid hyperthyroxinemia‡
3 Corneal microdeposits (reversible)
4 Peripheral neuropathy (irreversible)
5 Liver damage (irreversible)
6 Photosensitivity
7 Bradycardia, idioventricular rhythm
   Hypotension if rapidly infused
8 Nightmares, sleep disturbance

* Thyroid toxicity reflects high (37%) iodine content
‡ Due to impaired deiodination of T_4 to T_3

DIGOXIN THERAPY

Side-effects of digoxin
1 Gastrointestinal
   — Diarrhea, abdominal pain, ulceration (local effect)
   — Nausea, vomiting (central effect)
2 Central
   — Confusion, convulsions, depression
   — Commoner in elderly patients

3 Visual (dose-related)
  — Xanthopsia, haloes, blurring
4 Rare
  — Facial pain; gynecomastia; hyperkalemia
  — Muscle necrosis

Contraindications to digoxin therapy
1 Wolff–Parkinson–White syndrome*
2 AV block
3 HOCM (or severe aortic stenosis) in sinus rhythm
4 Constrictive pericarditis; acute myocarditis
5 Prior to elective cardioversion (relative‡)

* Antedromic (with tachycardias)
‡ cf. do *not* cardiovert in digoxin toxicity

Metabolic predispositions to digoxin toxicity
1 General
  — Old age, low body weight
  — Pre-existing myocardial disease
2 Renal impairment
3 Metabolic abnormality
  — Hypoxia (esp. cor pulmonale)
  — Hypokalemia
  — Hypomagnesemia
  — Hypercalcemia
  — Hypothyroidism
4 Cardiac amyloidosis

Arrhythmias in digoxin toxicity
1 'Classical'
  — AV block plus junctional/ventricular arrhythmia
2 Common in elderly patients: ↑ automaticity
  — Frequent ventricular ectopic beats (in 50%)
  — Ventricular bigeminy
  — Ventricular tachycardia (in 5%); VF
3 Common in young patients (esp. overdoses):
  ↑ AV block
  — Junctional rhythm (seen in 20%)
  — Atrial tachycardia + varying block ('SVT with
    block')
  — Sinus bradycardia, sinoatrial nodal block, sinus
    arrest

Management of digoxin toxicity*
1 Cease digoxin administration
2 Correct electrolyte imbalance
  — Aim to maintain serum K^+ at 4.5–5.5 mmol/L
  — Do *not* administer KCl in presence of AV block
  — Infuse potassium in saline (not in dextrose)
3 AV block
  — Atropine, phenytoin
  — Temporary pacing
4 Supraventricular tachycardia
  — Propranolol
5 Ventricular arrhythmias
  — Phenytoin
  — Temporary pacing
  — (Emergency) cardioversion
6 Rarely needed therapies
  — Antidigoxin antibodies (Fab fragments)
  — Dialysis

* *Most* patients can be managed with the first two measures
alone

SYMPATHOLYTIC AND SYMPATHOMIMETIC THERAPY

Physiological manifestations of adrenergic stimulation
1 α_1 (postsynaptic) stimulation
  — Peripheral vasoconstriction, pressor effects
  — Catecholamine agonists
    • Dopamine, (nor)adrenaline
  — Peripheral α_1 antagonist
    • Prazosin
2 α_2 (presynaptic) stimulation
  — Sympathetic inhibition
  — Central α_2 agonist
    • Clonidine
3 β_1 (predominantly cardiac) stimulation
  — Tachycardia, positive inotropy
  — Increased AV conduction
  — Catecholamine agonists
    • (Nor)adrenaline, isoprenaline
    • Dopamine, dobutamine
  — Cardioselective blockers:
    • Metoprolol, atenolol, acebutolol
4 β_2 (predominantly peripheral) stimulation
  — Peripheral vasodilatation
  — Bronchodilatation
  — Catecholamine agonists
    • Adrenaline, isoprenaline
    • Dopexamine, dobutamine
5 Dopaminergic
  — Low-dose: coronary/cerebral/renal *vasodilatation*
  — Moderate-dose: mainly β_1 effects
  — High-dose: mainly α_1-mediated *vasoconstriction*

Hazards of combining β-blockers with other therapy
1 Verapamil*
  — Depression of myocardial contractility and
    conduction
2 Ergotamine, dopamine
  — Non-selective block of β_1-mediated vasodilatation
    (→ severe vasoconstriction and necrosis)
3 Prazosin
  — Accentuation of 'first-dose' hypotension
4 Adrenaline
  — Immediate severe hypertension
5 Indomethacin
  — Antagonism of hypotensive effect
6 Cimetidine
  — Potentiation of hypotensive effect
7 Antianginal therapy of coronary artery spasm
  — Antagonism by β-blockade

* especially parenteral administration
NB: Even when used as *eyedrops* (e.g. timolol)
β-blockers are contraindicated in asthmatics

Rationâle of β-blockade in myocardial infarction
1 IV (within 4 h of infarct ± streptokinase/angioplasty)
  — May reduce chest pain
  — May reduce infarct size (and ?cardiogenic shock)
  — May prevent some arrhythmias (incl. SVT, VF)
2 Oral (post-infarct maintenance)
  — Reduced mortality/reinfarction rate, esp. if
    • Modest LV dysfunction
    • Positive exercise test prior to discharge (may
      indicate need for catheterization ± CABG)

ANGIOTENSIN-CONVERTING ENZYME (ACE) INHIBITORS

Currently available ACE inhibitors
1 Captopril
   — Rapid onset of action, short half-life
   — Requires b.d./t.d.s. dosage regimen (on empty stomach)
2 Enalapril
   — Hepatically bioactivated to enalaprilat
   — Slower onset of action; once-daily dosage
3 Lisinopril
   — Substitution of lysine for proline in enalaprilat
   — 24-hour duration of action; once-daily dosage
4 Others
   — Alecapril (prodrug for captopril)
   — Pentopril, ramipril (long duration of action)

Proposed mechanisms of action of ACE inhibitors
1 Reduction of angiotensin II levels
   — Vasodilatation
   — ↓ Renin release
   — ↓ Aldosterone secretion
2 Increased bradykinin, prostacyclin, prostaglandin E_2 levels
   — Vasodilatation

Indications for ACE inhibition
1 Refractory heart failure
   — incl. Congestive cardiomyopathy‡
2 Severe hypertension (esp. high-renin), incl.
   — Renovascular hypertension*
   — Hypertension in scleroderma
3 Controversial indications
   — Left ventricular hypertrophy
   — Cardioprotection in acute myocardial infarction
4 Diabetic nephropathy
5 Unacceptable toxicity using multidrug regimens

* NB: Risk of precipitating acute renal failure if *bilateral* renal artery stenosis
‡ NB: *β-blockers* may also be useful in dilated cardiomyopathy (ref. 2.5); cf. most *calcium blockers* should be avoided in LV dysfunction

Therapeutic benefits of ACE inhibitors in hypertension
1 Peripheral vascular resistance is reduced
2 Renal, cardiac and cerebral perfusion is maintained or increased due to selective vasodilating activity
3 No effect on myocardial conductivity or contractility
4 No effect on metabolism of glucose, urate, lipids or electrolytes; safe to use in diabetes and gout
5 Reduce proteinuria, nephropathy in hypertensive diabetics
6 Safe to use in asthma and depression
7 Do not cause fatigue or impotence; hence, high compliance

Benefits of ACE inhibitors in refractory heart failure
1 Improved hemodynamics
   — No reflex tachycardia (reflecting ↓ preload)
2 Improved exercise tolerance and angina threshold
   — ↓ Myocardial oxygen use despite ↑ cardiac output
3 Improved renal function and electrolyte balance
   — No secondary hyperaldosteronism
4 Regression of LV hypertrophy
5 Improved survival

Side-effects of ACE inhibitors
1 Sulfhydryl moiety-related (i.e. seen with captopril/ alecapril)
   — Rash (dose-related; commoner in renal failure)
   — Taste disturbance
   — Mouth ulcers
   — Neutropenia/agranulocytosis ⎫ Unusual at
   — Proteinuria/nephrosis ⎬ doses now
   — Euphoria ⎭ used
2 'Class' effects (→ longer-acting ACE inhibitors)
   — Hypotension (see below)
   — Hyperkalemia (esp. in renal failure)
   — Cough (see below)
   — Angioedema (in 0.1%; may be fatal)
   — Renal insufficiency (esp. in bilateral renal artery stenosis or concurrent loop diuretic therapy)

Cough associated with ACE inhibition
1 Affects 10–20% patients
   Causes change of therapy in up to 5%
2 Affects mainly female non-smokers
3 Probably rises due to potentiation of ACE substrates such as bradykinin (or substance P, prostaglandins)
4 Diagnosis
   — Stops within 4 days of ceasing medication
   — Recommences within a week (usually within hours) of restarting same or different ACE inhibitor
5 May respond to cromoglycate (vagolytic) prophylaxis

Risk factors for 'first-dose' hypotension with ACE inhibitors
1 Advanced cardiac failure, esp. if
   — Hyponatremia (± salt restriction)
   — Diuretic therapy
2 High-renin hypertension
3 Hemodialysis

VASODILATOR THERAPY

Indications for vasodilator therapy
1 Cardiac failure*
   — Cardiogenic shock, cardiomyopathy
   — Acute valvular incompetence; septal rupture
   — Hypertensive heart failure
2 Hypertension
   — Crisis (incl. encephalopathy)
   — Refractory hypertension
3 Angina‡

* Hypotension and/or reflex tachycardia do not usually occur when vasodilators are used appropriately for CCF
‡ Best vasodilator in this context: glyceryl trinitrate

Predominant preload reducers
1 Nitrates
2 Frusemide

3   Morphine (in pulmonary edema)

NB: Frusemide causes initial rapid venodilatation, followed by slower off-loading effect due to diuresis

Predominant afterload reducers
1   Hydralazine
2   Nifedipine
3   Nitroprusside
4   Prostacyclin (PGI_2)*

* Particularly useful as a vasodilator in Buerger's disease

Pre- and afterload reducers
1   Prazosin
2   ACE inhibitors, e.g. captopril
3   Sodium nitroprusside ('SNIP')
4   Atrial natriuretic peptide (ANP)

NB: Nitroprusside best for 'forward failure', e.g. in septal/chordal rupture, acute mitral/aortic incompetence due to endocarditis

Toxicity of prolonged (> 48 h) nitroprusside infusions
1   Cyanide intoxication*
2   Lactic acidosis
3   Hypothyroidism

* Plasma CN^- levels can be monitored

THROMBOLYTIC THERAPY

Potential indications for thrombolytic therapy
1   Hyperacute phase (< 6 h) myocardial infarction (p. 74)
2   *Massive* pulmonary embolism (> 40% vascular bed) or *any* life-threatening pulmonary embolism
    — i.e. Patient is hypotensive and sick
3   Massive iliofemoral thrombosis*

* Thrombolytic therapy reduces incidence of post-phlebitic syndrome (p. 80)

Contraindications to thrombolytic therapy
1   Absolute
    — Recent prolonged/traumatic cardiac resuscitation
    — Active bleeding, e.g from peptic ulcer
    — Increased risk of hemorrhagic stroke
        • Cerebral hemorrhage in last 2 months
        • Recent skull trauma
        • Brain tumor
    — Retinal hemorrhages, e.g. diabetic*, hypertensive
    — Blood pressure > 200/120 mmHg
    — Surgery within the last 2 weeks
    — Pregnancy/puerperium
    — Previous allergic reaction to SK or APSAC‡
2   Relative
    — History of CVA, peptic ulcer or severe hypertension
    — Recent surgery or trauma (but > 2 weeks ago)
    — Suspected intracardiac thrombus (e.g. MS with AF)
    — Coagulopathy or severe chronic liver disease
    — Prior thrombolytic treatment with SK or APSAC‡

* controversial
‡ In this situation, treat instead with urokinase or tPA

Monitors of thrombolytic therapy
1   PTTK/APTT, (pro)thrombin time, euglobulin lysis time
2   Resolution of condition requiring treatment
    — As determined by lung scan, blood gases, etc.
3   Overdosage may be corrected by aprotinin or FFP

CORONARY THROMBOLYSIS

Indications for post-infarct thrombolytic therapy
1   No known contraindication to thrombolysis
2   Symptom duration less than 6 h
3   Patient younger than 65
4   No previous infarcts
5   Anterior (or inferior) infarct

Coronary recanalization efficiency
1   Intravenous streptokinase   — 50%
2   Intracoronary streptokinase   — 70%
3   Intravenous TPA   — 70%

TPA or streptokinase? Points to consider
1   TPA is a recombinant human protein which binds fibrin in clots then activates (cleaves) plasminogen to plasmin, causing localized thrombolysis. Streptokinase (or urokinase) similarly binds fibrin in clots, but also degrades fibrinogen, leading to *generalized* fibrinolysis
2   Despite the apparently greater specificity of TPA, neither its efficacy nor its safety record have been proven superior to those of streptokinase; both are complicated by cerebral hemorrhage in 0.5–1.0% of cases
3   Clinical trials of TPA have shown 50% (the TIMI-1 study) and 26% (the ASSET study) reductions in death from myocardial infarction
4   Clinical trials of streptokinase have shown 25% (the ISIS-2 study) and 18% (the GISSI study) reductions in death from myocardial infarction, the latter increasing to 50% if given in the first hour of symptoms
5   TPA is far more expensive than streptokinase

UNDERSTANDING CARDIOVASCULAR DISEASE

TACHYARRHYTHMIAS

Management of atrial flutter
1   Slow ventricular rate
    — Digoxin (*if* digoxin toxicity excluded)
2   If *tachycardia* persists despite digitalization, consider
    — Adenosine (p. 64), *or*
    — β-blocker, *or*
    — Verapamil
3   If *sinus rhythm* does not occur despite digitalization, add
    — Quinidine (in CCU)*, *or*
    — Disopyramide
4   If above measures fail
    — Prepare for elective synchronized cardioversion

— Commence heparin infusion 48 h before
— Cease digoxin 24 h prior to version
— Commence quinidine after; maintain for
  3 months

* If quinidine is commenced, the maintenance dose of digoxin should be reduced by 50% pending attainment of a new steady state

Cardioversion: indications and contraindications

1 Indications
   — Coarse ventricular fibrillation
   — Ventricular tachycardia or rapid atrial fibrillation of recent onset with hemodynamic deterioration
   — Atrial flutter or paroxysmal atrial tachycardia resistant to medical therapy
2 Relative contraindications
   — Suspected intracardiac thrombus
   — Digoxin toxicity and/or hypokalemia
   — Low anticipated success rate
     • Long-standing atrial fibrillation or
     • AF with thyrotoxicosis*, or
     • AF with left atrial diameter > 50 mm on echo

* Best treated with β-blocker

Rapid atrial fibrillation resistant to digoxin?

1 Inadequately treated CCF + myocardial infarction
2 Thyrotoxicosis*
3 Wolff–Parkinson–White syndrome
4 Mitral stenosis
5 Pulmonary embolism
6 Myocarditis, congestive cardiomyopathy
7 Intracardiac (or pericardial) metastases

NB: Digoxin toxicity *rarely* causes lone atrial fibrillation
* Even in the absence of overt hyperthyroidism, low or undetectable TSH levels can indicate patients at risk of atrial fibrillation

Indications for warfarinization in atrial fibrillation*

1 Age 65–80, *plus*
2 Stroke risk factors from history
   — Previous TIA/thromboembolism, *or*
   — Hypertension, heart disease, diabetes, *or*
3 Stroke risk factors from echocardiogram
   — Left atrial enlargement (± thrombus), *or*
   — Mitral annulus calcification, *or*
   — LV dysfunction

* Fibrillators not meeting these criteria should receive aspirin

Diagnostic considerations in recurrent palpitations

1 Normal electrophysiologic study
   — Idiopathic
   — Anxiety
   — Thyrotoxicosis
   — Pheochromocytoma
2 Abnormal electrophysiologic study
   — Intranodal bypass tract (commonest*)
   — Wolff–Parkinson–White syndrome
   — Atrio-His bypass (Lown–Ganong–Levine syndrome)
   — Intraatrial/sinus node reentry

* Palpitations distinctively associated with sensation of pounding in neck

Indications for electrophysiologic study in tachyarrythmias

1 Wide-complex tachycardias unable to be distinguished from ventricular tachycardia
2 Ventricular tachycardia
3 Recurrent symptomatic supraventricular tachycardia with
   — Hemodynamic compromise ('presyncope')
   — Syncopal episodes
   — Wolff–Parkinson–White syndrome on resting ECG

Differential diagnosis of wide-complex tachycardia

1 Ventricular tachycardia (VT)
   — Usually regular
   — No effect of adenosine
2 Wolff–Parkinson–White with anterograde conduction
   — May be regular *or* irregular
   — Slowing of ventricular response by adenosine
3 *Torsade de pointes* (p. 57)
   — Irregular
   — Terminated by $MgSO_4$ (2 g IV over 3 min)
4 Supraventricular tachycardia (SVT) with aberrant conduction
   — Termination by adenosine

ECG characteristics of common paroxysmal SVTs

1 Atrioventricular nodal reentrant SVT
   — Hidden P waves, pseudo-R (V_1), pseudo-S (II or III)
2 Orthodromic* atrioventricular reentrant SVT
   — Inverted P waves; QRS alternans
3 WPW with atrial fibrillation
   — Irregular rhythm, variable QRS conformation
4 Multifocal atrial tachycardia
   — Variable P, P-R and rate

* i.e. accessory pathway-mediated, not antidromic conduction

VT or SVT with aberrancy? Factors favoring VT*

1 Past history of ventricular disease (e.g. aneurysm)
2 Heart rate < 170/min; no effect of carotid sinus massage
3 Clinical evidence of AV dissociation
   — Cannon waves in JVP; 'a' waves slower than
   — *Beat-to-beat variation* in systolic blood pressure
   — Varying intensity of S_1
4 ECG evidence of AV dissociation
   — Dissociated P waves
   — Fusion beats, capture beats
   — Left axis deviation
   — QRS duration > 140 ms
   — QRS morphology different to previous tracings
5 No benefit from adenosine

* NB: Do *not* give verapamil (dangerous in VT) to *any* patient with broad-complex tachycardia of unknown cause; try adenosine, procainamide or (if urgent) cardiovert

Antiarrhythmic role of IV adenosine

1 Action
   — A purine nucleoside which slows AV nodal conduction by activating adenosine (A_1) receptors
   — Half-life of only a few seconds ($\rightarrow \downarrow\downarrow$ adverse effects); hence, administered as a rapid IV bolus

2 Diagnostic use
  — Differentiates SVT from VT *safely*
    • Arrhythmia terminated? Junctional origin
    • Transient AV block induced? Atrial origin
    • No effect? Ventricular origin or WPW
3 Therapeutic use
  — Paroxysmal junctional tachycardia (drug of choice)
4 Side-effects and interactions
  — Transient chest discomfort, flushing, headache
5 Contraindications
  — Asthma
  — second-/third-degree heart block
  — Concurrent R_x (may potentiate adenosine)
    • Dipyridamole, disopyramide

WOLFF–PARKINSON–WHITE SYNDROME (WPW)

Associations of WPW
1 Mitral valve prolapse
2 Hypertrophic cardiomyopathy (uncommonly)
3 Ebstein's anomaly; secundum ASD

Arrhythmias encountered in WPW
1 Paroxysmal atrial tachycardia (in 70%)
2 Atrial fibrillation (in 10–15%)
3 Atrial flutter (in 5%)*

* Development of one-to-one conduction is highly suggestive of the diagnosis

Subtypes of WPW
1 Type A (left-sided)
  — QRS above the isoelectric line in V_1
  — Simulates posterior or inferior infarction
  — Accessory pathway connects left atrium and ventricle
2 Type B (right-sided)
  — QRS below the isoelectric line in V_1
  — Simulates anterior or inferior infarction
  — Pathway connects right atrium and ventricle (e.g. in Ebstein's anomaly)

Management of WPW
1 Observe if asymptomatic
2 Refer for electrophysiologic study at first *hint* of symptoms
3 Medical therapy
  — Amiodarone
  — Disopyramide
  — β-blockers/verapamil
4 Avoid
  — Digoxin
  — Carotid sinus massage (if high risk of AF)
5 Radiofrequency ablation of accessory AV pathways
6 Surgical division of bundle of Kent (following His bundle studies) if refractory to medical measures

BRADYARRHYTHMIAS

Causes of bradyarrhythmias
1 Primary (e.g. ischemic) heart disease:
  — Sinoatrial dysfunction ('sick sinus')

  — Nodal rhythm
  — Complete heart block
2 β-blockade
3 Increased intracranial pressure
4 Metabolic
  — Hypothyroidism
  — Hypothermia
  — Hyperbilirubinemia (profound)

ECG manifestations of sick sinus syndrome
1 Prolonged episodes of sinus bradycardia
  — Absolute (< 40/min)
  — Relative (e.g. < 50/min going up stairs)
2 Marked sinus arrhythmia with symptoms of hypoperfusion
3 Periods of sinus arrest (> 2 sec)
4 Junctional escape rhythms
5 'Brady-tachy' syndrome: background bradycardia punctuated by paroxysmal bursts of rapid atrial flutter/fibrillation
6 Chronic atrial fibrillation (end-stage sinus node dysfunction)

Diagnosis and management of sick sinus syndrome
1 Resting ECG
  — Slow AF
  — Marked, atropine-resistant bradycardia (following β-blockade or digoxin therapy esp.)
2 Holter study (see above)
3 Stress test
  — Excessive tachycardia at submaximal load
4 Management
  — Atrial fibrillation
    • Warfarinization (INR ~ 1.5)
  — Syncope associated with bradycardias
    • Ventricular demand pacing

AORTIC DISSECTION

Predispositions to aortic dissection
1 Hypertension
2 Coarctation
3 Marfan's syndrome
4 Pregnancy

Acute severe chest pain: is it thoracic aortic dissection?
1 Ascending aorta dissection
  — Marfanoid habitus
  — Continuous severe chest/back pain
  — New aortic incompetent murmur
  — Signs of cardiac tamponade
  — ECG: acute infarct (right coronary occlusion) in 1–2%*
2 Aortic arch dissection
  — Reduced pulse in left arm
  — Asymmetric blood pressure readings
  — Carotid occlusion, esp. left
3 Descending aortic dissection
  — Reduced femoral pulse, esp. on left
  — Microhematuria (renal infarction)
  — Left basal dullness (hemothorax)

* NB: Classically the ECG is normal in aortic dissection.

Management priorities in thoracic aortic dissection
1 General measures
 — Confirm diagnosis:
  • Echo (esp. transesophageal: best test), *or*
  • MRI (best for stable dissections), *or*
  • CT, *or*
  • Aortography
2 Ascending (type 1 dissection)
 — Reduce aortic filling pressure
  • Glyceryl trinitrate
  • IV propranolol ± nitroprusside infusion
  • Nifedipine ± nitroprusside infusion
 — Urgent thoracotomy to prevent
  • Intrapericardial rupture
  • Aortic incompetence
  • Carotid artery involvement
 — Vascular graft ± aortic valve replacement
3 Descending (type II) dissection
 — Urgent treatment of hypertension + negative inotrope
 — Non-operative management *unless*
  • Major arterial involvement (e.g. renal)
  • Uncontrolled hypertension
  • Continued pain
 — Long-term β-blockade

AORTIC COARCTATION

Congenital associations of coarctation
1 Bicuspid aortic valve (→ ~ 90%)
2 Congenital aortic valvular stenosis
3 Ventricular septal defect
4 Patent ductus arteriosus (differential cyanosis)
5 Male sex (M:F = 2:1); Turner's syndrome

Radiological features of aortic coarctation
1 Rib notching affecting inferior aspects of posterior ribs (3–8) due to collateralizing anastomoses between internal mammary and inferior epigastric arteries (Dock's sign); not usually present until adolescence.
2 Rib notching confined to right hemithorax indicates coarctation proximal to left subclavian
3 Dilatation of ascending aorta and left subclavian artery visible at the left mediastinal border
4 Post-stenotic aortic dilatation ('reverse-3' sign)

Complications of coarctation
1 Intracranial hemorrhage (subarachnoid or intracerebral)*
2 Refractory hypertension (normoreninemic) ± IHD
3 Aortic dissection/rupture (esp. during pregnancy)
4 Infective endarteritis (rare)
5 Perioperative catastrophes
 — Mesenteric infarction
 — Renal ischemia
 — Paraplegia (due to anterior spinal artery occlusion); more likely if absent collaterals on angiography

* Due to associated berry aneurysms

ATRIAL SEPTAL DEFECT (ASD)

Murmurs encountered in ASD
1 Pulmonary flow murmur
2 Tricuspid flow murmur (usually implies large shunt)
3 Pulmonary incompetent (Graham–Steell) murmur of pulmonary hypertension
4 Associated lesions
 — Late systolic murmur (MVP + secundum ASD)
 — Mitral incompetence (primum lesion: cleft valve)
 — Mitral stenosis (Lutembacher's syndrome)
 — Tricuspid incompetence (pulmonary hypertension)
  • Primum defect
  • Ebstein's anomaly (with secundum defect)

NB: Auscultatory hallmark of ASD is fixed splitting of the second sound, though slight respiratory variation can occur

Diagnostic work-up of suspected ASD
1 CXR
 — Pulmonary plethora
 — Right ventricular/pulmonary artery enlargement
 — 'Hilar dance' on fluoroscopy
2 ECG
 — Right axis deviation + incomplete RBBB (secundum)
 — Left axis deviation + complete RBBB (primum)
 — First-degree heart block (sinus venosus type)
3 Echo
 — Paradoxical septal motion
 — Right ventricular enlargement
 — Shunt visualization using bubble contrast
4 'First-pass' nuclear scan → shunt quantification
5 Cardiac catheterization
 — Shunt size (oximetry, dye dilution curve)
 — Pulmonary hypertension
 — Associated lesions

Indications for surgery in ASD
1 Pulmonary:systemic blood flow > 1.5:1.0
2 Pulmonary:systemic vascular resistance < 0.7:1.0

Determinants of shunt magnitude in ASD
1 Relative ventricular compliance
 — ↑ LV dysfunction may *increase* shunt
2 Relative resistance of pulmonary and systemic vasculature
 — ↑ Pulmonary hypertension may *decrease* shunt

COMPLICATIONS OF CONGENITAL HEART DISEASE

Common left-to-right shunts
1 VSD (30%)
2 ASD (10%)
3 PDA (10%)

Indications for surgery in ventricular septal defect
1 Pulmonary:systemic blood flow > 1.5:1.0
2 Pulmonary:systemic vascular resistance < 0.5:1.0

Signs of a developing Eisenmenger complex
1 Decreasing intensity of pulmonary/tricuspid flow murmurs
2 Increasing intensity of P_2 (palpable)
3 Development of right parasternal heave
4 Development of single S_2
5 Appearance of Graham–Steell murmur
6 Development of central cyanosis; clubbing (late)

Eisenmenger's syndrome: causes of death
1 Right ventricular failure
2 Massive hemoptysis
3 Cerebral embolism/abscess
4 Pregnancy
5 Anesthesia

NB: Infective endocarditis *rarely* occurs in patients with Eisenmenger's

Congenital causes of left axis deviation on ECG
1 Ostium primum atrial septal defect
2 Tricuspid atresia
3 AV communis (endocardial cushion defect)
4 Myotonic dystrophy
5 VSD, PDA

Congenital lesions prone to endocarditis
1 Bicuspid aortic valve, esp.
   — With significant stenosis or regurgitation
   — Post-surgery
2 Patent ductus arteriosus
3 *Small* VSD (*maladie de Roger*)*
4 Ostium primum ASD
5 Cyanotic congenital heart disease
   — e.g. Tetralogy of Fallot
6 Hypertrophic cardiomyopathy with mitral regurgitation
7 Aortic coarctation

* 'Jet lesion': jet damages RV wall → prone to endocarditis

Congenital lesions at negligible risk of endocarditis
1 Mitral valve prolapse without murmur
2 Isolated secundum ASD

INFECTIVE ENDOCARDITIS

High-risk scenarios for infective endocarditis
1 Rheumatic valve damage
2 Congenital heart disease
3 Prosthetic valve
4 Intravenous narcotic abusers

Features of endocarditis in IV drug abusers
1 Predominant valve involvement
   — Tricuspid
   — Valve damaged initially by starch/lactose contaminants
   — Subsequently colonized by needle-borne bacteria/fungi
2 Predominant microorganisms
   — *Staph. aureus*
   — Enterococci (group D streptococci. e.g. *Str. fecalis*)

— *Pseudomonas* spp. (e.g. *Ps. cepacia, Ps. aeruginosa*)
— *Candida parapsilosis, B. cereus, Serratia marcescens*

Predispositions to various organisms
1 Normal valve (+ bedsores, IV drug abuse)
   — *Staph. aureus*
   — Poor oral hygiene/dentition
2 Rheumatic heart disease (+ dental surgery)
   — *Str. viridans* (α-hemolytic)
3 Sigmoidoscopy/cystoscopy/intrauterine device
   — *Str. fecalis*
4 Cardiac surgery, valve prosthesis
   — *Staph. albus* (> 50%)*
   — Fungi, esp. *Candida* spp.
   — *Pseudomonas* spp.
   — JK organism
5 Colonic carcinoma
   — *Str. bovis* (classically)
6 Homelessness, alcoholism
   — *Bartonella* spp.

* 80% penicillin-resistant; R_x vancomycin + rifampicin ± gentamicin

Streptococcal endocarditis: organisms implicated
1 Viridans streptococci, esp, *Str. mitior, Str. sanguis*
   — Account for 50% of strep endocarditis
2 *Str. mutans, Str. bovis* (GI tract commensals)
   — Account for 30% of strep endocarditis
3 *Str. milleri* (anerobic strep), enterococci
   — Account for 15% of strep endocarditis
4 Group A, group B, pneumococci
   — Account for < 1% each

Factors worsening prognosis of infective endocarditis
1 Prosthetic valve as nidus
2 Cultures negative (40% mortality)
3 *Staph. aureus* isolated from blood cultures

Negative blood cultures? Some considerations
1 Prior antibiotic therapy
2 Fastidious organism or inappropriate culture medium
   — HACEK organisms*
   — *Brucella* spp., *Legionella* spp.
   — *Chlamydia psittaci*
   — Rickettsiae, esp. Q fever (*Coxiella burneti*)
   — Pyridoxine-dependent streptococci
   — L-forms, anaerobes, fungi
3 Right-sided endocarditis
4 Sampling error (cultures taken in abacteremic phase)
5 Misdiagnosis
   — Atrial myxoma
   — Non-bacterial thrombotic endocarditis‡

* *hemophilus-actinobacillus-cardiobacterium-eikenella-kingella*
‡ Associated with mucinous adenocarcinomas (esp. lung, stomach, ovary)

Reasons for fever recrudescence in treated endocarditis
1 Antibiotic inappropriate
   Antibiotic levels subtherapeutic

Antibiotic resistance
Antibiotic allergy
Antibiotic use complicated by superinfection (e.g. fungal)
2   Extensive valve ring infection
3   Metastatic abscesses (splenic, cerebral, myocardial)
4   Pulmonary emboli (septic or bland)
5   Phlebitis, esp. infected central line

Indications for surgery in infective endocarditis
1   Suspected extensive valve ring infection
2   Refractory heart failure, esp. with aortic incompetence
3   Repeated septic emboli. e.g. due to *H. parainfluenzae*
4   Persistent bacteremias/fevers despite optimal therapy
5   Prosthetic valve involvement (esp. fungal or early post-op)

Monitors of established endocarditis
1   Symptoms
2   Temperature
3   Daily physical examination
4   Urinalysis
5   White cell count, hemoglobin, ESR
6   Blood cultures during antibiotic therapy and on cessation
7   Weekly estimations of minimum bactericidal concentration (MBC) of antibiotic (see below); *Staph.* titres (etc.)
8   Neutrophil alkaline phosphatase if abscess suspected

Determination of antibiotic dosage in infective endocarditis*
1   Streptococcal endocarditis
    — Maintain peak antibiotic level > 8 x MBC
2   Neutropenic patients
    — Maintain peak antibiotic level > 16 x MBC
3   Staphylococcal or pseudomonal endocarditis
    — Maintain trough antibiotic level > 16 x MBC
    — Maintain peak antibiotic level > 32 x MBC

* In practice, consult the microbiologists

Presumptive antibiotic therapy if organism unknown*
1   'Community-acquired' endocarditis
    — Ampicillin + gentamicin
2   Prosthetic valve or drug addict
    — Ciprofloxacin + rifampicin, *or*
    — Ampicillin + gentamicin + flucloxacillin
3   Elderly patient and/or renal impairment
    — Ampicillin + netilmicin
4   Major penicillin allergy
    — Vancomycin‡

* In practice, consult the microbiologists
‡ cf. prophylaxis: *clindamycin* may be better tolerated (p. 217)

Patients requiring procedural antibiotic prophylaxis
1   Past medical history of infective endocarditis
2   Prosthetic heart valves
3   Rheumatic heart disease
4   Most congenital heart disease (exception: secundum ASD)

5   Mitral valve prolapse with incompetence (i.e. with murmur)
6   Hypertrophic cardiomyopathy

Procedures for which prophylaxis recommended*
1   Dental surgery with expected gingival bleeding
2   Tonsillectomy, adenoidectomy, cholecystectomy
3   Rigid bronchoscopy or esophagoscopy
4   Esophageal dilatation
5   Variceal sclerotherapy
6   Cystoscopy and most genitourinary surgery (incl. TURP)
7   Colonoscopy and most lower gastrointestinal surgery
8   Any surgery involving incision of septic tissue

* For examples of antibiotic scheduling, see p. 217

Procedures for which prophylaxis may be unnecessary*
1   Dental fillings above the gingival margin ± intraoral injection of local anesthetic
2   Flexible bronchoscopy ± biopsy
3   Endoscopy ± biopsy (i.e. fibreoptic gastroduodenoscopy)
4   Cardiac catheterization
5   Cesarean or vaginal delivery
6   Laparoscopy, D&C, abortion, IUD insertion/removal

* *Unless* (i) patients are 'high-risk'(p. 71) for endocarditis, or (ii) sepsis is anticipated

---

CARDIAC FAILURE

Concepts and definitions
1   Cardiac failure
    — A condition in which adequate cardiac output can only be maintained by elevated venous filling pressure
2   Preload
    — Left ventricular end-diastolic pressure
3   Afterload
    — Left ventricular systolic wall tension

Cardiac syndromes of systolic or diastolic dysfunction
1   Predominant diastolic dysfunction ('stiff heart')
    — Mitral or tricuspid stenosis
    — Cardiomyopathy
      • Hypertrophic
      • Restrictive
    — Pericardial disease
      • Constriction
      • Tamponade
2   Predominant systolic dysfunction ('weak heart')
    — Ischemic heart disease
    — Congestive cardiomyopathy
3   Combined systolic/diastolic dysfunction
    — Valvular heart disease (except MS/TS)
    — Hypertensive heart disease

Clinical implications of systolic vs diastolic dysfunction
1   Diastolic dysfunction
    — Clinical course
      • Onset typically sudden, deterioration rapid

- Edema and/or cardiomegaly are unusual
— Drugs used
  - Nifedipine, β-blockers, ACE inhibitors
2 Systolic dysfunction
  — Clinical course
    - Onset and decline typically gradual
    - Edema and/or cardiomegaly are common
  — Drugs used
    - Diuretics, digitalis

Radiological signs associated with cardiac failure
1 Dilated upper lobe veins
2 Kerley B lines
3 Perihilar alveolar opacities
4 Cardiomegaly
5 Effusion(s), esp. on right

Very high JVP plus a 'normal' chest X-ray?
1 Constrictive pericarditis
2 Tricuspid stenosis
3 Pulmonary embolism
4 Restrictive cardiomyopathy
5 Right ventricular infarction

Pulmonary edema with normal cardiac size on CXR
1 Myocardial infarction
2 Mitral stenosis
3 Constrictive pericarditis
4 Toxic
  — Chlorine inhalation
  — Heroin use
  — Oxygen toxicity
5 Intracranial catastrophe
6 Pneumonia; aspiration; septicemia; fat emboli

Precipitants of cardiac failure in valvular disease
1 Onset of atrial fibrillation
2 Infective endocarditis
3 Recrudescence of rheumatic fever
4 Acute myocardial infarction
5 Pregnancy; anemia; lack of compliance with medication

Diagnostic considerations in refractory heart failure
1 Silent myocardial infarction
2 Pulmonary emboli
3 High-output failure in elderly: thyrotoxicosis, Paget's disease
4 Left ventricular aneurysm
5 Silent valvular stenosis
6 Thiamine deficiency
7 Anemia
8 Myocarditis
9 Cardiac tamponade; constrictive pericarditis
10 Iatrogenic
  — Overvigorous diuresis
  — Tachyarrhythmia due to digoxin toxicity

CXR correlation with pulmonary capillary wedge pressure
1 CXR → Dilated upper lobe veins
  — PCWP = 15 mmHg
2 CXR → Kerley B lines
  — PCWP = 20 mmHg
3 CXR → Pulmonary edema
  — PCWP ≥ 25 mmHg

NB: Therapeutic changes of PCWP precede CXR changes by up to 48 h

Therapy according to PCWP
1 Elevated PCWP + normal cardiac output
  — Preload reduction
  Elevated PCWP + *low* output
  — Pre- *and* afterload reduction
2 Optimal PCWP (18–20 mmH) + low output
  — Afterload reduction, positive inotropes
3 Low PCWP + low output*
  — Intravenous fluids + positive inotropes

* e.g. in right ventricular infarction or overvigorous diuresis

An outpatient approach to treating heart failure
1 Begin with a diuretic (e.g. frusemide)*
2 If still symptomatic, add an ACE inhibitor
3 If still symptomatic, add digoxin (even if sinus rhythm)
4 Symptomatic arrhythmia? Consider amiodarone

* Assuming here that the diagnosis is clear and that conservative measures have not helped

Differential diagnosis of low central venous pressure (< - 3 cm)
1 Warm extremities
  — Drug overdose
  — Brainstem lesion
  — Septic shock
2 Cool extremities, low hemoglobin
  — Hemorrhage
3 Cool extremities, normal/high hemoglobin
  — Gastrointestinal fluid losses (diarrhea, vomiting)
  — Renal fluid loss (e.g. diabetic ketoacidosis)
  — Third spacing (e.g. rapid accumulation of ascites)

NB: CVP is *not* accurate in determining LV filling pressure (and hence guiding treatment), e.g. in cardiogenic shock

Differential diagnosis of nocturnal dyspnea
1 Cardiac
  — Left ventricular failure
  — Coronary spasm
2 Pulmonary
  — Asthma
  — Extrinsic allergic alveolitis; emboli
3 CNS/pharyngeal
  — Sleep apnea
4 Anxiety

ATRIAL NATRIURETIC PEPTIDE

Atrial natriuretic peptide (ANP) in cardiac failure
1 Compensatory ↑ ANP seen in heart failure and edema states
2 Increased atrial filling pressure → increased ANP secretion
3 ANP levels are inversely proportional to left ventricular function; LV deterioration → further ANP elevation

4 Reduction in ANP follows successful treatment of failure

Functions of atrial natriuretic peptide
1 Diuretic function
   — Inhibits distal tubular reabsorption of sodium
   — Promotes excretion of sodium and water (not K^+)
   — May also increase GFR (see below)
2 Vasodilator function
   — Inhibits vasoconstriction mediated by angiotensin II and noradrenaline
   — Secondarily inhibits renin–aldosterone axis and ADH
   — Does *not* lead to reflex tachycardia despite lowering BP

CARDIOMYOPATHY

Restrictive cardiomyopathy > constrictive pericarditis?
1 Pulse
   — No paradox
2 Jugular venous pulse
   — Normal 'y' descent, no Kussmaul's sign
3 Apical impulse
   — Prominent
4 Auscultation
   — Associated AV valvular incompetence (often)
5 Extra sounds
   — S_3 (low-pitched)
6 CXR
   — No pericardial calcification; cardiomegaly
7 ECG
   — LVH, Q waves, ventricular conduction disturbances
8 Echo
   — No pericardial thickening/effusion; LV thickening
9 Catheter
   — LV end-diastolic pressure > RV end-diastolic pressure
   — RV systolic pressure > 60 mmHg
10 Endomyocardial biopsy
   — Abnormal

Hypertrophic cardiomyopathy > aortic valvular stenosis?
1 Family history
   — Premature sudden death
2 Pulse
   — Jerky (steeply rising)
3 Apex beat
   — Double impulse (due to S_4)
4 A_2
   — Normal intensity and splitting
5 Murmur
   — Late systolic (ejection) ± mitral regurgitation
   — Maximal at sternal edge, inaudible in carotids
   — ↑ Valsalva/standing/nitrates; ↓ squatting/isometrics
6 CXR
   — No valvular calcification or post-stenotic dilatation

7 ECG
   — Septal Q waves; WPW (rarely)
8 Echo

Features favoring myocarditis over cardiomyopathy*
1 Young patient
2 Recent history of fevers/myalgias prior to cardiac symptoms
3 Minor cardiomegaly only

* i.e. acute myocarditis *vs* chronic congestive (dilated) cardiomyopathy

Reversible causes of dilated cardiomyopathy
1 Ischemic heart disease
   — 'Hibernating' myocardium (p. 75)
   Valvular heart disease
   — Aortic stenosis
2 Infiltration by systemic disease
   — Sarcoidosis
   — Amyloidosis
   — Lymphoma
3 Infectious
   — Viral, e.g. CMV*
   — Bacterial, esp. *C. diphtheriae*
   — Parasitic, e.g. *T. gondii*‡
4 Poisoning
   — Alcohol (± thiamine deficiency)
   — Lead, mercury
   — Cocaine
   — Antiretroviral drugs, e.g. AZT
5 Nutritional
   — Thiamine deficiency (± alcohol); beri-beri
   — Selenium deficiency (Keshan disease)
6 Endocrinopathy
   — Thyrocardiac disease (hypo- or hyper-)
   — Acromegaly, pheochromocytoma
   — Peripartum

* cf. Coxsackie: commoner but not reversible
‡ cf. Chagas', trichinosis: probably irreversible

HYPERTROPHIC CARDIOMYOPATHY (HOCM)

Associations of hypertrophic cardiomyopathy
1 Familial (↑ penetrance in males)
2 Friedreich's ataxia
3 Pompe's disease
4 Familial lentiginosis

Echocardiography of hypertrophic cardiomyopathy
1 Asymmetric septal hypertrophy (septum > 12 mm thick *and* > 130% posterior wall thickness)
2 Systolic anterior motion of anterior leaflet of mitral valve
3 Premature closure of the aortic valve
4 Reduced EF slope due to reduced ventricular compliance

Features of catheterization in hypertrophic cardiomyopathy
1 Distorted left ventricular cavity with systolic obliteration
2 Elevated left ventricular end-diastolic pressure

3 Associated thickening of papillary muscles
4 Post-ectopic reduction in intraaortic pressure

Drugs contraindicated in hypertrophic cardiomyopathy

1 Digoxin (unless in atrial fibrillation)
2 Other positive inotropes
3 Atropine; other positive chronotropes
4 Nitrates; other vasodilators
5 Diuretics (unless in cardiac failure)

Principles of management in hypertrophic cardiomyopathy

1 Echocardiographic screening of all family
< 18 years
2 Detection (Holter) and therapy (amiodarone*) of arrhythmias
3 Minimization of strenuous activity
4 Prophylaxis against infective endocarditis
5 Symptoms: β-blockers (do *not* reduce risk of sudden death)
6 Symptoms refractory to medical therapy: septal myomectomy

* Reduces morbidity if VT has occurred

ISCHEMIC HEART DISEASE

Reversible independent risk factors for premature heart disease

1 LDL-hypercholesterolemia (± low HDL-cholesterol)
2 Hypertension
3 Smoking

Irreversible risk factors for ischemic heart disease

1 Age
2 Male sex
3 Positive family history
4 Elevated lipoprotein (a) level

Unstable angina: definition(s)

1 Recent symptomatic progression
— Increasing frequency and/or duration of angina
— Development of pain at rest/at night/after meals
— Development of nitrate-resistant angina
2 Recurrent angina despite maximal medical therapy
3 Clinically suspected infarct with negative ECG and enzymes

Clinical features of coronary artery spasm (variant angina)

1 Symptoms (e.g. dizziness)
— Often occur at rest or at night
2 ECG (classically)
— ST elevation before and during pain
3 Stress ECG
— Typically negative if no associated coronary disease
4 Angiography
— Absent collateralization, varying stenotic sites

SMOKING

Plasma and urinary markers of cigarette smoke exposure

1 Cotinine (and/or nicotine)
2 Carbon monoxide
3 Thiocyanate
4 Urinary mutagenesis assays

Physiological sequelae of cigarette smoking

1 ↑ Platelet adhesion/aggregation/whole blood viscosity
2 ↑ Heart rate; ↑ catecholamine sensitivity/release
3 ↑ Carboxyhemoglobin level, ↑ hematocrit
4 ↓ HDL-cholesterol/vascular compliance
5 ↓ Threshold to ventricular fibrillation

Cardiovascular sequelae of cigarette smoking

1 Increased incidence of
— Sudden death*
— Coronary artery disease
— Malignant hypertension
— Subarachnoid hemorrhage
— Ischemic stroke
2 Increased mortality due to aortic aneurysm
3 Increased morbidity from peripheral vascular disease
4 Increased thromboembolism if taking oral contraceptives

* Note that using 'low-tar' cigarettes does *not* substantively reduce the incidence of cigarette-related myocardial infarction

PASSIVE SMOKING

Passive smoking: characteristics of sidestream smoke

1 Contributes 85% of cigarette smoke in an average 'smoking' room (cf. 15% from exhaled 'mainstream' smoke)
2 Exposure of non-smoking individual living or working with smokers averages 1–2 cigarettes/day
3 Sidestream smoke is of higher pH and contains smaller particles than does mainstream smoke
4 Sidestream smoke contains higher carbon monoxide concentrations than does mainstream smoke

Childhood disease associations of passive (parental) smoking

1 Exacerbation of asthma
2 Impairment of lung function
— ↓ FEV_1 and forced midexpiratory flow rate
3 ↑ Bronchitis /glue ears/tonsillectomy/adenoidectomy

CARDIAC ARREST

Cardiac arrest: emergency intervention

1 Precordial 'thump' *if* definitely pulseless
— May revert asystole or VT (but only 2% of VF)
2 Crash cart arrives: → 'blind' cardioversion
— May revert VF (but not asystole)

3   Get ECG trace
    — If VF, defibrillate again
    — Intubate and ventilate with 100% O_2
    — Get IV line in
    — If still in VF, shock again @ 360 J
4   Commence CPR
    — 10 cycles of 5:1 compression:ventilation
5   Repeat cardioversion cycle (see below)

ECG concomitants of cardiac arrest
1   Asystole
2   Ventricular fibrillation
3   Pulseless sinus rhythm (electromechanical dissociation)

ECG-guided management of cardiac arrest
1   Asystole
    — Check leads
    — Give IV adrenaline 1 mg IVI (10 mL 1:10,000)
    — Can't exclude VF? Shock @ 200 J
    — Definitely no VF? Atropine 2 mg IV*
    — Consider transvenous pacing *if* electrical activity‡
2   Ventricular fibrillation
    — Shock @ 200 J
    — Still fibrillating? Repeat shock @ 200–300 J ± @ 360 J
    — Fine VF can be 'coarsened' with IV adrenaline*
    — Still fibrillating? Lignocaine 100 mg (1.5 mg/kg) IV*
    — Shock again, and give (say) bretylium 5 mg/kg‡
    — Continued resuscitation
      • CPR for 1–2 min between each drug
      • Repeat adrenaline every 5 min
      • Bicarbonate (50 mL 8.4%) every 20 min
3   Documented hyperkalemia? (rare)
    — Calcium chloride IV
    — More frequent (incl. initial) bicarbonate

NB: Effective chest compression and hyperventilation between countershocks is *vital* to prospects of success
* Things are fairly desperate at this point
‡ *very* desperate

Hazards of indiscriminate bicarbonate administration
1   Pulmonary edema
2   Paradoxical worsening of intracellular acidosis*

* Acidosis is best managed with hyperventilation alone; bicarbonate is only routinely indicated in prolonged resuscitation

Positive prognostic associations of cardiac arrest*
1   Presence of a witness
2   Ventricular fibrillation on initial ECG

* cf. asystole or electromechanical dissociation: < 5% survival

Guidelines for judging when to terminate resuscitation
1   Once commenced, 10 min is usual minimum*
    — Usually continue while VF remains recognizable
    — Persistent asystole usually indicates failure
2   Should mentally exclude important contingencies
    — Defibrillator malfunction
    — Electromechanical dissociation
3   Prolonged (> 60 min) resuscitation justified in

    — Hypothermia or drowning (esp. children)
    — Drug overdose

* Assuming that patient's overall condition does not make resuscitation inappropriate

---

MYOCARDIAL INFARCTION

Preventive initiatives relevant to myocardial infarction*
1   Smoking cessation
    — 50% ↓ risk within 5 years of stopping
2   Reduction of hypertension
    — 2% ↓ risk for each 1 mmHg ↓ diastolic BP
3   Reduction of hyperlipidemia
    — 2% ↓ risk for each 1% ↓ plasma cholesterol
4   Exercise
    — 40% ↓ risk for active vs. sedentary lifestyle
5   Ideal body weight
    — 30% ↓ risk for ideal weight vs. obese
6   Estrogen replacement therapy (in menopause)
    — 40% ↓ risk compared to unreplaced women
7   Low-dose aspirin prophylaxis
    — 30% ↓ risk compared with non-users
8   Mild alcohol consumption‡
    — 25% ↓ risk compared to teetotallers

* Risk reductions are not additive and do not imply reductions in overall (non-disease-specific) mortality; moreover, associations may not be causal
‡ See reference 2.2

Acute myocardial infarction: early serologic diagnosis
1   Myoglobin
    — Levels rise within 2 h post-infarct
    — Low specificity
2   Cardiac troponin I and troponin T
    — Levels rise within 4 h post-infarct
    — High specificity
3   CK-MB (total creatine kinase)
    — Levels rise within 6 h post-infarct
    — Moderate specificity
4   $CK\text{-}MB_2$ (isoform of CK-MB)
    — Levels rise within 6 h post-infarct
    — High specificity

Bad prognostic indicators in acute myocardial infarction
1   Advanced age, female sex
2   Previous infarct, recent pain
3   Heart rate > 100, systolic BP < 100
4   CK-MB > 2000 IU/mL
5   ECG
    — Heart block
    — New conduction defects, complex arrhythmias
6   CXR
    — Pulmonary edema (cardiogenic shock)

'Cardiogenic shock': could it be anything else?
1   Hypovolemia
    — Overvigorous diuresis
    — Third-spacing
    — Hemorrhage
2   Electromechanical dissociation
    — Cardiac tamponade*
    — Cardiac rupture‡

— Massive pulmonary embolism
— Tension pneumothorax
3 Other causes of shock
— High output failure
— Adrenal failure
— Septic shock
— Anaphylaxis

* NB: Tamponade may be associated with ↑ BP due to increased peripheral vascular resistance; may fall after pericardiocentesis
‡ Ruptured interventricular septum or papillary muscle

Common mechanisms of death following myocardial infarction
1 First few hours — Ventricular fibrillation
2 First few days — Pump failure
3 First few months — Reinfarction

Myocardial infarction: pathogenesis and extent
1 Anterior infarct
— Due to occlusion of left anterior descending coronary
— Extent of jeopardized myocardium indicated by
• Number of 'acute' precordial leads
• Degree of ST elevation
• RBBB*
2 Inferior infarct
— Caused by occlusion of right coronary or left circumflex
— ↓↓ Jeopardized myocardium; hence, ↓ CCF (see below)

* Signifies LAD occlusion proximal to first septal branch

Myocardial infarction: complications by site
1 Anterior infarct
— Ventricular arrhythmias (incl. late-onset VF)
— Left ventricular aneurysm or thrombus formation
— Cardiac rupture/VSD
2 Inferior infarct
— Atrial/junctional arrhythmias
• Bradycardia
• High-degree AV block
• Complete heart block
— Papillary muscle dysfunction
— Associated right ventricular infarction (in 40%)

Diagnosis of right ventricular infarction
1 Clinical suspicion: 'inferior' infarct + arrhythmias
— High-degree AV block indicates need for RV pacing
— Atrial fibrillation: may require cardioversion
— Ventricular arrhythmias → ? Complete heart block
2 Signs/CXR
— Elevated JVP *but* clear lung fields
3 ECG
— 1 mm ST elevation in *right* precordial lead V_{4R}*
4 Hemodynamic monitoring
— Low/normal PCWP despite low output failure
— Right atrial pressure:PCWP > 0.86
5 Therapeutic response
— Improve with preload enhancement
• IV saline
• Dobutamine (if no response to saline)

— Deteriorate with preload reduction
• Nitrates
• Diuretics
• Morphine

NB: Such patients have a high mortality (30% vs. 5% for uncomplicated inferior infarct) and should receive thrombolysis or angioplasty
* i.e. this lead should be recorded in patients presenting with classical 'inferior' infarcts (ST elevation in II, III, aVF)

Features of non-Q-wave (non-transmural) myocardial infarction
1 Fewer acute occlusions demonstrable, but overall extent of (chronic) coronary disease similar to transmural infarcts
2 Less myocardial necrosis
Less marked enzyme elevations
3 Fewer acute complications
Lower short-term mortality
4 *Higher* incidence of reinfarction
Long-term prognosis equivalent or worse
5 Aspirin (and perhaps diltiazem) improves outlook

Myocardial infarction without coronary artery block?
1 Coronary microvascular disease
Coronary artery spasm
Coronary angiography-induced
2 Acute plaque rupture
3 Recanalized coronary thrombosis (endogenous thrombolysis)
4 Aortic stenosis
Ascending aortic dissection (very rare)
Arteritis: Takayasu's, PAN

Drugs reducing mortality after myocardial infarction
1 Proven benefit
— β-blockers
• IV (acute): mortality reduction 0.5%
• Oral (long-term): mortality reduction 1.5%
— Aspirin*
• Acute: mortality reduction 2%
• Long-term: mortality reduction 1.5%
— Thrombolytic therapy (p. 64)
• Preadmission: mortality reduction 3%
• Inpatient: mortality reduction 2%
— ACE inhibitor‡ (begin after nitrates ceased; → years)
• AMI → LV failure: mortality reduction 4%
• AMI → LV dysfunction: mortality reduction 1%
2 Suspected benefit, but *not* proven
— Nitrates‡ (use in first 24 h)
— Magnesium sulphate¶
— Heparin (may administer subcutaneously)
• Net value uncertain (i.e with tPA, aspirin R_x)
• Consider in large anterior infarcts
— Amiodarone
3 *No* benefit
— Calcium antagonists

* Also maintains patency of CABG
‡ Limit infarct size
¶ May prevent myocardial 'stunning' (p. 75)

Contraindications to magnesium therapy* post-infarct
1 Preexisting high magnesium levels (e.g. renal failure)

2 Hypotension or bradycardia
3 AV block
4 More than 6 h since infarct

* Believed by some to prevent reperfusion injury of 'stunned' myocardium, though results of ISIS-4 do not support this (see ref. 2.8)

REPERFUSION INJURY

Myocardial definitions in acute infarction
1 'Jeopardized' myocardium
   — Myocardium 'at-risk' of infarction during early (reversible) period of coronary occlusion
   — Extent of jeopardized myocardium represents potential benefit of thrombolytic intervention
2 'Hibernating' myocardium
   — Myocardium which is persistently (but reversibly) impaired in function by reduced oxygenation due to coronary artery disease; an autoregulatory mechanism of myocardial self-preservation
3 'Stunned' myocardium
   — Myocardium which requires a time lag (often several weeks) to improve functionally following revascularization; a retrospective characterization

Pathophysiology of post-infarction reperfusion injury
1 Intracellular calcium overload
2 Osmotic myocyte swelling
3 Free radical-induced microvascular damage

Clinical manifestations of reperfusion injury
1 Reperfusion arrhythmias
   — Common after intracoronary thrombolysis or PTCA
   — Include ventricular fibrillation (→ 6–7% post-PTCA)
   — Early reperfusion (< 30 min) potently causes VF
2 Myocardial stunning
   — Reversible ventricular dysfunction
   — Systolic performance may improve up to 6 months
3 Lethal myocyte injury
   — Contraction band necrosis may lead to cardiac rupture
   — Rupture commoner following thrombolysis

Therapeutic prevention of reinfarction
1 Stop smoking
2 β-blockade
3 Aspirin
4 Coronary artery bypass grafting for patients found to have left main disease following positive convalescent stress ECG
5 Angioplasty

HYPERLIPIDEMIA

Macroscopic appearance of hyperlipidemic serum
1 Chylomicronemia   — Lipemic supernatant
2 Increased VLDL/IDL   — Diffusely lipemic
3 Increased LDL   — Clear

Incidence and genetics of primary hyperlipidemias
1 Common hyperlipidemias
   — Autosomal dominant transmission (familial)
   — WHO types IIa, IIb, IV
   — Major excesses of *cholesterol* and *triglycerides*
      • IIa: cholesterol (↑ LDL)
      • IIb: cholesterol (↑ LDL) + triglyceride (↑ VLDL)
      • IV: triglycerides (↑ VLDL) + cholesterol
2 Uncommon hyperlipidemias
   — Autosomal recessive transmission
   — WHO types I, III, V
   — Major (primary) excesses of *lipoproteins*
      • I: chylomicrons (↑ triglycerides, cholesterol)
      • III: IDL 'remnants' (↑ cholesterol, triglycerides)
      • V: VLDL (↑ triglycerides/cholesterol/chylomicra)

Clinical characterization of hyperlipidemias
1 Fasting hypertriglyceridemia
   — Chylomicronemia (I, V) due to
      • Lipoprotein lipase deficiency
      • Apo C-II deficiency
   — Excess VLDL (IIb, IV, V)
   — *Not* associated with atherosclerosis
   — Symptoms and signs of hypertriglyceridemia
      • Eruptive xanthomata (usually *resolve* with R_x)
      • Abdominal pain ± pancreatitis
      • Hepatosplenomegaly
      • Lipemia retinalis (whitish arterioles)
2 Hypercholesterolemia with excess LDL (IIa, IIb)
   — Due to 1° LDL receptor defect or LDL overproduction
   — Strongly associated with atherosclerosis
   — Symptoms and signs of hypercholesterolemia
      • Tendinitis, polyarthritis
      • Tendon xanthomata (usually *persist* despite R_x)
      • Planar xanthomata (in homozygotes only)
      • Arcus senilis: pathological *if* younger than 40
      • Xanthelasma
3 Broad-β 'remnant' hyperlipidemia with excess IDL (III)
   — Strongly associated with accelerated atherosclerosis
   — Responds well to fibrates (xanthomata regress)
   — Symptoms and signs of excess IDL
      • Tuberous xanthomata (esp. elbows, knees)
      • Linear palmar-crease (planar) xanthomata
      • Peripheral vascular disease (p. 47)

Secondary hyperlipidemias
1 Predominantly increased cholesterol
   — Hypothyroidism
   — Cholestasis (esp. PBC)
   — Anorexia nervosa
2 Predominantly increased triglycerides
   — Alcohol abuse
   — Diabetes mellitus
   — Chronic renal failure
3 Increased cholesterol and triglycerides
   — Nephrotic syndrome
   — Paraproteinemic states (rarely)
   — High-dose steroid therapy

Drugs adversely affecting blood lipids*
1 Thiazides‡
2 Non-selective β-blockers‡
3 Isotretinoin (for acne)
4 Norgestrel-containing oral contraceptives

* Increased triglycerides and/or reduced HDL-cholesterol
‡ Clinical significance is probably nil: both continue to be of
value in reducing cardiovascular morbidity

Factors affecting HDL-cholesterol levels
1 Factors associated with low levels
   — Obesity, dietary sugar, diabetes
   — Progestogens, androgens, male sex
   — Cigarette smoking
   — Nephrotic syndrome
   — Drugs (see above), incl. probucol
   — Tangier disease, familial LCAT deficiency
2 Factors associated with high levels
   — Regular exercise ($\uparrow$ HDL-2)
   — Estrogens, female sex
   — Moderate alcohol intake ($\uparrow$ HDL-3)
   — Increasing age/education status
   — Phenytoin use
   — Fish oil (e.g. cod liver oil; see below)

Hypolipidemic states in clinical medicine
1 Bassen–Kornzweig syndrome
   — $\downarrow$ Apolipoprotein B and all lipid fractions except
     HDL
   — Characterized by acanthocytosis, ataxia, retino-
     pathy, steatorrhea and death before middle life
   — R_x: vitamin E (A, D, K) + medium-chain
     triglycerides
2 Tangier disease
   — $\downarrow$ HDL but *no* cardiovascular disease; no
     treatment
   — Manifests with orange tonsils, neuropathy,
     splenomegaly and corneal opacities
3 LCAT deficiency
   — $\downarrow$ HDL, $\uparrow$ VLDL
   — Manifests with atheroma, uremia, hemolysis

APOLIPOPROTEINS

Apolipoproteins in cardiovascular disease
1 Apolipoproteins are the polypeptide components
   which make up lipoproteins; these apolipoproteins
   include A-I, A-II, A-IV; B48, B100; C-I, C-II, C-III; D, E, F
2 Lipoproteins are water-soluble protein complexes
   which transport lipids (cholesterol and triglycerides)
   in plasma; they comprise LDL, VLDL, HDL, IDL and
   chylomicrons
3 Lipoprotein (a) antigen [Lp(a)] is a variant LDL
   associated with coronary artery disease*
4 Apolipoprotein B is the main lipid transport protein
   — Apo B100 is the sole protein constituent of LDL
     and the major protein constituent of VLDL
   — Apo B48 is the major protein of chylomicrons
   — $\uparrow$ Apo B → coronary artery disease
   — $\downarrow$ Apo B → Bassen–Kornzweig syndrome
5 Apo A-I is the major protein constituent of HDL
   — $\downarrow$ Apo A-I → hypertriglyceridemia (#IV, V)
   — $\downarrow$ Apo A-I, apo B → coronary artery disease

6 Apo C-II is an activator of lipoprotein lipase
   — $\downarrow$ Apo C-II → fasting chylomicronemia (#I, V)
7 Apo E consists of three isoforms: E3, E4, E2
   — Apo E3 is the commonest allele
     • An abnormal apo E3 → IDL 'remnants' (#III)
   — $\uparrow$Apo E4 → high LDL and cholesterol
   — $\uparrow$ Apo E2 (uncommon) → low LDL and cholesterol

* Despite its strong association with atherogenesis, reduction of
Lp(a) levels by apheresis does *not* correlate well with regression
of atheroma

HYPOLIPIDEMIC DRUGS

Mechanisms underlying hypolipidemic therapy
1 Statins: lovastatin, simvastatin, pravastatin
   — HMG CoA reductase (cholesterol synthesis)
     inhibitors
   — Cause 30% $\downarrow$ plasma LDL levels
   — Also enhance LDL receptor expression
   — Well tolerated (occasional myalgias, $\uparrow$ CK)
   — Use in hypercholesterolemia
2 Fibrates: bezafibrate, gemfibrozil ($\pm$ clofibrate)
   — Isobutyric acid derivatives activating lipoprotein
     lipase
   — Reduce VLDL ($\pm$ LDL, fibrinogen); $\uparrow$ HDL
   — Clofibrate reduces IDL but *increases* LDL
   — Use in type III or mixed hyperlipidemias
3 Cholestyramine, colestipol
   — Non-absorbable anion-exchange resins; bind bile
     acids
   — Reduce LDL (but *increase* VLDL/triglycerides)
   — Use in familial hypercholesterolemia
4 Acipimox, nicofuranose
   — Nicotinic acid derivatives inhibiting lipolysis
   — Reduce VLDL mainly, but also reduce LDL and
     IDL
   — Use in hypertriglyceridemia or as adjunctive
     therapy
5 Probucol (an antioxidant)
   — Lowers LDL cholesterol (but may also lower HDL)
   — May lower LDL levels by 30% when used with
     resin
   — Also an antioxidant, but therapeutic value
     unclear
6 Fish oils (omega-3 fatty acids), e.g. eicosapentoic
   acid
   — Substitute for essential fatty acids in cell
     membranes
   — Metabolized by cyclooxygenase to prosta-
     glandins
   — Reduce platelet aggregation, triglycerides

NB: *No* drug treatment is effective for hypertriglyceridemia due
to primary deficiency of apoprotein C-II or lipoprotein lipase

Side-effects of hypolipidemic therapy
1 Statins
   — Gastrointestinal upset
   — Liver dysfunction (asymptomatic transaminitis)
   — Myositis (esp. in patients who exercise heavily)
   — Rhabdomyolysis, esp. if also receiving
     • Cyclosporin A (→ 5-fold $\uparrow$ plasma level)
     • Gemfibrozil, nicotinic acid

2   Fibrates
— Nausea, abdominal discomfort
— Gallstones, cholecystitis; also transaminitis
— Loss of libido, alopecia, weight gain
— Myopathy (esp. if hypoalbuminemic or azotemic)
— Potentiation of warfarin (cf. cholestyramine)
• Displacement from plasma protein (transient)
• Inhibits hepatic metabolism
3   Resins
— Constipation (usual), abdominal distension (common); steatorrhea (only with large doses)
— Nausea, vomiting
— Reduced absorption of digoxin, thyroxine, warfarin, folate and fat-soluble vitamins (A,D,E,K)
4   Nicotinates
— Flushing; headaches
— Nausea, abdominal pain, diarrhea
— Hepatotoxicity; gout; glucose intolerance

NB: Aggressive hypocholesterolemic therapy has been associated with an increased risk of *hemorrhagic stroke*; hence, improvements in *all-cause mortality* are necessary to justify routine usage

Rhabdomyolysis due to hypolipidemic drugs
1   Fibrates
— Clofibrate
— Bezafibrate
— Gemfibrozil
2   Statins
— Simvastatin
— Pravastatin

Which hypolipidemic?*
1   Predominant hypercholesterolemia
— Start with a statin ($\rightarrow \uparrow$ HDL, $\downarrow$ TGs; $\downarrow$ LDL-chol.)
— Maximum statin dose *not tolerated*? Substitute
• A resin (e.g. colestipol; less well tolerated)
• A fibrate (e.g. gemfibrozil)
• Nicotinic acid
— Maximum statin dose *ineffective*? Add
• A resin
2   Predominant hypertriglyceridemia
— Start with a fibrate ($\downarrow$ TGs by 30%)
— Alternatives
• Nicotinic acid (less well tolerated)
• Fish oil (see below)
3   Mixed hyperlipidemia
— Start with a fibrate
— Second-line
• Nicotinic acid, *or*
• A statin‡

* i.e. assuming dietary measures (e.g. stopping alcohol) and appropriate patient selection
‡ Do *not* combine fibrates and statins (increased risk of myopathy)

Therapeutic targets in treating hypercholesterolemics
1   Aim to keep *total cholesterol* < 6.0 mmol/L
2   Aim to keep *LDL-cholesterol* < 4.0 mmol/L
3   Aim to keep *total:HDL cholesterol ratio* < 5

Observations suggesting cardiovascular benefits of fish oils
1   Fish oils, esp. those containing the n-3 (ω-3) poly-unsaturated acids eicosapentenoic acid (EPA; C20:5) and docosahexenoic acid (DHA; C22:6), are abundant in the diet of populations with little coronary disease, e.g. Eskimos, Japanese, Greenland Inuits
2   High membrane n-3:n-6 fatty acid ratios are associated with reduced incidence of coronary disease
3   Dietary n-3 polyunsaturated fatty acids are associated with the following alterations in atherogenic risk factors
— $\downarrow$ Plasma cholesterol/triglycerides, $\downarrow$ VLDL/LDL
— $\uparrow$ HDL$_2$
— $\downarrow$ Blood pressure
4   Dietary n-3 polyunsaturated fatty acids are associated with the following alterations in thrombogenic risk factors
— $\uparrow$ Bleeding time (reduced platelet aggregation)
— $\downarrow$ Platelet thromboxane A$_2$
— $\uparrow$ Vascular prostacyclin
— $\downarrow$ Platelet reactivity to ADP/adrenaline/thrombin

Fish oil: putative mechanisms of action
1   Antiatherogenic action ($\downarrow$ coronary artery disease)
— $\downarrow$ Cholesterol, LDL/VLDL, triglycerides; $\uparrow$ HDL
2   Antithrombotic action ($\downarrow$ incidence of vascular 'events')
— Competitive inhibition of arachidonic acid
— Cyclooxygenase inhibition
— $\downarrow$ Thromboxane A$_2$-mediated platelet aggregation
3   Antiinflammatory action (?$\downarrow$ severity of arthritis, migraine)
— Competitive inhibition of arachidonic acid
— $\downarrow$ Lipooxygenase inhibition; $\downarrow$ IL-I
— $\downarrow$ TNF/leukotriene B$_4$-induced neutrophil chemotaxis

Differential diagnosis of hypertension
'RECAP'
1   'R' — **R**enal
• Renal artery stenosis
• Chronic renal failure with fluid overload
• Unilateral parenchymal renal disease
• Polycystic kidneys
2   'E' — **E**ssential
— **E**ndocrine
• Pheochromocytoma
• Primary hyperaldosteronism
• Cushing's syndrome
• Thyrotoxicosis
• Acromegaly
• Hyperparathyroidism
3   'C' — **C**ollagen-vascular diseases (e.g. polyarteritis nodosa)
— **C**erebral (e.g. raised intracranial pressure)

— **C**ontraceptive pill
— **C**lonidine withdrawal
4 'A' — **A**lcohol
— **A**ortic coarctation
— **A**cute intermittent porphyria
5 'P' — **P**regnancy-associated hypertension
— **P**olycythemia rubra vera

Causes of malignant phase
1 Essential hypertension
2 Rapidly progressive glomerulonephritis
3 Pregnancy-associated hypertension
4 Renovascular*
5 Polyarteritis; scleroderma
6 Pheochromocytoma
7 Iatrogenic
— Interaction with MAO inhibitor
— Clonidine withdrawal

* Onset may be *acute* if hemorrhage occurs into atheromatous plaque or if aortic aneurysm expands over renal artery origin

Alternating hypotension and hypertension
1 Iatrogenic
— e.g. Diuretics, methyldopa
— Hemodialysis
2 Pheochromocytoma (esp. if secreting adrenaline)
3 Hyponatremic hypertensive syndrome
— Seen in renovascular hypertension of recent origin
4 Syndrome of baroreflex failure
— Hypertensive attacks prevented by clonidine

* cf. syndrome of baroreflex failure: labile hypertension but *little* orthostasis

Non-pharmacological management of mild hypertension
1 Stop smoking (reduces morbidity; does not reduce BP)
2 Ideal body weight
3 Low salt diet
4 Alcohol restriction
5 Biofeedback/relaxation/hypnotherapy
6 Regular exercise

Efficacy of antihypertensive treatment
1 Therapy reduces mortality in *moderate/severe* hypertension*
2 Less effective in *mild* hypertension‡ or in elderly patients
3 Reduces risk of *stroke* (>> myocardial infarction)
4 Does not *reverse* ischemic heart/peripheral vascular disease
5 Smoking may negate benefits of antihypertensive therapy
6 Clinical efficacy depends critically on patient *compliance*

* diastolic BP > 100 mmHg
‡ diastolic BP < 95 mmHg

Indications for treatment of 'mild' hypertension* in elderly
1 History of coronary or cerebrovascular disease
2 Development of fourth heart sound
3 Retinopathy (grade III or IV)

4 Elevated serum creatinine
Elevated urinary microalbumin excretion
5 ECG: left ventricular hypertrophy/strain
6 CXR: cardiomegaly

* BP < 180/95

An approach to antihypertensive prescribing
1 Commence with a β-blocker
— Increase as necessary, pending side-effects
2 If still uncontrolled, add *either*
— Diuretic, *or*
— Calcium blocker (e.g. nifedipine)
3 If still uncontrolled
— Discontinue β-blocker/calcium blocker
— Substitute an ACE inhibitor (± diuretic)
4 If still uncontrolled
— Investigate

Drug therapy of orthostatic hypotension
1 Fludrocortisone + pindolol
2 Octreotide

RENOVASCULAR HYPERTENSION

Hypertension: indications for further investigation*
1 Age < 35
2 Associated postural hypotension
3 Hypertensive retinopathy
4 Abnormal urinalysis (proteinuria/hematuria/glycosuria)
5 Hypokalemia without diuretic therapy, esp. if marked
6 Azotemia (esp. if recent onset)
7 Severe hypertension poorly controlled by multiple drugs

*NB: Experienced radiologists and vascular surgeons are a prerequisite

Investigational modalities in renovascular hypertension
1 Plasma renin activity ± captopril 'challenge'
2 Pre- and post-captopril renal isotopic uptake of ^{99m}Tc-DTPA*
3 Rapid-sequence intravenous pyelography
4 Venous digital subtraction angiography
5 Selective venous sampling for renal vein renins*
6 Renal arteriography ± immediate angioplasty (best approach)

*↓ In stenosed kidney, ↓ post-captopril; *lateralization* indicates improved chance of successful BP control following revascularization

Varieties of renovascular disease
1 Fibromuscular dysplasia (age < 30 years)
2 Atheromatous (age > 60 years)

Diagnostic potential of arteriography in hypertension
1 Renal artery stenosis
2 Aortic coarctation
3 Polyarteritis nodosa
4 Pheochromocytoma

NB: Severe uncontrolled hypertension contraindicates elective angiography

Abnormal plasma renin activity: differential diagnosis
1 Elevated, no hypertension
   — Addison's disease
   — Hemorrhage
   — Liver disease
   — Pregnancy
   — Bartter's syndrome
   — Drugs
     • Diuretics, vasodilators
     • Estrogens
     • Sympathomimetics; lithium
2 Elevated, hypertensive
   — Malignant hypertension
   — Essential hypertension (in 15% of cases)
   — Renovascular disease or end-stage renal failure
   — Hemangiopericytoma (reninoma)
3 Low, no hypertension
   — Old age
   — Drugs
     • β-blockers
     • Clonidine, methyldopa; guanethidine
4 Low, hypertensive
   — Essential hypertension (85%. esp. if elderly)
   — Conn's/Cushing's syndromes
   — Congenital adrenal hyperplasia
     • 17-hydroxylase deficiency
   — Drugs
     • Corticosteroids

Therapeutic options in 'renal' hypertension
1 Salt and fluid restriction
2 Drug therapy
   — ACE inhibitors* (e.g. captopril)
   — β-blockers (e.g. metoprolol)
   — Vasodilators (e.g. prazosin)
3 If refractory, treat 'operable' renovascular disease by
   — Percutaneous angioplasty
   — Vascular surgery
4 If refractory and no operable extrarenal vascular lesion
   — Consider bilateral nephrectomy (a desperation move)

* Unless bilateral renal artery stenosis (p. 63)

Surgical intervention in renovascular hypertension: indications
1 Percutaneous transluminal angioplasty
   — Fibromuscular dysplasia
   — Single atheromatous plaque in arterial midportion
   — Intrarenal arterial stenosis inaccessible to surgery
   — Transplant artery stenosis
   — Contraindication to surgery
2 Surgical revascularization
   — Ostial lesions
   — Extensive atheromatous plaques

Renovascular hypertension: predictors of surgical cure
1 Young patient
2 Recent onset of hypertension
3 Normal serum creatinine
4 Homolateral:contralateral renal vein renin ratio > 1.5
5 Captopril challenge → ↓ BP, ↑ plasma renin activity

Indications for emergency drug therapy of severe hypertension
1 Sodium nitroprusside infusion + arterial monitor (urgent)
   — Hypertensive encephalopathy
     • Avoid β-blockers, methyldopa
   — ↑ BP + myocardial infarct and/or pulmonary edema
     • Avoid hydralazine
   — Dissecting aortic aneurysm (plus β-blocker)
     • Avoid hydralazine
   — Contraindicated in uremia, raised intracranial pressure
2 Sublingual nifedipine 10 mg or captopril 25 mg
   — Hypertensive retinopathy without encephalopathy
     • Avoid β-blockers, methyldopa
   — Severe hypertension + acute renal failure*
     • Avoid β-blockers
3 Phentolamine or labetalol infusion
   — Clonidine withdrawal (rare now)
   — Pheochromocytoma
   — MAOI interaction (e.g. with dietary tyramine)
     • Avoid β-blockers
   — Labetalol contraindicated in acute LVF
4 Hydralazine (or nifedipine)
   — Eclampsia
     • Avoid diuretics, ACE inhibitors, β-blockers
   — Contraindicated in angina
5 Enalapril
   — Acute LVF

NB: Diazoxide is now obsolete
* Unless bilateral renal artery stenoses, stenosis in a solitary functioning kidney, or severe renal failure, in which cases avoid captopril

ESTROGENIC STATES AND CARDIAC DISEASE

Cardiac conditions commonly exacerbated by pregnancy
1 Stenoses
   — Mitral stenosis
   — Aortic stenosis
   — Aortic coarctation
2 Pulmonary hypertension
   — Primary
   — Eisenmenger's syndrome

Treatment options in pregnancy-associated hypertension
1 Oral treatment*
   — Hydralazine
   — Methyldopa
2 Emergency treatment (e.g. for eclampsia)
   — Diazoxide
   — Labetalol, nifedipine
3 Prophylaxis during third trimester
   — Low-dose aspirin

* β-blockers may also be used, but beware of fetal bradycardia/hypoglycemia

Metabolic alterations in oral contraceptive users
1 ↑ Fibrinogen/plasminogen/FDPs/factors VII, VIII, X

2   ↓ Antithrombin III; ↓ albumin, haptoglobin
3   ↑ Transferrin, ceruloplasmin (↑ *total* serum iron, copper)
4   ↑ Triglycerides (VLDL), insulin, aldosterone, cortisol
5   ↓ Renin, ACTH

Clinical concomitants of estrogen replacement therapy
1   Reduced incidence of coronary artery disease
2   Reduced mortality from coronary artery disease
3   *No* change in stroke risk

PULMONARY HYPERTENSION

Mechanisms of pulmonary hypertension
1   Increased pulmonary blood flow
    — Left-to-right shunt
2   Elevated pulmonary venous pressure
    — Mitral stenosis
3   Obliteration of vascular bed
    — Pulmonary emboli
    — Emphysema
    — Primary pulmonary hypertension
    — Collagen-vascular diseases

Diseases involving pulmonary arteries
1   Primary pulmonary hypertension
2   Churg–Strauss syndrome (cf. PAN)
3   Wegener's granulomatosis
4   Takayasu's arteritis
5   Systemic sclerosis

Associations of primary pulmonary hypertension
1   Raynaud's phenomenon, SLE*, scleroderma
2   Familial
3   Pregnancy
4   Iatrogenic: oral contraceptives, metformin
5   Ingestion of aminorex or crotolaria alkaloids

* esp. if anticardiolipin antibody positive

Diagnosis of primary pulmonary hypertension
1   CXR
    — Peripheral oligemia ('pruned' peripheral vasculature)
    — Proximal-dilated pulmonary arteries ('deer's antlers')
    — Pulmonary arterial calcification if long-standing
2   Pulmonary angiography*
    — No emboli
    — No peripheral arterial stenosis
    — No intracardiac shunt
    — Normal PCWP (excludes MS, cor triatriatum)

* Choriocarcinoma growing down the pulmonary arteries is a rare, curable cause of 'primary' pulmonary hypertension; diagnose by plasma β-HCG

VENOUS THROMBOSIS

Differential diagnosis of the swollen calf
1   Deep venous thrombosis
2   Cellulitis

3   Ruptured plantaris
4   Ruptured Baker's cyst
5   Popliteal artery aneurysm (incl. mycotic)
6   Hematoma (esp. in patient on anticoagulants)

'Post-phlebitic syndrome': pathogenesis, features and diagnosis
1   Previous venous thrombosis irreversibly damages venous valves (esp. in perforators) and distorts drainage
2   Gradual onset of symptoms worsened by upright posture
    — Tense ankle edema (implies deep vein incompetence)
    — Calf pain, esp. on exercise ('venous claudication')
    — Cyanosis, pigmentation, induration and ulceration
3   Essentially a diagnosis of exclusion
    — Negative venogram*
    — Negative impedance plethysmography
    — Negative radiofibrinogen scan
    — Doppler → deep venous reflux

* Misleading if thrombus has organized

ETIOLOGY OF VENOUS THROMBOSIS

Classical predispositions to thrombosis: Virchow's triad
1   Abnormal blood flow
    — e.g. Intrapelvic obstruction
2   Abnormal blood
    — e.g. Polycythemia vera, factor V mutation
3   Abnormal vessel wall
    — e.g. Coronary atherosclerosis

Non-specific predispositions to venous thrombosis
1   **H**istory
    — Previous thrombosis or embolism
2   **H**ypomobility
    — Cerebrovascular accident
    — Myocardial infarction, cardiac failure
    — Post-operative, esp. hip/pelvic/abdominal surgery
3   **H**ypovolemia
    — Nephrotic syndrome
    — Dehydration, esp. in elderly
4   **H**ypercoagulability
    — Malignancy*, esp. disseminated
    — Cigarette smoking
5   **H**ormones
    — Estrogens
    — Puerperium

* Cytotoxic chemotherapy per se may cause additional hypercoagulability

Specific conditions associated with thromboembolism
1   Hereditary causes of thrombophilia*
    — Common
      • Factor V Leiden mutation‡
      • Hyperhomocysteinemia¶
      • Elevated Lp(a)
    — Uncommon
      • Antithrombin III deficiency (1/2000)
      • Protein C (or S) deficiency
      • Heparin co-factor II deficiency

2 Specific diseases causing acquired hyper-coagulability
— SLE and/or lupus anticoagulant (anticardiolipin; p. 191)
— Paroxysmal nocturnal hemoglobinuria
— Polycythemia vera, essential thrombocythemia
— 'Warm' autoimmune hemolytic anemia
— Sickle-C disease
3 Drugs
— e.g. Rifampicin

* Most DVT patients do *not* have any identifiable coagulation abnormality
‡ Mutation → resistance to activated protein C; occurs in up to 7% population
¶ Important diagnosis since condition responds to vitamins (folate, pyridoxine, hydroxocobalamin)

Clinical sequelae of resistance to protein C*
1 Increased thrombosis, esp.
— When taking oral contraceptives
— When pregnant
2 Increased incidence of myocardial infarction
— esp. In homozygotes

* i.e. due to factor V Leiden

INVESTIGATING THROMBOSIS

Indications for investigating thrombotic tendency
1 Venous or arterial thrombosis in young patient (< 40 yrs)
2 Recurrent thromboembolic events and/or family history
3 Recurrent abortion
4 Skin necrosis while taking warfarin*

* Affects individuals with protein C or S deficiency

Techniques of detecting thrombi
1 Venography
— Advantages
• Quick, accurate ('gold standard')
— Disadvantages
• May be painful and/or cause phlebitis
• Risk of contrast hypersensitivity
• Radioactivity exposure
• False-negative: recanalized thrombus
2 Duplex B-mode ultrasound/color Doppler
— Advantages
• Quick, painless, non-invasive and cheap
• Sensitive/specific for proximal thrombi
• Currently the most popular approach
— Disadvantages
• Insensitive for distal (calf) thrombi
• False-negative: non-occlusive proximal thrombi
• False-positives possible in CCF
3 ^{125}I-labelled fibrinogen scanning
— Advantages
• Non-invasive, painless
• Accurate for actively extending calf thrombi

— Disadvantages
• Slow (results take 24–72 h) and expensive
• Radioactivity exposure
• Insensitive for iliofemoral thrombus
• False-negative: non-extending thrombus
• False-positives: hematoma or inflammation
4 Impedance plethysmography
— Advantages
• Non-invasive, painless, no radioactivity
• Sensitive for proximal occlusive thrombi
• Good when combined with ^{125}I-fibrinogen
— Disadvantages
• May require serial studies
• Insensitive for calf thrombi
• False-negative: non-occlusive proximal thrombi
• False-positive: cardiac failure
5 Miscellaneous
— D-dimer
• Absence in plasma may *exclude* fresh thrombus
— Edema fluid protein concentration
• Levels > 10 g/L suggest cellulitis > thrombosis
— Thermography
• False-positives with any inflammation

PERIPHERAL ARTERIAL DISEASE

Cardiogenic sources of systemic emboli
1 Mitral stenosis
2 Post-infarct
3 Atrial fibrillation (alone)
4 Prosthetic valve (p. 59)
— Mitral > aortic
— Mechanical > biological
5 Other
— Sick sinus syndrome
— Mitral valve prolapse
— Infective endocarditis
— Left atrial myxoma

Digital gangrene with normal pulses
1 Diabetes mellitus
2 Vasculitis; cold agglutinins
3 Thromboembolism
4 Hyperviscosity
5 Iatrogenic
— Excess ergot or dopamine
— Intraarterial thiopentone or adrenaline

Claudication of the upper limb
1 Atheroma
2 Buerger's disease
3 Takayasu's arteritis
4 Proximal coarctation
5 Thoracic outlet syndrome
6 Polymyalgia rheumatica

REVIEWING THE LITERATURE: CARDIOLOGY

2.1   Lakka TA et al (1994) Relation of leisure-time physical activity and cardiorespiratory fitness to the risk of acute myocardial infarction in men. N Engl J Med 330: 1549–1554

Study of 1453 men aged 42 to 60 showing a 65% reduction in risk of myocardial infarction for the fittest one-third of the study population.

2.2   Gronbaek M et al (1994) Influence of sex, age, body mass index, and smoking on alcohol intake and mortality. Br Med J 308: 302–306

Doll R et al (1994) Mortality in relation to consumption of alcohol: 13 years' observations on male British doctors. Br Med J 309: 911–918

Two studies tending to confirm the controversial association of low-level alcohol consumption (~ 1 unit/day) and improved cardiovascular and overall mortality.

2.3   Meisel SR et al (1991) Effect of Iraqi missile war on incidence of acute myocardial infarction and sudden death in Israeli civilians. Lancet 338: 660–661

Yeung AC et al (1991) The effect of atherosclerosis on the vasomotor response of coronary arteries to mental stress. N Engl J Med 325: 1551–1556

Two studies supporting a link between stress and cardiovascular morbidity.

Carroll D et al (1995) Pressor reactions to psychological stress and prediction of future blood pressure: data from the Whitehall II study. Br Med J 310: 771–776

Reactivity of blood pressure to stressful stimuli did *not* predict later occurrence of hypertension, thus tending to blur the above conclusion.

2.4   Uretsky et al (1993) Randomized study assessing the effect of digoxin withdrawal in patients with mild to moderate chronic congestive heart failure: results of the PROVED study. JACC 22: 955–962

Packer M et al (1993) Withdrawal of digoxin from patients with chronic heart failure treated with angiotensin converting enzyme inhibitors. N Engl J Med 329: 1–7

These two studies, PROVED and RADIANCE, supported (but have not quite 'proved') the notion that digoxin benefits around 20% of non-fibrillating CCF patients.

2.5   Waagstein F et al (1993) Beneficial effects of metoprolol in idiopathic dilated cardiomyopathy. Lancet 342: 1441–1446

Placebo-controlled randomized study of 383 cardiomyopathics showing major benefits in the metoprolol-treated cohort with respect to ejection fraction, pulmonary wedge pressure, exercise time and transplantation frequency.

Atkison P et al (1995) Hypertrophic cardiomyopathy associated with tacrolimus in paediatric transplant patients. Lancet 345: 894–896

Fascinating report of five reversible HOCM cases occurring in children receiving the cyclosporin-like immunosuppressant drug tacrolimus (formerly FK506).

2.6   Watts GF et al (1992) Effects on coronary artery disease of lipid-lowering diet, or diet plus cholestyramine, in the St Thomas' Atherosclerosis Regression Study (STARS). Lancet 339: 563–569

Law MR et al (1994) By how much and how quickly does reduction in serum cholesterol concentration lower risk of ischaemic heart disease? Br Med J 308: 367–373

The former study was one of several randomized studies

documenting active regression of atheroma induced by blood lipid reduction (esp. LDL-cholesterol) due to either diet or drugs. The latter article is an overview of similar studies involving 500,000 men and 18,000 cardiovascular events and confirms that a 5-year plasma cholesterol reduction of 10% (0.6 mmol/L) lowers risk of cardiac death by 50% at age 40 and 20% at age 70.

2.7   RITA Trial (1993) Coronary angioplasty versus coronary artery bypass surgery: the Randomised Intervention Treatment of Angina (RITA) trial. Lancet 341: 573–580

King SB et al (1994) A randomized trial comparing coronary angioplasty with coronary bypass surgery. N Engl J Med 331: 1044–1050

Both RITA and EAST confirmed no difference in myocardial infarction rates or survival following PTCA or CABG. However, both suggested that angina and subsequent therapeutic procedures were commoner in the PTCA group.

2.8   SOLVD Investigators (1992) Effect of enalapril on mortality and the development of heart failure in asymptomatic patients with reduced left ventricular ejection fractions. N Engl J Med 327: 685–691

One of many studies to trumpet the virtues of ACE inhibitors in ischemic heart disease.

ISIS-4 (1995) A randomised factorial trial assessing early oral captopril, oral mononitrate, and intravenous magnesium sulphate in 58,050 patients with suspected acute myocardial infarction. Lancet 345: 669–685

No benefit of post-infarct magnesium demonstrated in this study and perhaps some hazard (more hypotension). Use of nitrates during the first month also failed to improve mortality; but ACE inhibition for the first month reduced 1-year mortality by about five per 1000 infarcts.

2.9   GUSTO Angiographic Investigators (1993) The effects of tissue plasminogen activator, streptokinase, or both on coronary artery patency, ventricular function, and survival after acute myocardial infarction. N Engl J Med 329: 1615–1622

Randomized study of 2431 patients confirming the survival benefits of thrombolytic therapy following acute myocardial infarction.

2.10   Antiplatelet Trialists' Collaboration (1994) Collaborative overview of randomised trials of antiplatelet therapy: prevention of death, myocardial infarction, and stroke by prolonged antiplatelet therapy in various categories of patients. Br Med J 308: 81–106

Overview of 145 randomized trials showing substantial improvements in death, infarct and stroke rates of all 'risk' patients taking aspirin 75–325 mg/day. However, no evidence on benefit in low-risk individuals is yet available.

2.11   den Heijer M et al (1995) Is hyperhomocysteinaemia a risk factor for recurrent venous thrombosis? Lancet 345: 882–885

Ridker PM et al (1995) Mutation in the gene coding for coagulation factor V and the risk of myocardial infarction, stroke and venous thrombosis in apparently healthy men. N Engl J Med 332: 912–917

Two studies describing two newly recognized – but surprisingly common – hereditary predispositions to venous thrombosis.

Selhub J et al (1995) Association between plasma homocysteine concentrations and extracranial carotid-artery stenosis. N Engl J Med 332: 286–291

Another study showing that arterial disease is also linked to hyperhomocystinemia (a 2-fold excess risk of carotid stenosis) – as well as to low levels of folate and pyridoxine, two enzymes involved in homocysteine metabolism.

2.12 Glynn RJ et al (1995) Evidence for a positive linear relation between blood pressure and mortality in elderly people. Lancet 345: 825–829

Community study of 3657 elderly Americans, documenting major increases in morbidity and mortality for elderly patients with uncontrolled hypertension; the authors conclude that hypertension should be actively treated in the elderly.

CHAPTER 3
Endocrinology

Physical examination protocol 3.1 You are asked to assess a patient for clinical evidence of hypopituitarism

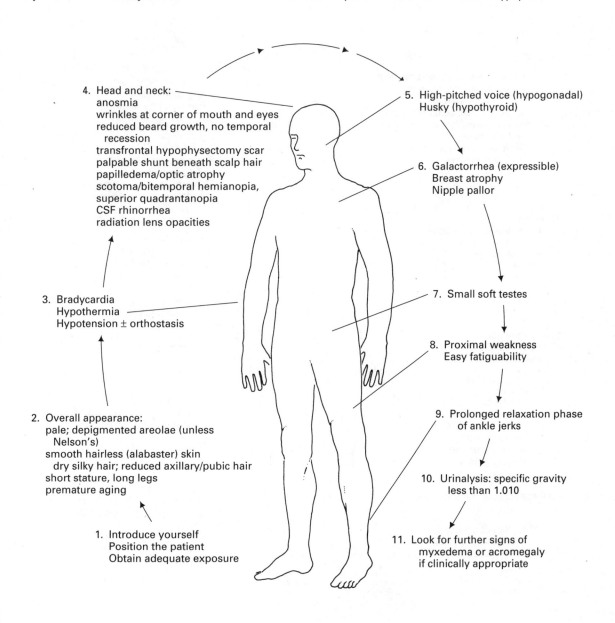

4. Head and neck:
   anosmia
   wrinkles at corner of mouth and eyes
   reduced beard growth, no temporal
     recession
   transfrontal hypophysectomy scar
   palpable shunt beneath scalp hair
   papilledema/optic atrophy
   scotoma/bitemporal hemianopia,
   superior quadrantanopia
   CSF rhinorrhea
   radiation lens opacities

5. High-pitched voice (hypogonadal)
   Husky (hypothyroid)

6. Galactorrhea (expressible)
   Breast atrophy
   Nipple pallor

3. Bradycardia
   Hypothermia
   Hypotension ± orthostasis

7. Small soft testes

8. Proximal weakness
   Easy fatiguability

2. Overall appearance:
   pale; depigmented areolae (unless
     Nelson's)
   smooth hairless (alabaster) skin
   dry silky hair; reduced axillary/pubic hair
   short stature, long legs
   premature aging

9. Prolonged relaxation phase
   of ankle jerks

10. Urinalysis: specific gravity
    less than 1.010

1. Introduce yourself
   Position the patient
   Obtain adequate exposure

11. Look for further signs of
    myxedema or acromegaly
    if clinically appropriate

Physical examination protocol 3.2 You are asked to examine a patient who has recently noticed increasing hat size

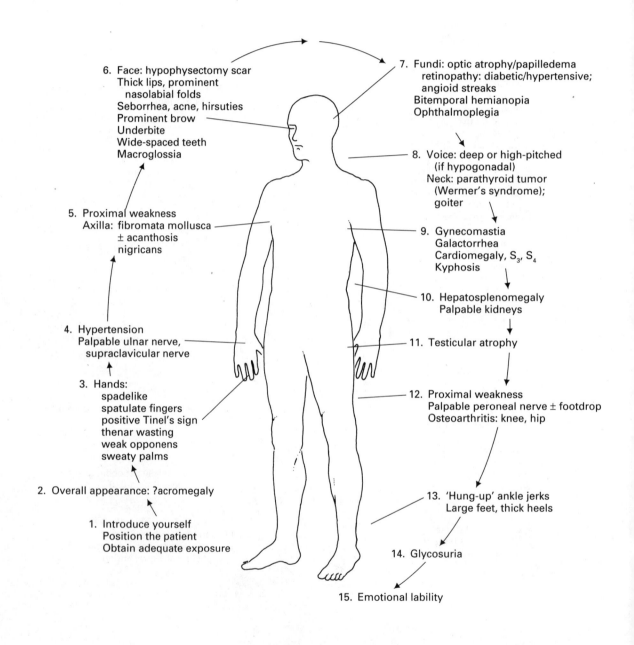

6. Face: hypophysectomy scar
   Thick lips, prominent
      nasolabial folds
   Seborrhea, acne, hirsuties
   Prominent brow
   Underbite
   Wide-spaced teeth
   Macroglossia

7. Fundi: optic atrophy/papilledema
      retinopathy: diabetic/hypertensive;
      angioid streaks
   Bitemporal hemianopia
   Ophthalmoplegia

5. Proximal weakness
   Axilla: fibromata mollusca
      ± acanthosis
      nigricans

8. Voice: deep or high-pitched
      (if hypogonadal)
   Neck: parathyroid tumor
      (Wermer's syndrome);
      goiter

9. Gynecomastia
   Galactorrhea
   Cardiomegaly, S_3, S_4
   Kyphosis

4. Hypertension
   Palpable ulnar nerve,
      supraclavicular nerve

10. Hepatosplenomegaly
    Palpable kidneys

3. Hands:
      spadelike
      spatulate fingers
      positive Tinel's sign
      thenar wasting
      weak opponens
      sweaty palms

11. Testicular atrophy

12. Proximal weakness
    Palpable peroneal nerve ± footdrop
    Osteoarthritis: knee, hip

2. Overall appearance: ?acromegaly

1. Introduce yourself
   Position the patient
   Obtain adequate exposure

13. 'Hung-up' ankle jerks
    Large feet, thick heels

14. Glycosuria

15. Emotional lability

Physical examination protocol 3.3   You are asked to examine a patient with recent onset of lethargy and cold intolerance

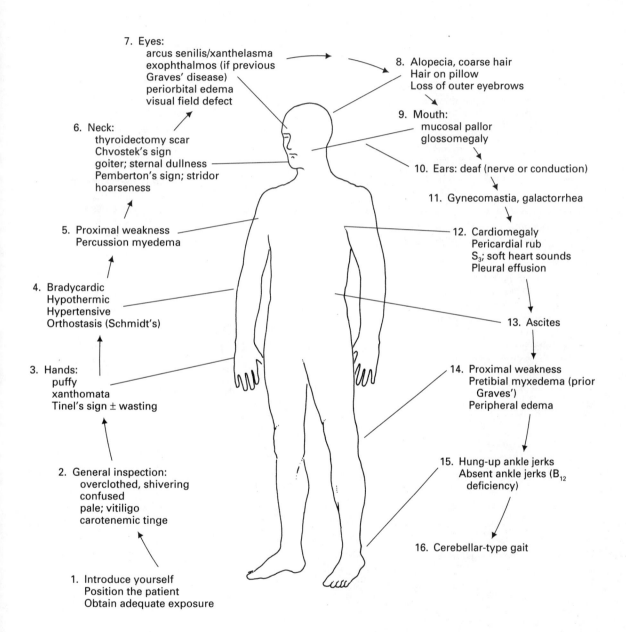

7. Eyes:
   arcus senilis/xanthelasma
   exophthalmos (if previous
   Graves' disease)
   periorbital edema
   visual field defect

8. Alopecia, coarse hair
   Hair on pillow
   Loss of outer eyebrows

6. Neck:
   thyroidectomy scar
   Chvostek's sign
   goiter; sternal dullness
   Pemberton's sign; stridor
   hoarseness

9. Mouth:
   mucosal pallor
   glossomegaly

10. Ears: deaf (nerve or conduction)

11. Gynecomastia, galactorrhea

5. Proximal weakness
   Percussion myedema

12. Cardiomegaly
    Pericardial rub
    S_3; soft heart sounds
    Pleural effusion

4. Bradycardic
   Hypothermic
   Hypertensive
   Orthostasis (Schmidt's)

13. Ascites

3. Hands:
   puffy
   xanthomata
   Tinel's sign ± wasting

14. Proximal weakness
    Pretibial myxedema (prior
       Graves')
    Peripheral edema

2. General inspection:
   overclothed, shivering
   confused
   pale; vitiligo
   carotenemic tinge

15. Hung-up ankle jerks
    Absent ankle jerks (B_{12}
       deficiency)

1. Introduce yourself
   Position the patient
   Obtain adequate exposure

16. Cerebellar-type gait

Physical examination protocol 3.4   You are asked to begin by examining the neck of a patient who looks possibly thyrotoxic

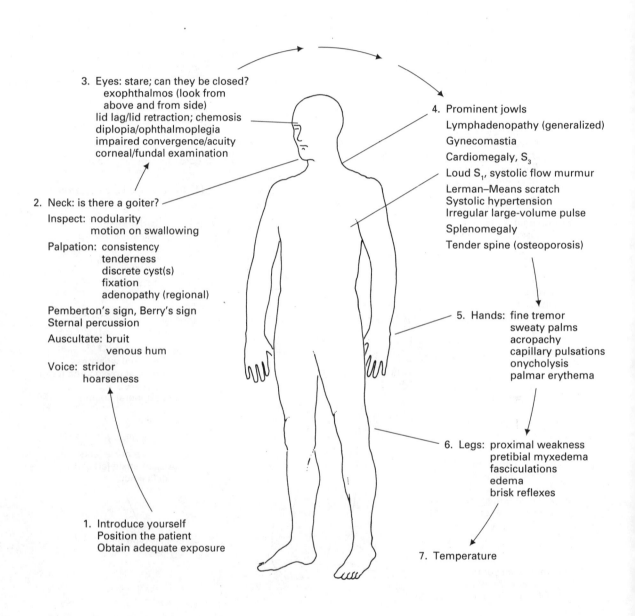

3. Eyes: stare; can they be closed?
   exophthalmos (look from
   above and from side)
   lid lag/lid retraction; chemosis
   diplopia/ophthalmoplegia
   impaired convergence/acuity
   corneal/fundal examination

2. Neck: is there a goiter?
   Inspect: nodularity
            motion on swallowing
   Palpation: consistency
              tenderness
              discrete cyst(s)
              fixation
              adenopathy (regional)
   Pemberton's sign, Berry's sign
   Sternal percussion
   Auscultate: bruit
               venous hum
   Voice: stridor
          hoarseness

1. Introduce yourself
   Position the patient
   Obtain adequate exposure

4. Prominent jowls
   Lymphadenopathy (generalized)
   Gynecomastia
   Cardiomegaly, S_3
   Loud S_1, systolic flow murmur
   Lerman–Means scratch
   Systolic hypertension
   Irregular large-volume pulse
   Splenomegaly
   Tender spine (osteoporosis)

5. Hands: fine tremor
          sweaty palms
          acropachy
          capillary pulsations
          onycholysis
          palmar erythema

6. Legs: proximal weakness
         pretibial myxedema
         fasciculations
         edema
         brisk reflexes

7. Temperature

Physical examination protocol 3.5   You are asked to examine a patient who is known to have diabetes mellitus

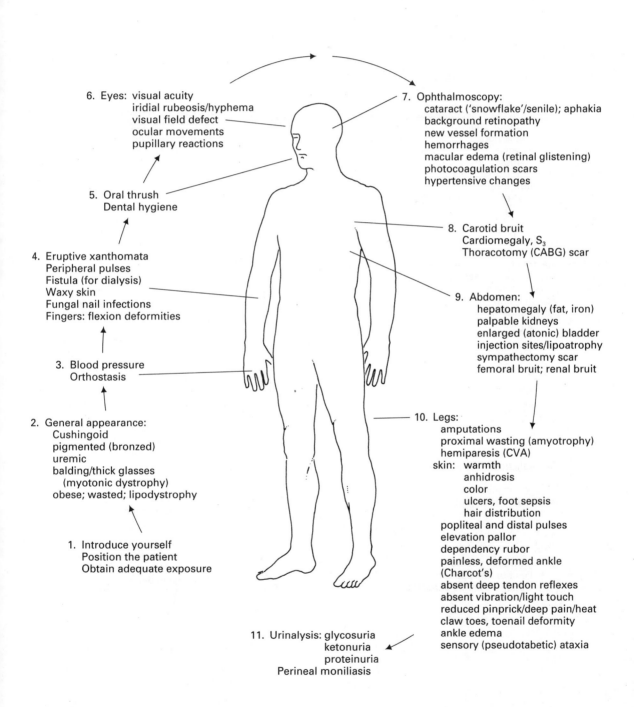

6. Eyes: visual acuity
   iridial rubeosis/hyphema
   visual field defect
   ocular movements
   pupillary reactions

7. Ophthalmoscopy:
   cataract ('snowflake'/senile); aphakia
   background retinopathy
   new vessel formation
   hemorrhages
   macular edema (retinal glistening)
   photocoagulation scars
   hypertensive changes

5. Oral thrush
   Dental hygiene

8. Carotid bruit
   Cardiomegaly, S₃
   Thoracotomy (CABG) scar

4. Eruptive xanthomata
   Peripheral pulses
   Fistula (for dialysis)
   Waxy skin
   Fungal nail infections
   Fingers: flexion deformities

9. Abdomen:
   hepatomegaly (fat, iron)
   palpable kidneys
   enlarged (atonic) bladder
   injection sites/lipoatrophy
   sympathectomy scar
   femoral bruit; renal bruit

3. Blood pressure
   Orthostasis

10. Legs:
    amputations
    proximal wasting (amyotrophy)
    hemiparesis (CVA)
    skin: warmth
           anhidrosis
           color
           ulcers, foot sepsis
           hair distribution
    popliteal and distal pulses
    elevation pallor
    dependency rubor
    painless, deformed ankle
    (Charcot's)
    absent deep tendon reflexes
    absent vibration/light touch
    reduced pinprick/deep pain/heat
    claw toes, toenail deformity
    ankle edema
    sensory (pseudotabetic) ataxia

2. General appearance:
   Cushingoid
   pigmented (bronzed)
   uremic
   balding/thick glasses
   (myotonic dystrophy)
   obese; wasted; lipodystrophy

1. Introduce yourself
   Position the patient
   Obtain adequate exposure

11. Urinalysis: glycosuria
    ketonuria
    proteinuria
    Perineal moniliasis

Physical examination protocol 3.6 You are asked to examine a patient suspected of having Cushing's syndrome

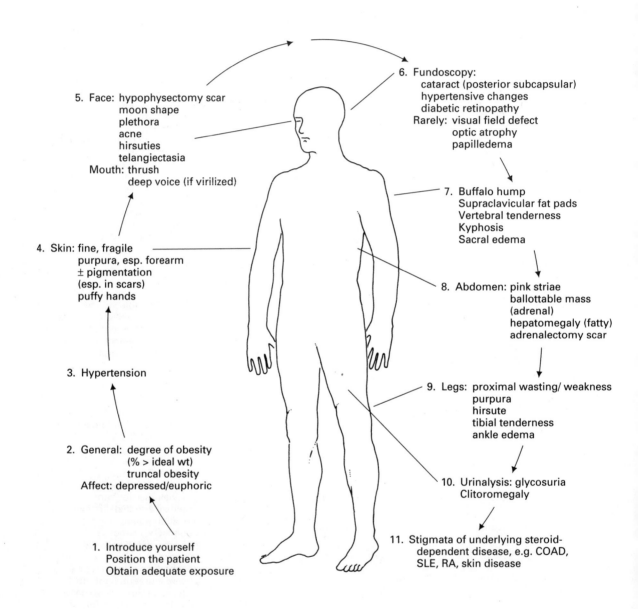

5. Face: hypophysectomy scar
   moon shape
   plethora
   acne
   hirsuties
   telangiectasia
   Mouth: thrush
   deep voice (if virilized)

4. Skin: fine, fragile
   purpura, esp. forearm
   ± pigmentation
   (esp. in scars)
   puffy hands

3. Hypertension

2. General: degree of obesity
   (% > ideal wt)
   truncal obesity
   Affect: depressed/euphoric

1. Introduce yourself
   Position the patient
   Obtain adequate exposure

6. Fundoscopy:
   cataract (posterior subcapsular)
   hypertensive changes
   diabetic retinopathy
   Rarely: visual field defect
   optic atrophy
   papilledema

7. Buffalo hump
   Supraclavicular fat pads
   Vertebral tenderness
   Kyphosis
   Sacral edema

8. Abdomen: pink striae
   ballottable mass
   (adrenal)
   hepatomegaly (fatty)
   adrenalectomy scar

9. Legs: proximal wasting/ weakness
   purpura
   hirsute
   tibial tenderness
   ankle edema

10. Urinalysis: glycosuria
    Clitoromegaly

11. Stigmata of underlying steroid-
    dependent disease, e.g. COAD,
    SLE, RA, skin disease

Diagnostic pathway 3.1   This patient has a goiter. What is the differential diagnosis?

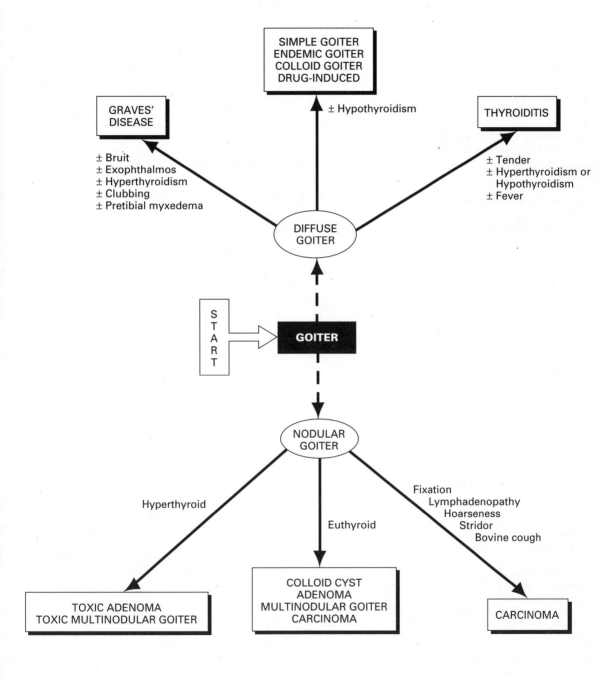

CLINICAL ASPECTS OF ENDOCRINE DISEASE

Commonest endocrine short cases
1 Diabetic retinopathy
2 Graves' disease/goiter
3 Acromegaly

PITUITARY DISORDERS

Principal features of hypopituitarism
1 Hypothyroidism (without goiter)
2 Hypoadrenalism (with pallor: 'alabaster skin')
3 Hypogonadism (with fine wrinkled skin: 'crows feet')
4 Hyposthenuria* (diabetes insipidus)

* Note that *serum* osmolality or sodium concentration may be normal (i.e. not increased) if water intake has been adequate

Acromegaly: indicators of disease activity
1 Severity of
   — Seborrhea, sweating, skin tags*
   — Hypertension, edema
   — Glucose intolerance
2 Serial measures of
   — Visual fields
   — Visual acuity
3 Plasma insulin-like growth factor-1 (IGF-1) level‡

* Fibromata mollusca
‡ 'Somatomedin C', the peripheral hormonal effector of growth hormone

Common causes of morbidity/mortality in acromegaly
1 Hypertension
2 Cardiomyopathy
3 Cerebrovascular disease

NB: These complications may respond dramatically to octreotide therapy

Mechanisms of polydipsia in acromegaly
1 Dehydration secondary to hyperhidrosis
2 Osmotic diuresis (in 10%) due to glucose intolerance (in 50%)
3 Diabetes insipidus

Mechanisms of galactorrhea in acromegaly
1 Concomitant adenomatous secretion of prolactin (in 30%)
2 Compression of posterior pituitary stalk by adenoma, causing reduced ingress of prolactin-inhibitory factor (PIF)
3 Reduced pituitary TSH secretion → compensatory elevation of hypothalamic TRH secretion → prolactin release

Prolactinomas: clinical presentations in females
1 Galactorrhea (in 50% *only**)
2 Hypogonadism‡ (↓ FSH/LH)
   — Reduced libido
   — Amenorrhea due to ovulatory failure
   — Infertility: regular anovulatory menstrual cycles
3 Dysfunctional uterine bleeding

4 Visual field defect (in 5%)
   — If macroadenoma present (in 30%)
5 Osteoporosis
   — If *long-term* reduction of E_2 results

* Conversely, most cases of non-puerperal lactation do *not* have ↑ prolactin
‡ Indication for active treatment

Distinguishing features of prolactinomas in males
1 Less common; later age of presentation
2 Galactorrhea distinctly unusual
3 Hypogonadism in 90%: impotence, obesity, infertility
4 Visual symptoms common due to high frequency (80%) of macroadenomas (usually associated with ↑↑ prolactin)

HYPERTHYROIDISM

Pointers to the diagnosis of Graves' disease
1 Smooth diffuse goiter
   — Esp. with bruit
2 Ophthalmopathy (see below)
   — Clinically apparent in 40%
3 Classical but rare
   — Localized mucinous edema (pretibial myxedema)
   — 'Acropachy'*
4 Non-specific
   — Splenomegaly
   — Lymphadenopathy
5 Laboratory (see also p. 98–99)
   — Thyroid-stimulating immunoglobulin (TSI)
   — Low or undetectable TSH (i.e. hyperthyroidism)

* = Clubbing + subcutaneous fibrosis + phalangeal periosteal proliferation

Clinical manifestations of Graves' ophthalmopathy
1 Primary ('autoimmune') manifestations
   — Proptosis, exophthalmos
   — Ophthalmoplegia
      • Lymphocytic infiltration of external eye muscles
      • Inferior recti most affected → vertical diplopia
2 Secondary (mechanical) complications
   — Optic nerve compression
      • Often occurs insidiously with *mild* proptosis
      • ↓ Acuity, central scotoma
      • ↓ Color vision; Marcus–Gunn pupil
      • Variable disc appearance on fundoscopy
   — Impaired convergence
   — Corneal ulceration
      • Occurs with *marked* proptosis of acute onset
   — Chemosis, lid edema, glaucoma
3 'Sympathetic' manifestations (*if* thyrotoxic*)
   — Lid-lag
   — Lid retraction ('stare')
      • Sclera visible above and below iris
      • Due to overactivity of Müller's muscle

* These signs also occur in non-autoimmune hyperthyroidism

Bilateral exophthalmos: differential diagnosis
1 Graves' disease
2 Uremia

3 Alcoholism
4 Malignant hypertension
5 Carcinomatosis
6 SVC obstruction

Unilateral exophthalmos: differential diagnosis
1 Graves' disease (commonest cause)
2 Contralateral Horner's syndrome (i.e. misdiagnosis)
3 Cavernous sinus pathology
— Cavernous sinus thrombosis
— Caroticocavernous fistula (pulsating)
— Rhinocerebral mucormycosis
4 Intraorbital pathology
— Histiocytosis X
— Wegener's granulomatosis
— Riedel's thyroiditis with pseudotumor oculi
— Tumor (e.g. optic nerve glioma)

Neuromyopathies in thyroid disease
1 Proximal myopathy
— Seen in thyrotoxicosis, less in hypothyroidism
— Affects mainly upper limbs; reverts when euthyroid
2 Hypokalemic periodic paralysis
— Seen in association with toxic multinodular goiter
— Commonest in Asian males, esp. in hot season
— Linked to hyperinsulinemia; treated with propranolol
3 Myasthenia gravis
— Affects 5% Graves' patients; suspect if bulbar weakness
— Exacerbated by thyrotoxicosis or hypothyroidism
4 Graves' ophthalmoplegia
— Seen also in euthyroid patients
— Predominant weakness of upward and lateral gaze
5 Hoffmann's syndrome
— Pseudomyotonia of myxedematous muscles
— Manifests with muscle aching following exertion

HYPOTHYROIDISM

Signs suggesting severe hypothyroidism
1 Hoarseness
2 Profound bradycardia or hypothermia
3 Mental confusion or coma
4 Markedly prolonged relaxation phase of deep tendon reflexes

Differential diagnosis of 'hung-up' tendon jerks
1 Myxedema
2 Other (rare) causes
— Diabetes mellitus
— Sarcoidosis
— Syphilis
— Profound hypothermia
— Post-partum
— Anorexia nervosa
— β-blockade

Factors favoring secondary (pituitary) hypothyroidism
1 No goiter

2 No soft-tissue (myx)edema
3 Stigmata of hypopituitarism (pale areolae, hyposthenuria)
4 Normal plasma cholesterol
5 Enlargement of sella turcica
6 TSH not elevated despite low free T_4

Pathogenetic mechanisms of thyroid enlargement
1 **T**hyroiditis (Hashimoto's)
2 **T**SI (thyroid-stimulating immunoglobulin; → Graves')
3 **T**SH (multinodular goiter)
4 **T**umor

DIABETES MELLITUS

Abdominal pain in diabetic patients: differential diagnosis
1 Gastric dilatation
— Acute (ketoacidosis)
— Chronic (autonomic neuropathy)
2 Pancreatitis
— Acute (a complication of type IV hyperlipidemia)
— Chronic (precedes development of diabetes)
3 Infarction
— Mesenteric
— Myocardial (painless in autonomic neuropathy)
4 Genitourinary
— Urinary tract infection
— Bladder retention (painless in early stages)
5 Hepatobiliary
— Cholecystitis
— Hepatic capsular distension due to steatosis, esp. in poorly controlled patients receiving high insulin
6 Thoracolumbar radiculopathy (amyotrophy; see below)
— Due to nerve root ischemia

Clinical features of diabetic amyotrophy
1 Presents acutely in a poorly controlled type II diabetic with ↑↑ HbA_{1c} but no known microvascular disease
2 Initially manifests with asymmetric weakness of hip/knee
3 Radicular pain and/or other sensory symptoms may be associated; almost always accompanied by hyporeflexia
4 Often complicated by contralateral pelvic girdle weakness, wasting, weight loss, incontinence and impotence
5 Occasionally associated with extensor plantar response and/or ↑ CSF protein
6 Excellent long-term prognosis: partial recovery usual within 1–2 years, though recurrence not uncommon

The diabetic foot: factors contributing to morbidity
1 Ischemia
— Microvascular disease (esp.)
— Macrovascular disease (atheroma) ± thrombosis

2 Infection (incl. osteomyelitis)
  — Stiff (glycosylated) collagen
    • → Ulcers (cellulitis)
  — Hyperglycemic leukocyte dysfunction
    • → Poor wound healing
3 Neuropathy (in 80%)
  — Sensory loss (incl. Charcot joint development)
    • → Trauma, burns
  — Motor loss
    • Weak intrinsics → 'claw toe' → plantar ulcers
  — Visual loss
    • Reduced visual acuity (→ poor foot care)
4 Deformity
  — Callus, bunion, hammer-toe → ↑ trauma

The infected diabetic foot: bacteriology and therapy
1 Mild infections (tend to be Gram-positive)
  — *Staph. aureus*
  — Streptococci
2 Serious infections
  — Gram-negative aerobes
  — Anaerobes
3 Empirical (preculture) treatment options
  — Non-limb-threatening infection
    • Oral flucloxacillin *or* IV cefazolin
  — Limb-threatening infection
    • Ciprofloxacin + clindamycin (oral/IV)
  — Life-threatening infection
    • Vancomycin + metronidazole (IV)

Patterns of fetal morbidity in gestational diabetes
1 Mild (newly diagnosed) diabetes
  — Macrosomia (→ dystocia)
2 Severe (known microvascular disease)
  — Small-for-dates
3 Spontaneous abortions*
  — Intrauterine fetal death
4 Malformations (esp. anencephaly)
  — Increased with maternal ketosis
5 Neonatal morbidity
  — Jaundice, respiratory distress
  — Hypoglycemia (maternal hyperglycemia → ↑ insulin)
6 Reduced childhood intelligence
  — IQ inversely proportional to third-trimester ketosis

* Incidence reduced if blood glucose levels tightly controlled in first trimester

DIABETIC EYE DISEASE

Differential diagnosis of ocular pain in diabetic patients
1 Third nerve palsy
2 Iridial rubeosis
3 Mucormycosis
4 Secondary glaucoma
5 Poor visual acuity → eyestrain

Characteristics of a diabetic third nerve palsy
1 Sudden onset
2 Painful
3 Pupillary sparing

4 Probably reflects microvascular disease of vasa nervorum
5 Diplopia usually improves within 12 months

Common causes of impaired visual acuity in diabetic patients
1 Macular edema in acute hyperglycemia
2 Retinopathy impinging on macula
3 Retinal detachment or vitreous hemorrhage
4 Hyphema secondary to iridial rubeosis
5 Cataract (classical, rare 'snowflake' type in type I diabetes)
6 Cerebrovascular accident

Diabetic retinopathy: characterizing the lesions
1 Maculopathy (commonest cause of diabetic blindness)
  — Macular edema
  — Macular exudates
  — Macular ischemia
2 'Background' retinopathy (i.e. acuity unimpaired)
  — Microaneurysms
  — Hemorrhages (dot and blot)
  — Hard exudates (lipid deposits)
  — Soft exudates ('cotton wool' spots = infarcts)
  — Venous calibre changes: beading, looping, dilatation
  — Arteriolar changes: narrowing, tortuosity, AV nipping
3 Proliferative retinopathy (→ type I diabetes)
  — New vessels (from disc or periphery)
  — Fibrous patches
  — Vitreous hemorrhage
  — Retinal detachment
  — Rubeosis iridis

COMPLICATIONS OF DIABETES

Key prognostic variables influencing diabetic complications
1 Major predictive factors in *macrovascular* complications
  — Age
  — Duration of diabetes
2 Major predictive factors in *microvascular* complications
  — Hyperglycemia severity
  — Plasma prorenin activity
3 Retinopathy
  — Smoking
  — Hyperglycemia
4 Nephropathy
  — Hypertension
  — Family history of cardiovascular disease*
  — Hyperglycemia
5 Neuropathy/amyotrophy
  — Hyperglycemia
  — Incidence correlates with HbA_{1c} level and inversely with plasma insulin

* Serum Lp(a) concentrations correlate with proteinuria

Pathogenetic phases of diabetic nephropathy
1 Preclinical phase
   — GFR normal or high
   — Blood pressure normal
   — Urinary albumin excretion elevated but undetectable by routine tests (i.e. 'microalbuminuria')
2 Clinically overt nephropathy
   — Declining GFR
   — Hypertension
   — Frank proteinuria

Clinical presentations of nephropathy
1 Worsening of hypertension
2 Development of nocturia
3 Unexplained ↓ glycosuria (i.e. 'threshold' elevation)
4 Increase in microalbuminuria
5 Decrease in insulin requirement
6 Increase in hypoglycemic frequency

Causes of premature death in insulin-dependent diabetes
1 Macrovascular disease
   — Ischemic heart disease (35%)
   — Cerebrovascular disease (15%)
2 Microvascular disease
   — Renal failure (25%)
3 Ketoacidosis (20%)
4 Hypoglycemia (15%)

Causes of insulin resistance in treated diabetics
1 Common
   — Poor compliance with insulin regimen
   — Obesity (→ downregulation of endogenous receptors)
2 Acute
   — Acidemia (e.g. in ketoacidosis)
   — Profound hypokalemia
3 Circulating antagonists
   — Acromegaly
   — Cushing's syndrome
   — Pregnancy
4 Rare
   — Insulin receptor abnormalities (p. 114)
   — Pathogenic insulin antibodies (*very* rare)
5 Iatrogenic, e.g.
   — Thiazide administration
   — Steroid therapy

CLINICAL DIAGNOSIS OF ADRENAL DISORDERS

Pathophysiologic prevalence in Cushing's syndrome
1 Cushing's disease — 70%
2 Ectopic ACTH
  Adrenal adenoma — 10% each
3 Adrenal carcinoma — 5%
4 Adrenal hyperplasia
  Depression, alcohol — 1% each

Cushing's syndrome: features of discriminative value
1 Cushing's (benign ACTH-dependent) disease
   — Atrophic livid striae (skin atrophy)

— Proximal myopathy } → 'lemon-on-sticks'
— *Truncal* obesity } habitus
— Spontaneous purpura
— Osteoporosis (esp. males, premenopausal females)
2 Adrenal carcinoma
   — Childhood onset
   — Hirsutism/virilism/acne
   — Abdominal mass
3 Ectopic ACTH (paraneoplastic)
   — Hypokalemia → weakness
   — Pigmentation *if* survival sufficient (e.g. thymoma)
4 Iatrogenic
   — Posterior subcapsular cataracts
   — Aseptic necrosis of bone
   — Glaucoma; papilledema (pseudotumor)
5 Simple obesity*/polycystic ovaries
   — Pale striae
   — Generalized (may be massive) > truncal
   — 'Buffalo hump'
   — Oligomenorrhea
   — Hypertension, glucose intolerance

* i.e. these features are of *poor* diagnostic value

Hypoadrenalism: primary or secondary?
1 Primary (adrenal failure)
   — Pigmentation
   — Hyperkalemia
   — Metabolic acidosis
2 Secondary (pituitary failure)
   — Depigmented areolae
   — Despite normal aldosterone secretion, symptomatic hypovolemia *may* still occur due to vomiting/diarrhea or diabetes insipidus
   — Similarly, hyponatremia *may* still occur due to concomitant hypothyroidism or SIADH
3 The above may be distinguished by
   — Plasma ACTH assay
   — Tetracosactrin (Synacthen) test*

* Unless *long-term* pituitary failure → adrenal atrophy → false-positive

Differential diagnosis of grossly elevated plasma ACTH
1 Addison's disease
2 Nelson's syndrome
3 Ectopic (neoplastic) ACTH production

PHEOCHROMOCYTOMA

Common sites of extraadrenal pheochromocytoma
1 Organ of Zuckerkandl (aortic bifurcation)
2 Paraspinal sympathetic ganglia
3 Bladder wall (symptoms on micturition)
4 Spermatic cord
5 Glomus jugulare (usually non-secreting tumors)

Clinical aspects of pheochromocytoma
1 **H**eadache
  Hypertension
   — Non-paroxysmal in 50%
   — May paradoxically *worsen* following β-blockade

Hypotension (orthostatic in 50%)
Heartbeat awareness (palpitations)
Hyperhidrosis (sweating)
2 10% are malignant (histology not predictive)
   10% are extraadrenal (greater risk of malignancy)
   10% are familial (often bilateral): usually non-secretory
   10% are multiple (30% in children)
3 Noradrenaline-secreting type
   — May mimic essential hypertension
   — Absent tachycardia
   — Pallor
   — *Angor animi*
4 Adrenaline-secreting type
   — May mimic acute anxiety attacks
   — Orthostasis
   — Flushing *may* follow initial upper body pallor
5 Aspects distinguishing diagnosis from carcinoid syndrome
   — Pallor > flushing
   — Hypertension > hypotension
   — Constipation > diarrhea
   — Cardiomyopathy > valve defects
6 **C**omplications
   — **C**onstipation
   — **C**ardiomyopathy
   — **C**erebral hemorrhage
   — **C**holelithiasis
   — **C**hronic renal failure
   — **C**arcinoma (medullary) of thyroid (MEN2; p. 115–116)
   — **C**ushing's syndrome (ACTH secretion by tumor)

DISORDERS OF GROWTH AND SEXUAL DEVELOPMENT

Presentations of congenital adrenal hyperplasia
1 21-hydroxylase deficiency
   — Commonest (90%) subtype; allele → 1: 50*
   — ↓ Aldosterone/cortisol → hypotension, salt-wasting
   — Secondary ↑ ACTH → ↑ androgens (incl. testosterone)
     • Precocious puberty in males (but *atrophic* testes)
     • Virilization in females
   — ↑ Urinary 17-hydroxysteroids
   — ↓ Plasma renin activity
2 3-β-hydroxysteroid dehydrogenase‡ deficiency
   — ↓ Cortisol/aldosterone → hypotension, salt-wasting
   — ↓ Testosterone (primary) → sexual infantilism
     • Male pseudohermaphroditism
   — Secondary ↑ ACTH → ↑ DHEA (weak androgen) →
     • Female virilization
   — ↑ Urinary 17-ketosteroids
3 11-β-hydroxylase deficiency
   — ↓ Cortisol/aldosterone → ↑ DOC¶
     • Hypertension (in 70%)
   — ↑ ACTH → ↑ androgens (like 21-hydroxylase deficiency)
     • Precocious puberty, virilization
   — ↑ Urinary 17-hydroxy- *and* 17-ketosteroids

4 17-α-hydroxylase deficiency
   — ↓ Cortisol → 2° ↑ aldosterone → hypertension, ↓ K⁺
   — ↓ Testosterone → sexual infantilism
     • Male pseudohermaphroditism
     • Primary amenorrhea in females
   — Urinary 17-hydroxysteroids and 17-ketosteroids
5 18-hydroxylase deficiency (very rare)
   — ↓ Aldosterone → salt-wasting
   — Normal cortisol/ACTH/androgens; no genital defects
   — Normal 17-hydroxysteroids and 17-ketosteroids
   — ↑ Plasma renin activity

* Heterozygotes detectable by post-ACTH ratio of 17-hydroxyprogesterone to 11-desoxycorticosterone (<12 in normals, >12 in heterozygotes)
‡ Inhibited by licorice ingestion (causes transient hypertension)
¶ 11-desoxycorticosterone

Phenotypes of abnormal sexual development
1 Klinefelter's syndrome
   — Karyotype: XXY (due to chromosomal non-dysjunction)
   — Eunuchoid male with small firm (hyalinized) testes
2 Turner's syndrome
   — Karyotype: XO (due to chromosomal non-dysjunction)
   — Prepubertal female with streak (vestigial) ovaries
3 True hermaphroditism
   — Karyotype: XX/XY (due to dizygotic fusion)
   — Ambiguous genitalia with ovary + testis (or ovotestis)
4 Male pseudohermaphroditism: *androgen insensitivity syndrome* (complete or partial)
   — Formerly designated 'testicular feminization'
   — Due to mutations affecting androgen receptors
   — Karyotype: XY (X-linked defective androgen receptor)
   — ↑ LH, testosterone levels (end-organ insensitivity)
   — Physical features
     • 'Normal' breasts
     • Short vagina (absent uterus/oviducts)
     • ↓↓ Axillary/genital hair
     • Clitoromegaly, 'bulging groins'
   — Presents with
     • Inguinal herniae (containing testes)
     • Primary amenorrhea in adolescence/adulthood
   — R_x: Castrate after puberty (prevents gonad neoplasia)
5 Male pseudohermaphroditism: *5-α-reductase deficiency*
   — Karyotype: XY (autosomal recessive, but signs → males)
   — Failure to activate testosterone to dihydrotestosterone
   — Causes 'penis-at-twelve' syndrome: masculinization occurs at puberty due to ↑↑ testosterone secretion
   — Prepubertal phenotype: male with hypospadias, epispadias or vagina, impalpable prostate, cryptorchidism, micropenis
6 Female pseudohermaphroditism
   — Karyotype: XX

— Seen in congenital adrenal hyperplasia: 21-hydroxylase, 11-β-hydroxylase or 3-β-dehydrogenase deficiency
— *Partial* enzyme defects may manifest only with hirsutism or menstrual irregularities

Differential diagnosis of dwarfism
1 Dwarfism with normal limb proportions
   — Growth hormone deficiency (e.g. hypopituitarism)
   — Severe systemic disease
2 Dwarfism with disproportionately short limbs
   — Achondroplasia
   — Ellis van Creveld syndrome
   — Hereditary hypophosphatasia

Diseases associated with gynecomastia
1 Paraneoplastic β-HCG production
   — Testicular germ-cell tumor, choriocarcinoma
   — Adrenal tumors
2 Primary or secondary hypogonadism
   Androgen insensitivity syndromes
3 Systemic disease
   — Chronic liver disease
   — Thyrotoxicosis
   — Renal failure ± hemodialysis
4 Drugs (p. 116)

Headaches associated with bilateral testicular enlargement?
1 Mumps
2 FSH-secreting pituitary adenoma

Differential diagnosis of cryptorchidism
1 Hypothalamic disease
   — e.g. Kallmann's syndrome (↓ GnRH)
2 Pituitary disease
   — e.g. Anencephaly (↓ LH)
3 Testicular (Leydig cell) insufficiency
   — 5-α-reductase deficiency (↓ DHT)
   — 3-β-dehydrogenase deficiency (↓ testosterone)
4 Testicular (Sertoli cell) insufficiency
   — e.g. Hernia uteri inguinalis (↓ AMH*)
5 Spermatic cord defects
   — e.g. Testicular feminization (androgen resistance)

* Anti-Müllerian hormone

INVESTIGATING ENDOCRINE DISEASE

THE PITUITARY AND HYPOTHALAMUS

Tests of hypothalamic integrity
1 Insulin tolerance (hypoglycemia) test →
   — ↑ Cortisol (i.e. implies ↑ CRH → ↑ ACTH*)
   — ↑ Growth hormone (GH; due to ↑ GHRF)
   — ↑ Somatostatin, dopamine
2 Clomiphene stimulation →
   — ↑ LH, FSH (GnRH)
3 Metyrapone (11-β-hydroxylase inhibitor) test →
   — ↑ ACTH (CRH)

— ↑ Urinary 17-hydroxysteroids
— *Exaggerated* response in (pituitary) Cushing's disease
4 Water deprivation test‡ →
   — ↑ ADH (synthesized in hypothalamus)

* In *long-standing* hypoadrenalism, give tetracosactrin (synthetic ACTH, 'Synacthen') for 2 weeks to prevent false-positives due to adrenal atrophy
‡ *Inappropriate* (dangerous) for diagnosis of *acute* diabetes insipidus, e.g. post-microadenomectomy

Contraindications to insulin tolerance testing*
1 Hypoadrenalism (unless pretreated with dexamethasone)
2 Ischemic heart disease
3 Epilepsy

* Note that for assessing HPA axis integrity following long-term steroids, a CRH stimulation test (or short 'Synacthen' test) is almost as good as ITT

Tests of pituitary reserve post-hypophysectomy
1 TRH stimulation
        → ↑ TSH, ↑ prolactin
2 GnRH stimulation
        → ↑ LH, ↑ FSH
3 Arginine vasopressin stimulation
        → ↑ GH (in children)
4 Tetracosactrin/ACTH stimulation
        → ↑ Cortisol*

* Indirectly confirming normal *long-term* ACTH release; see above

Investigating pituitary function*
1 Screening: serum levels of *target* hormones
   — e.g. T_4, cortisol
2 Serum levels of *pituitary* hormones
   — e.g. TSH, prolactin
3 Pituitary hormone suppression (if *excess* suspected), e.g.
   — Dexamethasone suppression (↑ ACTH: Cushing's)
   — Glucose tolerance test (fail to suppress GH: acromegaly)
4 Pituitary hormone stimulation (if *deficiency* suspected), e.g.
   — 'Synacthen' test
   — GnRH stimulation (see below)

* NB: So-called 'non-functioning' (clinically silent) pituitary tumors may be detectable by measuring the α-subunit of glycoprotein hormones (FSH, LH, TSH) in peripheral blood

Common endocrine deficiencies post-hypophysectomy
1 ↓ GH increment on stimulation (80%)
2 ↓ FSH/LH (75%)
3 ↓ ACTH/TSH (40%)
   — *Always* signifies need for replacement

Imaging the pituitary gland
1 Lateral skull X-ray with coned views of the pituitary fossa
   — Sellar enlargement (pituitary tumor, empty sella)
   — Double floor of dorsum sellae (may be normal variant)
   — Erosion of posterior clinoid processes
   — Suprasellar calcification (craniopharyngioma)

2 High-resolution coronal-plane CT with contrast
   — Obviates need for pneumoencephalography to
     demonstrate suprasellar tumor extension
   — Metrizamide cisternography excludes empty sella
3 Magnetic resonance imaging (MRI)
   — Investigation of choice for suspected pituitary
     disease
   — More sensitive than CT for microadenomas
   — Clearly localizes tumor microanatomy
   — Reliably excludes giant aneurysm

Differential diagnosis of an enlarged sella turcica
1 Pituitary tumor
2 Primary hypothyroidism (hyperplasia of TSH-
   secreting cells)
3 Pregnancy
4 Empty sella syndrome

Features of empty sella syndrome
1 Reflects arachnoid herniation via sellar diaphragm
   Pituitary is flattened against sellar floor; pituitary
   stalk may be laterally deviated
2 May be primary (congenital) or secondary to
   — Surgery, radiotherapy
   — Tumor infarction; classically affects obese
     hypertensive multipara
3 Most have normal pituitary function 15% have mild
   hyperprolactinemia
4 Degree of sellar enlargement correlates with
   probability of pituitary dysfunction
5 Factors making the diagnosis unlikely
   — Visual field defect
   — Erosion of posterior clinoids/dorsum sellae on
     SXR

Laboratory diagnosis of acromegaly
1 Diagnostic serology
   — Failure to suppress plasma GH with oral glucose
     load*
   — ↑ Plasma IGF-1 level
2 Supportive serology
   — ↑↑ Fasting morning GH (10% false-negative rate)
   — Paradoxical GH elevation following TRH, GnRH
   — Loss of GH circadian rhythm
   — ↑ Prolactin (in 30%)
3 Supportive radiology
   — Enlarged sella turcica (in 90%)
   — Enlarged frontal sinuses; increased skull thickness
   — Macrognathia, underbite, wide-spaced teeth
   — 'Arrowhead' tufting of fingertips; ↑ jointspace
   — Heelpads > 22 mm thick (female), > 25 mm thick
     (male)
4 Confirmatory (post-operative) histology
   — Eosinophilic pituitary adenoma

* Currently the best test; normally suppresses to < 4 mU/L.
Random level < 1 mU/L effectively excludes acromegaly. Levels < 5
mU/L throughout GTT, or on multiple random samples, indicate
satisfactory treatment of acromegaly

Screening tests for growth hormone deficiency
1 Overnight urinary GH levels
2 Plasma levels of IGFBP-3*
3 Combined IGF-1 and IGF-2 plasma levels

* One of the IGF-binding proteins in serum

Diagnostic confirmation of growth hormone deficiency
1 Failure of GH rise following insulin hypoglycemia*
2 Failure of GH rise following physiologic stimuli
   — Exercise
   — Sleep
3 Failure of GH rise following pharmacologic stimuli
   — Arginine infusion
   — Clonidine

* Glucose < 2.2 mmol/L plus sweating, tachycardia; associated
with significant mortality and long-term neurologic damage

THYROID FUNCTION TESTS

A quick approach to excluding thyroid dysfunction
1 Suspected thyrotoxicosis? Order
   — TSH, *plus*
   — Free T_4, *plus*
   — Free T_3 (*if* free T_4 normal)
2 Suspected hypothyroidism? Order
   — TSH* (if *primary* hypothyroidism suspected)
   — Free T_4

* cf. plasma ACTH in Addison's disease – *no* use in monitoring
cortisol replacement (*unless* elevation occurs during post-
adrenalectomy cortisol replacement, indicating development of
Nelson's syndrome)
NB: Elevated TSH in patient receiving T_4 replacement may
indicate *non-compliance* (esp. if TSH fluctuates from test to test)
rather than under-replacement

Specific indications for T_3 radioimmunoassay
1 Suspected hyperthyroidism (T_3-toxicosis), esp. in
   elderly
2 Monitoring of thyroid status following
   discontinuation of antithyroid drugs
3 Diagnosis of amiodarone-induced thyrotoxicosis
   — To exclude euthyroid hyperthyroxinemia (p. 99)

NB: T_3 is produced by TSH-stimulated thyroid gland; hence,
typically *not* elevated in (say) factitious T_4-toxicosis

Clinical spectrum of thyroid dysfunction
1 T_3-toxicosis
   — Clinically toxic
   — ↑ T_3, normal free T_4
   — Commoner
     • In iodine-deficient communities
     • In toxic adenomas
     • Following ablative therapy for toxicosis
2 T_3-euthyroidism
   — Clinically euthyroid
   — ↓ T_4, normal/↑ T_3
   — Occurs in
     • Compensated (early) hypothyroidism
     • Ophthalmic Graves'
     • Functioning adenoma
3 T_4-toxicosis
   — Clinically toxic in 50% ('sick hyperthyroid')
   — ↑ T_4, ↓ T_3
4 Sick euthyroid
   — Clinically euthyroid (but sick)
   — ↓ T_3, ↑ rT_3 (reverse-T_3); ↑ T_3 receptors
   — ↓ T_4 (often), normal TSH

5 Euthyroid hyperthyroxinemia
   — Clinically euthyroid
   — $\uparrow T_4$ (total or free): variable TBG and total T_3
   — *Normal* TSH rise in response to TRH stimulation

Elevated T_3/T_4 with detectable TSH?

1 Euthyroid hyperthyroxinemia (see below)
   — T_3, T_4 *normal* by equilibrium dialysis assay
2 TSH-secreting pituitary tumor
   — Associated with $\uparrow\uparrow$ SHBG ($\pm$ abnormal CT)
3 Thyroid hormone resistance syndrome*
   — $\uparrow\uparrow$ Free α-subunit:total TSH ratio

* Usually due to mutant ligand-binding domain of thyroid hormone receptor

Differential diagnosis of euthyroid hyperthyroxinemia

1 Elevated thyroid-binding globulin (any cause)
2 Familial dysalbuminemic hyperthyroxinemia
3 Hyperemesis gravidarum
4 Iatrogenic
   — Iodine-rich drugs, e.g. amiodarone
   — High-dose propranolol

Thyrotoxicosis with low radioactive iodine uptake

1 Thyroiditis (see p. 115)
   — Subacute granulomatous (de Quervain's) thyroiditis
   — Subacute lymphocytic ('silent') thyroiditis
     • Post-partum painless thyroiditis
     • Spontaneously resolving hyperthyroidism
   — Chronic lymphocytic thyroiditis ('Hashitoxicosis')
2 Iatrogenic
   — Recent iodine exposure (Jod–Basedow phenomenon)
   — Incompletely radioiodine-treated Graves' disease
   — Thyrotoxicosis factitia* (self-administration of T_4)
3 Neoplastic
   — *Struma ovarii*
   — Functioning metastases from follicular thyroid Ca
   — Extrinsic compression of normal gland by tumor mass

* Characterized by low thyroglobulin levels

Indications for a TRH stimulation test*

1 Investigation of symptomatic patients with inappropriately normal (or elevated) plasma TSH
   — TSH-induced hyperthyroidism (pituitary adenoma)
   — Thyroid hormone resistance syndromes
2 Assessment following pituitary surgery or irradiation
   — Documentation of adequate thyrotropin (TSH) reserve following pituitary irradiation and/or surgery
   — Documentation of adequate treatment of acromegaly; i.e. TRH does *not* cause $\uparrow$ GH
   — Documentation of adequate excision of prolactinoma; i.e. TRH $\rightarrow$ *no change* in serum prolactin
3 Evaluation of hypogonadism with borderline LH/FSH
   — Delayed puberty (TRH $\rightarrow$ $\uparrow$ prolactin) *vs.*
   — Hypogonadotropic hypogonadism (TRH $\rightarrow$ *no change* in prolactin)

4 Characterization of 'non-functioning' pituitary adenomas
   — LH/FSH (or β-subunit) rise indicates cell of origin

* NB: The advent of highly sensitive TSH assays has now almost eliminated this test

Abnormalities of the TRH stimulation test

1 'Flat' TSH response
   — Thyrotoxicosis (primary)
   — 'Euthyroid' patients with
     • Ophthalmic Graves' disease
     • Functioning adenoma
     • Recently treated toxicosis
     • Multinodular goiter
   — Other: acromegaly, Cushing's, L-DOPA use
2 Exaggerated or prolonged TSH rise
   — Primary hypothyroidism
   — Pregnancy

INVESTIGATING THE DIABETIC PATIENT

Indications for a glucose tolerance test

1 Pregnancy
   — Glycosuria
   — Risk factors for diabetes mellitus
2 Non-diagnostic elevation of blood glucose *plus* glycosuria
3 Investigation of peripheral neuropathy

Abnormalities of the glucose tolerance test

1 Pronounced glycemia
   — Diabetes mellitus
2 'Flat' response
   — Malabsorption
   — Addison's disease
3 'Lag storage' curve
   — Post-gastrectomy
   — Thyrotoxicosis
   — Chronic liver disease

Indications for home blood glucose monitoring (HBGM)

1 Stabilization of any young or insulin-dependent diabetic
2 Gestational diabetes
3 Abnormal renal threshold for glucose (e.g. renal failure)
4 Impaired color vision (e.g. due to retinopathy + photocoagulation; hinders urinalysis interpretation)
5 Unexplained insomnia, anxiety attacks, angina or epilepsy

Factors elevating the glycosylated hemoglobin (HbA$_{1c}$) level

1 Hyperglycemia (in previous 8 weeks), esp. ketoacidosis
2 Hypertriglyceridemia
3 Pregnancy (first and second trimester)
4 Renal failure
5 Iron deficiency
   Hereditary spherocytosis (post-splenectomy)
   Elevated HbF (e.g. thalassemia): mimics HbA$_{1c}$
6 Aspirin/alcohol ingestion

Factors depressing the HbA$_{1c}$ level
1 Reticulocytosis (e.g. hemolysis, hemorrhage) + anemia
2 Pregnancy (third trimester)
3 Assay performed in hot environment

Practical limitations of HbA$_{1c}$ measurement
1 Only reflects glycemic control over previous 8 weeks*. Hence, *not* useful in monitoring short-term therapy; home blood glucose monitoring (HBGM) is essential for this
2 Fasting glucose measures may be more reliable in diagnosing and monitoring patients with type II diabetes

* cf. serum *fructosamine*: reflects shorter-term glycemic control, thus may be useful during (say) pregnancy

Technical considerations in diabetic monitoring
1 *Arterial* glucose levels are higher than venous; capillary blood samples are intermediate
2 *Plasma* glucose is 10% higher than whole blood
3 Glucose metabolism continues (i.e. levels decline) in vitro at ~ 3–4% per hour (esp. in heparinized whole blood), making it imperative to use inhibitors (e.g. NaF, Li) and process samples promptly
4 Urine glucose monitoring is useless in patients with normal renal thresholds, since good diabetic control should keep glucose below the glycosuric level

Urinary ketone detection and significance
1 Urinary dipstick tests detect reaction of only one ketone body (acetoacetate) with nitroprusside
2 Other ketones (acetone, β-hydroxybutyrate) may predominate in hypoxic patients, yet be undetected by dipstick
3 Heavy ketonuria combined with glycosuria indicates developing ketoacidosis
4 Mild ketonuria can occur during fasting or pregnancy

HYPOGLYCEMIA

Predispositions to recurrent hypoglycemia
1 Inappropriate insulin regimen, e.g.
   — 'Sliding scale' urinalysis with renal glycosuria
   — Somogyi effect (p. 101)
   — Inadvertent IM injections
   — Low renal threshold, patient monitoring urinalysis*
2 Insulin sensitivity
   — Renal failure
   — Celiac disease; diabetic gastroparesis
   — Hypothyroidism
3 Alcohol abuse
4 Absence of neuroglycopenic 'warning signs'
   — Recurrent hypoglycemia, e.g. due to insulinoma
   — Coexisting hypoadrenalism ± hypopituitarism‡
   — Autonomic neuropathy
   — β-blockade (esp. non-selective)
5 Factitious hyperinsulinism or sulphonylurea ingestion
   Non-compliance, manipulative behavior (esp. adolescents)

* Largely a theoretical hazard these days
‡ e.g. post-hypophysectomy for retinopathy

Hypoglycemia without hyperinsulinemia?
1 Alcohol ingestion
   — Inhibits hepatic gluconeogenesis (as does lactic acidosis)
   — Usually presents as hypothermic coma in semi-starved alcoholics with depleted hepatic glycogen
2 Non-islet cell tumors (release IGF-2)
   — Bulky mesenchymal tumors (e.g. fibrosarcoma)
   — Hepatoma, adrenal carcinoma
3 Sepsis
   — esp. *P. falciparum*
4 Physiologic
   — Starvation
   — Prolonged exercise
   — Post-prandial (rare)
5 Iatrogenic
   — Oral hypoglycemics
   — Post-Polya gastrectomy (late dumping)
   — Salicylism (in children)
   — Propranolol (inhibits hepatic glycogenolysis)

Insulinoma: making the diagnosis
1 Clinical
   — Symptoms (syncope, amnesia) on fasting or exercise
   — Symptoms accompanied by low plasma glucose
   — Symptoms relieved by glucose
2 Screening test: three overnight 16-hour fasts
   — Blood sugar abnormally low in 90% of insulinomas
   — Non-suppression of insulin (> 6 μU/mL) and C-peptide
   — ↓ C-peptide/proinsulin? Factitious hypoglycemia
3 Supporting tests
   — Elevated fasting insulin: glucose ratio
   — High proinsulin (> 20% total insulin)
   — Stimulation of insulin secretion by calcium infusion
4 Insulin (or tolbutamide) tolerance test
   — Non-suppression of proinsulin and/or C-peptide
   — Non-suppression excludes post-prandial hypoglycemia
5 Tumor localization and biopsy
   — CT and/or angiography (initial work-up)
   — Endoscopic or intraoperative ultrasonography

NB: Paradoxically, insulinoma may be associated with post-prandial hyperglycemia, since normal post-prandial ↑ insulin may be suppressed

Factitious hypoglycemia
1 Clinical: recurrent hypoglycemia in a (para)medically employed patient or member of diabetic patient's family
2 Grossly elevated plasma insulin during attacks
3 Low proinsulin and/or C-peptide levels (cf. insulinoma)
4 Insulin antibodies may be assayed if porcine insulin used
5 Sulfonylurea abuse may lead to elevated insulin and C-peptide levels, normal proinsulin levels and positive urine/serum drug screens

NB: Most iatrogenic hypoglycemia is *inadvertent*; cf. thyrotoxicosis factitia

NOCTURNAL HYPOGLYCEMIA

Nocturnal hypoglycemia: diagnostic considerations
1 Clinical
   — Nocturnal distress, nightmares
   — Mental dullness/depression
   — Morning headaches and/or hypothermia
   — Onset of idiopathic epilepsy
2 Overnight voided urine sample
   — ↑ Cortisol/creatinine ratio
3 Confirm hypoglycemia
   — 3 a.m. (inpatient) blood sugar

Nocturnal hypoglycemia: the Somogyi effect
1 Suggested by confirmation of nocturnal
   hypoglycemia associated with a.m. urinalysis →
   glucose + ketones
2 Pathogenesis: nocturnal hypoglycemia due to insulin
   overtreatment causes compensatory release of
   glucose-mobilizing hormones (e.g. cortisol, catecholamines) resulting in paradoxical waking
   hyperglycemia
3 For diagnosis, distinguish
   — *Dawn effect* (greater endogenous a.m. insulin
     requirement) from
   — *Somogyi effect* (where hyperglycemia occurs due
     to reactive, rather than circadian, excess of
     counter-regulatory hormones)

Nocturnal hypoglycemia: therapeutic approach
1 Supper late
   — Complex carbohydrate, protein
2 Extra supper if
   — Heavy evening exercise, *or*
   — Glucose < 6.5 mmol/L
3 Give intermediate-acting insulin
   — At bedtime instead of with the evening meal
   — In thigh, not in abdominal wall
4 Use longer-acting evening insulin
   — e.g. Isophane, ultralente

DIAGNOSING DIABETES AND ITS COMPLICATIONS

Rapid assessment of glucose tolerance using single plasma levels
1 Random glucose < 8 mmol/L
   Fasting glucose < 6 mmol/L
   — Normal
2 Random glucose 8–11 mmol/L
   Fasting glucose 6–8 mmol/L
   — Impaired glucose tolerance
3 Random glucose > 11 mmol/L
   Fasting glucose > 8 mmol/L
   — Diabetes mellitus

Assessing diabetic treatment using glycosylated hemoglobin*
1 HbA_{1c} < 10%
   — Reasonable control
2 HbA_{1c} 10–14%
   — Control can be improved: ?compliance ?regimen

3 HbA_{1c} > 15%
   — Treatment plan needs major overhaul

* HbA_{1c} normal range = 5–8.5%

Hyperosmolar coma: making the diagnosis
1 Blood glucose level > 50 mmol/L
   Serum osmolality < 340 mosmol
2 Minimal or absent ketonuria and acidosis
3 Azotemia and/or hypernatremia (if severe or
   prolonged)
4 Plasma insulin usually detectable; lactate/alcohol
   usually not

Indications for renal biopsy in diabetes mellitus
1 Red cell casts or persistent (micro)hematuria (sterile
   urine)
2 Unusually early (e.g. no retinopathy) or rapid
   nephropathy

INVESTIGATING ADRENAL DISEASE

Diagnostic sequence in suspected Cushing's syndrome
1 Overnight dexamethasone (1–2 mg) suppression test
   — 10–30% false-positive results (see below)
2 Extended low-dose dexamethasone suppression
   — 0.5 mg q 6 h for 48 h; collect urine for free cortisol
   — Best single screening test
3 24-h urinary free cortisol
   — Unless renal impairment
4 Plasma ACTH
5 8 a.m. and midnight cortisol levels
6 CRH stimulation test
   — Establishes ACTH dependency (see below)
   — Distinguishes pituitary and ectopic ACTH
7 MRI of sella with gadolinium and T1-weighted
   images
8 CT of adrenals (± thorax, abdomen if ectopic ACTH)

NB: No *single* test should be relied upon

False-positive 1 mg dexamethasone suppression tests*
1 Simple obesity (cf. false-negatives: rare)
2 Non-compliance (check dexamethasone level)
3 Depression
4 Alcoholism
5 Iatrogenic
   — Estrogens
   — Antiandrogens: spironolactone, cyproterone
   — Phenytoin, alcohol, other enzyme inducers

* Occur in up to 20% of tests

Features of alcohol-induced pseudo-Cushing's syndrome
1 Vaguely 'Cushingoid' appearance
   — Central adiposity
   — Bruising
   — Myopathy
   — Osteoporosis, rib fractures
   — Hypertension; impaired glucose tolerance
   — Depression, psychosis
2 Typical biochemical abnormalities
   — Increased free plasma or urinary cortisol*

— Decreased circadian rhythm of plasma cortisol‡
— Overnight (1 mg) dexamethasone → no suppression

3 Spironolactone treatment for ascites may underlie some false-positive tests

4 Distinguished from 'true' Cushing's by
— Extended (2-day) dexamethasone suppression followed by CRH stimulation test
— Naloxone stimulation test: detects pseudo-Cushing's CRH *hyper*secretion (cf. true Cushing's: ↓ CRH)

* esp. following (1) ethanol withdrawal or (2) liver damage leading to impaired production of cortisol-binding globulin (CBG)
‡ *Poor* sensitivity and specificity for diagnosis of Cushing's

Features of 'food-dependent' Cushing's syndrome

1 Arises due to aberrant adrenal *sensitivity* to GIP (glucose-dependent insulinotrophic polypeptide; p. 141), presumably reflecting 'illicit' adrenal gland expression of GIP receptors

2 GIP hypersensitivity leads to *ACTH-independent* bilateral adrenal hyperplasia (may be nodular)

3 Ingestion of meals leads to elevated cortisol levels paralleling rises in GIP; *no* abnormality of GIP regulation or secretion

4 Responsive to octreotide (p. 105)

ACTH dependence of Cushing's syndrome

1 ACTH-dependent
— ↑ ACTH on CRH stimulation
• Cushing's disease*
• Ectopic ACTH (or CRH) syndrome

2 ACTH-independent
— *No* ↑ ACTH on CRH stimulation
• Food-(GIP receptor) dependent Cushing's
• Adrenocortical tumors (cortisol-secreting)

* NB: Peripheral plasma ACTH levels are often in the normal range – rather than elevated – in pituitary Cushing's. ACTH levels from the inferior petrosal sinus may be of greater sensitivity here (see below)

Etiological clues in established Cushing's syndrome

1 Pituitary Cushing's ('disease')
— High-dose (8 mg/day) dexamethasone → cortisol *suppression* (< 10% basal levels)
— CRH test → *normal* ↑ ACTH (in 90%)
— Inferior petrosal sinus ACTH at least double plasma ACTH (cf. in ectopic ACTH: < 1.8)
— Petrosal sinus sampling also *lateralizes* pituitary lesion following CRH stimulation

2 Primary adrenal adenoma
— Plasma ACTH undetectable; no rise with CRH
— ⁷⁵Se/NP59 scanning: lateralizes lesion (cf. hyperplasia)

3 Primary adrenal carcinoma
— Urinary cortisol excretion may exceed 5000 nmol/ 24 h
— Plasma ACTH undetectable
— ↑ DHEA/urinary 17-ketosteroids
— ↑ Testosterone in females
— ⁷⁵Selenium scanning if lesion not visible on CT*

4 Ectopic ACTH secretion
— Absolute plasma ACTH level may exceed 500 ng/L

— Urinary cortisol excretion may exceed 5000 nmol/ 24 h
— Metyrapone/CRH test → no (further) ↑ ACTH‡

5 Alcohol- or depression-induced pseudo-Cushing's syndrome
— Normal insulin hypoglycemia test (p. 97)

* Adrenal nodular hyperplasia may occur in pituitary Cushing's; hence, visualization of adrenal nodule is *not* diagnostic of primary adrenal tumor. Note also that NP59 scan is often *negative* in adrenal carcinoma
‡ Exception: ACTH-secreting bronchial carcinoids. Note also that tumors may secrete 'big ACTH' which can be missed by some ACTH assays

Diagnostic approach to the patient with an adrenal mass

1 Key symptoms and signs
— Hypertension
• Absent? Pheo-, Conn's, Cushing's *unlikely*
— Hirsuties, virilization
• Assay plasma androgens (DHEA, testosterone)
— Obesity
• Absence makes Cushing's unlikely

2 Key investigations
— Hypokalemia
• Absence virtually excludes Conn's
— CT mass > 6 cm diameter
• Favors carcinoma over other lesions
— Urinary VMA, metanephrines, catecholamines
• To exclude pheochromocytoma

Conn's syndrome (primary hyperaldosteronism): diagnosis

1 Suggestive presentations
— Unexpected occurrence of severe hypokalemia in a mild hypertensive on diuretic therapy
— *Untreated* hypertensive with hypokalemia and urinary potassium excretion > 30 mmol/24 h*

2 Proposed screening tests
— High-salt diet (→ *persistent* hypokalemia)
— Lack of aldosterone suppressibility despite
• High-salt diet or intravenous sodium loading
• Oral fludrocortisone or captopril
— Aldosterone elevation following IV metoclopramide
— Plasma aldosterone:renin ratio > 30:1

3 Dexamethasone suppression test *if* screening test positive
— Glucocorticoid-suppressible hyperaldosteronism‡
— Suppressibility contraindicates laparotomy

4 Tests distinguishing aldosterone-producing adenomas (70%) from bilateral adrenal hyperplasia (30%)
— Angiotensin II → *no* ↑ aldosterone if adenoma
— Selenocholesterol (or NP59) scan
— Venous catheterization + effluent analysis
— Biopsy (cf. excision: *only* indicated for adenoma)

* NB: Untreated renovascular or 'malignant' hypertension may also be associated with hypokalemia due to secondary hyperaldosteronism
‡ Dominant disorder associated with 8q22 genetic locus, family history of CVA, variable blood pressure and increased urinary excretion of 18-oxocortisol (cf. adrenal hyperplasia); hyperaldosteronism here is ACTH-driven

Bartter's syndrome (primary hyperreninemia): diagnosis
1 Usually presents in childhood with failure to thrive, enuresis (due to potassium-depletion nephropathy) and weakness
2 Normotensive (intravascular hypovolemia); no edema
3 Low serum potassium, elevated urinary potassium Hypochloremic metabolic alkalosis
4 Elevated urinary chloride*
5 Insensitivity to IV angiotensin or vasopressin Hypersensitivity to IV saralasin‡ or captopril
6 Therapeutic response to indomethacin

* cf. diuretic abuse, laxative abuse, surreptitious bulimic vomiting; p. 300
‡ an angiotensin II inhibitor

Liddle's syndrome (pseudohyperaldosteronism): diagnosis
1 Hypertension
2 Low aldosterone levels
3 Responds to salt restriction or triamterene

Pheochromocytoma: how to diagnose your first
1 24-h urinary free catecholamines/VMA
2 Plasma adrenaline/noradrenaline: sample taken at rest via an indwelling needle inserted 30 min previously
3 Pentolinium (or clonidine) catecholamine suppression test
4 Whole-body ^{131}I-MIBG scanning*
5 Abdominal CT scanning
6 Selective venous sampling or angiography (premedicate with the β-blocker phenoxybenzamine for 3 days first)

NB: No *single* investigation excludes the diagnosis
* esp. useful for extraadrenal, multiple or metastatic pheos

Secondary adrenal insufficiency after long-term steroids?
1 Short 'Synacthen' (tetracosactrin) test
2 CRH stimulation test
3 Insulin tolerance test (p. 97)

DISORDERS OF SEXUAL FUNCTION

Approach to investigation of amenorrhea
1 Measure urinary HCG to exclude pregnancy
2 ↑ FSH
— Proceed to karyotyping if 'primary' amenorrhea
— Consider diagnosis of premature menopause
3 ↓ FSH: perform
— Serum prolactin
— Thyroid function tests (esp. TSH)
— Skull X-ray + coronal CT/visual field mapping
4 ↓ FSH and ↑ LH: perform GnRH stimulation to confirm Stein–Leventhal syndrome (→ exaggerated LH response)
5 ↑ Testosterone: consider
— Testicular feminization
— 5-α-reductase deficiency*

* cf. 17-ketoreductase deficiency → ↓ testosterone

Laboratory features of anorexia nervosa
1 ↓ FSH/LH/17β-estradiol/DHEA
2 Normal serum prolactin
3 'Sick euthyroid' (p. 98)
Delayed peak following TRH- and GnRH-stimulation
4 ↑ GH/ACTH/cortisol
5 Hyposthenuria

Hirsutism: clinical and laboratory characterization
1 Exclude racial or familial causes
2 Exclude drug-induced causes
— Phenytoin
— Minoxidil, diazoxide
— Steroids, cyclosporin A; androgens
3 ↑ Plasma DHEA/urinary 17-ketosteroids
— Adrenal origin (e.g. tumor)
↑ ACTH-inducible rise in 17-hydroxyprogesterone
— Late-onset 21-hydroxylase deficiency (p. 96)
4 ↑↑ Testosterone, normal DHEA
— Ovarian origin (e.g. Sertoli–Leydig cell tumor*)
5 LH:FSH > 2.5 *plus* ↑ free testosterone
— Stein–Leventhal syndrome (see below)

* 'arrhenoblastoma' (term no longer used)

Gonadotrophic characterization of amenorrhea
1 ↑ FSH
— Ovarian failure (1°/2°)
2 ↑ LH, ↓ FSH
— Polycystic ovary (Stein–Leventhal) syndrome
3 ↑ LH, normal FSH
— Pregnancy
4 ↓ FSH, ↓ LH
— Hypopituitarism
5 ↓ FSH, ↑ prolactin
— Hyperprolactinemia + prolactinoma

Differential diagnosis of hyperprolactinemia
1 Pregnancy or puerperium
2 Pituitary tumor
3 Myxedema
4 Renal failure
5 Drugs, esp. phenothiazines

Elevated prolactin levels: quantitative significance
1 Plasma prolactin > 5000 mU/L (200 ng/mL)
— Prolactinoma (diagnostic)
2 Plasma prolactin < 1500 mU/L
— Non-prolactinoma hyperprolactinemia
3 Intermediate levels
— Prolactinoma (consistent)
— 'Pseudo-prolactinoma'*

* 'Non-functioning' pituitary tumor compressing pituitary stalk

Investigating infertility in the menstruating female
1 Check ovulation
— Chart basal body temperature for several months
— Measure midluteal phase serum progesterone
2 Serum prolactin
3 Laparoscopy in secretory phase with diagnostic curettage

— Diagnosis
  • Endometriosis
  • Polycystic ovaries
  • Unruptured luteinized follicles
— Therapy
  • Hydrotubation (tubal insufflation)

Features of polycystic ovaries (Stein–Leventhal syndrome)

1 Symptoms due to abnormal metabolism of
  — Androgens (and related steroid hormones)
  — Insulin
2 Common symptoms
  — Progressive hirsutism (often since adolescence), acne
  — Irregular periods (± infertility, amenorrhea)
  — Weight gain, obesity (due to hyperinsulinemia)
3 Supportive investigations
  — Abnormal glucose tolerance test
    • Subclinical insulin resistance common
  — Abnormal pelvic ultrasound*
    • Polycystic ovaries in 80%
  — Abnormal lipids
    • esp. ↓ HDL_2
4 Sex hormones
  — ↑ Free testosterone
  — ↑ Plasma LH; LH:FSH ratio > 2.5

* NB: The sonographic finding of polycystic ovaries is non-specific (i.e. found in up to 20% of 'normal' women – including some young children – as well as in other hyperandrogenic anovulatory conditions) and hence of little diagnostic value. It is also insensitive, being false-negative in 10–20% of women with polycystic ovaries. Hence, pelvic ultrasound is typically of little value in assessment of infertility or hirsutism

Investigation of males with abnormal sexual phenotype

1 Small (firm) testes, hypogonadal, ↑ FSH
  — Karyotype (?Klinefelter's)
2 Small testes, virilized
  — 17-OH-progesterone (?congenital adrenal hyperplasia)
3 Normal testicular size, ↑ FSH
  — Irreversible azoospermia (e.g. tubular hyalinization)
4 Normal testicular size, azoospermia, normal FSH
  — Varicocele
  — Epididymal/vas obstruction (e.g. Young's syndrome)
5 Normal testicular size, azoospermia, ↓ FSH
  — Exclude pituitary tumor
6 Absent pubic hair*
  — Investigate for gonadal failure

* cf. females: absent pubic hair implies *adrenal* failure

Criteria for normal semen analysis

1 Ejaculate volume ≥ 1.5–6 mL
2 Number ≥ 20×10^6/mL*
3 Motility ≥ 60% active forward progression
4 Morphology ≥ 60% normal oval shapes

NB: Evaluate three times over a 6–12 week period before concluding azoospermia
* Number may drop during (hot) summer; 'contraceptive' azoospermia may also be inducible by weekly testosterone injections

Pituitary tumors: therapeutic considerations

1 Transsphenoidal microadenomectomy
  — Good results in Cushing's disease, esp. in children
  — Complications: CSF rhinorrhea, diabetes insipidus
  — 10 year recurrence rate averages 25%
2 Transfrontal hypophysectomy
  — Treatment of choice for patients with macro-adenomas and/or visual symptoms or signs
  — Usual first-line treatment for craniopharyngioma
3 Radiotherapy (incl. ⁹⁰yttrium implantation)
  — Reduction of adenoma size/function may take *years**
  — High incidence of subsequent hypopituitarism
  — Occasionally complicated by (late) pituitary apoplexy
4 Medical management
  — Somatostatin analogues
    • Octreotide (SMS 201-995), esp. for acromegaly → tumor shrinkage in up to 50%
    • Add UDCA (p. 138) to prevent gallstones
  — D_2 receptor agonists‡
    • Cabergoline; lisuride, pergolide, quinagolide
    • Bromocriptine (less effective than cabergoline in reducing prolactin levels)
  — Metyrapone (11-β-hydroxylase inhibitor)
    • For Cushing's disease presurgery
5 Bilateral adrenalectomy
  — For Cushing's disease *not* cured by adenomectomy
  — Must also irradiate pituitary to prevent Nelson's

* Hence, *inappropriate* for patients with visual symptoms or infertility
‡ *First-line* therapy for prolactinomas or hyperprolactinemic hypogonadism

Replacement therapy in panhypopituitarism

1 Cortisone acetate 25 mg mane 12.5 mg nocte*
2 Thryoxine 100–150 µg/day
3 Intranasal dDAVP 2–6 times per day
4 Conception not desired
  — Females: daily combined oral contraceptive pill
  — Males: IM testosterone enanthate every 2–3 weeks
5 Conception desired: short-term administration of either
  — FSH, *or*
  — HCG, *or*
  — Low-dose pulsatile GnRH analogues

* May monitor adequacy of replacement with plasma renin activity

Metabolic effects of growth hormone replacement

1 Increased lean body mass (anabolic effect)*
2 Increased basal metabolic rate
3 Increased muscle strength, heart and exercise capacity
4 Increased bone mass, density (and turnover)
5 Increased GFR, renal plasma flow
6 Increased plasma glucose (catabolic effect)
7 Reduced plasma LDL-cholesterol‡

8 Sodium retention, edema
9 Improved sleep, social functioning, well-being

* Note that in *adults* no change in *total* body weight usually occurs
‡ But ? also ↑ Lp(a)

SOMATOSTATIN ANALOGS

Main physiologic actions of somatostatin*
1 Effects on anterior pituitary
— Inhibits GH secretion (and thus IGF-1)
— Inhibits LH release
2 Effects on gut and peripheral hormones
— Inhibits insulin release
— Inhibits gastrin and CCK release
— Inhibits secretin release
— Inhibits motilin release
— Inhibits pancreatic polypeptide release
— Inhibits VIP release

* A hypothalamic tetradecapeptide also present in gut – gastric D cells and small intestine, by far the most abundant source – pancreatic islets and in the nervous system (myenteric and submucosal neural plexuses)

Indications for octreotide therapy
1 Acromegaly
2 Other pituitary adenomas
— ACTH-secreting tumors
— TSH-secreting tumors
— 'Non-secreting' pituitary adenomas*
3 Other hypersecreting endocrine tumors
— VIPoma
— Carcinoid syndrome
— Glucogonoma, insulinoma
4 GIP-receptor-dependent Cushing's (p. 102)
5 Variceal bleeding
— Safer and cheaper than vasopressin
6 Anecdotal indications
— Polycystic ovary syndrome
— Pancreatic pseudocysts
— Pancreatic and enterocutaneous fistulae
— Secretory diarrhea (e.g. cholera)
— Dumping syndrome
— Psoriasis
— Intestinal pseudoobstruction‡

* May relieve headache within minutes
‡ e.g. due to scleroderma; R_x may reduce bacterial overgrowth

Problems with octreotide therapy
1 Need for b.d. subcutaneous injections; expense
2 Impaired glucose tolerance
Diabetics receiving insulin or oral hypoglycemics may require close monitoring (glucagon release also inhibited)
3 May precipitate cholelithiasis (reduced gallbladder motility)
Biliary colic (rare)
4 Reduces gut absorption of cimetidine, cyclosporin
5 Thyroid function may be altered
6 Abdominal cramps, tenesmus, flatulence (common)
Steatorrhea (rare)

GOITER

Non-toxic multinodular goiter: management considerations
1 Reduction of nodule size using T_4 suppression (150–200 µg/day)* may be *less* effective if
— Goiter is long-standing
— TRH-stimulation test is 'flat'‡
2 Antithyroid drugs (thionamides) confer no benefit
3 Biopsy and/or thyroidectomy should be undertaken if no shrinkage within 3 months of conservative therapy
4 Carcinoma occasionally complicates multinodular goiter

* First ensure that goiter is not *already* associated with TSH suppression
‡ i.e. subclinical autonomous T_4 production (p. 99)

Approach to thyroid nodules
1 Clinical characterization
— Multiple nodules? fixed? nodes? bruit? euthyroid?
2 ^{99m}Tc scan
— 'Hot' nodule (1% cancer risk; exclude thyrotoxicosis)
— 'Cold' nodule (20% cancer risk*)
3 Ultrasound
— Smooth thin-walled cyst‡ → lower cancer risk
4 T_4-suppression
— Therapeutic trial for up to 3 months¶
5 Fine needle aspiration (FNA) cytology
— Negative cytology does *not* exclude malignancy (up to 25% of FNA results are indeterminate)
6 Thyroidectomy: partial or total
— Pending frozen section and operative findings

* i.e. increased malignancy risk; but *most* are benign
‡ Note, however, that cystic nodules per se are often malignant; i.e. ultrasound examination provides strictly limited reassurance on this score
¶ In practice, most solitary thyroid nodules *rarely* shrink in response to TSH suppression

Cytological diagnoses possible with fine needle aspiration
1 Thyroid cancer, esp. papillary*
2 Colloid goiter
3 Hashimoto's thyroiditis

* cf. follicular or Hürthle cell tumors: often require large-bore needle biopsy or excision for diagnosis

Complications of thyroidectomy
1 Short-term
— 'Thyroid storm' (if thyrotoxic preop)
— Hypocalcemia (hypoparathyroidism)
— Recurrent laryngeal nerve palsy; hemorrhage
2 Long-term
— Hypothyroidism (may be late or insidious)

THERAPY OF THYROTOXICOSIS

Thyroid storm: approach to management
1 Prevention
— Treat possible precipitating factors (e.g. sepsis)
— Render euthyroid prior to elective surgery

2   IV fluids as required to maintain BP; tepid sponge, fan
3   Propylthiouracil (PTU) 200 mg p.o. q 6 h
4   Potassium iodide 200 mg IV over 15 min (give 1 h post-PTU)
5   Propranolol 1 mg IV, then 2 mg IV q 4 h p. r. n.*
6   Dexamethasone in supraphysiological ('shock') dosage

* NB: β-blockers may *not* be contraindicated in rate-dependent thyrocardiac failure; use short-acting IV esmolol or combine propranolol with digoxin

Rationâle of dexamethasone therapy in thyroid storm
1   Prevents Addisonian crisis in patients with associated (albeit unrecognized) autoimmune hypoadrenalism
2   Inhibits glandular release of T_4
3   Inhibits peripheral conversion of $T_4 \rightarrow T_3$

Drugs inhibiting glandular release of thyroxine
1   Dexamethasone
2   Lithium
3   Iodine*

* cf. the *Wolff–Chaikoff effect,* where iodine inhibits organification/coupling

Pharmacological actions of propylthiouracil
1   Inhibits organification of tyrosine
2   Inhibits coupling of MIT (monoiodotyrosine) and DIT
3   Inhibits peripheral conversion of $T_4 \rightarrow T_3$

Management of thyrotoxicosis
1   Antithyroid drugs (carbimazole/methimazole, PTU)
    — Usually given for 12–18 month therapeutic trial
    — 60% patients relapse (99% of toxic adenoma patients)
    — Occasionally used long-term in elderly patients
2   Radioiodine (^{131}I)
    — Takes 2–3 months to achieve response
    — Teratogenic; contraindicated if pregnancy possible*
    — *Not* carcinogenic (cf. external thyroid radiation)
    — 30% will still be thyrotoxic after a single treatment
    — 60% will be hypothyroid within 20 years of treatment
    — Risk of deteriorating ophthalmopathy may be greater than with other antithyroid therapies
3   Subtotal thyroidectomy
    — Undertaken after thyrotoxicosis controlled, e.g. after 6 weeks' carbimazole + 1 week's iodine ± propranolol
    — 30% will be hypothyroid within 10 years of treatment
    — Losing popularity now to ^{131}I

* No longer contraindicated in young patients per se

Clinical monitors of response to antithyroid therapy
1   Slowing of heart rate
2   Weight gain
3   Goiter shrinkage

Factors predictive of prolonged remission to thionamides*
1   Small goiter

2   Reduction in goiter size on treatment
3   Mild thyrotoxicosis
4   T_3-toxicosis
5   Low or absent TSI titer
6   HLA-DRw3 negative

* Methimazole/carbimazole, propylthiouracil; inhibit organification of iodide and coupling of iodothyronine

Relative indications for PTU > methimazole/ carbimazole*
1   Thyroid storm
2   Pregnancy
3   Puerperium

* NB: In other circumstances methimazole is to be preferred; longer plasma half-life and lower risk of agranulocytosis

Potential indications for β-blockers
1   Rapid control of symptoms during initial treatment
2   Thionamide hypersensitivity or toxicity
3   Preparation for surgery

Factors contributing to high-output thyrotoxic heart failure
1   Factors contributing to volume overload
    — Reduced systemic vascular resistance
    — Increased blood volume*
    — Increased diastolic relaxation
2   Factors contributing to reduced diastolic filling
    — Increased heart rate
    — Increased stroke volume
    — Atrial fibrillation‡

* Treat with diuretics, but note that high-dose frusemide may compete with T_3/T_4 for TBG binding
‡ Slow ventricular rate with digoxin ± propranolol; larger than usual doses may be needed

Relative indications for ablative therapy in Graves' disease
1   Elderly patient
2   Poor compliance
3   Large goiter
4   Nodular change in goiter
5   Recurrent disease despite conservative therapy

Prerequisites for radioiodine therapy
1   Patient is not pregnant
2   Patient has been *already* rendered *euthyroid*

Relative indications for radioiodine therapy
1   Thyrotoxic patient relapsing following thionamide therapy
2   Thyrotoxic patient relapsing following thyroidectomy
3   Thyrotoxic patient normally treatable with surgery (e.g. toxic adenoma) but unfit for anesthesia
4   Euthyroid patient with metastatic differentiated thyroid cancer (esp. lung metastases from follicular cancer)

Indications for total thyroidectomy
1   Medullary thyroid carcinoma (± MEN2; p. 115)
2   Anaplastic thyroid carcinoma
3   Differentiated thyroid carcinoma involving both lobes

Indications for subtotal thyroidectomy in thyrotoxicosis

1 Thyrotoxic patient with large symptomatic goiter
   — e.g. SVC obstruction, thoracic outlet syndrome
2 Young thyrotoxic patient unable to tolerate thionamides
3 Young thyrotoxic woman desiring pregnancy

Graves' disease in pregnancy: management considerations

1 The placenta is crossed by
   — TSI (but not T_4) → fetal goiter
   — Thionamides: → fetal goiter*; teratogenic (PTU least)
   — ^{131}I (→ cretinism; teratogenic)
   — Propranolol (→ fetal bradycardia)
2 *Neonatal* hyperthyroidism (suggested by persistent fetal tachycardia) may pose greater risks than hypothyroidism‡
   — Intrauterine hyperactivity
   — Growth retardation, craniosynostosis
   — Increased perinatal mortality
3 If ultrasound reveals fetal goiter, fetal hypothyroidism may be confirmed by percutaneous umbilical blood sampling and treated by amniotic fluid injection of T_4
4 Thyrotoxic maternal Graves' disease may be treated with the smallest possible dose of thionamide and/or propranolol
5 Neonates may require thionamides for up to 2 months even if maternal antithyroid treatment has ensured fetal euthyroidism at delivery (TSI may persist in the neonate)

* Due to fetal TSH; may obstruct labor
‡ In contrast, mild non-autoimmune *maternal* hyperthyroidism may be less hazardous in pregnancy (to mother and child) than hypothyroidism; elevated maternal and fetal TBG elevations may 'mop up' excess

Therapeutic approach to Graves' ophthalmopathy

1 Assess severity
   — Clinical examination (p. 92)
   — MRI (or CT) scanning; B-scan ultrasound
2 Conservative therapy
   — Lubricating eyedrops, for
     • Corneal protection
   — Fresnel prisms, for
     • Diplopia
3 Medical therapy
   — Oral/IV prednisone and/or cyclosporin A
   — Retroorbital steroids
   — Botulinum toxin injected into affected muscle(s)
4 Radiotherapy
   — 20 Gy to retroocular tissues
5 Palliative surgical therapy
   — Lateral tarsorrhaphy, for
     • Exposure keratopathy
   — Muscle transposition/recessing, for
     • Ophthalmoplegia
6 Definitive surgery
   — Orbital decompression, for
     • Optic nerve compression
     • Impaired retinal function

HYPOTHYROIDISM

Treatment of myxedema associated with ischemic heart disease

1 Begin replacement with low-dose L-thyroxine (e.g. 25 µg/day: probably safer than T_3 in this context)
2 Increase to full dose by 25 µg/day every 2 weeks; monitor symptoms (of angina, arrhythmia or failure) and ECG
3 Reduce digoxin if toxicity suspected (despite plasma levels)
4 Avoid β-blockers if bradycardic or borderline CCF

Common perioperative complications in hypothyroid patients

1 Intraoperative
   — Hypotension
   — Cardiac failure (esp. during cardiac surgery)
2 Post-operative
   — Lack of fever despite documented infection
   — Constipation, ileus
   — Neuropsychiatric disorder, esp. confusion

Rationâle for monitoring thyroxine replacement

1 Clinical assessment correlates poorly with TFTs
2 Chronic underreplacement accelerates atherogenesis*

* cf. evidence that chronic overreplacement accelerates *osteoporosis* is weak

MANAGEMENT OF DIABETIC KETOACIDOSIS

Potential hazards in ketoacidosis

1 Insulin-induced *hypophosphatemia* may enhance oxygen–hemoglobin affinity and thus aggravate tissue hypoxia; phosphate supplementation is not routine, however
2 Severe *acidemia* may
   — Impair cardiac and respiratory (@ pH < 6.9) function
   — Reduce ventricular threshold to fibrillation
   — Increase ventilatory work
   — Lead to insulin resistance
3 *Rapid* correction of acidemia with intravenous *bicarbonate* may be associated with the following hazards
   — Alkalemia, as correction of CSF acidosis (which controls ventilatory rate) 'lags' behind periphery
   — Paradoxical worsening of CSF acidosis as CO_2 (but not HCO_3) equilibrates across the blood–brain barrier
   — CSF hyperosmolality leading to cerebral edema
   — Exacerbation of tissue hypoxia due to Bohr effect*
4 Intracellular potassium depletion may result if supplements not prescribed when K^+ falls below 5.0 mmol/L

* i.e. rapid correction of acidosis enhances oxyhemoglobin affinity, accompanied by a slower increase in red cell 2,3-DPG

An approach to managing diabetic ketoacidosis
1 Insulin
— Administer via pump at 0.1 U/kg/h initially
— Aim to lower blood glucose by 3 mmol/L/h
— Increase rate by 2 U/h if no improvement after 2 h
2 Potassium
— Give about 20 mmol/h if K$^+$ <6 mmol/L
— Withhold if anuric *or* K$^+$ > 6 mmol/L *or* ECG →↑ K$^+$
— If serum K$^+$ < 3 mmol/L, give 30–40 mmol/h
— Aim to maintain K$^+$ > 4 mmol/L during insulin
3 Fluids
— Must be clinically assessed
— A typical regimen in a dehydrated DKA patient
might be: normal saline 1 litre IV stat, 1 litre over
1 h, 1 litre over 2 h, then 1 litre q 4 h as needed*
4 Bicarbonate
— Consider giving 50 mmol NaHCO$_3$ *if* pH < 7.0
5 Tapering off
— When blood glucose < 10 mmol/L, change saline
to 5% dextrose; monitor glucose and potassium
hourly

* cf. hyperosmolar coma: fluids and insulin are more
conservatively administered; aim for complete rehydration and
normoglycemia only after 36–72 h

Managing the acutely ill diabetic: a few tips
1 An acutely ill insulin-dependent diabetic may need to
increase (rather than reduce) insulin dose
2 Even if meals have been missed due to illness,
elevated blood or urine glucose indicates an increase
in insulin dosage
3 Vomiting may indicate severe ketosis, therefore
requiring urgent insulin supplementation
4 Heavy ketonuria and/or severe vomiting constitute
indications for hospitalization in any ill diabetic
patient

INNOVATIONS IN INSULIN

Basic ingredients of insulin management
1 Regular self-monitoring of blood glucose
2 Short- and long-acting insulin
3 Infusion pumps; pen injectors (in UK)

Tight blood glucose control: benefits and uncertainties
1 Measures of 'tight control'
— Mean amplitude of glucose excursion
— Mean plasma glucose < 8.5 mmol/L
— HBA$_{1c}$ ≤ 7%
2 Benefits
— Prevention/regression of retinopathy
— Reduced microalbuminuria, ↑ GFR
— Improved neuropathy
3 Problems
— Increased frequency of severe hypoglycemia
— No proven reduction of ketoacidosis
— Retinopathy may *initially* deteriorate

Indications for using recombinant human insulin
1 Newly diagnosed diabetes
2 Lipoatrophy at porcine insulin injection sites
3 Proven allergy to porcine insulin

4 Diabetic pregnancy (? prevents fetal pancreatic
insulitis)
5 Insulin resistance due to antibody production (rare)

RETINOPATHY

Diabetic retinopathy: indications for photocoagulation
1 Proliferative retinopathy*
— New vessels within one disc diameter of optic
disc
— Fibrosis, retinal detachment
2 Fresh hemorrhages
— Preretinal and/or vitreous hemorrhages, esp.
3 Maculopathy
— *Focal* photocoagulation controls early exudative
maculopathy
— *Peripheral* ('panretinal') photocoagulation is
needed to control maculopathy due to edema or
ischemia

NB: Do *not* photocoagulate macula or optic disc
* may also be treated with vitrectomy if no severe macular
ischemia

Efficacy of retinal laser photocoagulation
1 Renders hypoxic retina anoxic, thus preventing
further secretion of putative neovascularizing factors
2 Central visual acuity remains normal if therapy
undertaken early, but visual fields constrict and night
vision worsens
3 New vessels atrophy within a month of treatment
4 In general, argon laser is better for focal
photocoagulation, while xenon laser is better for
peripheral lesions

Indications for fluorescein angiography
1 To evaluate and follow up patients with significant
retinopathy evident on fundoscopy
2 To evaluate patients with known retinopathy in
whom visual deterioration occurs
3 To evaluate major changes in fundoscopic signs
4 To direct laser treatment in patients with
maculopathy or proliferative retinopathy

NB: Fluorescein angiography is *not* indicated in patients without
fundoscopic abnormality

Potential indications for vitrectomy
1 Retinitis proliferans
2 Bilateral vitreous hemorrhages with visual acuity
< 6/60
3 Failure of laser photocoagulation to preserve visual
acuity

SURGERY IN THE DIABETIC PATIENT

**Perioperative management of insulin-dependent
diabetes**
1 Admit at least 2 days preop to assess glycemic control
2 Cease long-acting insulin and stabilize on short-
acting and intermediate-acting insulin

3 Schedule operation for first thing in the morning
4 On day of operation, commence infusion of dextrose, soluble insulin (1–2 U/h at first) and KCl at least 1 h preop
5 Measure blood glucose q 2 h initially; aim for 5–10 mmol/L level; measure serum potassium q 6 h
6 Post-op, continue insulin infusion until first meal, then recommence preprandial subcutaneous soluble insulin in lieu of infusion and commence intermediate-acting insulin prior to evening meal

Perioperative management of sulfonylurea-treated diabetics
1 Omit tablets on morning of surgery
2 If preoperative blood glucose > 15 mmol/L, cancel surgery and reschedule while stabilization underway
3 If preoperative blood glucose > 12 mmol/L, commence 'sliding scale' insulin titrated against blood/urine glucose
4 If glucose drops below 10 mmol/L while receiving insulin, commence dextrose infusion
5 Cease insulin when euglycemic
6 Once eating, recommence tablets if hyperglycemia recurs

ORAL HYPOGLYCEMICS

Postulated mechanisms of action of oral hypoglycemic agents
1 Sulfonylureas
   — Main effects
     • Stimulate pancreatic insulin release
     • Reduce glucagon secretion
   — Controversial effects
     • Increase number of insulin receptors
     • Reduced hepatic extraction of insulin
2 Biguanides (metformin)
   — Reduce hepatic gluconeogenesis (mainly)
   — Induce anorexia (and hence weight loss)
   — Reduce intestinal glucose absorption

Clinical problems with sulfonylurea therapy
1 High failure rate
   — 80–90% overall
   — 40% failure within first 3 months
   — Of those 'successfully' controlled, 25% per annum will need to be changed to insulin
   — Of those successfully controlled in the longer term, 50% can cease drug treatment if challenged
2 Hypoglycemia (cf. metformin), esp. with chlorpropamide
3 Leukopenia/thrombocytopenia
4 Cholestasis
5 Photosensitivity
6 Weight gain (increased insulin availability)

Metabolic associations of oral hypoglycemic therapy
1 Drugs undergoing predominant renal excretion
   — Chlorpropamide
   — Metformin
     Drugs undergoing predominant hepatic metabolism

— Glibenclamide
— Tolbutamide*
2 Drugs with long half-life (once-daily administration)
   — Chlorpropamide‡
     Drugs with medium half-life (up to b.d. administration)
   — Glibenclamide
     Drugs with short half-life (up to three times daily)
   — Metformin
   — Tolbutamide*
3 Effects on water metabolism
   — Chlorpropamide → ↑ ADH sensitivity (mimics SIADH)
   — Glibenclamide → diuretic effect
4 Chlorpropamide → alcohol-induced flushing, esp. if
   — Family history of non-insulin-dependent diabetes
   — No microangiopathic complications
5 Metformin-induced lactic acidosis: commoner if
   — Renal failure, cardiac failure
   — Liver failure, alcohol abuse
   — Perioperative (or other cause of hypoxia)
   — > 2 g/day dosage
   — Associated cimetidine therapy

* Virtually superseded by glibenclamide now
‡ Drugs with long half-lives are most likely to cause hypoglycemia. Drugs with short half-lives are thus particularly suitable for elderly patients

OTHER MANAGEMENT MODALITIES IN DIABETES

Principles of dietary management
1 Non-insulin-dependent diabetes
   — 2000 kCal/day
   — Regular exercise
2 Insulin-dependent diabetes
   — Caloric restriction as required for ideal body weight
   — Balanced diet: a variety of foods enjoyed by the patient
   — Protein intake averaging 1 g/kg/day
   — Approximately 50% of total caloric intake should consist of complex carbohydrate (high fibre)
   — Restrict alcohol, refined sugar, saturated fats, salt
   — Regular exercise program

Pros and cons of antihypertensive prescribing in diabetes
1 ACE inhibitors
   — Advantages
     • No hyperglycemic/hyperlipidemic effects
     • *Improve* proteinuria/nephropathy
   — Disadvantages
     • Hyperkalemia
     • May *impair* renal function in renovascular hypertension (reversible)
2 β-blockers
   — Advantages
     • Cardioprotective
   — Disadvantages
     • Impotence
     • Hypoglycemia (↓ awareness; prolongation)
     • Worsening of peripheral vascular disease
     • ↑ Triglycerides, ↓ HDL

3 Thiazides
   — Advantages
     • Cheap
   — Disadvantages
     • Hyperglycemia, hypercholesterolemia
     • Impotence; postural hypotension
4 Calcium antagonists
   — Advantages
     • No hyperglycemic/hyperlipidemic effects
   — Disadvantages
     • Postural hypotension

Useful drugs in diabetic autonomic neuropathy
1 Gustatory facial sweating
   — Tricyclics
2 Gastroparesis
   — Metoclopramide
3 Diarrhea
   — Tetracycline

Anticipated problems in uremic diabetics
1 If managed with hemodialysis
   — Vascular access
   — Worsening of retinopathy
2 If managed with peritoneal dialysis
   — Hyperglycemia
   — Recurrent peritonitis
3 If managed with transplantation
   — Steroid-induced worsening of diabetic control
   — Severe and/or recurrent infections

CUSHING'S DISEASE

Treatment modalities in Cushing's disease
1 For adults, transsphenoidal microadenomectomy is best
2 Best indicator of surgical cure is post-op hypocortisolism
3 Bilateral adrenalectomy now only for failed transsphenoidal microadenomectomy in women desiring pregnancy
4 Nelson's syndrome (ACTH-secreting pituitary tumor) occurs in 10% adults (30% children) after bilateral adrenalectomy
5 ^{60}Co (heavy-particle) pituitary irradiation is used primarily in children; ocular nerve palsies may result
6 Medical management alone (e.g. cyproheptadine) may suffice

PREGNANCY

Physiologic changes during pregnancy
1 Cardiovascular changes*
   — Increased cardiac output ($\uparrow$ heart rate/stroke volume)
     • Ventricular hypertrophy
   — Increased blood volume ($\rightarrow$ hemodilution, $\downarrow$ Hb)
     • S_3, systolic ejection murmur
   — Decreased peripheral resistance
     • $\uparrow$ Pulse pressure

   — Aortic unfolding
     • Inverted T wave in $V_{2/3}$
2 Respiratory changes
   — Increased tidal volume (progesterone effect)
   — Decreased residual volume (diaphragm elevation)
3 Renal changes
   — Increased renal blood flow and GFR
   — Increased tubular reabsorption
   — Decreased plasma urea/creatinine
4 Genitourinary changes
   — Uterine enlargement
     • Myometrial cell hypertrophy (E_2 effect)
     • Increased blood supply (1–1.5 L/min)
   — Collecting tract dilatation (progesterone effect)
     • Bladder relaxation
     • Ureteric reflux, stasis, infection
   — Frequency of micturition
     • Increased urine production (early)
     • Uterine compression of bladder (late)
5 Endocrine changes
   — Adrenocortical hyperfunction
     • Increased ACTH *and* cortisol
     • Increased renin (esp. first trimester)
   — Hypothalamic hyperfunction
     • Increased oxytocin release (posterior pituitary)
   — Anterior pituitary changes
     • Increased prolactin, placental lactogen (HPL)
     • Reduced FSH/LH (due to $\uparrow E_2$, progesterone)
     • Reduced growth hormone (due to $\uparrow$ HPL)

* Reflect increased oxygenation requirement

Diseases often improved by pregnancy
1 Rheumatoid arthritis*
2 Graves' disease
3 Sarcoidosis
4 Migraine
5 Chronic renal failure

* But prone to 'flare' in puerperium

Diseases often worse in pregnancy
1 Diabetes mellitus
   — Glucose intolerance
   — Microvascular disease
2 Diabetes insipidus
   — Pituitary
   — Nephrogenic
3 Nerve entrapment syndromes
   — Carpal tunnel*
   — Meralgia paresthetica
4 Intracranial lesions (may enlarge)
   — Pituitary macroadenoma, esp. prolactinoma
   — Suprasellar meningioma
   — Arteriovenous malformation
5 Infections
   — Viruses: varicella, measles, polio, influenza, HCV
   — Malaria
6 Miscellaneous
   — SLE
   — Epilepsy
   — Sickle-cell anemia
   — Cardiovascular disorders (p. 79)

* Note that this may also *respond* to hormone replacement therapy in post-menopausal women

Factors implicated in recurrent miscarriages
1 Poor oocyte quality (e.g. age-related)
 — Tends to be more important than implantation failure
2 LH hypersecretion (mid- to late-cycle)
 — incl. Polycystic ovary syndrome
 — Impairs fertilization
3 Phospholipid antibodies
4 Low prostacyclin:thromboxane ratio
5 Chromosomal abnormalities

INFERTILITY TREATMENT

Pathogeneses of infertility
1 Oligospermia — 30%
2 Ovulatory dysfunction — 30%
3 Tubal disease — 20%
4 Uterine disease — 10%
5 Cervical disease — 3%
6 Unidentifiable causes — 5%

Prime indications for assisted reproduction*
1 Tubal disease
 — Main indication for IVF
2 Endometriosis
3. Male subfertility
 — Main indication for GIFT

* Certain diagnoses must be *excluded*, e.g. hyperprolactinemia

'Test-tube' pregnancies: what's the success rate?*
1 Extracorporeal fertilization
 — In vitro fertilization (IVF)‡
 • Embryos cultured to 4–8 cell stage, then replaced ('embryo transfer – ET')
 • 15% deliveries per operation
2 Intrafallopian transfer
 — Gamete intrafallopian transfer (GIFT)
 • 20% deliveries per operation
 — Zygote intrafallopian transfer (ZIFT)
 • 24% deliveries per operation

* NB: The most critical factor determining success is the *number* of eggs (or embryos) transferred, not the therapeutic technique. Keep in mind that the natural fecundity rate is only 25%
‡ 30% embryos harbor lethal chromosomal anomalies

Factors reducing probability of successful assisted pregnancy
1 Asymmetrical, poorly defined blastomeres
2 Advanced age of egg donor
3 Parental smoking (either partner)

Infertility treatment in polycystic ovary syndrome
1 Fertility drugs, e.g.
 — Clomiphene
 — Pulsatile (stimulatory) GnRH therapy
2 Ovarian cyst electrocautery
 — Performed at laparoscopy
3 Wedge resection (i.e. of the ovaries)
 — Now largely abandoned; adhesions → infertility

Complications of fertility drug therapy
1 Multiple pregnancy

2 Increased miscarriage rate
3 Ovarian hyperstimulation syndrome
 — Massive ovarian enlargement (stromal edema)
 — Third-space fluid accumulation*
 — Severity parallels ↑ plasma estradiol
 — Renin levels also elevated
 — Increased risk in polycystic ovary syndrome

* Ascites, pleural and pericardial effusions – occasionally fatal

Therapeutic options in endometriosis
1 Danazol (synthetic androgen)*
2 Progestogens (e.g. norethisterone, medroxyprogesterone)
3 Gestrinone (an antiprogestogen and weak androgen)
4 GnRH agonists‡
5 Surgical ablation

* Duration of treatment limited by hyperlipidemia
‡ Duration of treatment limited by bone demineralization

ORAL CONTRACEPTIVES

Beneficial effects of combined oral contraceptives
1 Contraception (incl. fewer ectopic pregnancies; cf. IUDs)
2 Less dysmenorrhea or menorrhagia; less endometriosis
3 Less benign breast disease
4 Fewer follicular and luteal ovarian cysts
5 Lower risk of endometrial and ovarian cancer

Patient evaluation prior to (estrogenic) oral contraception
1 Past history of neoplasia
 — Breast cancer
 — Endometrial cancer
 — Hydatidiform mole
 — Uterine leiomyomata (fibroids)
 — Hepatic tumors
 — Prolactinoma
2 History of disorder worsening during pregnancy
 — Pruritus
 — Jaundice
 — Herpes gestationis (*not* a viral infection)
 — Otosclerosis
3 History of vascular disorder
 — Thromboembolism
 — Cardio- or cerebrovascular condition
 — Hypertension (incl. pulmonary)
 — Cigarette smoking
 — Migraine (esp. 'classical', focal, basilar)
4 Examination
 — Weight, urinalysis, blood pressure
 — Breasts, liver, fundi
 — Vaginal examination
5 Baseline investigations
 — Cervical smear
 — Urine HCG
 — Serum lipids (fasting)
 — Liver function tests
 — ECG if indicated

Drug interactions with oral contraceptives (OCs)

1 Drugs reducing OC efficacy due to hepatic enzyme induction
  — Rifampicin (contraindicated in OC users); griseofulvin
  — Phenytoin, carbamazepine, barbiturates
2 Drugs antagonizing OCs due to ↓ enterohepatic recirculation
  — Tetracycline, ampicillin, purgatives
3 Hepatic enzyme inhibition by OCs → potentiation of
  — Imipramine
  — Barbiturates
  — Chlordiazepoxide; pethidine
4 Reduction of epileptic threshold by OCs (i.e. seizure activity may worsen despite increased anticonvulsant levels)

Pharmacologic strategies for opposing estrogen

1 Antiestrogens (e.g. tamoxifen)
  — Compete for binding of estrogen receptors
  — May have some (weak) estrogenic effects
2 Progestogens (e.g. norethisterone, megestrol)
  — Enhance hypothalamic negative feedback on estrogen
3 Androgens (esp. danazol)
  — Suppress HPA axis by reducing GnRH pulses
4 Aromatase inhibitors (e.g. aminoglutethimide)
  — Prevent peripheral production of active estrogen metabolites
5 GnRH agonists
  — Downregulate LH/FSH receptors if used continuously, thus suppressing estrogen release from ovary
  — May cause initial 'flare' of estrogen release

GONADOTROPHIN-RELEASING HORMONE THERAPIES

Classification and mechanisms of GnRH therapies

1 GnRH agonists
  — e.g. LHRH agonists
    • Buserelin, goserelin
    • Leuprolide
  — Stimulate gonadotrophin (FSH/LH) secretion
  — *Pulsatile* therapy → ↑ gonadal hormone secretion (i.e. simulates physiologic GnRH action)
  — *Continuous* therapy* → ↓ gonadal hormone secretion (via downregulation of GnRH receptors)
2 GnRH antagonists (investigational)
  — Competitively inhibit GnRH by binding receptors
  — Do *not* cause LH/FSH secretion
  — Advantages
    • Immediate effect (cf. agonist suppression)
    • No 'flare' of neoplastic disease activity

* e.g. given by depot intramuscular injection

Indications for pulsatile (stimulatory) GnRH therapy

1 Anovulatory infertility (any cause)*
  — e.g. Prior to egg harvest for assisted reproduction
2 Hypogonadotrophic hypogonadism (e.g. Kallmann's)
  — e.g. For initiation of puberty

* Alternatives to GnRH analogs include clomiphene, HMG (human menopausal gonadotrophin) and HCG

Indications for continuous (suppressive) GnRH therapy

1 Females
  — Endometriosis
  — Polycystic ovary syndrome
  — Uterine fibroids, dysfunctional uterine bleeding
  — Premenopausal breast cancer (adjuvant, metastatic)
2 Male
  — Metastatic prostate cancer
3 Both sexes
  — Contraception (potentially)
  — Precocious puberty (if hypergonadotrophic)

Problems with suppressive GnRH therapy

1 Expense
2 Hot flushes, loss of libido (both sexes)
3 Bone demineralization
  — Density falls 2–5% every 6 months
  — May be reversible on periodic cessation

SEX HORMONE REPLACEMENT THERAPY

Physiologic effects of estrogen

1 Menstruation
2 Vaginal cornification
3 Cervical mucus formation
4 Breast development
5 Axillary hair

Undisputed indications for estrogen replacement

1 Gonadal dysgenesis
2 Premature menopause (e.g. Wertheim's hysterectomy)

Benefits of post-menopausal low-dose estrogen replacement

1 Improvement of vasomotor instability (hot flushes)
2 Prevention/reversal of atrophic vaginitis
3 Reduced morbidity and mortality from osteoporotic fractures
4 Reduced cardiovascular mortality*
  — 15% ↓ LDL
  — 15% ↑ HDL_2
  — ↓ Lp(a)

* Clinically relevant to women at high cardiovascular risk

Neoplastic hazards of hormone replacement

1 Endometrial cancer (due to unopposed E_2)‡
  — Absolute risk 1% per year; relative risk about six-fold
  — Risk reduced by concomitant progestogen therapy*
2 Hepatic adenoma (due to E_2; p. 146)
  — Prone to intraperitoneal hemorrhage
3 Breast cancer
  — Long-term estrogens slightly increase risk
  — Progestogens may further increase risk

‡ Risk also increased with long-term adjuvant tamoxifen therapy
* Similar protective effect of combined therapy claimed for ovarian cancer

MIFEPRISTONE (RU 486)

Effects of mifepristone*
1 Blocks progesterone (and glucocorticoid) receptors
2 Induces endometrial sloughing
3 Softens the cervix
4 Disinhibits endometrial contraction
5 Teratogenicity uncertain

* A semisynthetic steroid similar to norethisterone; weakly antiandrogenic

Potential indications for mifepristone
1 Termination of early (≤ 9 weeks) pregnancy*
   — i.e. 'Abortion pill' (like methotrexate; p. 29)
   — May obviate suction termination and anesthesia
   — Single dose (600 mg) effective in ~ 75%; addition of prostaglandin pessary increases efficacy to 95%‡
2 Facilitation of protracted labor
   — i.e. May help avoid Cesarean
3 Dilatation and softening of cervix to expedite
   — Endometrial biopsy, D&C
   — Difficult IUD insertion
4 Unproven indications
   — Cushing's disease, adrenal tumors
   — Glaucoma
   — Meningioma
   — Breast cancer
   — Endometriosis

* Sometimes combined for this purpose with the antiulcerogenic prostaglandin misoprostol; do not confuse the two when treating ulcers
‡ NB: Appropriate clinic observation, instruction and follow-up is essential; 1% require emergency transfusion or evacuation, while ~ 30% need opiates

Contraindications to mifepristone as abortifacient
1 Absolute contraindications
   — Pregnancy unproven
   — Adrenal insufficiency (incl. steroid use)
   — Bleeding diathesis
   — Unwillingness to proceed to suction termination if medical abortion unsuccessful or incomplete
2 Relative contraindications
   — Heavy smoking > 35 yrs, cardiovascular disease
   — Renal failure; asthma
   — Alcohol abuse, liver failure
   — Current (last week) aspirin/NSAID use
3 Avoid due to lack of efficacy
   — Ectopic pregnancy

Alternative methods of post-coital contraception*
1 High-dose ethinylestradiol (or other estrogen)
   — Effective, but nauseating
2 Short-course estrogen/progestogen oral contraceptive
   — Two 'full-dose' tablets (ethinylestradiol 100 μg + levonorgestrel 500 μg) repeated 12 h later
   — 2% still become pregnant
3 Danazol
   — Less effective than estrogens

4 Prompt insertion of copper IUD
   — May be recommended only to mothers

* Within 72 h; not referred to as 'abortion' since implantation has not occurred
NB: None of the above treatments are quite as effective emergency contraceptives as mifepristone

SEXUAL DISORDERS AND DRUG THERAPY

Treatment options in idiopathic hirsutism
1 Mild hirsutism
   — Reassurance
2 Moderate hirsutism, pregnancy desired
   — Shaving, waxing, depilatory creams, electrolysis
3 Moderate hirsutism, pregnancy not desired
   — Combined oral contraceptive
     • Reduces free testosterone by increasing SHBG and reducing LH
4 Severe hirsutism, pregnancy desired
   — Dexamethasone 0.25 mg nocte
     • Reduces ACTH → ↓ adrenal androgens
5 Severe hirsutism, pregnancy not desired
   — Cyproterone acetate, spironolactone
     • Block interaction of DHT with androgen receptor
6 Polycystic ovary syndrome
   — Octreotide

Major drug classes causing male sexual dysfunction*
1 Alcohol/narcotic addiction
2 Estrogens, corticosteroids
3 'Antiandrogens': spironolactone, cimetidine
4 Antihypertensives: methyldopa, propranolol
5 Phenothiazines, tricyclics

* Loss of libido; impotence; ejaculatory impairment

Clinical relevance of anabolic steroids
1 Include
   — Oxymethalone, nandrolone decanoate, stanozolol
2 Established use
   — Aplastic anemia (→ erythropoiesis)
3 Commonest use
   — Bodybuilding amongst athletes (illicit)
4 Hazards
   — Testosterone suppression (testis atrophy, impotence)
   — Liver tumors (hepatoma, angiosarcoma)

UNDERSTANDING ENDOCRINE DISEASE

Characteristics of hormonal action
1 Steroid and thyroid hormones
   — Lipid-soluble; require plasma carrier protein
   — Long plasma $t^{1/2}$; easily measured in serum
   — Actions are gradual in onset (hours to days)
   — Hormone binding induces conformational change in nuclear receptor which then binds DNA
2 Polypeptide hormones and catecholamines
   — Water-soluble; circulate free, bind membrane receptors
   — Short plasma $t^{1/2}$; serum levels hard to interpret

— Actions are rapid in onset (minutes to hours)
— Binding to membrane receptor proteins activates cytoplasmic 'second messenger' (e.g. cAMP) which transduces signals to nucleus

Prohormones: hormone precursors requiring activation
1 T_4
— Prohormone for T_3
2 Testosterone
— Prohormone for dihydrotestosterone (DHT)
3 (Dietary) vitamin D_2 = ergocalciferol
(Skin-derived *or* dietary) vitamin D_3 = cholecalciferol
— Prohormones for 1,25-dihydroxyvitamin D

Peptide hormones with structural similarities
1 Glycoproteins with identical β-subunits
— LH, FSH
— TSH
— HCG*
2 Large single-chain polypeptides with amino acid homology
— Growth hormone (GH)
— Prolactin (PRL)
— Human placental lactogen (HPL)
3 CNS neurotransmitters
— Melatonin
— Serotonin
4 Receptor tyrosine kinase ligands
— Insulin
— Insulin-like growth factors (IGF)-1 and -2
— Relaxin
5 Serine/threonine kinase ligands
— Inhibin
— Activin
— Transforming growth factor-β
— Bone morphogenetic proteins

* NB: Weak TSH agonism may rarely cause thyrotoxicosis in choriocarcinoma patients with grossly elevated β-HCG

Circadian rhythmicity of hormone release
1 Late afternoon
— Prolactin*
2 Early phase of sleep
— Growth hormone
3 Late phase of sleep
— ACTH/cortisol
— TSH, LH

* Hence, to demonstrate hyperprolactinemia, test in morning

Stress-inducible peptide hormones
1 ACTH/cortisol
2 ADH*
3 Prolactin
4 Growth hormone (in lean patients)
5 Glucagon

* Potently induced by nausea

Melatonin secretion: regulation and function
1 Secreted by pineal gland* during the night (darkness) Inhibited by light (even in some consciously blind patients)
2 Influences circadian sleep–wake rhythms

3 Implicated in 'jet-lag' pathogenesis; may have therapeutic value in this context
4 High levels may cause hypogonadotrophic hypogonadism
Increased levels also seen in anorexia nervosa

* Pineal calcification may indicate secretory hyperfunction

Predominant estrogens in the human life cycle
1 E_1 (estrone)
— Post-menopausal
2 E_2 (estradiol)
— Child-bearing years
3 E_3 (estriol)
— Pregnancy
— Fetal life

Diseases caused by end-organ resistance to hormones*
1 Testicular feminization syndrome, Reifenstein's syndrome
— Defective androgen receptors
— Causes feminization or pseudohermaphroditism
— Androgen resistance also due to 5-α-reductase defects
2 Albright's hereditary osteodystrophy
— Associated with apparent resistance to PTH‡
— Linked to constitutively activating mutations of adenyl cyclase-stimulatory G-protein subunit (G_s)
3 X-linked nephrogenic diabetes insipidus (XR)
— Resistance of distal nephron to ADH
— Due to mutated vasopressin V2-receptor
4 Type II vitamin D-dependent rickets
— End-organ resistance to 1,25 dihydroxyvitamin D
5 Laron dwarfism (AR)
— ↓↓ GH receptors → ↓↓ IGF-1 release
— Treatable with IGF-1
Pygmy dwarfism
— ↓↓ Plasma GH-binding protein (GHBP)
— May reflect loss of GH receptors
6 Type A insulin receptor abnormality (AR)
— Reduced number of insulin receptors
— Linked with Stein–Leventhal (polycystic ovaries; p. 104)
7 Familial hypocalciuric hypercalcemia (AD; p. 238)
— Failure of PTH suppression by calcium due to mutations affecting a calcium-sensing receptor
8 Familial thyroid hormone resistance (AD)
— Due to dominant-negative mutant T_3 receptors
— Most mutations affect T_3-binding domain of c-*erb*A
9 Familial male-limited precocious puberty (AD)
— Null mutations affect the LH receptor
10 Familial isolated GH deficiency (AD)
— Some cases due to GH receptor gene mutations

* i.e. all such diseases may be associated with *high* hormone levels
‡ (Pseudo)pseudohypoparathyroidism; some may respond to vitamin D

UNDERSTANDING DIABETES

Antibodies detectable in diabetes mellitus
1 Insulin antibodies

— Usually seen in patients treated with porcine insulin
— IgE type may mediate allergic reactions
— Rarely associated with insulin resistance
2 Islet cell antibodies
— May play a pathogenetic role in type I diabetes
— Predicts young family members at high risk of IDDM
3 Islet cell insulin receptor-blocking antibodies (p. 190)
— IgG-mediated reduction in receptor affinity for insulin
— Associated with SLE-like phenotype
4 Islet cell insulin receptor-stimulating antibodies
— May play a role in disturbed glucose homeostasis

Factors correlating with severity of microvascular disease
1 Duration of diabetes
2 Degree of long-term hyperglycemia
3 Hypertension

Anomalies of diabetic adiposities
1 Lipodystrophy
— Associated with insulin-resistant diabetes, i.e. type A insulin receptor abnormality (see above)
2 Lipoatrophy
— Occurs at sites of porcine insulin injection; responds to injection of monocomponent insulin
3 Lipohypertrophy
— Commoner with monocomponent insulin use, esp. if injection sites not rotated

Clinical features of syndrome X (Reaven's syndrome)
1 Insulin resistance (hyperinsulinemia)
— Clinical diabetes unusual
2 Central/upper body obesity
— Worsens insulin resistance
3 Hypertension
— Severity proportional to hyperinsulinemia
4 Hyperlipidemia
— ↑ VLDL* (esp. males)
— ↓ HDL (esp. females)
5 Females often have polycystic ovaries (p. 104)
— No increase in coronary disease in these patients

* cf. LDL: usually *normal*

Infections increased in poorly controlled diabetics
1 Rhinocerebral mucormycosis
2 Emphysematous cholecystitis (*Clostridia* spp.)
3 Necrotizing cellulitis/fasciitis (mixed aerobes and anaerobes)
4 Malignant otitis externa (*Ps. aeruginosa*)
5 Oral or vulvovaginal candidiasis
6 Furunculosis (staphylococcal)
7 Abscesses, e.g. perinephric
8 Influenza/*Staph.* pneumonia
9 Tuberculosis

NB: Infection may either complicate or precipitate ketoacidosis

UNDERSTANDING THYROID DISEASE

Clinical varieties of thyroiditis
1 Chronic lymphocytic (Hashimoto's) thyroiditis

— Common
— Female:male = 20:1
— Onset: gradual, painless
— Transient 'Hashitoxicosis' unusual
— Signs: diffuse painless goiter, no bruit
— Biopsy: lymphocytic infiltrate, Askanazy cells
— Associations: thyroid autoantibodies, HLA DR5
— Sequelae: persistent hypothyroidism in 80%
2 Subacute granulomatous (de Quervain's) thyroiditis
— Uncommon
— Female:male = 2:1
— Onset: acute, painful, transient thyrotoxicosis usual
— Signs: small goiter, extremely tender
— Biopsy: giant cell infiltrate, granulomata
— Associations: viral infection
— Sequelae: transient hypothyroidism in 10%
3 Subacute lymphocytic ('silent') thyroiditis
— Common
— Female:male = 5:1
— Onset: acute (often peripartum), painless
— Transient thyrotoxicosis usual
— Signs: goiter usually absent
— Biopsy: similar to Hashimoto's
— Associations: thyroid autoantibodies, HLA DR5
— Sequelae: transient hypothyroidism in 25%
4 Chronic fibrosing (Riedel's) thyroiditis
— Rare
— Onset: gradual
— Signs: woody (ligneous) indurated thyroid
— Biopsy: widespread fibrosis
— Associations: retroperitoneal fibrosis, sclerosing cholangitis, Peyronie's disease
— Sequelae: persistent hypothyroidism in 50%

Cardiac manifestations of thyroid disease
1 Hypothyroidism
— Hypercholesterolemia, ischemia*
— Pericarditis, pericardial effusion
— Cardiomyopathy, cardiac failure
— Hypotension *or* hypertension
— Bradycardia; low-voltage ECG
2 Thyrotoxicosis
— Sinus tachycardia; AF ± thromboembolism
— Bounding pulse, widened pulse pressure
— Angina, myocardial infarction
— High-output CCF; cardiomyopathy
— Sudden death (presumed VF)

* ↓ LDL clearance, ↓ hepatic lipase activity

POLYGLANDULAR ENDOCRINE DISORDERS

Multiple endocrine neoplasia (MEN): the clinical spectrum
1 Multiple endocrine neoplasia type I (MEN1)
— **P**arathyroid adenoma/hyperplasia (90%)
— **P**ituitary adenoma (60%)
— **P**ancreatic islet cell tumor (e.g. gastrinoma)
— Other: lipomata, carcinoids, thymoma
2 Multiple endocrine neoplasia type IIa (MEN2a)
— Pheochromocytoma*
— Medullary carcinoma of the thyroid

— Parathyroid hyperplasia (in 50%; generally subclinical)
— Gliomas, meningiomas
3 Multiple endocrine neoplasia type IIb (MEN2b)
— Similar to IIa, though hyperparathyroidism rare
— Marfanoid habitus
— Mucosal neuromas, protruding lips, gut gangliomas

* Also seen in von Hippel–Lindau syndrome

Other polyglandular endocrine syndromes
1 Schmidt's syndrome
— Addison's + Hashimoto's
— Hypoparathyroidism
— Primary gonadal failure
— Diabetes mellitus
2 Candidiasis/endocrinopathy syndrome
— Hypoparathyroidism
— Addison's disease
— Pernicious anemia
3 Lipodystrophies
— Diabetes mellitus
— Stein–Leventhal syndrome
— Acromegaly, Cushing's
4 Albright's syndrome
— Precocious puberty in girls (predominantly)
— Cushing's syndrome, acromegaly (±)
5 Pinealoma
— Diabetes insipidus (ectopic location)
— Precocious puberty in boys (only 10%)

Endocrine causes of proximal weakness
1 Thyroid dysfunction
— Thyrotoxicosis (myopathy or periodic paralysis)
— Hypothyroidism
2 Adrenal dysfunction
— Cushing's disease
— Corticosteroid therapy (esp. triamcinolone)
3 Diabetic amyotrophy (p. 93)
4 Acromegaly
5 Primary hyperparathyroidism
6 Primary hyperaldosteronism
7 Vitamin D deficiency (osteomalacia)

DRUG INTERACTIONS IN ENDOCRINE DISORDERS

Alcohol abuse and glucose homeostasis
1 Hypoglycemia may occur due to
— Prolonged fasting
— Reduced hepatic glycogen storage capacity

— Impaired gluconeogenesis due to high NADH levels
— 'Reactive' to carbohydrate diet (i.e. ↑ insulin release)
— Acute potentiation of drug-induced hypoglycemia
2 Hyperglycemia may occur due to
— Obesity
— Chronic pancreatitis
— Insulin resistance due to elevated free fatty acid levels
— Induced hepatic metabolism of sulfonylureas with chronic ingestion (i.e. worsening of diabetic control)

β-blockers and glucose homeostasis
1 May predispose to hypoglycemia due to prevention of catecholamine-induced hepatic glycogenolysis
2 May lead to potentiation and prolongation of sulfonylurea-induced hypoglycemia due to lack of negative feedback on insulin release (esp. if α-agonism, e.g. labetalol)
3 Impair awareness of developing (systemic) hypo-glycemia, with attendant risk of profound neuro-glycopenia, esp. with non-selective β-blockade

Drug-induced gynecomastia and/or galactorrhea
1 Gynecomastia alone (± impotence); normal prolactin
— Alcohol (± chronic liver disease)
— Estrogens; androgens, progestogens (→ estrogens)
— Antiandrogens
  • Cyproterone acetate, flutamide
  • Spironolactone
  • Cimetidine
— Weak estrogens
  • Digitoxin
  • Ketoconazole
2 Gynecomastia and/or galactorrhea (↑ prolactin)
— Methyldopa, reserpine
— Heroin, morphine, marijuana
— Tricyclics, haloperidol, phenothiazines

Drug-induced azoospermia: causes
1 Cytotoxics (esp. MOPP, alkylators)
2 Sex steroids (incl. high-dose androgens; → ↓ FSH)
3 'Antiandrogens'
— Danazol, etc. (→ ↓ LH → ↓ testosterone)
— Cimetidine
— Spironolactone
4 Sulfasalazine
5 Colchicine, phenytoin, nitrofurantoin; major tranquillizers
6 Alcohol, marijuana

REVIEWING THE LITERATURE: ENDOCRINOLOGY

3.1   Daneshdoost L et al (1991) Recognition of gonadotroph adenomas in women. N Engl J Med 324: 589–594

Eleven of 16 women with 'non-secreting' pituitary adenomas were found to have TRH-inducible increases in LH/FSH (or β-subunits thereof) secretion, suggesting that most 'non-functioning' tumors originate from gonadotrophin-secreting cells.

3.2   Hashizume K et al (1991) Administration of thyroxine in treated Graves' disease. N Engl J Med 324: 947–953

Coadministration of T_4 during methimazole treatment reduced TSH receptor antibody titers, as well as the subsequent frequency of hyperthyroidism.

3.3   Schlaghecke R et al (1992) The effect of long-term glucocorticoid therapy on pituitary–adrenal responses to exogenous corticotropin-releasing hormone. N Engl J Med 326: 226–230

Study of 279 patients on steroid therapy concluding that pituitary–adrenal function cannot be reliably inferred from steroid dose, duration or plasma cortisol levels; CRH testing is recommended as being comparable in value to insulin tolerance testing.

3.4   Patrick AW et al (1991) Human insulin awareness of acute hypoglycaemic symptoms in insulin-dependent diabetes. Lancet 338: 528–532

Colagiuri S et al (1992) Double-blind crossover comparison of human and porcine insulins in patients reporting lack of hypoglycaemia awareness. Lancet 339: 1432–1435

Mitrakou A et al (1993) Reversibility of unawareness of hypoglycemia in patients with insulinomas. N Engl J Med 329: 834–839

The first two studies refute the notion that human insulin causes more hypoglycemia (less forewarning thereof) than porcine insulin. The third study indicates that recurrent hypoglycemia can itself lead to progressive unawareness of neuroglycopenia.

3.5   Helmrich SP et al (1991) Physical activity and reduced occurrence of non-insulin-dependent diabetes mellitus. N Engl J Med 325: 147–152

Prospective questionnaire study of 6000 college graduates suggesting that increased exercise reduces risk of type II diabetes, esp. in 'at-risk' individuals.

3.6   Björck S et al (1992) Renal protective effect of enalapril in diabetic nephropathy. Br Med J 304: 339–343

Lewis EJ et al (1993) The effect of angiotensin-converting-enzyme inhibition on diabetic nephropathy. N Engl J Med 329: 1456–1462

Two studies indicating a nephroprotective effect of ACE inhibitors, perhaps not directly related to their antihypertensive effects.

3.7   Wang PH et al (1993) Meta-analysis of intensive blood-glucose control on late complications of type I diabetes. Lancet 341: 1306–1309

Reichard P et al (1993) The effect of long-term intensified insulin treatment on the development of microvascular complications of diabetes mellitus. N Engl J Med 329: 304–309

Powrie JK et al (1994) Role of glycemic control in development of microalbuminuria in patients with insulin dependent diabetes. Br Med J 309: 1608–1612

Three studies indicating that the rate of progression of microvascular disease in type I diabetes can be reduced by about 50% by tight glycemic control, albeit at the cost of increased hypoglycemic morbidity.

3.8   Sauer MV et al (1990) A preliminary report on oocyte donation extending reproductive potential to women over 40. N Engl J Med 323: 1157–1160

First report showing that old ladies can still bear children provided that they receive young eggs.

Auger J et al (1995) Decline in semen quality among fertile men in Paris during the past 20 years. N Engl J Med 332: 281–285

Intriguing study from a French sperm bank suggesting a progressive year-by-year decline in sperm concentration and morphology for the last two decades.

3.9   Czeisler CA et al (1995) Suppression of melatonin secretion in some blind patients by exposure to bright light. N Engl J Med 332: 6–11

Study of a small cohort of blind patients showing that insomnia improved in three patients whose melatonin levels dropped in response to light; thus confirming the role of melatonin in governing circadian rhythms.

3.10 Glasier A et al (1992) Mifepristone (RU 486) compared with high-dose estrogen and progestogen for emergency postcoital contraception. N Engl J Med 327: 1041–1044

Scottish study documenting the 'morning-after' contraceptive efficacy of the oral abortifacient.

CHAPTER 4

Gastroenterology

Physical examination protocol 4.1   You are asked to examine the gastrointestinal system

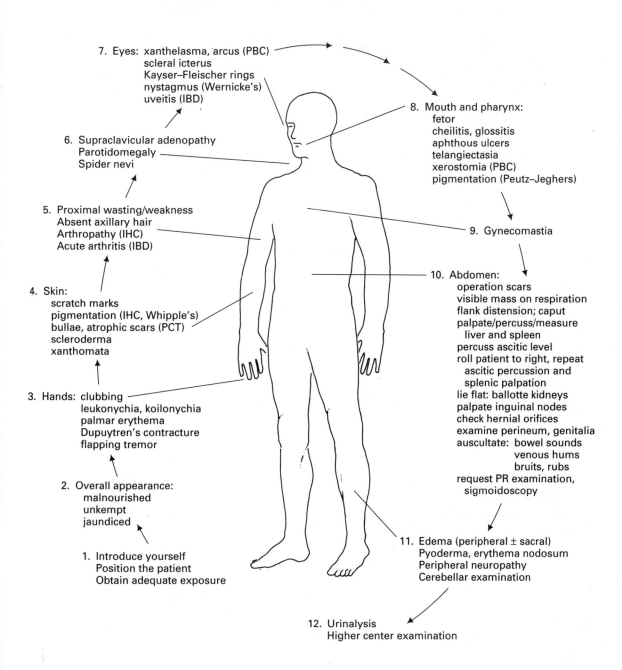

7. Eyes: xanthelasma, arcus (PBC)
    scleral icterus
    Kayser–Fleischer rings
    nystagmus (Wernicke's)
    uveitis (IBD)

8. Mouth and pharynx:
    fetor
    cheilitis, glossitis
    aphthous ulcers
    telangiectasia
    xerostomia (PBC)
    pigmentation (Peutz–Jeghers)

6. Supraclavicular adenopathy
    Parotidomegaly
    Spider nevi

5. Proximal wasting/weakness
    Absent axillary hair
    Arthropathy (IHC)
    Acute arthritis (IBD)

9. Gynecomastia

4. Skin:
    scratch marks
    pigmentation (IHC, Whipple's)
    bullae, atrophic scars (PCT)
    scleroderma
    xanthomata

10. Abdomen:
    operation scars
    visible mass on respiration
    flank distension; caput
    palpate/percuss/measure
       liver and spleen
    percuss ascitic level
    roll patient to right, repeat
       ascitic percussion and
       splenic palpation
    lie flat: ballotte kidneys
    palpate inguinal nodes
    check hernial orifices
    examine perineum, genitalia
    auscultate: bowel sounds
                venous hums
                bruits, rubs
    request PR examination,
       sigmoidoscopy

3. Hands: clubbing
    leukonychia, koilonychia
    palmar erythema
    Dupuytren's contracture
    flapping tremor

2. Overall appearance:
    malnourished
    unkempt
    jaundiced

1. Introduce yourself
    Position the patient
    Obtain adequate exposure

11. Edema (peripheral ± sacral)
    Pyoderma, erythema nodosum
    Peripheral neuropathy
    Cerebellar examination

12. Urinalysis
    Higher center examination

Diagnostic pathway 4.1   The patient is jaundiced. Why do you think this might be?

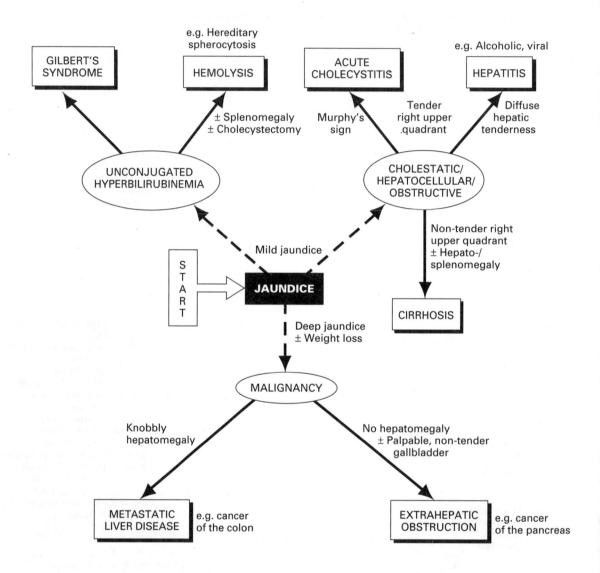

Diagnostic pathway 4.2   This patient is noted to have hepatomegaly. What is your provisional diagnosis?

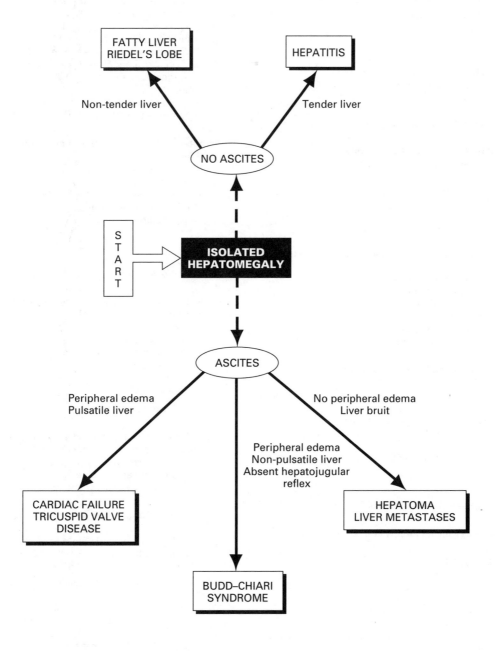

CLINICAL ASPECTS OF GASTROINTESTINAL DISEASE

Commonest gastrointestinal short cases
1 Hepatosplenomegaly
2 Ascites
3 Jaundice

Precipitants of morning vomiting
1 Pregnancy (rarely, trophoblastic tumors)
2 Alcoholic gastritis
3 Migraine
4 Intracranial space-occupying lesion

Diagnostic significance of macroglossia
1 In adults
   — Amyloidosis
   — Acromegaly
2 In children
   — Hypothyroidism
   — Down's syndrome

Recurrent alcohol-induced abdominal pain? Causes
1 Common
   — Alcoholic hepatitis
   — Alcoholic gastritis/peptic ulcer
   — Acute pancreatitis
2 Classical
   — Hodgkin's disease
   — Acute intermittent porphyria

Recurrent acute abdomen of obscure cause
1 Narcotic addiction (malingering)
2 Familial Mediterranean fever (± narcotic addiction)
3 Sickle-cell anemia
4 Acute intermittent (or variegate) porphyria
5 C_1-esterase inhibitor deficiency (p. 188)
6 Lead poisoning
7 Iatrogenic (digoxin, anticholinergics, erythromycin)

GASTROINTESTINAL BLEEDING

Local lesions causing recurrent gastrointestinal bleeding
1 Angiodysplasia (telangiectasia)
   — Often multiple
   — Tend to affect right colon
   — Higher incidence in elderly patients
   — Angiography may be required for visualization
2 Hemangioma
   — Tend to affect stomach, small bowel or rectum
   — Typically gross (visible) lesions; cf. angiodysplasia
3 Telangiectasia
   — e.g. Hereditary hemorrhagic telangiectasia
4 Diverticulitis
   — incl. Meckel's
5 Hemorrhoids
6 Colorectal cancer

Rare systemic causes of recurrent gastrointestinal bleeding
1 Polycythemia rubra vera
2 Vasculitis
   — Polyarteritis nodosa
   — Henoch–Schönlein purpura
3 Behçet's syndrome
4 Amyloidosis
5 Inherited collagenoses
   — Pseudoxanthoma elasticum
   — Type IV Ehlers–Danlos syndrome
   — Degos disease
6 Other
   — Peutz–Jeghers syndrome (± intussusception)
   — Gardner's syndrome

Hematemesis in the alcoholic: pathogenetic considerations
1 Variceal hemorrhage
2 Peptic ulcer
3 Alcoholic gastritis (or esophagitis)
4 Mallory–Weiss syndrome
5 Coagulopathy

LIVER DISEASE

Clinical signs of portal venous hypertension
1 Specific signs
   — Caput medusae
   — Venous hum (rare)
   — Anorectal varices (*not* hemorrhoids)
2 Non-specific signs
   — Ascites
   — Splenomegaly*

* Insensitive sign; absent in 50%

Clinical variables affecting esophageal varices
1 Prediction of variceal development
   — Portal pressure (> 12 mmHg)
2 Prediction of variceal bleeding
   — Variceal size (> 5 mm diameter)

Natural history of patients with symptomatic varices
1 One-third will die during the first bleed
2 One-third will rebleed within 6 weeks
3 One-third will remain alive after 12 months

Direction of abdominal venous flow: diagnostic significance
1 Outwards (i.e. from umbilicus)
   — Portal hypertension (caput medusae)
2 Upwards
   — Budd–Chiari syndrome or IVC thrombosis
3 Downwards
   — SVC obstruction

Clinical signs associated with alcohol abuse
1 Dupuytren's contracture
2 Parotidomegaly
3 Wernicke's syndrome (pp. 233, 295)

Differential diagnosis of palmar erythema/spider nevi
1 Less than five spider angiomata may be normal
2 Chronic liver disease
3 Pregnancy/oral contraceptive use
4 Thyrotoxicosis
5 Rheumatoid arthritis

Massive hepatomegaly: some causes
1 Fatty infiltration
2 Metastatic liver disease
3 Polycystic disease

Differential diagnosis of hepatomegaly and heart failure
1 Right ventricular failure ± tricuspid incompetence
2 Constrictive pericarditis
3 Alcoholic cardiomyopathy with fatty liver
4 Hemochromatosis
5 Amyloidosis
6 Carcinoid syndrome

Liver disease and splenomegaly without portal hypertension?
1 Chronic active hepatitis
2 Alcoholic hepatitis
3 Idiopathic hemochromatosis
4 Primary biliary cirrhosis
5 Infiltrations: sarcoid, amyloid

Helpful clinical features in characterizing chronic liver disease
1 Fever
  Ascites, edema
  Gynecomastia
  Dupuytren's — Alcoholic cirrhosis
  Parotidomegaly
2 Pigmentation
  Hepatomegaly
  Testicular atrophy
    and hypogonadism
  Gynecomastia — Hemochromatosis
  MCP arthropathy (jaundice/ascites
  Cardiac failure uncommon)
  Glycosuria
  Usually male
3 Splenomegaly (often with- — Chronic active
    out portal hypertension) hepatitis
  Prominent spider nevi (pigmentation
  Often young (15–30) uncommon)
4 Scratch marks
  Xanthelasma — Primary biliary
  Pigmentation cirrhosis
  Usually female

Fever and abnormal liver function? Differential diagnosis
1 Acute viral hepatitis
2 Alcoholic hepatitis
3 Cholangitis
4 Liver abscess

LIVER FAILURE

Features of hepatic encephalopathy
1 Grade I

— Fluctuating confusion ± euphoria/depression
— Inversion of sleep pattern
— Slow, slurred speech
2 Grade II ('hepatic precoma')
— Drowsiness, inappropriate behavior
— Fetor hepaticus
— Flapping tremor
— Constructional apraxia
3 Grade III
— Incoherent
— Sleeps all day, but rousable
— Hyperreflexia, myoclonus, extrapyramidal signs
4 Grade IV
— Unrousable (comatose)
— Extensor plantar responses

The flapping tremor: differential diagnosis
1 Hepatic precoma
2 Uremia
3 CO_2 narcosis

ASCITES

Ascites: sudden worsening in stable cirrhosis
1 Spontaneous bacterial peritonitis*
— e.g. Coliforms, *Flavobacterium* spp., TB
— Predisposition: ascitic protein < 10 g/L
— R_x cefotaxime; prophylaxis with norfloxacin
2 Hepatic vein thrombosis
— Budd–Chiari syndrome (p. 127)
3 Hepatoma
— Associated with high AFP
4 Acute deterioration of hepatocellular function
— e.g. Due to sepsis, alcoholic binge, gut hemorrhage
5 Rupture of dilated abdominal lymphatics
— Causes chylous ascites

* Positive ascitic culture *and* WCC > 250/μL; cf. *bacterascites* (positive culture but WCC < 250/μL) and *culture-negative neutrocytic ascites* (WCC > 250/μL but negative culture)

Differential diagnosis of chylous ascites
1 Intraabdominal lymphoma or carcinoma
2 Hepatic cirrhosis
3 Nephrotic syndrome
4 Tuberculosis
5 Trauma (incl. surgery, e.g. distal splenorenal shunt)

Further examination of the patient with ascites
1 Abdominal signs suggesting primary liver disease
— Ballottable spleen
— Caput medusae, venous hum, testicular atrophy
2 Signs suggesting intraabdominal malignancy
— Absent ankle edema
— Palpable supraclavicular nodes
— Hepatic bruit
— Palpable tumor (e.g. on rectal examination)
3 Signs suggesting cardiac etiology
— Elevated jugular venous pressure ± 'v' waves
— Pulsatile tender hepatomegaly
— Cardiomegaly, S_3, tricuspid murmur
— Pulsus paradoxus (constriction)

4   Signs suggesting hepatic vein/IVC thrombosis
  — Ascites > edema
  — Absent hepatojugular reflux (patient lying flat)
  — Upward-draining lower abdominal wall veins
  — Non-pulsatile tender hepatomegaly

INTESTINAL DISEASES

Chronic diarrhea*: factors favoring organic bowel pathology
1   Nocturnal diarrhea (interrupting sleep)
2   Passage of blood per rectum
3   Weight loss; fever; anemia
4   Age of symptom onset > 50 years

* i.e. duration > 4 weeks

Differential diagnosis of chronic diarrhea
1   Inflammatory bowel disease
2   Malabsorption
3   Infection
  — Giardiasis
  — Amebiasis
  — *Cl. difficile*
  — AIDS-associated gut infections (p. 228)
4   Endocrinopathy
  — Thyrotoxicosis*
  — Adrenal insufficiency
  — Diabetes mellitus
5   Spurious
  — Ca colon
  — Stricture
  — Ischemic colitis
  — Fecal incontinence
6   Iatrogenic, e.g.
  — Antibiotics, antacids
  — Post-gastrectomy
  — Radiation enteritis
  — Laxative abuse
7   Irritable bowel syndrome
  — Diagnosis of exclusion

* Also a rare cause of constipation

Diarrheal syndromes responsive to fasting
1   Osmotic diarrhea
  — Carbohydrate malabsorption
  — Laxative abuse
2   Non-osmotic malabsorption
  — Steatorrhea
  — Bile acid malabsorption
    • After ileal resection
    • After cholecystectomy
3   Incontinence

Inflammatory bowel disease (IBD): indicators of severity
1   Extent of colonic disease
  — May not be ascertainable during relapse
2   Number of stools/day
  — esp. If bloody; < 4 = mild, > 8 = severe
3   Constitutional
  — Fever, tachycardia, pain, distension
4   Weight loss
  — esp. If > 5 kg

5   Blood
  — $\downarrow$ Hb, $\uparrow$ WCC/platelets/ESR
  — $\uparrow$ Leukocyte adhesion/aggregation
6   Biochemistry
  — $\downarrow$ K$^+$/albumin
  Acute phase reactants
  — $\uparrow$ CRP/orosomucoid IL-6
  — $\uparrow$ Fecal lactoferrin
7   AXR
  — Colon diameter (> 6.5 cm = severe)
  — Subphrenic gas (?asymptomatic on steroids)
  — Mucosal 'islands' (pseudopolyps)

Diagnostic clues in chronic diarrhea
1   Fever
  — IBD, Whipple's
  — TB, amebiasis
2   Neuropathy
  — Amyloidosis
  — Diabetic diarrhea
3   Wasting
  — Malabsorption
  — Thyrotoxicosis
  — Uncontrolled IBD
  — Cancer
4   Lymphadenopathy
  — Lymphoma, Whipple's
  — HIV
5   Skin rash
  — Celiac disease (dermatitis herpetiformis)
  — Ulcerative colitis (pyoderma)
  — Carcinoid syndrome (flushing)

Common sites of ischemic colitis
1   Splenic flexure
  — Watershed of inferior/superior mesenteric arteries
2   Rectosigmoid junction
  — Watershed of inferior mesenteric/internal iliac arteries

IRRITABLE BOWEL SYNDROME

Common presentations of irritable bowel syndrome*
1   Abdominal pain relieved by defecation
2   Chronic or recurrent abdominal distension
3   'Morning rush' (urgency, loose stools)
4   Sensation of incomplete evacuation
5   Passage of mucus in stool

* diagnosis of exclusion, prob. pathologically heterogeneous

Differential diagnosis of irritable bowel syndrome
1   Psychological precipitant
  — Depression
  — Stress-related
  — Laxative abuse
2   Endocrinopathy
  — Thyrotoxicosis
  — Hypothyroidism
  — Addison's disease

3 Neuropathy
— Autonomic (p. 267–268)
— Lead poisoning
— Porphyria
4 Malabsorption, dietary intolerance
— Alactasia
— Gluten-induced enteropathy
5 Inflammatory bowel disease
6 Colorectal cancer (if recent onset)

Features favoring functional bowel disorders
1 Long-standing symptoms (years)
2 Vague or variable localization of discomfort
3 Symptomatic failure of all therapeutic measures
4 Non-specific accompaniments
— Tiredness, headache, insomnia
— Nausea, flatulence, easy satiety
5 Affective disturbance

INVESTIGATING GASTROINTESTINAL DISEASE

GASTROESOPHAGEAL DISORDERS

Investigation of dysphagia
1 Barium swallow*
— Good for confirming
• Web
• Pouch
• Stricture
• Achalasia
• Spasm
— Reduces risk of endoscopic perforation in these disorders, esp. pouch
2 Endoscopy‡ ± biopsy
— Proceed to this even if swallow is negative

* Limited diagnostic utility for patients without dysphagia
‡ In general, this investigation is hard to beat

Investigation of non-dysphagic esophageal dysfunction
1 Is reflux present?
— Best test: 24-h esophageal pH monitoring
— Positive if pH < 4, esp. during sleep
2 Are symptoms due to reflux?
— Best test: acid perfusion (Bernstein) test
— Correlates with symptoms (not with esophagitis)
3 Is there a peptic stricture/erosion?
— Best test: barium swallow then endoscopy
4 Is esophagitis present?
— Best test: endoscopy and biopsy
5 Is there a dysmotility syndrome?
— Best test: esophageal manometry

Clinical varieties of esophageal dysmotility syndromes
1 Diffuse spasm
2 'Nutcracker' esophagus
3 Achalasia

Applications of radionuclide esophageal transit studies
1 May provide a non-invasive alternative to endoscopy in patients (esp. children) with suspected esophagitis

2 Correlates well with manometry in assessment of dysmotility
3 Supplements ambulatory esophageal pH monitoring by demonstrating reflux *volume* (and hence severity)

ENDOSCOPY

Absolute indications for endoscopy
1 Gastrointestinal blood loss
— Hematemesis, hematochezia, melena
— Unexplained iron-deficiency anemia and/or positive fecal occult blood
2 Suspected esophageal disease without tissue diagnosis
— Progressive dysphagia or odynophagia
— Suspicious barium swallow
3 Suspected gastric pathology without tissue diagnosis
— Gastric ulcer on barium meal
— Follow-up of gastric ulcer
— Progressive weight loss, epigastric pain or vomiting

The dyspeptic patient: to endoscope or not to endoscope?
1 Endoscopy generally not indicated
— Self-limiting dyspepsia
— Known duodenal ulcer responding to therapy
— Typical symptoms of reflux or irritable bowel syndrome manageable with conservative measures
2 Endoscopy generally indicated
— Severe or persistent symptoms
— Refractory symptoms in a young (< 40 yrs) patient
— Recent onset of symptoms in patients > 40 years

HYPERGASTRINEMIA

Indications for fasting serum gastrin estimation
1 Family history of peptic ulceration
2 Multifocal peptic ulceration
Peptic ulceration of distal duodenum or jejunum
Recurrent post-operative peptic ulceration
3 Peptic ulceration with hypercalcemia (i.e. ?MEN1; p. 115)
4 Intractable watery diarrhea or steatorrhea
5 Radiologic/endoscopic evidence of gastric rugal hypertrophy

Gastric hyperacidity without elevated gastrin?
1 Duodenal ulcer
2 Elevated plasma histamine
— Systemic mastocytosis
— Mast cell (basophilic) leukemia

Hypergastrinemia: differential diagnosis
1 *Gross* elevation (> 600 ng/L)
— Achlorhydria

— Gastrinoma
— Renal failure
2 Minor elevation
  — Failure of patient to fast
  — Antral G-cell hyperplasia/retained antrum
  — Gastric outlet obstruction and/or gastric ulcer
  — Small bowel resection and/or Crohn's disease
  — Hepatic insufficiency
  — Hypercalcemia
  — H$_2$-receptor antagonist therapy, omeprazole

Gastrinoma: diagnostic confirmation
1 Fasting hypergastrinemia (*plus* gastric acid)
2 *Paradoxical* rise* in serum gastrin after secretin infusion
3 Nasogastric intubation followed by pentagastrin infusion
4 Barium studies (incidental)
  — Ectopic ulceration (e.g. post-bulbar, esophageal)
  — Rugal hypertrophy, duodenal nodularity
  — Increased secretions; hyperperistalsis
5 Percutaneous transhepatic portal venous sampling
6 Tumor visualization by CT or angiography‡ (→ biopsy)
  Tumor localization by endoscopic ultrasonography
  Tumor localization by examination of proximal duodenum¶

* Or failure of serum gastrin to fall; or supranormal rise after calcium infusion
‡ Up to 50% failure rate
¶ Duodenal tumors may be ≤ 2 mm diameter

PEPTIC ULCER DISEASE

Pathogenesis of peptic ulcers
1 *H. pylori**
2 NSAIDs
3 Gastrinoma
4 Rare causes: Crohn's disease, herpes simplex

* NB: Causative organism of antral (type A) gastritis; whether it is directly ulcerogenic in duodenal ulcer remains contentious. *No* known role in esophagitis or non-ulcer dyspepsia

Diagnostic utility of gastric acid secretory testing
1 Normal basal acid output (BAO)
  — 0–10 mmol/h HCl
  Normal maximal* acid output (MAO)
  — 10–30 mmol/h HCl
  BAO normally < 20% MAO
2 MAO = 0 mmol/h HCl
  — Achlorhydria
3 ↑ BAO (± ↑ MAO)
  — Duodenal ulcer disease
  — Hyperhistaminemia (see above)
4 ↑↑ BAO, ↑ MAO; BAO:MAO > 30%
  — Gastrinoma

* i.e. after stimulation with pentagastrin, histamine

Associations of achlorhydria
1 Type A (atrophic) gastritis ± pernicious anemia
2 Vagotomy

3 Gastric cancer
4 VIPoma, somatostatinoma

HELICOBACTER PYLORI INFECTIONS

Epidemiology of *H. pylori*
1 Progressively acquired from childhood at a rate ~ 1% per year
2 Higher prevalence in lower socioeconomic communities
3 Fecal–oral transmission implicated in spread
4 Implicated in pathogenesis of gastric MALT (mucosa-associated lymphoid tissue) lymphoma, and perhaps adenocarcinoma
5 Decline in seropositivity appears to parallel decline in incidence of gastric cancer

Diagnosis of gastric *H. pylori* infection
1 Serology (IgG)*
2 ^{14}C-urea breath test (p. 131)
3 Endoscopic biopsy and culture
4 PCR of biopsy, gastric fluid, feces

* Also useful for monitoring eradication therapy

DIAGNOSTIC ASPECTS OF LIVER DISEASE

True liver 'function' (> damage) tests
1 Albumin
2 Prothrombin time

Elevated alkaline phosphatase: features favoring liver origin
1 Heat-stable isoenzyme ('bone burns')
2 ↑ GGT
3 ↑ Serum bile acids

Investigation of suspected alcoholic liver disease
1 ↑ γ-glutamyl transpeptidase (GGT)*
  — Induced by alcohol ingestion
  — May also reflect intrahepatic obstruction in cirrhosis
2 Blood film
  — Round macrocytes (*unless* coexisting folate deficiency)
  — Target cells (*non-specific* indicator of liver disease)
3 Biochemical profile
  — AST:ALT > 2:1, AST < 500 IU/L (cf. viral hepatitis)
  — ↑ Urate, ↑ triglycerides, ↓ Mg^{2+}, ↓ albumin (less specific)
4 ↑ Blood alcohol
  — If drinking within last 24 h suspected
5 ↑ Plasma AFP; gallium scan
  — If hepatoma suspected
6 Liver biopsy (see below)

* Alkaline phosphatase is also inducible, but less sensitive

Investigation of occult gastrointestinal blood loss
1 Fecal occult blood testing
  — For confirmation of bleeding

— Negative testing does *not* reliably exclude bleeding
2 Endoscopy
— Gastroduodenoscopy and colonoscopy
3 Angiography
— Detects angiodysplasias and small bowel bleeding
4 Barium follow-through*
5 Radionuclide studies
— ^{59}Fe (oral) whole body counting
• Good for assessing intermenstrual blood loss
— ^{99m}Tc-labelled sulfur colloid (IV)
• Detects *active* hemorrhage (> 0.5 mL/min)
— ^{51}Cr-RBC or ^{99m}Tc-RBC labelling (IV 'blood pool scan')
• May also be of value in intermittent bleeding
— ^{99m}Tc pertechnate (IV)
• → ectopic gastric mucosa (Meckel's diverticulum)
6 Exploratory laparotomy
— A last resort

* NB: Angiography *impossible* for days if barium studies performed first

Laboratory diagnosis of idiopathic hemochromatosis
1 Transferrin saturation > 80% (*plus* ↑ serum Fe, ↓ TIBC)
2 Serum ferritin > 1000 µg/L (best screening test)
Serum ferritin increases following desferrioxamine
3 Desferrioxamine-chelatable urinary Fe excretion > 7.5 mg/24 h
4 Quantitative phlebotomy > 7.5 g Fe
5 Liver biopsy: stainable Fe grade 3 or 4
6 Hepatic Fe quantitation: > 100 µmol/g dry weight (diagnostic)

Distinction of hemochromatosis from alcoholic liver disease
1 Ferritin > 1000 µg/L (normal range < 300 µg/L)
— cf. Alcoholics: often 300–1000 µg/L
2 *Massive* iron overload on liver biopsy
— cf. Alcohol: moderate only
3 Elevated ferritin levels
— In first-degree relatives as well as patient
4 HLA-A3 linkage
— An association only; *not* a diagnostic test

Diagnosis of hepatic vein thrombosis (Budd–Chiari)
1 Confirmatory investigations
— Ultrasound of hepatic veins and IVC
— Hepatic venography
• Thrombosis (± inferior vena caval thrombosis)
2 Supportive investigations
— Isotope liver scan
• Selective caudate lobe uptake (hypertrophied)
— Liver biopsy
• Centrizonal venous congestion

Biochemical characterization of jaundice
1 Conjugated hyperbilirubinemia
↑ GGT/alkaline phosphatase
Bilirubinuria, absent urobilinogen*
— Common bile duct obstruction

2 Conjugated (± unconjugated) hyperbilirubinemia
AST/ALT > 1000 IU/L
Bilirubinuria
— Acute hepatitis
3 Unconjugated hyperbilirubinemia
— Gilbert's, Crigler–Najjar
— Hemolysis

* NB: Urobilinogen *not* routinely measured now

HEPATITIS

Serologic investigation of acute hepatitis
1 IgM anti-HAV
2 HBsAg *and* IgM anti-HBc
3 Anti-HCV
4 If above are *negative*, request
— IgM anti-HEV (or rising IgG anti-HEV)
— EB viral capsid antigen IgM
— CMV serology

Hepatitis B serology made easy
1 Presence of HBsAg implies active infection
Appearance of anti-HBs implies recovery and immunity
2 Presence of HBeAg implies patient is infective to others
Anti-HBe generally (not invariably) implies loss of infectivity
3 HBcAg (core antigen) cannot be detected in peripheral blood
High-titer IgM anti-HBc implies acute (severe) hepatitis B
IgM anti-HBc appears after HBsAg disappears; may be the *only* detectable marker of recent HBV infection at this time
4 Persistence of IgM anti-HBc implies chronic HBV (esp. CAH)

Variant hepatitis B infections
1 Precore mutant
— Endemic in Mediterranean
— Negative HBeAg due to mutations of precore region
— Liver disease progresses despite anti-HBe, perhaps indicating cross-recognition of HBcAg by anti-HBe
— Positive HBV DNA
2 Surface gene 'escape mutants'
— Occurs post-vaccination, post-transplant
— Point mutation in 'a' determinant of surface gene leads to loss of immune recognition → reactivated HBV

Diagnosis of hepatitis C
1 History of 'at-risk' behavior
— IV drug abuse, skin tattooing
— Blood transfusion, organ transplant
2 Anti-HCV serology
— Immunoenzymatic (ELISA-3) 99% specific
— May take up to 6 months to become positive (average 3 months)

— False-negatives in transplant patients; occasional false-positives in blood donors
— ELISA results are confirmed by immunoblot (RIBA)
3 Plasma RNA PCR
— Sensitive, but many false-positives
— Mainly used for
• HCV diagnosis post-transplant
• Early diagnosis of acute hepatitis
• Perinatal transmission detection
• Monitoring of antiviral therapy
4 HBsAg and IgM anti-HAV negative
5 Abnormal liver function tests ± symptoms

Investigation of the patient with chronic hepatitis
1 If HBsAg and anti-HCV negative
— Request anti-HBc and anti-HBs
2 If HBsAg or anti-HBc positive > 6 months (chronic hepatitis)
— Request HBeAg and anti-HBe
3 If chronic HBsAg carrier deteriorates, request
— δ agent antibody
— IgM anti-HAV
— AFP
4 If patient is *not* proven to have hepatitis B or C, request
— Autoantibodies: smooth muscle/mitochondrial/ ANA
— Serum ceruloplasmin, 24-h urinary copper
— $α_1$AT level; E8V VCA IgG (p. 215)
5 Liver biopsy is *always* requested in the initial work-up

The stages of chronic hepatitis B infection
1 Active replicative phase (→ acute, or chronic active, hepatitis)
— HBeAg +, anti-HBe
— HBV DNA + (most sensitive marker)
— HBV DNA polymerase +
— ↑ AST/ALT (T cell-dependent liver necrosis)
2 Intermediate phase
— Cessation of HBV replication
— Acceleration of hepatocyte damage
3 Integrative phase (→ chronic persistence hepatitis/ hepatoma)
— HBeAg −, anti-HBe +
— HBsAg remains + usually (but not invariably)
— HBV DNA becomes integrated into hepatocyte genome

LIVER BIOPSY

Abnormal enzymes? Treatable diagnoses on liver biopsy
1 Chronic active hepatitis (esp. autoimmune)
2 Hemochromatosis
3 Wilson's disease
4 Granulomatous liver disease (esp. TB)

Provisional diagnoses contraindicating liver biopsy*
1 Hemangioma, angiosarcoma
2 Amyloidosis with prolonged bleeding time
3 Hydatid disease

4 Extrahepatic biliary obstruction‡
5 *Any* liver disease with uncorrected coagulopathy

* Associated with 0.01% mortality rate
‡ Predisposes to post-biopsy biliary leak

How to biopsy a chronically diseased liver
1 If prothrombin time, Hb and platelet count are normal, group and hold, then proceed with caution
If abnormal platelet function suspected, may be worthwhile to check bleeding time (debatable)
2 If prothrombin time abnormal and patient *not* jaundiced, give vitamin K 10 mg/day (IM for 3 days or orally for 5 days) and repeat prothrombin time; if index < 1.3, proceed
3 If prothrombin time abnormal and patient jaundiced, give vitamin K (usually IM with anaphylactic kit ready) and check PT the next day; if normal, proceed
4 If prothrombin time remains > 4 sec prolonged after vitamin K (indicating major hepatic parenchymal damage) and if biopsy required urgently, cover with fresh frozen plasma (FFP). Check the prothrombin time following completion of FFP infusion, then biopsy. Further FFP may be needed post-biopsy
5 If FFP ineffective, dispense with percutaneous biopsy altogether and opt for a transjugular biopsy catheter if the diagnosis is still regarded as absolutely necessary

HEPATIC HISTOPATHOLOGY

Differential diagnosis of hepatic granulomata
1 Sarcoidosis
2 Berylliosis
3 Primary biliary cirrhosis
4 Infection: TB, syphilis, Q fever, brucellosis, histoplasmosis
5 Drug-induced: allopurinol, phenylbutazone, sulfonamides

Liver histology in selected disorders
1 Alcoholic liver disease
— Mallory's hyaline (*not* pathognomonic)
— Centrilobular necrosis
— Giant mitochondria
— Ballooning degeneration of hepatocytes
— Pericellular fibrosis → 'chicken wire' appearance
2 $α_1$AT deficiency
— PAS-positive globules within hepatocytes
3 Chronic persistent hepatitis
— Preserved lobular architecture (intact limiting plate)
— Minimal fibrosis
— Mononuclear infiltrate confined to portal tracts
4 Chronic active hepatitis
— Disruption of lobular architecture
• Piecemeal necrosis (erosion of limiting plate)
• Bridging necrosis
• 'Rosette' and pseudolobule formation
— Mononuclear infiltrate extends into lobules
— Councilman bodies, Kupffer cell hyperplasia

Differential diagnosis of 'disappearing bile ducts' on biopsy
1 Primary biliary cirrhosis
— Affects biliary ductules
2 Sclerosing cholangitis
— Affects small and large bile ducts
3 Liver transplantation
— Graft vs. host disease
— Chronic rejection

INVESTIGATING PANCREATOBILIARY DISEASE

Laboratory diagnosis of acute pancreatitis
1 ↑ Serum amylase
— Good screening test, but frequent false-positives
— False-negatives → hyperlipidemia-induced pancreatitis
2 ↑ Serum lipase
— Most specific test
— Equally sensitive as amylase

Indicators of poor prognosis in acute pancreatitis
1 Clinical
— Age > 60; first attack
— Hypotension
— Ascites (esp. with high protein level)
2 Hemorrhagic pancreatitis
— Clinical signs
• Grey–Turner's sign (flank ecchymosis)
• Cullen's sign (periumbilical ecchymosis)
— Methemalbuminemia
— Low albumin Hb; anemia; leukocytosis (WCC > 15,000)
— Peritoneal lavage (hemorrhagic ascites)
3 Reduced blood levels
— ↓ Ca^{2+} *
— ↓ PaO_2
4 Increased blood levels
— ↑ Blood glucose
— ↑ BUN, ↑ AST
— ↑ Fibrinogen
5 Necrosis /abscess on contrast-enhanced CT

* When corrected for albumin; cf. *elevated* calcium: exclude causative hyperparathyroidism

Diagnosis of exocrine pancreatic insufficiency
1 Low plasma cholesterol, albumin, β-carotene*
— Non-specific screens for fat malabsorption
— 'False-positives' in liver disease
2 ^{14}C-triolein (triglyceride) breath test
— ↓ $^{14}CO_2$ production
— Indirect test of lipase secretion
— 90% sensitive/specific for fat malabsorption
3 PABA/^{14}C excretion
— Indirect test of chymotrypsin secretion
Fluorescein dilaurate test
— Index of esterase secretion
4 Nasoduodenal intubation
— Lundh test
— Secretin-pancreozymin test

5 3-day fecal fats
— Stool fat > 6 g/day (now outmoded)
— Sudan III stool fat easier to confirm
6 *Normal* ^{14}C-D-xylose absorption

* NB: *Folate* levels are normal in pure pancreatic insufficiency; low folate plus steatorrhea suggests jejunal biopsy

Investigations of choice for gallbladder disease
1 Oral cholecystography
— Cheap, available; assesses function and anatomy
— Confirms gallstones in anicteric patients
— Assesses gallstone composition and cystic duct patency
— Useful prior to gallstone dissolution or lithotripsy
— Side-effects: 25% diarrhea, 10% nausea, 10% dysuria
2 Real-time ultrasonography
— Quick, painless, non-invasive; difficult if obese
— Risk-free: no radiation, no contrast hypersensitivity
— High sensitivity for cholecystitis (incl. chronic)
— Distinguishes obstructive from hepatocellular jaundice
— May detect unsuspected non-biliary causes of pain
3 ERCP
— Investigation of choice for obstructive jaundice
— May be therapeutic (e.g. sphincterotomy, stenting)
— Useful in post-cholecystectomy jaundice
— Excludes false-negative ultrasound/ cholecystography
— Localizes obstruction in pancreatic/common bile duct
4 Percutaneous transhepatic cholangiogram (PTC)
— Uncommonly used for diagnostic studies now
— Localizes obstruction when intrahepatic ducts dilated*
— Useful for draining bile in inoperable obstruction‡
— Contraindicated in gross ascites or coagulopathy

* But ERCP better
‡ i.e. if stent placement proves impossible

Indications for ^{99m}Tc-HIDA hepatobiliary scintigraphy*
1 Morphine-enhanced cholescintigraphy
— Main indication: suspected cystic duct obstruction in acute cholecystitis
• Failure of gallbladder visualization within 30 min of morphine (contracts sphincter of Oddi) confirms diagnosis
• Gallbladder visualization within 1 h excludes diagnosis
— Also used to monitor post-operative biliary patency
— False-positives in alcoholics, hepatitis, pancreatitis, fasting, TPN, severe illness
— False-negatives in acalculous or chronic cholecystitis
2 Cholecystokinin-enhanced cholescintigraphy
— Main indication: assessment of 'biliary' pain in patients without demonstrable gallstones
— ↓ CCK-induced gallbladder ejection fraction in
• Biliary dyskinesia
• Sphincter of Oddi spasm
• Chronic acalculous cholecystitis

— Ejection fraction < 30% may predict successful symptomatic response to cholecystectomy

* DISIDA preferred to HIDA in jaundiced patients

Positive findings on oral cholecystography
1   Gallstones
2   Failure to opacify gallbladder despite second dose of contrast

Failure of gallbladder visualization by oral cholecystography?
1   Patient non-compliance
    — Tablets and/or contrast not taken
2   Gastric stasis, outlet obstruction; vomiting
3   Intestinal malabsorption or diarrhea
4   Liver disease
5   Gallbladder unable to concentrate dye
    — e.g. Chronic cholecystitis
6   Mechanical obstruction preventing entry of contrast
    — e.g. Acute cholecystitis

NB: In *jaundiced* patients the investigation of choice is biliary ultrasound

Indications for ERCP
1   Suspected choledocholithiasis
2   Persistent symptoms following biliary surgery
3   Cholestasis without intrahepatic bile duct dilatation*
4   For diagnosis (or preoperative assessment) of chronic pancreatitis or pancreatic carcinoma

* i.e. cholestasis due to suspected biliary tract disease

INVESTIGATING INTESTINAL DISEASE

Indications for colonoscopy
1   Bleeding per rectum *or* occult blood loss
2   Persistent bowel symptoms with normal sigmoidoscopy
3   Dysplasia monitoring in long-standing ulcerative pancolitis
4   Surveillance for recurrence following surgery for Ca colon
5   Abnormal barium enema (e.g. stricture, polyp)
6   Diagnostic or therapeutic removal of colonic polyps

Contraindications to colonoscopy
1   Peritonism
2   Toxic megacolon
3   *Any* acute severe inflammatory colonic process
4   Pregnancy
5   Recent (< 6/12) history of myocardial infarction

Advantages of colonoscopy over barium enema
1   More sensitive for tumor/polyp detection
2   More accurate, esp. in sigmoid colon and cecum
3   May detect vascular lesions such as angiodysplasia
4   May be useful in emergency assessment of PR bleeding
5   Enables tissue diagnosis

Rectal biopsy: diagnostic value
1   Ulcerative proctitis

2   Amyloidosis
3   Tay–Sachs; metachromatic leukodystrophy
4   Amebiasis (and other infective proctocolitides)
5   Pseudomembranous colitis (though may spare rectum)

GASTROINTESTINAL RADIOLOGY

Radiologic features of achalasia
1   Plain film
    — Intrathoracic air–fluid level
    — Absent gastric air bubble
    — Lower zone lung fibrosis (bronchiectasis)
2   Barium swallow
    — Tertiary contractions replacing peristaltic activity
    — Dilated, tapering lower esophagus ('beaked', 'rattail')

Giant gastric rugae: differential diagnosis
1   Malignancy (e.g. lymphoma, leiomyoma)
2   Gastrinoma
3   Ménètrier's disease*

* hypoproteinemic hypertrophic gastropathy

Jejunal ulcers: differential diagnosis
1   Ulcerative jejunitis (malignant histiocytosis)
2   Celiac disease, Crohn's disease
3   Gastrinoma
4   Meckel's diverticulitis (usually in boys; 5–10% bleed)
5   Mesenteric ischemia; polyarteritis
6   Lymphoma
7   Infection
    — Typhoid, dysentery, syphilis, TB, actinomycosis, fungi
8   Iatrogenic
    — Digoxin, potassium tablets

Multiple intestinal tumors? Differential diagnosis
1   Hereditary adenoma-carcinoma syndromes
    — Familial adenomatous polyposis (FAP)
    — Gardner's syndrome
    — Turcot's syndrome
2   Hereditary non-polyposis colorectal cancer (HNPCC)
    — DNA mismatch repair syndromes
    — Muir–Torre syndrome
3   Hereditary hamartoma syndromes
    — Peutz–Jeghers syndrome
    — Cowden's disease
    — Basal cell nevus syndrome
    — Sotos' syndrome
4   Non-hereditary polyposis syndromes
    — Cronkhite–Canada syndrome
    — Pneumatosis cystoides intestinalis

Space-occupying lesions on liver scan: clinical significance
1   Thick-walled cavity on ultrasound
    Gallium scan/^{111}In-WBC scan positive
    — Pyogenic liver abscess
    — R_x: aspiration + antibiotics
2   Thick-walled cavity on ultrasound
    Gallium negative; amebic serology positive (99%)

— Amebic liver abscess
— R_x: metronidazole
3 Thin-walled cyst on ultrasound
'Daughter' cysts
— Hydatid disease*
— R_x: open drainage (aspiration contraindicated)
4 Echodense lesion within cirrhotic parenchyma
AFP elevated
— Hepatoma‡
— R_x: excision/transplant
5 Multiple echodense lesions
Biopsy positive for malignancy
— Metastatic liver disease
— R_x: chemotherapy

* Serology often inconclusive
‡ AFP > 1000 ng/mL obviates need for CT-guided biopsy

Abdominal imaging techniques: ultrasound or CT?

1 Ultrasound
— Advantages
• No radiation dose
• Quick and relatively cheap
• Good resolution of luminal structures (e.g. biliary tree), cysts and abscesses
— Disadvantages
• Difficult in obese patients
• Less detail than CT
2 CT
— Advantages
• High quality images, esp. in obese patients
• Excellent delineation of retroperitoneal structures (e.g. pancreas, psoas)
— Disadvantages
• Difficult if lots of bowel gas
• Not very useful for biliary tree
• High radiation dose
• Time-consuming and expensive

MALABSORPTION

Diagnosis of bacterial overgrowth

1 High index of suspicion
— Crohn's
— Post-Polya
— Small bowel diverticulosis
— Hypomotility syndrome (e.g. scleroderma)
— Elderly
2 Low B_{12}
— Abnormal Schilling's test after intrinsic factor
3 ^{14}C-bile acid breath test (see below)
4 Duodenal aspiration and culture
— > 10^5 organisms/mL
5 Therapeutic trial of tetracycline

Diagnosis of lactose intolerance

1 History of milk-related diarrhea
2 Successful therapeutic trial of milk-free diet
3 Stool: pH < 6.5; Benedict's test positive
4 'Flat' lactose tolerance test (rarely used now)
5 Hydrogen breath test following oral lactose (best screen)

6 Small bowel biopsy with lactase quantitation (definitive)
— Primary alactasia: other disaccharidases normal
— Secondary lactose intolerance: all disaccharidases ↓

Breath testing: diagnostic value in malabsorption

1 ^{14}C-glycocholate (bile acid) breath test*
— Bacterial overgrowth
• ↑ Deconjugation (small bowel)
→ ↑ Breath/↓ fecal ^{14}C
— Ileal insufficiency
• ↑ Deconjugation (large bowel)
→ ↑ Breath/↑ fecal ^{14}C
2 Hydrogen breath test (e.g. after oral glucose, lactulose)
— Bacterial overgrowth
• Early H_2 peak (30 min; normally 2 h)
— Lactose intolerance (following oral lactose)
• 'Flat' H_2 response
— Indirect index of small intestinal transit time
• Early or late peak with ↑,↓ motility
3 ^{14}C-triolein breath test
— Steatorrhea (→ ↓ $^{14}CO_2$ excretion)
4 ^{14}C-galactose breath test
— Galactosemia (→ ↓ $^{14}CO_2$ excretion)
5 ^{14}C-urea breath test
— *Helicobacter pylori*‡
— Urea → ↑ NH_3 + $^{14}CO_2$

* Breath test now superseded by fecal bile acid estimation for diagnosis of bile acid malabsorption; ^{75}SeHCAT is used for this (p. 140)
‡ And other urease-positive gastric infections; not widely available

Small bowel biopsy: diagnostic value

1 Celiac disease
— Villous atrophy, crypt hypertrophy, mononuclears
2 Nodular lymphoid hyperplasia, hypogamma-globulinemia
— Villous atrophy but *no* plasma cells
3 Abetalipoproteinemia
— Lipid infiltration
4 Infections
— Parasites (*Giardia, Strongyloides, Coccidia*)
— Fungal (*Candida, Histoplasma*) infections
— Whipple's disease (*T. whippelii*; p. 133)
5 Other histopathologic diagnoses
— Crohn's disease
— Lymphoma, α heavy chain disease
— Intestinal lymphangiectasia

Measurement of gut permeability

1 D-xylose absorption (traditional test): false-positives in
— Renal failure
— Delayed gastric emptying
2 Alternatives
— Polyethylene glycol
— ^{51}Cr-EDTA
3 Lactulose/mannitol absorption ratio
— ↑ Disaccharide (lactulose) but ↓ monosaccharide (mannitol) absorption → celiac disease

AN APPROACH TO DIARRHEA

Watery diarrhea: secretory or osmotic?
1 Stool volume
   — Compare volume on normal diet with volume
     after 24-h nil by mouth (enforced) with IV fluids
     only
   — Volumes classically similar in secretory (cholera-
     like) diarrhea, but reduced in osmotic diarrheas
2 Stool electrolytes*
   — In secretory diarrhea
     • Fecal fluid Na^+/Cl^-/osmolality similar to plasma
     • Fecal fluid HCO_3^- and K^+ are 2–5 x plasma levels
     • Fecal fluid osmolality is *entirely* accounted for
       by (i.e. equal to) stool electrolytes ($Na^+ + K^+$)
   — In osmotic diarrhea
     • *Stool* osmolality ($2 \times [Na^+ + K^+]$) < *fecal fluid*
       osmolality (= 'osmotic gap')
3 Stool osmolality*
   — Virtually isotonic with plasma if secretory;
     osmotic gap < 50 mosm/L
   — Large osmotic gap (> 50) suggests laxative abuse

* NB: Laboratories generally *hate* doing these tests!

Investigating suspected laxative abuse
1 Hypokalemia
2 Stool volumes/electrolytes/osmolality
3 Urinary phenolphthalein
4 Fecal magnesium levels*
5 Sigmoidoscopy
   — Melanosis coli (if anthracene laxatives used)
   — Absent mucosal damage

* NB: Fecal magnesium may also be elevated in diarrheal
diseases other than those due to ingestion of magnesium-
containing laxatives

Diagnosis of giardiasis
1 Stool examination
   — Trophozoites (in unformed stools)
   — Cysts (in formed stools)
2 Endoscopic sampling of duodenal/jejunal fluid
  Endoscopic deep duodenal/jejunal biopsy
3 Therapeutic trial of metronidazole/tinidazole*

* Commonest and most practical 'diagnostic' approach

Bloody diarrhea: microbiological differential diagnosis
1 *Shigella* spp.
2 Enteroinvasive *E. coli*
3 *Campylobacter jejuni*
4 *Salmonella* spp.
5 *Entameba histolytica* (esp. if recent travel)
6 *Yersinia enterocolitica*
7 *Clostridium difficile* (if recent antibiotics)

Diarrhea with abundant fecal polymorphonuclear leukocytes?*
1 *Shigella* spp.
   — Classic cause of bacillary dysentery
2 Enteroinvasive *E. coli*
   — cf. Enterotoxigenic *E. coli* (few leukocytes)
3 *C. jejuni*
   — cf. *C. fetus* (mononuclears only)

4 *S. enteritidis*
   — cf. *S. typhi* (mononuclears only)
5 Amebic dysentery, yersiniosis
   — cf. Giardiasis (few leukocytes)
6 *V. parahemolyticus*
   — cf. *V. cholerae* (few leukocytes)
7 *Cl. difficile*

* i.e. *dysentery*; caused by *enteroinvasive* (not toxigenic)
organisms

INFLAMMATORY BOWEL DISEASE

Histologic hallmarks of inflammatory bowel disease
1 Ulcerative colitis
   — Crypts reduced in number; irregular; branched
   — Cryptabscesses +++
   — Loss of goblet cells
   — Paneth cell metaplasia +++
   — Thickening of muscularis mucosae
   — Infiltrate: polymorphs, eosinophils, plasma cells
2 Crohn's disease
   — Transmural involvement, fissuring
   — Glandular pattern relatively undisturbed
   — Non-caseating granulomata
   — Focal inflammation
   — Goblet cell preservation
   — Infiltrate: lymphocytes, macrophages, histiocytes
   — Cryptabscesses infrequent
   — Paneth cell metaplasia rare

Radiologic hallmarks of inflammatory bowel disease
1 Ulcerative colitis
   — Indicators of disease diagnosis
     • Fine, spiculating superficial ulcers, fuzzy
       contour
     • 'Collarstud' ulcers
   — Indicators of disease *severity*
     • 'Pseudopolyps' (luminal mucosal filling defects
       = inflammatory polyps between ulcers)
   — Indicators of disease *chronicity*
     • Tubular 'hosepipe' colon ($\downarrow$ haustration)
     • Shortened, narrowed colon
     • Retrorectal space > 2 cm
     • Barium reflux through patulous ileocecal valve
2 Crohn's disease
   — Early lesions
     • Thickening of valvulae coniventes
     • Aphthoid ulceration
   — Late lesions
     • 'Cobblestoning'
     • 'Rose-thorn' and 'collarstud' (deep) ulcers
     • Transmural fissuring
     • 'Skip lesions' (= involved segments)
   — Complications
     • Fistulae, sinuses, stenoses (on barium studies)
     • *Severe* colonic ulceration/edema may be
       evident on plain films
3 Ischemic colitis
   — Large asymmetric 'thumbprint' deformities (due
     to intramural edema), esp. at splenic flexure
   — Toxic dilatation

Radiographic stricture in Crohn's disease?
1 Transient bowel spasm
2 Inflammatory stenosis
3 Ischemic fibrosis
4 Pericolic abscess
5 Carcinoma

Diagnosis of Whipple's disease
1 Duodenal biopsy
— PAS-positive staining of foamy macrophages in lamina propria
2 Polymerase chain reaction (PCR)
— Primers specific for *T. whippelii* in infected tissues or peripheral blood
3 Electron microscopy
— Whipple bacillus visible in infected tissues
4 Therapeutic trial
— Penicillin/streptomycin; co-trimoxazole

MANAGING GASTROINTESTINAL DISEASE

ESOPHAGEAL DISEASE

Therapeutic measures in esophageal reflux
1 Minor disease
— Weight reduction, elevate bedhead
— Avoid alcohol/nicotine/caffeine/fat
— Post-prandial antacids
— Preprandial
• Metoclopramide*
• Domperidone‡
• Cisapride¶
— Nocturnal H_2-receptor antagonists
2 Major disease (incl. CREST, scleroderma)
— Omeprazole (treatment of choice)
— Surgery, e.g. Nissan fundoplication (now rare)

* Enhances gastric emptying/lower esophageal sphincter tone
‡ dopamine agonist
¶ myenteric plexus-selective cholinergic drug

Indications for surgery in esophageal reflux
1 Severe symptoms refractory to medical treatment
2 Penetrating ulcer unresponsive to medical treatment
3 Severe esophageal bleeding
4 Stricture requiring excessively frequent dilatation

Management of severe recurrent pain due to esophageal spasm
1 Endoscopy: exclude
— Intrinsic esophageal disease
— Peptic ulcer
2 Exclude non-gastroesophageal causes, e.g.
— Ischemic heart disease (ECG)
— Gallstones (OCG)
3 Nifedipine
4 Nitrates

MANAGEMENT OF PEPTIC ULCERATION

Medical modalities available for peptic ulcer
1 Antacids
— Sodium bicarbonate
• Absorbed; may cause alkalosis, fluid overload
— Magnesium salts, esp. trisilicate
• Tend to cause diarrhea
— Aluminium salts, hydroxide/silicate
• Tend to constipate
2 Cytoprotective agents ('coat' mucosa; no antacid properties)
— Colloidal bismuth
• Bactericidal to *H. pylori*
— Sucralfate (aluminium hydroxide and sucrose)
• Used as stress ulcer prophylaxis
3 Antisecretory agents
— H_2-receptor antagonists
• Ranitidine, cimetidine, famotidine, nizatidine
— H^+/K^+-ATPase (proton pump) inhibitors
• Omeprazole, lansoprazole
4 Antisecretory and cytoprotective agents
— Prostaglandin E_1/E_2 derivatives
• Misoprostol
5 Anticholinergics
— Pirenzipine (investigational)

Adverse effects of cimetidine*
1 Antiandrogenic effects
— Gynecomastia (in 1%)
— Impotence, oligospermia (in 1%)
2 Confusion, esp. if
— Elderly (esp. IV therapy)
— Renal impairment or liver disease
3 Reversible laboratory changes
— ↑ Serum creatinine
— ↑ Transaminases
— ↓ WCC and/or platelet count
4 Drug potentiation‡
— Inhibition of hepatic metabolism, e.g.
• Warfarin (↓ hydroxylation)
• Theophylline (↓ demethylation)
• Phenytoin (+ other anticonvulsants)
• Cyclosporin
— Competition for renal tubular secretion
• Procainamide (+ other antiarrhythmics)
5 Drug antagonism
— Reduced absorption due to ↑ gastric pH¶
• Ketoconazole

* Moderately unusual for these to be a problem in practice, however; diarrhea or headache are commoner
‡ Most of these interactions also occur with omeprazole
¶ Hence, also occurs with any other H_2-blocker

Advantages of ranitidine over cimetidine
1 More prolonged action (less frequent dosage: b.d.)
2 Binds cytochrome P_{450} less avidly (↓ drug interactions*)
3 Lower affinity for androgen receptors (less antiandrogenic)
4 Rarely causes confusional states
5 More potent (5–8 times) acid inhibitor on a molar basis

6 More effective for treating esophagitis
7 Fewer relapses during maintenance duodenal ulcer therapy

* Minor interactions still possible with warfarin, phenytoin, theophylline, procainamide

Indications for maintenance H_2-blocker therapy
1 *H. pylori* ruled out (present in 95% DU's), *plus*
2 Persistent symptomatic peptic ulceration*, *or*
3 Previous ulcer hemorrhage/bleeding, *or*
4 Post-surgical ulcer relapse, *or*
5 Necessity for concomitant NSAID treatment‡

* At least three symptomatic relapses per year
‡ If misoprostol contraindicated or not tolerated

Indications for omeprazole therapy
1 Gastrinoma (p. 142)
   — 60 mg/day in divided doses initially
   — Medical therapy of choice
2 Esophagitis (drug of choice)
   — Endoscopy confirms severe esophagitis, *or*
   — Failure of 8 weeks' H_2-blocker + antacids
   — Combine with cisapride for refractory disease
3 Refractory duodenal ulceration
   — *H. pylori* detected? Eradicated (but see below) with
      • Omeprazole + amoxicillin (80% success)
   — *H. pylori* not detected, but ulcer persists after 8 weeks' H_2-blocker therapy (0.5% patients only)
      • Try omeprazole 20 mg b.d. for 4–8 weeks
4 NSAID-associated gastric ulcer, *if*
   — NSAID must be continued, *and*
   — Misoprostol ineffective or toxic (diarrhea)

Advantages of proton pump inhibitors over H_2-blockers
1 More prolonged action
   — Once-daily dosage usually suffices
2 More potent acid inhibitor*; hence
   — More rapid ulcer healing

* Omeprazole improves its own bioavailability by reducing gut acidity

Sucralfate*: mechanisms of action
1 Physical barrier between lumen and mucosa
   Increases mucus viscosity/hydrophobicity
2 Binds and reduces pepsin activity
3 Increases mucosal prostaglandin and bicarbonate output
4 Trophic effects on mucosa (enhances blood flow)

* A water-insoluble salt of sucrose and aluminium hydroxide

Clinical use of misoprostol therapy
1 Action
   — *Cytoprotective* oral analog of prostaglandin E_1
   — *Antisecretory* effect (via histamine and prostaglandins)
2 Main indications
   — Prophylaxis* or R_x of NSAID-induced gastric damage
   — Permits ulcer healing in patients needing to continue NSAIDs; does not attenuate systemic NSAID effects
   — Second-line or adjunctive therapy for peptic ulcers unassociated with NSAID therapy

3 Toxicity
   — Diarrhea, cramps, flatulence (in 10%)
   — Dysmenorrhea, menorrhagia (↑ uterine contractility)
4 Contraindications
   — Pregnancy (promotes miscarriage)
5 Limitations
   — *Not* shown to reduce incidence of complications from NSAID therapy (hemorrhage, perforation, death)
   — Does *not* improve NSAID-induced dyspepsia

* In high-risk patients (e.g. past ulcer history) about to commence NSAIDs

Relative ulcerogenicity of NSAIDs
1 Least ulcerogenicity
   — Ibuprofen (< 1500 mg/day)
   — Diclofenac, sulindac
2 Intermediate ulcerogenicity
   — Indomethacin
   — Naproxen
3 Highest ulcerogenicity
   — Azapropazone
   — Piroxicam

Efficacy of antiulcer therapies
1 80% ulcers treated with H_2-receptor blockers heal in 6 weeks
   50–75% healed ulcers relapse within 1 year of ceasing therapy*
2 Healing is mediated primarily by nocturnal acid inhibition
   Maintenance cimetidine 400 mg nocte reduces relapse to 40%
   Ranitidine 150 mg nocte reduces relapse rates to 20%
3 Relapse rates following single-course treatment with colloidal bismuth (cheap; clears *H. pylori* from the gastric mucosa) are superior to single-course ranitidine
4 Highly selective vagotomy is associated with a 10% relapse rate and a 1% incidence of significant side-effects; but hardly ever indicated nowadays

* esp. smokers; duodenal more likely to relapse than gastric ulcers

MANAGEMENT OF *H. PYLORI* INFECTIONS

Clinical scenarios for considering anti-*Helicobacter* therapy
1 Duodenal ulcer
2 Gastric ulcer (some)
3 Chronic antral gastritis (perhaps)

Some *H. pylori* eradication regimens
1 'Triple therapy' (2 weeks)
   — Colloidal bismuth subcitrate 120 mg q.i.d., *plus*
   — Metronidazole 400 mg q.i.d., *plus*
   — Tetracycline 500 mg q.i.d.
2 If above fails
   — Substitute clarithromycin for metronidazole*
   — Can also substitute ranitidine for bismuth

3 Dual therapy (7–10 days)
— Omeprazole 20 mg b.d. *plus*
— Amoxicillin 500 mg t.d.s. (or clarithromycin)

* NB: Rapid *H. pylori* resistance to either drug used alone

A sequential approach to duodenal ulcer symptoms
1 Preliminary precautions
— Confirm diagnosis; exclude gastric ulcer, esophagitis
— Cease NSAIDs/cigarettes
— Exclude anemia/iron deficiency
2 Treat initially with
— Antacid + H_2-blocker for 6 weeks
3 No symptomatic improvement? Consider
— Serology or breath testing for *H. pylori*
Or switch medication empirically to
— Colloidal bismuth
4 In the light of these outcomes, consider
— *H. pylori* eradication (triple therapy; see above)
5 If *H. pylori* not suspected, consider
— Fasting serum gastrin
— Treating with sucralfate or omeprazole
— Maintenance H_2-blockers following symptom control

POST-GASTRECTOMY SYNDROMES

Anemia following gastric surgery: mechanisms
1 Iron deficiency ($\rightarrow$ anemia in 50%)
— Malabsorption due to duodenal bypass (Polya)
— Hypochlorhydria (Fe^{2+} less soluble than Fe^{3+})
— Recurrent bleeding (e.g. stomal ulcers, gastritis)
2 B_{12} deficiency ($\rightarrow$ anemia in 5%)
— $\downarrow$ Parietal cell mass (esp. in total gastrectomy)
— Bacterial overgrowth due to
• Blind loop (Polya): commonest cause
• Reduced motility (vagotomy)
• Hypochlorhydria
3 Folic acid deficiency ($\rightarrow$ anemia in 1%)

Mechanisms of post-Polya malabsorption
1 Inadequate luminal mixing of food and digestive secretions due to intestinal hurry (leading to steatorrhea)
2 Duodenal bypass $\rightarrow$ $\downarrow$ biliary and pancreatic secretions
3 Stagnant loop syndrome
4 Inadvertent gastroileostomy
5 'Unmasking' gluten sensitivity/pancreatic insufficiency
6 Stomal ulceration leading to formation of gastrocolic fistula

Possible significance of stomal ulcer development
1 Inadequate vagotomy/gastrectomy ('retained antrum')
2 Inadvertent gastroileal (or gastrocolic) anastomosis
3 Gastrinoma

Other complications of gastric surgery
1 Dumping ('early', 'late'); R_x octreotide

2 Biliary vomiting, biliary gastritis; alkaline reflux esophagitis
3 Osteomalacia, osteoporosis
4 Protein-losing enteropathy (cause unknown); diarrhea
Protein malnutrition (due to poor intake and absorption)
5 Reactivation of TB (cause unknown)
6 Development of malignancy in gastric remnant

UPPER GASTROINTESTINAL HEMORRHAGE

Acute management of upper gastrointestinal hemorrhage
1 Patients with known or suspected liver disease
— Correction of coagulopathy
— Encephalopathy regimen (p. 136)
2 Hemodynamic homeostasis
— Adequate transfusion (maintain Hb > 10 g/dL)
— IV fluid and electrolyte balance (central line if needed)
3 Emergency surgery, e.g.
— Oversewing of Mallory–Weiss tear
— Partial gastrectomy ± vagotomy for bleeding ulcer
— Total gastrectomy for erosive gastritis (last resort)

Effective drugs for gastrointestinal bleeding
1 Acute variceal bleeding
— Octreotide (drug of choice), somatostatin
— Vasopressin plus nitroglycerine
2 Portal hypertensive prophylaxis (gastropathy, varices)
— Propranolol
3 Stress ulcer prophylaxis
— Sucralfate
— High-dose intragastric antacids (in ICU)
— Acid suppression with H_2-blockade
4 Prevention of ulcer bleeding following initial healing
— Acid suppression (e.g. maintenance ranitidine)

Endoscopic management of bleeding peptic ulcers
1 Direct injection of adrenaline 1:20,000 or absolute alcohol
2 Uni- or multipolar electrocoagulation (diathermy)
3 Thermal coagulation using heater probe
4 Nd-YAG laser photocoagulation

Bleeding esophageal varices: specific therapeutic options
1 Continuous infusion
— Somatostatin or (intermittent) octreotide
— Vasopressin (+ nitrates)
2 Endoscopic injection sclerotherapy (standard acute R_x) ± octreotide
— Proven value in acute bleeding (not prophylaxis); mortality benefit unproven
— Complications: sepsis, esophageal ulceration
3 Staple-gun esophagogastric devascularization
4 Balloon tamponade (Sengstaken–Blakemore tube)
— Short-term measure only; must remove within 24 h

— Justified only if varices will be ablated on removal
5 Portocaval shunting
  — Not of proven value in acute bleeding
  — 50% mortality in emergency shunting
  — TIPS (transjugular intrahepatic portosystemic shunting) appears promising for sclerotherapy failures

HEMOCHROMATOSIS

Approach to presymptomatic hemochromatosis
1 Prevent complications by screening first-degree relatives
  — ↑ Serum ferritin
  — ↑ Transferrin saturation (> 55%)
2 Confirm suspected positives using
  — Liver biopsy
  — ± Quantitative phlebotomy, HLA-A3 phenotype
3 Venesection of affected patients
  — Until Hb = 10 g/dL
4 Annual monitoring of these patients*
  — Keep male ferritin levels < 350 µg/L
  — Keep female ferritin levels < 200 µg/L

* Effectively prevents liver/cardiac disease and skin bronzing

Efficacy of therapy for established hemochromatosis
1 Benefits
  — Prolongs life in symptomatic patients
2 Limitations
  — *Arthropathy* fails to improve
  — *Insulin requirement* in diabetics is rarely eliminated
  — *Hypogonadotrophic hypogonadism* (impotence, premature menopause) seldom improves*
  — *Risk of hepatoma* in cirrhotics is unaffected

* NB: Androgen therapy for impotence greatly increases hepatoma risk

MANAGEMENT OF ASCITES

Approach to managing ascites in chronic liver disease
1 Mild, minimally symptomatic ascites
  — Spironolactone
  — Low-salt diet
2 Tense, symptomatic ascites in patients with edema, normal renal function and serum sodium > 130 mmol/L
  — Hospital admission
  — Large-volume controlled paracentesis
  — Early discharge following stabilization on diuretics
3 Tense, symptomatic ascites in patients *without* edema, with renal impairment or serum sodium < 130 mmol/L
  — Hospital admission
  — Large-volume paracentesis *plus* albumin infusion
  — Early discharge following stabilization on diuretics

4 Recurrent ascites following paracentesis and diuretics
  — Culture ascites (bacteria, AFB)
  — Sudan III stain if fluid opalescent (chylous ascites)
  — Cytology (malignant cells)
  — Plasma AFP (hepatoma)
  — Liver scan (hepatoma, hepatic vein thrombosis)
5 Intractable ascites
  — TIPS*
    • ↓ Portal pressure, ascites, variceal bleeding
    • ↑ Risk of encephalopathy
  — IV reinfusion of ascitic ultrafiltrate (saves albumin)
  — Peritoneovenous (LeVeen) shunt

* Transjugular intrahepatic portosystemic shunting

Complications of peritoneovenous shunting
1 Disseminated intravascular coagulation*
2 Sepsis
3 Shunt blockage (very frequent)
4 Intravascular fluid overload (→ pulmonary edema)
5 Peritoneal fibromatosis (foreign body reaction)

* May be clinical or subclinical

HEPATIC ENCEPHALOPATHY

Inpatient monitoring of the patient in hepatic precoma
1 Higher centers
  — Regular close questioning by staff and relatives
2 Constructional apraxia
  — Handwriting chart
  — Five-pointed star chart
  — Reitan trail test (consecutive number connection)
3 Investigations
  — EEG (p. 269)
  — CT (if *any* diagnostic doubt)
  — Specific biochemistry (rarely done)
    • Plasma ammonia (sampled without tourniquet)
    • CSF glutamine

Hepatic encephalopathy: management of the 'at-risk' patient
1 Elimination of precipitants
  — Correction of hypothermia, ↓ K⁺, ↓ Mg²⁺
  — Withdrawal of loop diuretics, sedatives, alcohol
  — Active exclusion of sepsis
  — Treatment of gastrointestinal bleeding
  — Avoidance of surgery and general anesthesia if possible
2 Diet
  — High-calorie (incl. IV dextrose if necessary)
3 Bowel cleansing
  — Magnesium sulfate enemas
  — Lactulose (or lactilol)*
  — Consider gut sterilization‡ with oral neomycin
4 Consider steroids

* Acidifies gut lumen, thus converting liposoluble (absorbable) NH₃ to NH₄⁺ (less absorbable) while promoting bowel washout
‡ Promotes malabsorption of putative neurotoxin

PORTAL-SYSTEMIC SHUNTING

Relative contraindications to portal-systemic shunting
1 Age > 50 years
2 Previous episode(s) of encephalopathy
3 Jaundice
4 Ascites
5 Profound hypoalbuminemia
6 High IQ required for livelihood

Potential complications of portal-systemic shunting
1 Perioperative death ($\rightarrow$ 50% of 'poor-risk' patients)
2 Precipitation of hepatic encephalopathy
3 Development of hepatic nephropathy (hepatorenal failure)

DRUG-INDUCED LIVER DISEASE

Iatrogenic histopathologic mimics of primary liver disease
1 Viral hepatitis
— Halothane, isoniazid, ketoconazole
2 Alcoholic hepatitis
— Perhexiline maleate
3 Reye's syndrome
— Aspirin, valproate
4 Acute fatty liver of pregnancy
— Tetracycline
5 Cryptogenic cirrhosis/fibrosis
— Long-term methotrexate ($\rightarrow$ fibrosis esp.)
— Amiodarone
— Vitamin A intoxication, vinyl chloride monomer
6 Primary biliary cirrhosis
— Chlorpromazine
7 Chronic active hepatitis
— Methyldopa, isoniazid, nitrofurantoin, dantrolene
8 Granulomatous (hypersensitivity) hepatitis
— Allopurinol (+ many others)
9 Budd–Chiari syndrome (p. 127)
— Synthetic estrogens
10 Venoocclusive disease
— 6-thioguanine ± irradiation (for childhood tumors)
11 Cholestasis
— (Flu)cloxacillin
— Estrogens, anabolic steroids

Halothane hepatitis: occurrence and outcome
1 Incidence
— Clinically evident hepatitis: 1 in 10,000
— Asymptomatic $\uparrow$ AST/ALT: 10–25%
2 Predisposition
— 70% of affected patients are female
— 50% of affected patients are obese
3 Exposure frequency
— More than 80% patients have had at least two exposures
— Initial exposure is often followed by unexplained fever
— Toxic reexposure usually occurs within a month

4 Associated features
— Fever is seen in 75% of established hepatitis cases
— Eosinophilia is seen in 30% of cases
5 Mortality of established halothane hepatitis is 50%

PRIMARY LIVER DISEASE

Chronic active hepatitis: when to try steroid therapy
1 Symptoms causing reduced quality of life, *plus*
2 Severe histologic abnormalities on biopsy, *plus*
3 HBsAg *and* anti-HBc negativity, *plus*
4 Exclusion of reversible etiology
— Drug-induced chronic active hepatitis
— Wilson's disease
— α_1-antitrypsin deficiency

Therapeutic modalities in primary biliary cirrhosis
1 Ursodeoxycholic acid
2 Colchicine
3 Methotrexate
4 Cyclosporin
5 Liver transplantation

LIVER TRANSPLANTATION

Principal indications for liver transplantation
1 In children
— Congenital biliary atresia with persistent cholestasis despite Kasai procedure (1-year survival > 90%)
— Metabolic disease: Wilson's, α_1-antitrypsin deficiency, galactosemia, Crigler–Najjar, hypercholesterolemia
2 In adults with end-stage (but stable) liver disease
— Primary biliary cirrhosis
— Sclerosing cholangitis
— Budd–Chiari syndrome (p. 127)
— Cryptogenic cirrhosis, chronic active hepatitis
3 Neoplasms*
— *Small* hepatomas without $\uparrow\uparrow$ AFP
— Fibrolamellar tumors, hemangioendotheliomas
— Carcinoid or APUDoma metastases
4 Fulminant hepatic failure; hepatorenal syndrome

* Disappointing results in this context to date

Therapeutic outcome in liver transplantation
1 Overall 12-month survival — 75%
2 Primary biliary cirrhosis — 12-month survival 90%
3 Other causes of cirrhosis — 12-month survival 60%
4 HBV-induced liver disease — 12-month survival 50%
5 Hepatoma — 12-month survival 30%
6 Patients alive at 12 months— 80% 5-year survival

Contraindications to liver transplantation
1 Common
— Irreversible symptomatic liver failure
— Patient unfit for surgery
— No suitable donor

2 Absolute
— Active alcoholism*
— Systemic or biliary infection (incl. HIV)
— Extrahepatic malignancy
3 Relative
— Age > 60 years
— Portal vein thrombosis
— Portocaval shunt (→ uncontrollable surgical bleeding)
— Intrapulmonary AV shunting (> 50%)
— Multiple previous laparotomies
— HBeAg/HBV DNA+; δ agent infection
— Severe hepatic osteodystrophy

* Most centers require at least 6 months' abstinence; compliance can be assessed using carbohydrate-deficient transferrin. Similar post-graft prognosis

Complications of liver transplantation
1 Infection
— esp. *Pseudomonas* spp., *Candida* spp., CMV
2 Hepatic artery thrombosis (in up to 20%)
— May infarct graft → immediate retransplantation
— May → biliary peritonitis (bile duct infarct)
3 Acute rejection
— Almost invariable (day 4–10 post-transplant)
— Treated with steroids, cyclosporin A
4 Chronic rejection (in 10–20% patients)
— Causes 'vanishing bile duct syndrome' (jaundice)
— May respond to retransplantation
5 Cyclosporin A toxicity (p. 195–196)
— Nephrotoxicity, hypertension
— CNS: confusion, cortical blindness, pyramidal lesions, headaches, tremulousness
6 Death
— Affects up to 25% within 12 months

GALLSTONES: ALTERNATIVES TO CHOLECYSTECTOMY

Therapy of gallstones without open cholecystectomy
1 Oral dissolution using CDCA or UDCA
2 Laparoscopic cholecystectomy
Minilaparotomy cholecystectomy
3 Endoscopic sphincterotomy (during ERCP)
— For common bile duct stones
4 T-tube stone extraction using Dormia basket
5 Solvent infusion
— Via T-tube, nasobiliary or transhepatic catheter
• Bile acids/EDTA (calcium-containing stones)
• Methyl *tert*-butyl ether (MTBE; cholesterol stones)
6 Extracorporeal ultrasonic lithotripsy

Indications for endoscopic sphincterotomy > cholecystectomy
1 Elderly patients, *plus*
2 Patent cystic duct, *plus*
3 Common duct stone(s)

Prerequisites for extracorporeal lithotripsy
1 History of biliary colic (i.e. patient must be symptomatic)
2 Solitary radiolucent gallstone < 3 cm diameter (or < three stones with equivalent combined mass)
3 Functioning gallbladder on oral cholecystography
4 No recent cholecystitis/cholangitis, clotting defect, pregnancy

GALLSTONE DISSOLUTION THERAPY

Potential indications for bile acid therapy
1 Gallstones (see below)
2 Primary biliary cirrhosis
3 Sclerosing cholangitis
4 Benign cholestasis of pregnancy

Pharmacology and rationâle of gallstone dissolution
1 Cheno- and ursodeoxycholic acid (CDCA, UDCA) inhibit HMG-CoA reductase → ↓ biliary cholesterol concentration
2 Treatment best for patients unfit for cholecystectomy
3 Treatment does *not* dissolve pigment (radioopaque) stones
4 Treatment usually → ↑ plasma cholesterol, ↓ triglycerides
5 Treatment may be antagonized by phenobarbitone
6 CDCA is metabolized to lithocholic acid, a hepatotoxin, resulting in frequent ALT/AST elevation

Prerequisites for dissolution therapy
1 Functioning gallbladder (patent cystic duct) on OCG
2 Radiolucent (cholesterol) stones*
3 Stone diameter(s) < 1.5 cm
4 No common bile duct stones
5 No history of liver or pancreatic dysfunction
6 Not pregnant or morbidly obese

* Success likely if OCG shows stones *floating* within gallbladder, since this implies hypodense stones with large surface area for dissolution

Clinical aspects of gallstone dissolution
1 Main problems with this treatment are
— Stringent patient eligibility criteria (see above)
— Diarrhea
— Expense
2 In *highly selected* patients, dissolution rates reach 80%
Overall 12-month dissolution rates in patients with functioning gallbladders + radiolucent stones average 40%
3 Recurrences → 50% of 'successful' patients over 5–10 years
4 Treatment of hypercholesterolemic females → best results
5 Advantages of UDCA over CDCA
— More potent reduction of biliary cholesterol secretion
— More rapid onset of dissolution
— Less diarrhea, nausea, transaminitis
Disadvantage of UDCA
— Causes 'rim' calcification of gallstones (↓ dissolution)
6 Patients remaining symptomatic after 6 months medical therapy should be considered for surgery

LAXATIVE THERAPY

Indications for laxatives
1 Short-term therapy of constipation/painful defecation
2 Long-term therapy in elderly or debilitated patients with chronic abdominal/perineal muscular weakness
3 Prevention of iatrogenic constipation (esp. opiates)
4 Bowel preparation prior to investigation or surgery

Classifying laxatives
1 Bulking agents
— Bran, ispaghula husk, sterculia, methylcellulose
2 Fecal softeners
— Paraffin, docusate sodium
3 Osmotic laxatives
— Magnesium salts, lactulose, glycerol supp.
4 Stimulant laxatives
— Senna, bisacodyl, danthron, phenolphthalein

Individualizing laxative treatment
1 Rectal discomfort
— Glycerol suppositories
— Bisacodyl suppositories
2 Long-term therapy of constipation
— Bran (esp. unprocessed)
— Ispaghula husk
— Sterculia
— Methylcellulose
3 Short-term therapy of self-limiting constipation
— Senna
4 Second-line therapy of constipation
— Magnesium hydroxide
— Lactulose (expensive)
5 Refractory constipation
— Investigate to clarify cause

ANTIDIARRHEAL THERAPY

Infectious diarrhea: indications for antibiotics
1 Always
— Giardiasis (metronidazole 2 g/day for 3 days)
— Amebiasis *if* symptomatic
— Severe bacillary (*Shigella*) dysentery
2 Usually
— Pseudomembranous (antibiotic-associated) colitis*
3 Occasionally
— *Campylobacter* enterocolitis
— 'Traveller's diarrhea' (therapy or prophylaxis)

* Relapses may be due to loss of aerobic flora

Antibiotics relevant to pseudomembranous colitis
1 Frequent causes
— Ampicillin/amoxicillin
— Clindamycin/lincomycin
— Cephalosporins
2 Therapy*
— Oral metronidazole 250 mg q.i.d.
  • Cheap and effective first-line therapy

• Some systemic absorption, hence side-effects (nausea, metallic taste) may occur
— Oral vancomycin 125 mg q.i.d
  • Expensive but effective
  • Minimal systemic absorption
— Intravenous metronidazole
  • May be used in patients unable to tolerate oral therapy, e.g. post-operative, ileus
  • Biliary excretion ensures effective luminal concentrations in bowel‡
— Bacitracin (second-line therapy only)

* *Cholestyramine* 4 g q.i.d. may also be used to bind clostridial toxin
‡ cf. IV vancomycin: *not* recommended

INFLAMMATORY BOWEL DISEASE

Indications for surgery
1 Crohn's disease
— Persistent bowel obstruction
— Enteric fistulae with complications
— Perirectal suppuration
— Acute appendicitis; perforation
— Obstructive hydronephrosis
— Growth retardation (e.g. despite parenteral nutrition)
— Colonic cancer
2 Ulcerative colitis
— Severe colitis with failure to stabilize on intensive medical therapy (e.g. 5 days of IV steroids)
— Intractable pararectal or extraintestinal complications
— Acute complications, e.g. toxic megacolon, life-threatening bleeding, perforation
— Severe dysplasia
— Carcinoma (colonic or cholangiocarcinoma)
— Unacceptable medical side-effects

Colectomy: its effect on complications of ulcerative colitis
1 Complications responsive to colectomy
— Peripheral arthropathy (p. 349)
— Pyoderma gangrenosum
— Pararectal disease*
2 Complications resistant to colectomy
— Ankylosing spondylitis
— Sclerosing cholangitis

* NB: Uncommon in ulcerative colitis

Mechanisms of debility in inflammatory bowel disease
1 Anemia (normochromic *or* iron deficiency)
2 Portal pyemia
3 Liver disease
4 Fistulae (malabsorption)
5 Recurrent bowel obstruction (Crohn's)
6 Relapsing or refractory colitis

Therapeutic role of sulfasalazine
1 Drug = sulfapyridine (sulfonamide) and 5-acetylsalicylic acid (5-ASA) moieties joined by azo-bond (lysed in colon)

2 Induces remission in active ulcerative colitis and
   Crohn's
   Prevents flare-ups from quiescence in ulcerative
   colitis
3 Very little drug is absorbed in the small intestine
   Unabsorbed 5-ASA exerts topical therapeutic effect
   in colon
4 Dose-related toxicity is maximal in slow acetylators
   Hypersensitivity is usually due to the sulfapyridine
   moiety
5 5-ASA alone is now marketed in oral form (e.g.
   mesalazine, olsalazine) or as suppository/foam enema

Side-effects of sulfasalazine
1 Headaches
2 Gastrointestinal
   — Anorexia, nausea, vomiting
3 Hematologic
   — Hemolysis, methemoglobinemia
   — Agranulocytosis; folate deficiency
4 Male infertility
   — Oligospermia, reduced sperm motility
5 Neurologic
   — Peripheral neuropathy, tinnitus, vertigo
6 Other
   — Hepatitis, nephrosis, depression

Crohn's disease: approach to management
1 Acute ileitis
   — Steroids
   — Oral budesonide, a corticosteroid analog, is
     equally effective but less toxic (minimal
     absorption)
   — Methotrexate 25 mg/week
   — Azathioprine
2 Acute colitis
   — Sulfasalazine + steroids induce remission
3 Fistulae, perianal or colonic disease
   — Metronidazole (or surgery)
4 Cholorrheic enteropathy (= diarrhea due to ileal mal-
   absorption of bile acids, leading to colonic irritation)
   — Diagnose with fecal bile acids (^{75}SeHCAT*)
   — Treat with cholestyramine
5 Extensive ileal resection (> 100 cm) with frank
   steatorrhea
   — R$_x$: medium-chain triglycerides (MCT), low
     oxalate ± low lactose diet
   — Vitamin (A,D,E,K,B$_{12}$) supplements, TPN
6 Bacterial overgrowth
   — May underlie 'refractory' disease
   — Treat with broad-spectrum antibiotics (e.g.
     tetracycline)
   — May necessitate surgery
7 Post-surgical disease recurrence
   — Typically occurs proximal to anastomoses
   — Minimal surgical intervention is favored
8 Malignancy
   — Typically occurs in surgically excluded segments
     (increased duration of disease in such segments)
   — Routine surveillance not indicated
   — Excess of right-sided colonic Ca occurs in Crohn's
9 Maintenance prophylaxis
   — Sulfasalazine for colonic Crohn's

* ^{75}Se-labelled homocholic acid conjugated with taurine

Non-intestinal complications of Crohn's disease
1 Osteopenia
   Growth retardation*
2 Gallstones
3 Renal (oxalate) stones
   Ureteric obstruction
4 Psoas abscess
5 Amyloidosis
6 Thromboembolism

* May be *either* steroid-induced *or* disease-related

Use of continent ileorectal reservoirs ('Kock's ileostomy')*
1 Continence achievable in 80–95% patients
2 Anastomotic strictures occur in about 10%
3 Pouch failure occurs in 2–5%
4 Fecal stasis → anaerobic overgrowth → 'pouchitis' →
   diarrhea (responds to metronidazole)
5 'Primary' ileostomy diarrhea may respond to the
   long-acting somatostatin analog SMS-201-995
6 If pouch requires dismantling, further bowel
   shortening may exacerbate preexisting short bowel
   syndrome

* In ulcerative colitis

UNDERSTANDING GASTROINTESTINAL DISEASE

GASTRIC ACID REGULATION

Anatomic localization of acid-regulatory cells
1 Body of stomach* (corpus/fundus; proximal two-
   thirds)
   — Parietal (oxyntic) cells
     • Secrete HCl, intrinsic factor into lumen
   — Chief cells
     • Secrete pepsinogen into lumen
2 Gastric antrum (pyloric region; distal third)
   — G-cells (also found in proximal duodenum)
     • Secrete gastrin/somatostatin into bloodstream

* Site of atrophic gastritis

Factors regulating parietal cell acid output
1 Increased by
   — Vagal stimulation (e.g. food in stomach)
   — Gastrin (via blood)
2 Reduced by
   — Somatostatin
   — Anticholinergics, pirenzipine (block *vagal* activity)
   — H$_2$-receptor antagonists (block parietal cell
     activation)
   — Omeprazole (blocks acid *secretion*)

GUT HORMONES

Classification of regulatory peptides coexisting in gut and CNS
1 Paracrine (locally acting)
   — Somatostatin

2 Neurotransmitters
— VIP, substance P, bombesin, endorphins
3 Endocrine (distantly acting)
— Cholecystokinin (CCK), neurotensin

NB: All other gut peptides mentioned below exhibit mainly *endocrine* action

Gut peptides exhibiting structural similarities
1 Gastrin, CCK
2 Secretin, (entero)glucagon, VIP, GIP
3 Bombesin, substance P

Physiology and clinical significance of gastrin
1 Location
— Gastric antrum (also jejunum)
2 Released by
— Vagal stimulation (esp. gastric distension)
— Protein meals; alcohol
— Bombesin
3 Effects
— Stimulates gastric acid and pepsin secretion
— Inhibits gastric emptying
— Trophic to gastric mucosa
— Increases lower esophageal sphincter tone
4 Clinical significance
— Zollinger–Ellison (gastrinoma) syndrome
— Achalasia (cholinergic denervation hypersensitivity to gastrin implicated in pathogenesis of ↑ LES tone)

Physiology of cholecystokinin ('hormone of satiety')
1 Location: duodenum and jejunum
2 Released by protein/fat ingestion
3 Effects
— Stimulates gallbladder contraction
— Relaxes sphincter of Oddi
— Releases pancreatic proteolytic enzymes
— Trophic to pancreas
4 Clinical significance
— Used to assess pancreatic/gallbladder function

Physiology of secretin ('physiological antacid')
1 Location: duodenum and jejunum
2 Released by entry of acid into duodenum
3 Effects
— Stimulates pancreatic bicarbonate secretion
4 Clinical significance
— ↓ Secretion in celiac disease

Physiology of vasoactive intestinal polypeptide (VIP)
1 Location: post-ganglionic gut nerve cells
2 Released by direct neural mediation (*not* by meals)
3 Effects
— Inhibits gastric acid secretion
— Stimulates pancreatic bicarbonate secretion
— Stimulates gut secretion and insulin release
— Induces vasodilatation and hypotension
4 Clinical significance
— VIPoma
— ↓ Secretion in Chagas' and Hirschsprung's
— ↑ Secretion in Crohn's disease
— Implicated in post-gastrectomy 'dumping' (p. 135)

Physiology of substance P
1 Location: gut nerve cells
2 Released by unknown stimuli
3 Effects
— Inhibits pancreatic bicarbonate/amylase release
— Inhibits biliary secretion
— Inhibits insulin, stimulates glucagon release
— Stimulates salivation, vasodilatation, natriuresis
4 Clinical significance
— Implicated in nociception, asthma

Physiology of bombesin (gastrin-releasing peptide)
1 Location: gut nerve cells
2 Released by unknown stimuli
3 Effects
— Stimulates gastrin/gastric acid secretion
— Stimulates pancreatic enzyme secretion
4 Clinical significance
— Secreted in SCLC but no recognized syndrome

Physiology of glucose-dependent insulinotrophic polypeptide*
1 Location: throughout gut, esp. duodenum/jejunum
2 Released by *oral* glucose
3 Effects
— Stimulates insulin release‡
— Inhibits gastric acid secretion
4 Clinical significance
— ↓ Secretion in celiac disease

* GIP; formerly, 'gastric inhibitory polypeptide'
‡ NB: Oral glucose induces greater insulin release than does parenteral glucose per unit glycemia, due to ?presence of 'incretin' hormone (see GLP-1)

Physiology of motilin ('hormone of diarrhea')
1 Location: duodenum and jejunum
2 Released by meals (including drinking water; i.e. by vagally mediated gastric distension; also by fat)
3 Effects
— Stimulates gastric emptying
— Stimulates small intestinal motility
— Mediates gastrocolic reflex
4 Clinical significance
— ↑ Secretion in infective diarrheas, inflammatory bowel disease, and carcinoid syndrome
— *Erythromycin* (IV or oral) activates motilin receptors, causing abdominal cramps (toxicity), but also enhances motility in patients with hypomotility syndromes such as diabetic gastroparesis

Physiology of neurotensin
1 Location: ileum
2 Released by entry of food (esp. fat) to ileum
3 Effects
— Inhibits gastric emptying and acid secretion
— Stimulates intestinal secretion
— Induces hypotension
4 Clinical significance
— Implicated in post-gastrectomy 'dumping'

Physiology of enteroglucagon
1 Location: ileum and colorectum
2 Released by meals

3 Effects
— Trophic to small intestinal mucosa
— Inhibits gastric emptying and acid secretion
4 Clinical significance
— ↑ Secretion following bowel resection or bypass
— ↑ Secretion in celiac disease/cystic fibrosis
— Implicated in post-gastrectomy 'dumping'

Physiology of glucagon-like peptide 1 (GLP-1)
1 Location: terminal ileum and pancreatic α-cells
2 Released by oral glucose (gut), arginine (pancreas)
3 Effects
— Increases insulin secretion (? = 'incretin') if glucose is available
— Reduces plasma glucagon
4 Clinical significance
— Exaggerated post-prandial levels seen in post-gastrectomy dumping (together with excess insulin secretion)

Physiology of pancreatic polypeptide ('hormone of indigestion')
1 Location: pancreas
2 Released by vagal stimulation or (protein) meals
3 Effects
— Inhibits pancreatic and biliary secretion
4 Clinical significance
— Cosecreted in many gut endocrine tumor syndromes, esp: VIPoma (75%), glucagonoma (50%), gastrinoma (25%), carcinoid syndrome

Physiology of somatostatin (GH release-inhibiting hormone)
1 Location: pancreas ('D' cells) and throughout gut
2 Released by diverse stimuli
3 Effects
— Stimulates gastric emptying
— *Inhibits* almost everything else
  • Gastric acid and pepsin secretion
  • Pancreatic/biliary secretion, celiac blood flow
  • Release of GH, TSH, insulin, glucagon, gastrin, secretin, PP, GIP, motilin, enteroglucagon
4 Clinical significance
— Synthetic analogs successfully used in
  • VIPoma diarrhea control
  • Gastrinoma
  • Insulinoma, glucagonoma
  • Acromegaly (tumor sometimes reduces)
  • GI hemorrhage, pancreatitis

NB: *No* abnormality of gut hormones is linked to irritable bowel syndrome

GUT ENDOCRINE TUMOR SYNDROMES

General features of gut endocrine tumor syndromes
1 *All* may be due to malignant tumors and metastases are frequently evident at presentation (see below)
2 *Most* may cause diarrhea (see p. 143–144)
3 *Many* may be associated with secretion of other peptides (such as calcitonin, ACTH/CRH, PTH, adrenaline, noradrenaline, VMA), and clinical evolution from (say) VIPoma to insulinoma may occur

4 'Noisy' (clinically obvious) secreted hormones include
— Insulin
— Gastrin
— VIP
  'Quiet' hormones include
— Glucagon
— Somatostatin
— Pancreatic polypeptide
5 *Any* may be associated with multiple endocrine neoplasia (MEN1); this possibility should be regularly excluded by measuring plasma Ca^{2+} (plus PTH if Ca^{2+} elevated), performing lateral SXR and assaying pituitary hormones
6 Streptozotocin may be used to palliate unresectable disease, but response rates are modest (typically about 25%)

Gastrinoma: features
1 Primary G-cell tumors, usually found in pancreatic body/tail
2 50% develop parathyroid/pituitary adenoma (MEN1) Family history: renal stones, pituitary tumor, hypoglycemia
3 50% present with diarrhea or steatorrhea (see below)
4 95% present with duodenal ulceration, classically
— Young patient without risk factors (unless MEN1)
— Multiple large, deep ulcers
— Ectopic position (post-bulbar, jejunal, esophageal)
— Associated with pyloric stenosis or esophageal stricture
— Prone to perforation or hemorrhage, esp. post-op
— Healing resists normal-dose H_2-receptor antagonists
5 Management
— Medical
  • Omeprazole
  • *High*-dose (5 x normal) H_2-receptor antagonists
  • Addition of anticholinergics (if needed)
  • Pancreatic enzyme supplements (for steatorrhea)
  • Cholestyramine (for diarrhea)
— Surgical
  • If hypercalcemic: assess for parathyroidectomy
  • If no evidence of metastasis: laparotomy
  • If primary tumor localizable: resection
  • If disease unresectable *and* preoperative ulceration controllable with drugs, close up
  • If disease unresectable and difficulties in ulcer control, consider highly selective vagotomy
  • If disease unresectable and symptoms resistant to drugs, consider total gastrectomy (last resort)

VIPoma: features
1 Primary tumors are usually pancreatic in adults Children may develop benign ganglioneuroblastomas
2 Pancreatic origin (in 80%) is confirmed by coexisting elevation of pancreatic polypeptide
3 Causes watery diarrhea, dehydration, ↓ K^+
4 Associated
— Achlorhydria
— Flushing, hypotension (esp. on tumor palpation)

— Cholelithiasis and gallbladder dilatation
— Hypercalcemia (with or without MEN1)
— Glucose intolerance (usually subclinical)
5 Management
— **S**urgery if feasible
— **S**omatostatin analogs* (→ best symptom control)
— **S**ymptomatic
  • Opiates (codeine, loperamide)
  • Metoclopramide; indomethacin
  • Steroids
  • Fluid and electrolyte balance
— **S**treptozotocin (cytotoxic) for metastases

* e.g. octreotide (SMS 201-995): improves diarrhea by lowering VIP

Glucagonoma: features

1 Primary α-cell pancreatic tumors; commoner in females
2 Spontaneous symptomatic remissions characteristic
3 Sequelae
— Diarrhea (see below); hypercatabolic weight loss
— Stomatitis, glossitis, vulvovaginitis, nail dystrophy
— Thromboembolism
— Necrolytic migratory erythema (transient bullous or crusting rash, often involving perineum and leaving residual pigmentation)
— Glucose intolerance (often symptomatic)
— Hypocholesterolemia
4 Management
— Somatostatin analogs (for diarrhea)
— Insulin if required (for diabetes)
— Oral zinc (for rash)
— Anticoagulant prophylaxis (for thromboembolism)
— Tumor resection (for operable disease)
— Streptozotocin (for inoperable disease)

Other gut endocrine tumors: features

1 Somatostatinoma (D-cell tumor; rare)
— Diarrhea, steatorrhea (see below)
— Achlorhydria; dyspepsia
— Cholelithiasis, dilated gallbladder
— Glucose intolerance (usually subclinical)
2 Enteroglucagonoma (very rare)
— Small intestinal hypomotility
— Massive villous hypertrophy on jejunal biopsy
— Edema due to protein loss (see below)
3 PPoma/neurotensinoma (very rare)
— The only gut endocrine tumors which present with symptoms and signs of invasion or metastasis rather than of endocrine sequelae

Malignant potential of gut endocrine tumors

1 Insulinoma
— 5–10% are metastatic at presentation
2 Gastrinoma
— 30% are metastatic at presentation
3 Glucagonoma, VIPoma, somatostatinoma
— 50% are metastatic at presentation
4 Carcinoid syndrome
— > 98% are metastatic at presentation*

* cf. carcinoid tumors *without* syndrome: < 10% metastasize

CARCINOID SYNDROME

Symptoms and signs of carcinoid syndrome

1 *Acute* symptoms (induced by 5HT, kinins, etc.)
— Upper body flushing
— Dependent edema
— Pruritic wheals, serpentine flush (histamine-secreting)
— Wheezing, hypotension, fever, tachycardia
— Borborygmi, abdominal pain, diarrhea, vomiting
2 *Chronic* complications (indicative of disease duration)
— Telangiectasia; pellagra-like rash; arthropathy
— Hepatomegaly*; cirrhosis may also supervene
— Mesenteric fibrosis ('sclerosing peritonitis')
— Tricuspid incompetence (chordal fibrosis)
— Pulmonic stenosis (valvular adhesions)

* Rarely, bronchial or ovarian primaries may cause the syndrome in the absence of liver metastases

Symptoms of atypical carcinoid syndrome (lung primary)

1 Lacrimation
2 Parotid enlargement, salivation
3 Facial (not dependent) edema
4 Left-sided cardiac valve lesions

Benefits of octreotide in carcinoid syndrome

1 Effective in reducing *diarrhea*
2 Best available treatment for *flushing* (effective in 90%)
3 Infusion valuable for treating 'carcinoid crisis'

Other treatment modalities in carcinoid syndrome

1 Diarrhea (serotonin-induced)
— Non-specific: codeine, loperamide
— Serotonin blockers: cyproheptadine (cf. methysergide: *contraindicated* due to ↑ risk of fibrotic sequelae)
2 Flushing (due to kinins, substance P, serotonin)
— Phenoxybenzamine, corticosteroids
— Ketanserin (serotonin blocker)
3 *Serpentine* (histamine-induced) flushing of gastric carcinoids
— H_1 and H_2 histamine receptor antagonists
4 Hepatic pain
— Hepatic embolization
— Surgical debulking
5 Carcinoid crisis (e.g. perioperative)
— Corticosteroids
6 Pellagra
— Nicotinamide supplements (see p. 233)
7 Metastases
— Streptozotocin (limited efficacy)
— Interferon-α

HUMORAL DIARRHEA

Characteristics of diarrhea due to gut endocrine tumors

1 Gastrinoma
— Diarrhea not caused by ↑ gastrin but by ↓ intestinal pH

— This denatures pancreatic enzymes and precipitates bile salts with consequent ileal bile salt malabsorption
  • Dietary fat malabsorption (steatorrhea)
  • Colonic irritation by bile salts (watery diarrhea)
2 VIPoma ('pancreatic cholera')
  — 'Rice-water' (secretory) diarrhea (1–20 L/day)
  — Frequently nocturnal or fasting diarrhea
  — ± Colicky abdominal pain, dehydration, azotemia
  — Hypokalemic *acidosis**
3 Glucagonoma
  — Diarrhea, no steatorrhea
  — May be associated with hypokalemic alkalosis
  — Characteristic rash
  — Normochromic anemia
4 Somatostatinoma
  — Steatorrhea (↓ biliary secretion, intestinal absorption)
  — Associated with achlorhydria (↓ gastric acidity)
5 Enteroglucagonoma
  — Steatorrhea
  — No diarrhea (gut hypomotility)
  — Protein-losing enteropathy with edema (due to massive villous hypertrophy)
6 Carcinoid syndrome
  — Profuse secretory diarrhea (5HT-induced)
  — Associated borborygmi, abdominal pain, nausea

* VIP-induced achlorhydria → life-threatening loss of *alkaline* secretions

THE UPPER GASTROINTESTINAL TRACT

Pathogenetic mechanisms contributing to reflux esophagitis
1 ↓ Lower esophageal sphincter (LES) tone*
  — e.g. Scleroderma
2 ↓ Esophageal clearance of refluxed material
  — e.g. Esophageal spasm
3 ↑ Irritant content of refluxed material
  — e.g. Post-gastrectomy biliary gastritis; gastrinoma
4 ↑ Volume of gastric contents
  — e.g. Delayed gastric emptying, Ménètrier's disease

* cf. achalasia: increased LES tone due to cholinergic denervation hypersensitivity to acetylcholine

Barrett's esophagus*: what is its clinical significance?
1 Commoner in males
2 Found in 10% of patients undergoing biopsy for esophagitis
3 Found in 40% of patients with chronic peptic strictures
4 Carcinoma risk
  — Predisposes to about 5% of all esophageal cancer
  — Lifetime risk in a given patient is about 5%
  — This represents a 40-fold increase in risk
5 30% of patients presenting with carcinoma and Barrett's esophagus have no history of reflux symptoms

* Columnar-lined esophageal metaplasia above gastric cardia

Approach to the patient with Barrett's esophagus
1 Antireflux therapy (N.B. no evidence of metaplastic regression)
2 Endoscopic surveillance ± photodynamic R_x
3 Foci of high-grade dysplasia? Consider resection

Clinical features of hypertrophic gastropathies
1 Ménètrier's disease
  — Male predominance (3:1)
  — Presents with epigastric pain and peripheral edema
  — Barium meal/endoscopy: giant rugae, antral sparing
  — Achlorhydria (5% develop carcinoma)
  — Protein-losing enteropathy
2 Schindler's disease
  — Giant gastric rugae
  — Acid hypersecretion
  — Normal protein balance

VIRAL HEPATITIS: PATHOPHYSIOLOGIC ASPECTS

Predominant modes of transmission
1 Fecal–oral route
  — Hepatitis A virus (HAV)
  — Hepatitis E virus (HEV)
2 Parenteral (esp. via blood)
  — Hepatitis B virus (HBV)
  — Hepatitis C virus (HCV)
  — Hepatitis D virus (HDV)

Hepatitis A (HAV) pathophysiology
1 Picornavirus transmitted by fecal–oral route
2 Almost always self-limiting disease; most often subclinical
  Adult-onset disease tends to be more severe
3 Onset abrupt, fever higher, transaminitis shorter; but may be clinically *indistinguishable* from other viral hepatitides
4 Prominent cholestasis
5 IgM anti-HAV appears with symptoms, persists for 3–6 months

Hepatitis B (HBV) pathophysiology
1 Acute HBV (hepadnavirus) usually subicteric, 'flu-like
  10–20% get serum sickness prodrome due to HBsAg–HBsAb complexes depositing in skin and joints
2 Persistence of HBeAg beyond 12 weeks of symptom onset indicates possibility of disease chronicity
3 Interferon-α induces remission in 30%, esp. if
  — Female, heterosexual, non-Asian
  — Short duration of infection
  — Negative hepatitis D/HIV serology
  — High pretreatment ALT (> 1.3 x normal)
  — Low pretreatment serum HBV DNA
4 Remission marked by
  — Normalization of ALT
  — Conversion of HBeAg to HBeAb
  — Disappearance of serum HBV DNA
5 Combined foscarnet/ganciclovir may also have a role in treatment of severe HBV

6 Vaccination with recombinant HBsAg is revolutionizing the epidemiology of this disorder

Hepatitis C (HCV) pathophysiology

1 Non-A non-B hepatitis transmitted parenterally
   — Post-transfusion/-transplant (almost all cases)
   — IV drugs, tattoos; needle-stick (5–10% seroconvert)
   — Transplacental (vertical) transmission
   — Venereal transmission believed *rare*
2 Due to RNA flavivirus
   — Serologically detected; multiple serotypes
   — Incubation period intermediate between that of hepatitis A and hepatitis B (about 60 days)
3 Complicates 1% of transfusions
   — Implicated in 95% of transfusional hepatitis
   — 90% of anti-HCV-positive donors are infectious
   — Some infectious donors are anti-HCV-negative
4 Manifests as
   — Mild anicteric infection* ± large ALT fluctuations
   — HCV infection *persists* long-term in 80%
   — *Chronic* hepatitis in 50% (after 10 years)
   — *Cirrhosis* in 15% (after 15 years)
   — *Hepatoma*‡ in 5% (after 20 years)
   — Positive serology may be associated with essential mixed cryoglobulinemia
5 Genotype variants (at least 6 major and 12 minor)
   — Genotype 1 (esp. 1b) associated with more severe chronic liver disease, poor response to interferon
6 Management
   — Observation
   — Interferon-α (12-month course reduces viremia)
   — Ribavirin (oral guanosine analog)
   — Liver transplant (recurs, but OK in short term)

* NB: Chronic hepatitis may be confirmed on biopsy despite absent symptoms and persistently normal LFTs in patients who are anti-HCV-positive
‡ Synergistic tumorigenic effect of hepatitis B coinfection; hence, all anti-HCV patients should receive HBV vaccine

Hepatitis D (δ agent) pathophysiology

1 Defective RNA virus coated with HBsAg
   — Requires HBV to replicate but inhibits HBV replication
   — Mainly affects anti-HBe-positive patients
   — Minimally infective to HBsAg-negative individuals
2 Main reservoirs (incl. sexual partners of)
   — IV drug abusers
   — Polytransfused patients, esp. hemophiliacs
   — South Americans, Middle Easterns, Africans
3 Clinical scenarios
   — Coprimary infection with HBV (low morbidity)
   — Superinfection on chronic HBV (*high* morbidity)
   — Converts chronic persistent to chronic active hepatitis
   — May convert mild liver disease to cirrhosis in a year
4 *Persistence* of anti-δ IgM usually signifies development of chronic active hepatitis or cirrhosis
5 *No* link with hepatoma

Hepatitis E (HEV) pathophysiology

1 Due to single-stranded RNA virus (?togavirus)
   — May mimic hepatitis A

2 Implicated in epidemic waterborne non-A hepatitis reported in India in association with high fetal wastage and mortality in pregnant women
3 Acute illness indistinguishable from other forms of hepatitis, but no chronic sequelae (cf. HCV)

ACUTE AND CHRONIC HEPATITIS

Precipitants of fulminant hepatic failure*

1 Viral hepatitis (responsible for 50% of cases)
   — Hepatitis A (esp. in adults)
     • Relatively good prognosis
     • 60% survive; rarely need transplant
   — Acute hepatitis B, C, E (but may be seronegative)
   — Chronic hepatitis B with δ agent superinfection
2 Toxicity
   — Paracetamol overdose (responsible for 40% of cases)
     • *N*-acetylcysteine benefit up to 36 h post-ingestion
   — Halothane hepatitis
3 Other
   — Weil's disease (leptospirosis p. 207)
   — Wilson's disease (in children p. 232)
   — Acute fatty liver of pregnancy (AFLOP)
     • Best prognosis of all causes

* Defined as encephalopathy within 8 weeks of symptom onset; 80% mortality

Hepatitis in pregnancy

1 Most likely to transmit HBV if acquired in third trimester
2 HBeAg-positive mothers have an 85% chance of transmission (cf. anti-HBe-positive: 25% chance)
3 δ agent may also be transmitted at delivery
4 Cesarean section may reduce transmission (controversial)
5 Neonates at risk should be immunized (active and passive)
6 50% of infected male children die of cirrhosis or hepatoma

Chronic viral hepatitis: principal causes

1 Hepatitis B virus ± δ agent
2 Hepatitis C

Antigens implicated in pathogenesis of chronic active hepatitis

1 Autoimmune type I ('lupoid') hepatitis
   — Actin
2 Autoimmune type II hepatitis
   — $P_{450}db1$ (a hepatic microsomal P_{450} isozyme)
3 Tienilic acid-induced hepatitis
   — P_{450} isozyme metabolizing tienilic acid

SECONDARY CAUSES OF LIVER DISEASE

Alcohol-induced liver disease

1 Steatosis (fatty infiltration)
   — Dose-dependent, reversible

2 Hepatic siderosis
3 Alcoholic hepatitis
— 10–40% mortality
— Precursor lesion for cirrhosis
4 Central hyaline sclerosis
Pericellular fibrosis
5 Micronodular cirrhosis
6 Hepatocellular carcinoma

Hormone-induced liver disease
1 Pregnancy
— Benign cholestasis (recurs with pregnancy or OC use)
— Acute fatty liver (75% mortality; does *not* recur)
— Hepatic rupture (follows preeclamptic liver disease)
2 Oral contraceptive (OC) use
— Cholestasis (pruritus ± jaundice), cholelithiasis
— Hepatic vein thrombosis
— Adenoma(s) ± intraperitoneal rupture
— Focal nodular hyperplasia
3 Androgens (C-17 substituted testosterones)
— Cholestasis
— Peliosis hepatis
— Hepatoma, angiosarcoma

Cirrhosis: potential etiologies
1 Viruses
— HBV, HCV
2 Alcohol
— Chronic
3 Prolonged cholestasis
— Intra- or extrahepatic
4 Prolonged venous obstruction
— Budd–Chiari, constrictive pericarditis
5 Metabolic
— Idiopathic hemochromatosis
— Wilson's disease
— $\alpha_1 AT$ deficiency
6 Drugs (long-term)
— Methotrexate, INH, methyldopa, nitrofurantoin, vitamin A, dantrolene, oxyphenisatin

Liver dysfunction in inflammatory bowel disease
1 **C**holangitis
— Recurrent ascending cholangitis
— Sclerosing cholangitis (in ulcerative colitis only)
• No effective treatment, incl. colectomy
• May mimic hepatitis, PBC, cholangiocarcinoma
• May predispose to cholangiocarcinoma
Cholangiocarcinoma
Cholelithiasis (in Crohn's disease only)
2 **H**epatic vein thrombosis
Hepatic infiltration (fat, amyloid)

Amebic liver abscesses
1 Right lobe affected in 90%
Males affected in 80%
Single abscess only in 70%
2 Liver function tests usually normal

3 Formed stools may contain cysts (DD_x: leukocytes) and vegetative forms (usually early stages)
4 Secondary bacterial infection in 20%
5 Past history of amebic dysentery *rare*
6 Amebic serology positive in virtually 100%

Associations of hepatitis B surface antigenemia
1 Male homosexuality
2 Narcotic addiction
3 Hemophilia; hemodialysis; transplantation
4 Polyarteritis nodosa
5 Essential (mixed) cryoglobulinemia

Predispositions to hepatic vein thrombosis (Budd–Chiari)
1 Severe dehydration, esp. in early life
2 Post-partum; oral contraceptive use
3 Paroxysmal nocturnal hemoglobinuria
4 Malignancies
— Myeloproliferative disease (commonest cause)
— Hepatoma, renal cell carcinoma
5 Inflammatory bowel disease
6 Hepatic vein (or caval) webs*

* esp. in Orientals

Fatty liver? Differential diagnosis
1 Alcohol ingestion
2 Diabetes mellitus
— esp. High-dose insulin patients
3 Pregnancy
— Acute (fulminating) type
— High-dose intravenous tetracycline therapy*
4 Thyrotoxicosis; Cushing's syndrome
5 Inflammatory bowel disease
6 Morbid obesity; protein-calorie malnutrition; ileal bypass

* Should never be used in pregnancy in any case

Factors contributing to ethanolic hepatotoxicity
1 Increased oxidative stress
— ↑ NADH:NAD ratio
— ↑ Lactate:pyruvate ratio
2 Formation of acetaldehyde adducts
— Inhibition of enzyme activity
— Cytoskeletal dysfunction*
— Glutathione depletion
3 Free radical generation
— Lipid peroxidation
4 Immune system activation
— ↑ Interleukin-8 levels
5 Other effects
— Nutritional deficiencies
— Increased portal blood flow

* e.g. *Mallory bodies* are aggregated intermediate filaments

Management of alcoholic hepatitis
1 Abstention from alcohol
2 Nutritional support (does *not* prevent ethanolic damage)
   — Folate, B_{12}, B_6, thiamine
3 Adequate oxygenation and transfusion
4 Propylthiouracil
   — Improves hepatic redox state
5 Steroids
   — Anabolic steroids (oxandrolone)
      • In patients with mild-to-moderate malnutrition
   — Prednisone
      • In patients with abnormal prothrombin time and hyperbilirubinemia
      • Reduces mortality in encephalopathic patients who are not bleeding

HEPATIC ENCEPHALOPATHY

Pathogenesis of hepatic encephalopathy: general mechanisms
1 Hepatic insufficiency
   — Circulation of undetoxified metabolites (e.g. ammonia, aromatic amino acids) due to urea cycle breakdown
   — Abnormal cerebral metabolism
2 Urea cycle breakdown
   — ↓ Hepatic gluconeogenesis and insulin release
   — ↓ Uptake of branched-chain amino acids by muscle
3 Increased permeability of blood–brain barrier
4 Disturbed neurotransmitter balance
5 Impairment of cerebral Na^+/K^+-ATPase activity
6 Shunting via varices

Pathogenesis of hepatic encephalopathy: specific mechanisms
1 ↑ Blood ammonia → ↑ CNS ammonia
2 ↑ CNS ammonia → ↑ CNS (CSF) glutamine
3 CNS ammonia → abnormal α-ketoglutarate metabolism
4 ↑ Blood tryptophan (an aromatic amino acid) → ↑ CNS 5-hydroxytryptamine (serotonin)
5 ↑ Methionine → ↑ mercaptan (→ fetor)
6 ↓ CNS dopamine/noradrenaline
7 ↑ CNS octopamine (a 'false' neurotransmitter)
8 ↑ GABA (an inhibitory CNS neurotransmitter) activation
9 ?Endogenous benzodiazepine-like activity

PATHOPHYSIOLOGY OF INTESTINAL DISORDERS

Predispositions to giardiasis
1 Hypogammaglobulinemia, selective IgA deficiency
2 Celiac disease
3 Achlorhydria; post-gastrectomy
4 Chronic pancreatitis
5 Homosexuality
6 Institutionalized children
7 Travel/residence in developing countries

Malabsorptive mechanisms in bacterial overgrowth
1 Invasive mucosal damage (villous atrophy)
2 Mechanical barrier to absorption
3 Nutrient consumption by organisms (incl. B_{12} catabolism)
4 Production of abnormal gut motility
5 Deconjugation of bile acids leading to
   — Steatorrhea (jejunoileal malabsorption)
   — Colonic irritation → diarrhea

Mechanisms of diarrhea following ileal resection
1 Short bowel syndrome
   — Rapid transit → sodium/water malabsorption
2 Limited or recent resection
   — Cholorrheic diarrhea due to colonic irritation
3 Extensive resection
   — Frank steatorrhea due to biliary insufficiency
4 Loss of ileocecal valve
5 Gastric hypersecretion
   — Due to impaired gastrin inactivation

Gastrointestinal concomitants of panhypogammaglobulinemia
1 Infections
   — Giardiasis
   — Bacterial overgrowth
   — Viral and bacterial enteritides
2 Celiac disease
3 Nodular lymphoid hyperplasia
4 Pancreatic insufficiency
5 Pernicious anemia, gastric carcinoma

GLUTEN-INDUCED ENTEROPATHY (CELIAC DISEASE)

Clinical presentations of gluten-induced enteropathy
1 Common
   — Persistent non-specific gastrointestinal upset
   — Constitutional symptoms; symptomatic anemia
   — Minor abnormality detected on full blood count, e.g. mild macrocytic anemia, hyposplenism
2 Classical
   — Steatorrhea
   — Growth retardation
   — Osteomalacia
   — Dermatitis herpetiformis
3 Unusual
   — Amenorrhea, hypogonadism, infertility
   — Clubbing, bone pain, tetany, neuropathy
   — Edema, nocturia
   — Aphthous stomatitis
4 Rare
   — Fever of unknown origin
   — Lymphadenopathy; thrombocytosis
   — Recurrent pericarditis
   — Proctalgia fugax
   — Gastrointestinal lymphoma or adenocarcinoma

Diagnostic criteria in gluten-induced enteropathy
1 Best screening tests
   — Red cell folate (↓ in 70%)
   — Howell–Jolly bodies on film*

2 Definitive diagnosis (to justify lifelong dietary switch)
   — Subtotal villous atrophy on small bowel biopsy, *plus*
   — Symptomatic ± histologic resolution on diet, *plus*
   — Symptomatic *and* histologic relapse on gluten rechallenge

NB: Often *poor* correlation between symptomatic, biochemical and histologic improvement following gluten-free diet (biopsy may take *months* to improve)
* Highly specific finding in appropriate symptomatic context

Composition of the gluten-free diet
1 Excluded
   — Wheat
   — Rye
   — Barley
   — Oats
   — Malt
2 Not excluded
   — Rice
   — Corn
   — Soybean

Efficacy of the gluten-free diet
1 90% patients → clinical (symptomatic) remission
2 70% → 'biochemical' remission (e.g. normal red cell folate)
3 50% → 'mucosal' remission on rebiopsy

Failure of clinical remission with gluten-free diet
1 Inadequate dietary compliance
2 Undiagnosed complication or misdiagnosis
   — Lactose intolerance
   — Hypogammaglobulinemia
   — Bacterial overgrowth
   — Pancreatic insufficiency
   — Tropical sprue
3 Development of collagenous sprue (treatable with steroids)
4 Development of small bowel lymphoma

INTESTINAL PSEUDOOBSTRUCTION

Chronic intestinal pseudoobstruction: etiopathogenesis
1 Familial neuromyopathies
   — Familial myenteric plexus degeneration
   — Familial dysautonomia (Riley–Day syndrome)
   — Familial amyloidosis with autonomic neuropathy
   — Myotonic dystrophy
   — Acute intermittent porphyria
2 Acquired neuromyopathies
   — Systemic sclerosis (smooth muscle replaced by fibrosis)
   — Polymyositis
   — Parkinson's disease
   — Lead poisoning
   — Pelvic irradiation
3 Endocrinopathies
   — Diabetes mellitus (delayed gastric emptying)
   — Myxedema
   — Pheochromocytoma (long-standing)
   — Congenital hypoparathyroidism

4 Anticholinergic drugs
   — Phenothiazines
   — Tricyclics
   — Antiparkinsonian medication

Management modalities in pseudoobstruction
1 Cisapride
   — Prokinetic drug which promotes release of acetylcholine in the myenteric plexus
2 Erythromycin
   — Macrolide antibiotic which binds and activates motilin receptors in the proximal GI tract
3 Guanethidine plus neostigmine
   — For acute colonic pseudoobstruction
4 Colonoscopic decompression
   — Success rate of 75%, morbidity 3%, mortality 1%, in acute colonic pseudoobstruction
5 Conservative management

INTESTINAL NEOPLASIA

Histopathologic classification of polyps
1 Hyperplastic
   — No malignant potential per se, but may be associated with adenomas in proximal colon (controversial)
2 Juvenile
   — May be familial
3 Villous
   — Larger; hence, high neoplastic potential
4 Hamartomatous
   — e.g. Peutz–Jeghers
5 Inflammatory ('pseudopolyps')
   — True, non-neoplastic polyps occurring as post-inflammatory sequelae
   — Must be distinguished from carcinoma

Molecular events in the polyp–cancer sequence
1 Loss of heterozygosity on chromosome 5q*
2 DNA hypomethylation (→ chromatin activation)
3 Mutation on chromosome 17 (MCC)
4 *Ras* and p53 mutations
5 Deletion on chromosome 18 (DCC: adhesion molecule)
6 Mutation on chromosome 2 in hereditary non-polyposis colon cancer (DNA mismatch repair gene)

* Locus for adenomatous polyposis coli (APC) gene

MECHANISMS OF CIRRHOTIC SEQUELAE

Gynecomastia in alcoholic cirrhosis
1 ↑ Sex-hormone binding globulin (SHBG) levels
   → ↓ Free testosterone levels
2 Hypothalamopituitary axis suppression
   → ↓ Total testosterone levels
3 ↑ Estrogen production from precursors (e.g. DHEA)

Anemia in alcoholic liver disease
1 Hepatic insufficiency per se depresses erythropoiesis
2 Alcohol per se depresses erythropoiesis

3 Folate deficiency
4 Hypersplenism
5 Bleeding (see below)

Bleeding tendency in alcoholic cirrhosis
1 Reduced synthesis of coagulation factors
  Reduced activation of coagulation factors
2 Platelet function defect
  — Cirrhosis-induced von Willebrand's-type defect
  — Separate alcohol-induced platelet function defect
3 Thrombocytopenia
  — Hypersplenism
  — Marrow suppression
4 Local factors
  — Varices
  — Peptic ulceration
  — Gastritis
  — Mallory–Weiss

Coagulopathy in cirrhosis
1 Synthesis of all clotting factors except VIII may be reduced
2 Jaundiced patients may malabsorb vitamin K
  → ↓ activation of factors II, VII, IX, X, and proteins C and S
3 Prolongation of prothrombin time reflects reduced levels of factors II, V, VII, and X (cf. vitamin K dependence)
4 Since the half-life of factor VII is only 6 h, the pro-thrombin time is a sensitive index of hepatic function
5 Marked prolongation of both thrombin time and reptilase clotting time despite normal levels of fibrinogen antigen may reflect presence of abnormal fibrinogen*

* Dysfibrinogenemia; also associated with hepatoma

Ascitic tendency in cirrhosis
1 Activation of renin–angiotensin–aldosterone axis due to decreased effective central blood volume
  — Vasodilatation of splanchnic vascular bed
  — Peripheral vasodilatation (due to AV shunting)
  — High portal venous pressure
  — Low serum albumin
2 Perivenular hepatic fibrosis
  — Hepatic venous outflow obstruction
  — ↑ Sinusoidal pressure (intrahepatic hypertension) → fluid transudation
3 Other factors
  — ↑ Renal sympathetic tone/sodium retention
  — Reduced hepatic degradation of aldosterone
  — Excess thoracic duct lymph drainage

NB: Onset of refractory ascites signals 1-year mortality of 50%

BILE METABOLISM

Hepatobiliary defects predisposing to gallstone formation
1 Cholesterol-supersaturated bile
2 Increased tendency to cholesterol crystal nucleation
3 Impaired gallbladder contractility

Physiologic regulation of bilirubin metabolism
1 Bilirubin arises by cleavage of heme ring of hemoglobin, myoglobin, cytochromes. 70% of bilirubin originates from senescent RBC breakdown
2 Bilirubin binds tightly to albumin and may be displaced by drugs such as sulfonamides (leading to elevation of potentially neurotoxic free bilirubin → kernicterus)
3 Albumin-bound bilirubin is not renally filtered, but rather is exclusively metabolized by the liver and excreted in bile
4 On entering the hepatocyte, bilirubin is transported to the endoplasmic reticulum where it undergoes conjugation to the sugar molecule glucuronide. The enzyme regulating conjugation is called UDP-glucuronyltransferase. Hence, deficiencies of UDP-glucuronyltransferase cause unconjugated hyperbilirubinemia
5 Conjugated bilirubin is transferred to the canalicular membrane where it undergoes transport into the bile canalicular space. This is the rate-limiting step of bilirubin metabolism
6 Hepatocellular disease prevents canalicular transport of bilirubin into the bile, causing reflux of conjugated bilirubin back into the bloodstream

Familial non-hemolytic* hyperbilirubinemias
1 Gilbert's syndrome (autosomal dominant)
  — Affects 2–5% of the population, esp. slow acetylators
  — Mild unconjugated hyperbilirubinemia due to *minor* deficiency of UDP-glucuronyltransferase → ↓ conjugation/uptake (± ↓ RBC survival)
  — Jaundice precipitated by
    • Fasting (e.g. GTT)
    • Illness (e.g. 'flu)
    • Stress (e.g. surgery)
    • Alcohol ingestion
  — Liver function and histology *normal*
  — Phenobarbitone or rifampicin offer effective prophylaxis; but usually unnecessary
2 Crigler–Najjar syndrome type II (type I usually lethal)
  — Rare, relatively benign autosomal dominant condition
  — Unconjugated hyperbilirubinemia due to *major* deficiency of UDP-glucuronyltransferase
  — Phenobarbitone useful in management
3 Dubin–Johnson syndrome
  — Conjugated hyperbilirubinemia due to defective canalicular excretion; failure of OCG
  — Exacerbated by pregnancy, oral estrogens
  — BSP elimination: biphasic (late 2° rise)
  — Abnormal urinary coproporphyrin excretion
  — Biopsy: black centrilobular pigment
4 Rotor's syndrome
  — Conjugated hyperbilirubinemia due to defect in canalicular bilirubin excretion
  — *Normal* cholecystogram, biopsy, BSP test
  — Abnormal urinary coproporphyrin excretion

* Some patients with Gilbert's may have associated mild hemolysis

4.1 Daneshmend TK et al (1992) Omeprazole versus placebo for acute upper gastrointestinal bleeding. Br Med J 304: 143–147

Jensen DM et al (1994) A controlled study of rani-tidine for the prevention of recurrent hemorrhage from duodenal ulcer. N Engl J Med 330: 382–386

Slight reduction in endoscopic signs of intragastric bleeding, but no reduction of transfusion require-ment or mortality following omeprazole use in acute GI bleeders. Following ulcer healing, however, maintenance acid suppression (with ranitidine in this study) reduces the likelihood of rebleeding.

4.2 Perez-Ayuso RM et al (1991) Propranolol in prevention of recurrent bleeding from severe portal hyper-tensive gastropathy in cirrhosis. Lancet 337: 1431–1434

Poynard T et al (1991) Beta-adrenergic-antagonist drugs in the prevention of gastrointestinal bleeding in patients with cirrhosis and esophageal varices. N Engl J Med 324: 1532–1538

Long-term β-blockade appeared highly effective in reducing the rebleeding rate in both of these randomized studies.

Longstreth GF, Feitelberg SP (1995) Outpatient care of selected patients with acute non-variceal upper gastrointestinal haemorrhage. Lancet 345: 108–111

Non-randomized analysis of 141 patients with non-variceal upper GI bleeding treated as outpatients, none of whom died and only one of whom was admitted with rebleeding. Patients managed in this way tended to be younger, non-alcoholic and non-tachycardic.

4.3 Ramond M et al (1992) A randomized trial of prednisolone in patients with severe alcoholic hepatitis. N Engl J Med 326: 507–512

Randomized study of 61 alcoholics, showing 88% 2-month survival in steroid-treated patients but only 45% in controls.

4.4 Criqui MH, Ringel BL (1994) Does diet or alcohol explain the French paradox? Lancet 344: 1719–1723

Cross-cultural epidemiologic study showing that wine consumption correlated inversely with coronary disease, but that all-cause mortality was identical. The authors conclude that alcohol cannot be recommended as a public health measure.

4.5 Carson JL et al (1991) The low risk of upper gastrointestinal bleeding in patients dispensed corticosteroids. Am J Med 91: 223–229

Weil J et al (1995) Prophylactic aspirin and risk of peptic ulcer bleeding. Br Med J 310: 827–830

Provided that there was no past history of bleeding, the first study suggested a bleeding rate of only three per 10,000 patient months for steroid-treated dermatologic/asthma patients. The second, however, indicated that even low-dose (75 mg/day) aspirin was associated with a 2–3-fold increased risk of GI bleeding.

4.6 Patchett S et al (1991) Eradicating Helicobacter pylori and symptoms of non-ulcer dyspepsia. Br Med J 303: 1238–1240

Hentshcel E et al (1993) Effect of ranitidine and amoxicillin plus metronidazole on the eradication of Helicobacter pylori and the recurrence of duodenal ulcer. N Engl J Med 328: 308–312

Hosking SW et al (1994) Duodenal ulcer healing by eradication of Helicobacter pylori without anti-acid treatment. Lancet 343: 508–510

Dyspeptic patients without ulcers improve their gastritis, but not their symptoms, following H. pylori eradication. In contrast, eradication reduces recurrence rates of duodenal ulcer, suggesting a causative role. Moreover, ulcer healing appears inducible by eradicating H. pylori alone.

de Boer W et al (1995) Effect of acid suppression on efficacy of treatment for H. pylori infection. Lancet 345: 817–820

Study suggesting that acid suppression (using, in this case, omeprazole) further improves efficacy of an H. pylori eradication regimen – from 83% to 98%.

Sung J et al (1995) Antibacterial treatment of gastric ulcers associated with Helicobacter pylori. N Engl J Med 332: 139–142

Gastric ulcers healed as well in this study with antibacterial therapy alone as with the addition of omeprazole.

4.7 Nicholl JP et al (1992) Randomised controlled trial of cost-effectiveness of lithotripsy and open cholecystectomy as treatments for gallbladder stones. Lancet 340: 801–807

Barkun JS et al (1992) Randomised controlled trial of laparoscopic versus mini-cholecystectomy. Lancet 340: 1116–1119

The first study shows lithotripsy to be as effective and cost-effective as traditional cholecystectomy in patients with *small* stones. The second study suggested superior efficacy of laparoscopic cholecystectomy over the mini version.

4.8 Poupon RE et al (1994) Ursodiol for the long-term treatment of primary biliary cirrhosis. N Engl J Med 330: 1342–1347

Study of 145 PBC patients in which those treated with ursodiol experienced slower progression and less need for transplant.

4.9 Ekbom A et al (1990) Increased risk of large-bowel cancer in Crohn's disease with colonic involvement. Lancet 336: 357–359

The title says it all, really. Relative risk of 5–6 for those with colon-only disease.

De Mitri MS et al (1995) HCV-associated liver cancer without cirrhosis. Lancet 345: 413–415

Study of 19 HBsAg-negative non-cirrhotic hepatoma patients, showing PCR evidence of HCV (genotype 1b) gene expression in 11.

4.10 Gastinne H et al (1992) A controlled trial in intensive care units of selective decontamination of the digestive tract with nonabsorbable antibiotics. N Engl J Med 326: 594–599

No benefit from gut sterilization in this study of prophylactic antibiotic usage during mechanical ventilation; pneumonia occurred just as often. Fewer Gram-negatives grew, however.

4.11 Pasricha PJ et al (1995) Intrasphincteric botulinum toxin for the treatment of achalasia. N Engl J Med 322: 774–778

Study of 21 patients showing that botulinum toxin causes sustained remissions in achalasics who have their sphincters endoscopically injected.

CHAPTER 5

Hematology

Physical examination protocol 5.1   You are asked to examine the patient for signs of hematological disease

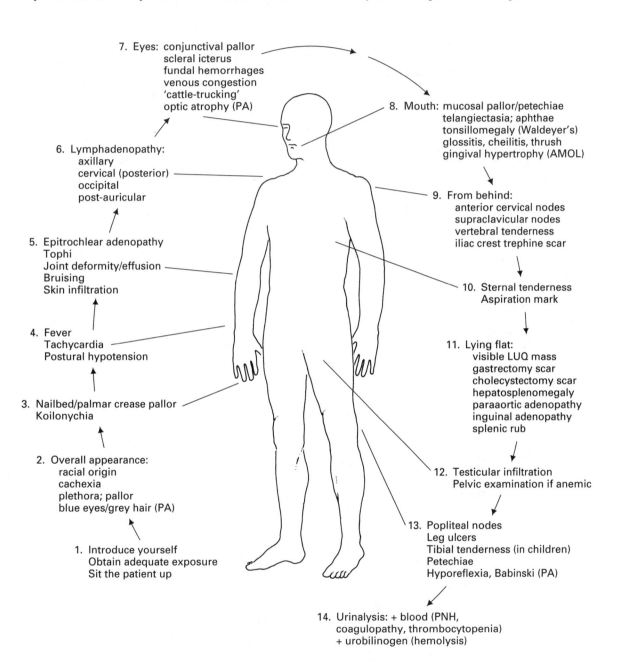

7. Eyes: conjunctival pallor
scleral icterus
fundal hemorrhages
venous congestion
'cattle-trucking'
optic atrophy (PA)

8. Mouth: mucosal pallor/petechiae
telangiectasia; aphthae
tonsillomegaly (Waldeyer's)
glossitis, cheilitis, thrush
gingival hypertrophy (AMOL)

6. Lymphadenopathy:
axillary
cervical (posterior)
occipital
post-auricular

9. From behind:
anterior cervical nodes
supraclavicular nodes
vertebral tenderness
iliac crest trephine scar

5. Epitrochlear adenopathy
Tophi
Joint deformity/effusion
Bruising
Skin infiltration

10. Sternal tenderness
Aspiration mark

4. Fever
Tachycardia
Postural hypotension

11. Lying flat:
visible LUQ mass
gastrectomy scar
cholecystectomy scar
hepatosplenomegaly
paraaortic adenopathy
inguinal adenopathy
splenic rub

3. Nailbed/palmar crease pallor
Koilonychia

12. Testicular infiltration
Pelvic examination if anemic

2. Overall appearance:
racial origin
cachexia
plethora; pallor
blue eyes/grey hair (PA)

13. Popliteal nodes
Leg ulcers
Tibial tenderness (in children)
Petechiae
Hyporeflexia, Babinski (PA)

1. Introduce yourself
Obtain adequate exposure
Sit the patient up

14. Urinalysis: + blood (PNH,
coagulopathy, thrombocytopenia)
+ urobilinogen (hemolysis)

Physical examination protocol 5.2   You are asked to examine a patient who has presented with bruising

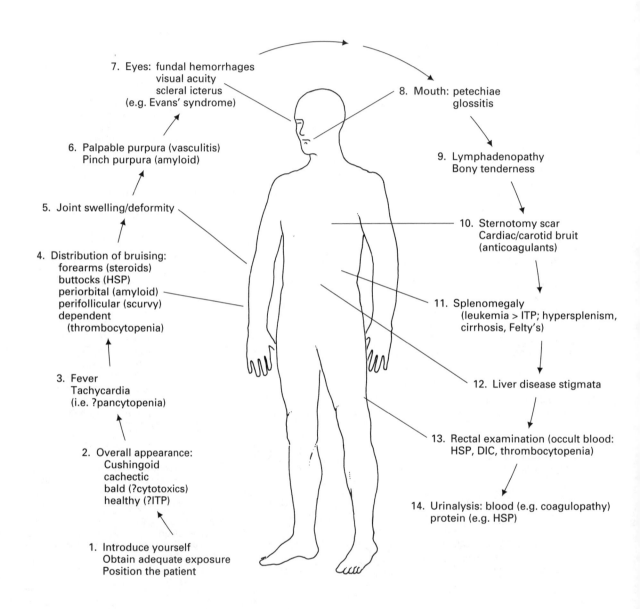

7. Eyes: fundal hemorrhages
   visual acuity
   scleral icterus
   (e.g. Evans' syndrome)

8. Mouth: petechiae
   glossitis

6. Palpable purpura (vasculitis)
   Pinch purpura (amyloid)

9. Lymphadenopathy
   Bony tenderness

5. Joint swelling/deformity

10. Sternotomy scar
    Cardiac/carotid bruit
    (anticoagulants)

4. Distribution of bruising:
   forearms (steroids)
   buttocks (HSP)
   periorbital (amyloid)
   perifollicular (scurvy)
   dependent
   (thrombocytopenia)

11. Splenomegaly
    (leukemia > ITP; hypersplenism,
    cirrhosis, Felty's)

3. Fever
   Tachycardia
   (i.e. ?pancytopenia)

12. Liver disease stigmata

2. Overall appearance:
   Cushingoid
   cachectic
   bald (?cytotoxics)
   healthy (?ITP)

13. Rectal examination (occult blood:
    HSP, DIC, thrombocytopenia)

1. Introduce yourself
   Obtain adequate exposure
   Position the patient

14. Urinalysis: blood (e.g. coagulopathy)
    protein (e.g. HSP)

Physical examination protocol 5.3   You are asked to examine a patient who has been found to have an enlarged spleen

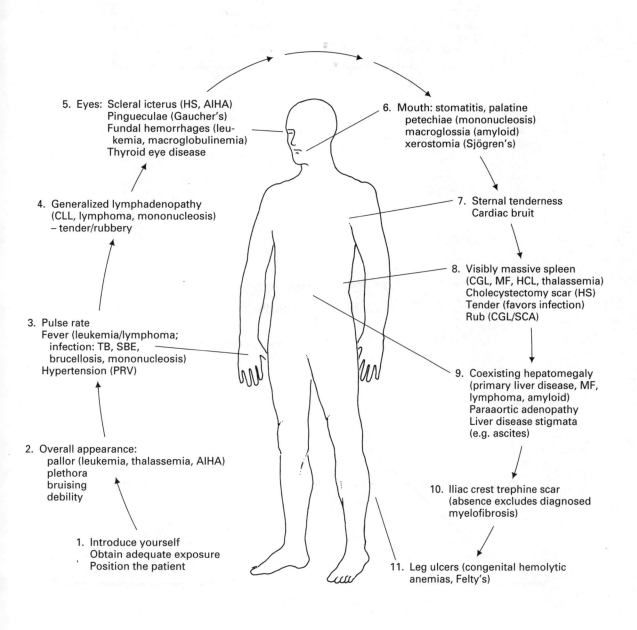

5. Eyes: Scleral icterus (HS, AIHA)
   Pingueculae (Gaucher's)
   Fundal hemorrhages (leu-
   kemia, macroglobulinemia)
   Thyroid eye disease

6. Mouth: stomatitis, palatine
   petechiae (mononucleosis)
   macroglossia (amyloid)
   xerostomia (Sjögren's)

4. Generalized lymphadenopathy
   (CLL, lymphoma, mononucleosis)
   – tender/rubbery

7. Sternal tenderness
   Cardiac bruit

8. Visibly massive spleen
   (CGL, MF, HCL, thalassemia)
   Cholecystectomy scar (HS)
   Tender (favors infection)
   Rub (CGL/SCA)

3. Pulse rate
   Fever (leukemia/lymphoma;
   infection: TB, SBE,
   brucellosis, mononucleosis)
   Hypertension (PRV)

9. Coexisting hepatomegaly
   (primary liver disease, MF,
   lymphoma, amyloid)
   Paraaortic adenopathy
   Liver disease stigmata
   (e.g. ascites)

2. Overall appearance:
   pallor (leukemia, thalassemia, AIHA)
   plethora
   bruising
   debility

10. Iliac crest trephine scar
    (absence excludes diagnosed
    myelofibrosis)

1. Introduce yourself
   Obtain adequate exposure
   Position the patient

11. Leg ulcers (congenital hemolytic
    anemias, Felty's)

Diagnostic pathway 5.1   This patient has presented with hepatosplenomegaly. What underlying disorders might be responsible?

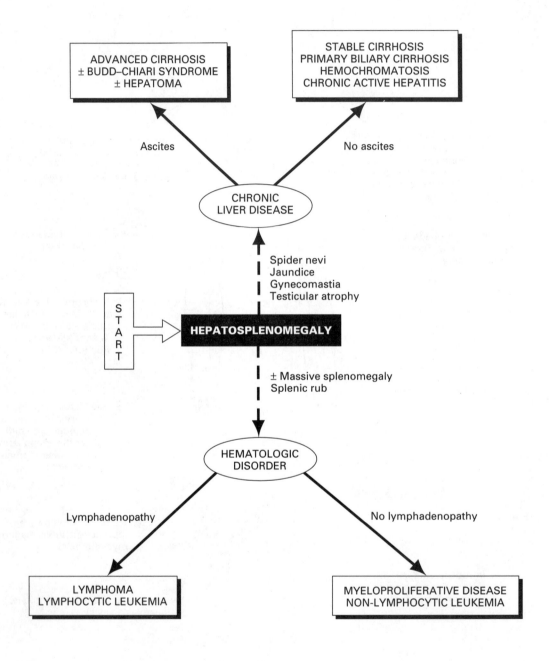

CLINICAL ASPECTS OF HEMATOLOGIC DISEASE

Commonest hematologic short cases
1 Splenomegaly
2 Cervical lymphadenopathy

PRESENTATIONS OF HEMATOLOGIC DISEASE

Abdominal pain in the hematologic patient
1 Biliary colic (e.g. hereditary spherocytosis)
2 Splenic infarct (e.g. chronic myeloid leukemia)
3 Vasoocclusive crisis (sickle-cell anemia)
4 Acute intermittent porphyria
5 Paroxysmal nocturnal hemoglobinuria
6 Hodgkin's disease (alcohol-induced pain)

History of the patient presenting with anemia
1 Duration of symptoms
2 Past history (e.g. ulcer, prosthetic valve, alcoholism)
3 Recent medications (e.g. NSAIDs, warfarin, steroids)
4 Operations (e.g. gastrectomy, ileal resection)
5 Menstrual history (esp. menorrhagia)
6 Diet (green vegetables, special restrictions)
7 Family history and racial background
8 Recent travel (e.g. to hookworm-endemic areas)
9 Toxic exposures (e.g. benzene, radiation)

Pathologic causes of epistaxis
1 Idiopathic thrombocytopenic purpura
2 Von Willebrand's disease
3 Hereditary hemorrhagic telangiectasia
4 Severe hypertension
5 Pertussis infection

Clinical manifestations of iron deficiency
1 Anemia
2 Koilonychia
3 Post-cricoid web (premalignant)
4 Atrophic glossitis
5 Angular stomatitis
6 Pica
7 Candidiasis

Infections in the leukemic host: clinical pitfalls
1 Fevers may arise due to non-infectious causes (e.g. drugs, transfusion reactions, graft-vs-host disease; p. 170)
2 Fevers may arise due to infection with multiple organisms, some of which may be difficult to identify
3 Fever may persist for the duration of neutropenia despite optimal antibiotic therapy
4 Fever may not occur at all in elderly or immunosuppressed patients with sepsis (± false-negative serologic responses)
5 Immunosuppressed febrile patients may fail to localize portal of sepsis due to poor inflammatory response

Clinical sequelae of hyperviscosity
1 CNS effects
— Lassitude, headache, deafness, nystagmus, convulsions
2 Visual loss
— Fundal hemorrhages, 'cattle-trucking', papilledema
3 Increased plasma volume
— Dilutional anemia, hypertension, heart failure
4 Platelet dysfunction*
— Bleeding, thrombosis, difficult venepuncture
5 Leukocyte dysfunction
— Sepsis, difficult crossmatch
6 Renal failure
— Plasmapheresis may minimize permanent damage

* esp. IgA myeloma

Complications of arteriovenous malformations
1 Spontaneous hemothorax
2 Cerebrovascular accident
3 Polycythemia, cyanosis

CLINICAL SIGNS OF HEMATOLOGIC DISEASE

Why do you think it's a spleen?
1 Can't get above it
2 Descends prominently on inspiration
3 Distinct edge + medial notch
4 Not ballottable
5 Percussion dullness over spleen/Traube's space
6 ± Audible rub

Differential diagnosis of epitrochlear lymphadenopathy
1 Non-Hodgkin's lymphoma, chronic lymphocytic leukemia
2 Infectious mononucleosis; secondary syphilis
3 Sarcoidosis
4 Intravenous drug abuse

Widespread retinal hemorrhages: differential diagnosis
1 Malignant hypertension
2 Diabetes mellitus
3 Hyperviscosity syndrome
4 Severe anemia, severe thrombocytopenia
5 Hb SC (sickle-C) disease

Clinical evaluation of bleeding tendency
1 Skin petechiae, epistaxes, purpura after minor trauma
Mucosal bleeding; menorrhagia
Immediate bleeding after lacerations
— Thrombocytopenia or platelet function defect*
— ↑ Bleeding time‡
2 Widespread intramuscular hematomas
Spontaneous hemarthroses
Delayed bleeding after lacerations
— Coagulation factor deficiency (90% in males)
— ↑ PTTK

* Incl. heterozygous von Willebrand's disease, even though platelets themselves are normal
‡ Clinical utility doubtful

POLYCYTHEMIA

Features common to primary and secondary polycythemia
1 Thrombotic tendency (esp. cerebral)
2 Hypertension
3 Headaches
4 Visual disturbances
5 Engorged retinal veins

Clinical features suggestive of polycythemia vera
1 Splenomegaly
2 Aquagenic pruritus
3 Bleeding (esp. gastrointestinal)
4 Gout
5 Peptic ulcer
6 Disease termination in myelofibrosis or leukemia (10%)

HODGKIN'S DISEASE

Clinical presentations of Hodgkin's disease
1 'B' symptoms (p. 164)
2 Pruritus *(not* a 'B' symptom)
3 Pel–Ebstein (cyclical) fever (p. 205): classic but *rare*
4 Alcohol-induced pain at sites of disease (incl. abdomen)
5 Infection (see p. 198)

Classical features of specific histologic subtypes
1 Lymphocyte predominant
   — Best prognosis
   — Usually early-stage (I, II) disease
2 Nodular sclerosing
   — Indolent chemosensitive but relapsing disease
   — Tends to affect young women
   — May cause bulky mediastinal adenopathy
   — Spreads by contiguity
   — Good prognosis *unless* bulky mediastinal disease
3 Mixed cellularity
   — Often associated with occult splenic involvement
   — Intermediate prognosis
4 Lymphocyte depletion
   — 'B' symptoms (e.g. fever of unknown origin)
   — Adenopathy more widespread than other subtypes
   — May present with visceral involvement, e.g. marrow fibrosis, osteoblastic bony disease ('ivory vertebrae')
   — Spreads by dissemination to distant sites
   — Worst prognosis

INVESTIGATING HEMATOLOGIC DISEASE

THE PERIPHERAL BLOOD FILM

Diagnosis suggested by blood film alone*
1 'Aleukemic' leukemia

— Circulating blasts, leukoerythroblastic precursors
2 Compensated 'warm' autoimmune hemolysis
   — Spherocytes, polychromasia, reticulocytosis
   Hereditary spherocytosis
   — (Micro)spherocytes, ↑ MCHC
3 Dysproteinemias
   — Rouleaux, bluish background
4 Disseminated intravascular coagulation
   Microangiopathic hemolysis
   — Red cell fragments
5 Infection
   — Infectious mononucleosis (atypical lymphocytes)
   — *M. pneumoniae* (autoagglutination)
   — Malaria (*P. vivax/ovale* -> Schüffner's dots), babesiosis
   — Relapsing fever (*Borrelia* spirochetes visible on film)
6 Thalassemia trait‡
   — Microcytosis, teardrops, targets
   Hb C disease
   — Target cells in abundance
7 Pyruvate kinase deficiency (→ ATP deficiency)
   — Xerocytes (dehydrated RBCs)

* i.e. ± normal blood count
‡ cf. sickle-cell trait: diagnosed by Hb electrophoresis (i.e. film normal)

Features of the post-splenectomy blood film
1 Howell–Jolly bodies
2 Pappenheimer bodies
3 Target cells
4 Spur cells, spherocytes
5 Thrombocytosis ± leukocytosis

Leukoerythroblastic blood film: diagnostic significance
1 **M**yelofibrosis
2 **M**arrow infiltration
   — Common causes
     • **M**etastatic cancer (e.g. breast, prostate)*
     • **M**yeloma
     • **M**alignant lymphoma
   — Uncommon causes
     • **M**arble bone disease (osteopetrosis)
     • **M**etabolic: Gaucher's disease

* bone scan usually positive; cf. myeloma, lymphoma

Infectious diseases mimicking leukemic blood films
1 Infectious mononucleosis
   — May mimic ALL
2 Pertussis, mycoplasma
   — May mimic CLL

Clues to underlying sepsis on the peripheral blood film
1 Neutrophilia
2 'Left shift': bandforms, (meta)myelocytes
3 Toxic granulation
4 Döhle bodies

Differential diagnosis of the dimorphic blood film
1 Sideroblastosis
2 Post-splenectomy
3 Post-transfusion

4 Iron loss combined with B$_{12}$/folate malabsorption
  — Post-gastrectomy
  — Pernicious anemia with gastric cancer
  — Celiac disease and/or intestinal lymphoma
  — Crohn's disease, Whipple's disease
5 Iron loss combined with hyposplenism
  — Celiac disease
  — Radical gastrectomy (incorporates splenectomy)

Pathologic significance of red cell inclusions
1 Howell–Jolly bodies
  Cabot's rings
  — Nuclear remnants seen in hyposplenic states
    (p. 199)
2 Heinz bodies*
  — Denatured globin chains in RBC periphery seen in
    unstable Hb, e.g. Hb Zürich/Köln, G6PD deficiency
  — Often associated with 'bite cells' on film
3 Pappenheimer bodies: iron granules in siderocytes
  — Positive Prussian blue reaction
  — Seen post-splenectomy and in lead poisoning
4 Basophilic stippling: implies dyserythropoiesis
  — Seen in lead poisoning (coarse stippling)
  — Also seen in thalassemia, 5'-nucleotidase
    deficiency

* Demonstrated using supravital stains, e.g. cresyl violet

Abnormal erythrocyte morphology: etiologic significance
1 Target cells
  — Chronic liver disease
  — Thalassemia; Hb C; Hb E*
  — Hyposplenism
  — Iron deficiency
2 Teardrop poikilocytes
  — Myelofibrosis
  — Dyserythropoiesis. e.g. thalassemia,
    megaloblastosis
3 Schistocytes
  — Microangiopathic hemolytic anemia (e.g. TTP)
  — Disseminated intravascular coagulation
4 Spur cells (acanthocytes)
  — Chronic liver disease (esp. Zieve's syndrome)
  — Abetalipoproteinemia
  — Renal failure, hyposplenism

* Asymptomatic condition (Hb $\alpha_2\beta_2^{26Glu \to Lys}$) even when
homozygous; but yields thalassemia major when crossed with β-
thal trait. Very common in Thailand, Cambodia, Laos

RBC distribution width (RDW) in anemia*
1 Normal RDW, ↑ reticulocyte count
  — α/β thalassemia minor
  — Hereditary spherocytosis
  — Severe hemolysis (> 10% reticulocytes)
2 Normal RDW, ↓ reticulocyte count
  — Anemia of chronic disease
  — Aplastic anemia
  — Myelodysplastic syndromes
3 ↑ RDW, ↑ reticulocyte count
  — Microangiopathic hemolytic anemia
  — Immune hemolysis; cold agglutinin disease
  — Sickle-cell anemia; sickle-β-thal, sickle-C
  — HbH disease
  — G6PD deficiency

4 ↑ RDW, ↓ reticulocyte count
  — Myelofibrosis
  — Sideroblastosis
  — Iron deficiency

* A quantitative measure of anisocytosis

IRON-DEFICIENCY ANEMIA

Abnormalities of plasma iron studies in hematologic disease
1 ↓ Fe, ↑ TIBC, ↓ ferritin – Iron deficiency
2 ↓ Fe, ↓ TIBC,↑ ferritin – Chronic disease
3 ↑ Fe, ↓ TIBC, ↑ ferritin – Chronic hemolysis

Temporal sequence of iron deficiency
1 Iron depletion
  — ↓ Marrow stainable iron
  — ↓ Stainable sideroblast ferritin
  — ↑ Red cell protoporphyrin
2 Iron deficiency
  — Absent marrow stainable iron
  — ↓ Fe, ↑ TIBC
  — Transferrin saturation < 15%
3 Iron deficiency anemia
  — Hypochromic microcytic film
  — ↑ RDW*
  — ↓ Hb

* cf. chronic disease: RDW (red cell distribution width) normal

Microcytosis disproportionate to anemia?
1 Thalassemia (incl. trait)
2 Venesected polycythemia vera

Investigation of unexplained hypochromic microcytic anemia
1 Blood film
  — Red cell morphology
  — Reticulocyte count
2 Iron studies
  — Serum iron, TIBC, transferrin saturation
  — Serum ferritin
3 Exclusion of gastrointestinal (or uterine) bleeding
  — Fecal occult blood testing and/or endoscopy
  — Angiography; ^{99m}Tc-labelled red cells
4 Marrow aspiration
  — Stainable iron stores
  — Ring sideroblasts
5 Urinary hemosiderin
  — ↑ In chronic intravascular hemolysis (e.g. PNH)
6 Hb EPG
  — Hb A$_2$ level (↑ in thalassemia trait)

Failure of microcytic anemia to respond to iron supplements
1 Wrong diagnosis
  — Thalassemia trait
  — Sideroblastosis (congenital)
2 Persistent bleeding
3 Malabsorption
  — Blind loop
  — Gastrectomy
4 Non-compliance

MEGALOBLASTIC ANEMIAS

Macrocytosis: factors favoring megaloblastosis
1 Oval (not round) macrocytes (esp. if > 3%)
2 Markedly elevated MCV (> 115 fL)
3 Hypersegmented (> 5 lobes) neutrophils
4 Marked poikilo-/anisocytosis
  Mild basophilic stippling
5 No target/spur cells, round macrocytes (cf. liver disease); no polychromatophilic macrocytes (cf. hemolysis)
6 ↑ Plasma 2-methylcitric acid (2-MCA) and/or cystathione

Clinicopathologic correlations in folate metabolism
1 Red cell folate is more informative than serum levels
2 Partial hematologic responses may be seen in (pure) B_{12} deficiency treated inadvertently with pharmacologic (5–15 mg/day) doses of folate*
3 Catastrophic progression of *neurologic* deficit may be seen in B_{12}-deficient patients treated inadvertently with folate. Hence, if in doubt, give both B_{12} and folate

* cf. primary folate deficiency, where maximal reticulocytosis follows physiologic – 200 μg/day – doses of folate

Clinicopathologic correlations in B_{12} deficiency
1 The microbiologic assay remains the 'gold standard' in determining B_{12} levels. Radioimmunoassay, though cheaper, has a higher false-negative and (occasionally) false-positive rate with respect to B_{12} deficiency, e.g. due to R-protein (see below) errors*
2 In B_{12} deficient patients, serum folate (and iron) levels are often elevated ('normal' levels may indicate coexisting folate, or iron, deficiency), while red cell folate levels may be reduced due to the 'folate trap' mechanism
3 Neurologic degeneration may occur without anemia
4 Transient ileal mucosal changes (analogous to macrocytosis) may lead to failure of normalization of the Schilling test following oral intrinsic factor in patients with pernicious anemia treated for less than (say) 6 weeks
5 Mean corpuscular volume may be normal in patients with coexisting iron deficiency (e.g. Crohn's, celiac disease, pernicious anemia with gastric cancer) or thalassemia trait
6 Blood transfusion is best avoided in initial management of severe megaloblastic anemia (risk of fluid overload)

* Elderly patients with normal RIA may thus still benefit from vitamin supplements

Investigations distinguishing primary B_{12} from folate deficiency*
1 Deoxyuridine suppression test
  — Deoxyuridine and tritiated thymidine added to patient's bone marrow in vitro
  — Megaloblastic marrow takes up ↑↑ thymidine
  — Corrects upon adding B_{12} (in B_{12} deficiency) or methyltetrahydrofolate (in folate deficiency)

2 24-h urinary methylmalonic acid (MMA) excretion
  — 10 g valine given as an initial loading dose
  — ↑ MMA excretion in B_{12} deficiency *only*
3 Serum MMA and 2-MCA
  — Elevated in B_{12} deficiency only

* i.e. if *both* B_{12} and folate levels low

Molecular regulation of B_{12} metabolism
1 Intrinsic factor (IF)
  — Synthesized by gastric parietal cells
  — Binds and transports dietary cobalamin (B_{12})
  — B_{12}-IF complex attaches to specific ileal receptors
2 R-proteins
  — Incl. transcobalamin (TC) I, III; made by leukocytes
  — Compete with IF for intragastric binding of cobalamin
  — Bind B_{12} more avidly than IF at low gastric pH
  — Facilitate hepatic storage and excretion of cobalamin
  — Degraded in jejunum by pancreatic enzymes, whereas IF resists proteolysis and binds liberated B_{12}
3 TC-II
  — Plasma protein synthesized by liver
  — Binds newly absorbed B_{12} in portal blood
  — Transports B_{12} to target tissues

Abnormalities of transcobalamin metabolism
1 ↓TC-II
  — Hereditary
  — Leads to ↓ B_{12} levels (with clinical deficiency)
2 ↑TC-I
  — Occurs secondary to CML/polycythemia vera
  — May cause ↑ B_{12} levels
3 ↑TC-III
  — Seen in benign leukocytosis (e.g. leukemoid reaction)
  — No change in B_{12} levels
4 ↑TC-II
  — Seen with macrophage activation (e.g. SLE, sarcoid)
  — No change in B_{12} levels

Some causes of vitamin B_{12} deficiency
1 Pernicious anemia
2 Gastrectomy (see p. 135)
3 Bacterial overgrowth (*E. coli, B. fragilis*)
4 Ileal resection (usually > 1 meter)
5 Pancreatic exocrine insufficiency (↓ R-protein proteolysis)
  Gastrinoma (low pH inactivates pancreatic proteases)
6 Imerslund's disease; *Diphyllobothrium latum* infestation*

* Both conditions endemic in Finland

Significance of clinical B_{12} deficiency in Crohn's disease
1 Bacterial overgrowth
2 Fistula
3 Ileal resection

NB: Major B_{12} deficiency is *unusual* in uncomplicated Crohn's

Differential diagnosis of an abnormal Schilling test
1 Corrects with addition of intrinsic factor
  — Pernicious anemia
2 Does not correct with intrinsic factor
  ↑ Fecal bile acids
  — Bacterial overgrowth
3 Does not correct with intrinsic factor
  ↓ Fecal bile acids
  — Ileal insufficiency (e.g. resection, severe Crohn's)
4 Does not correct with intrinsic factor
  Normal fecal bile acids
  — Renal failure*

* i.e. renal failure *spuriously* reduces Schilling test yield; B_{12} levels normal

Indicators of response following B_{12} replenishment
1 Erythroblastosis (bone marrow) within 12 h
  Reticulocytosis at 48 h, maximal at 1 week
2 ↑ Methylmalonic acid (MMA)
3 ↑ Serum alkaline phosphatase
4 ↑ Urate
5 ↓ K^+ (may be profound)
6 ↓ Folate; ↓ iron (usually subclinical)

Megaloblastic anemias with normal B_{12}/folate levels
1 Antimetabolite therapy (p. 29)
2 Erythroleukemia
3 Hereditary orotic aciduria (uridine-responsive)
  Lesch–Nyhan syndrome (adenine-responsive)

Etiology of non-megaloblastic macrocytosis
1 Alcohol ± liver disease
  Liver disease ± alcohol
2 Hypothyroidism (exclude coexisting pernicious anemia)
3 Acquired sideroblastosis*
4 Reticulocytosis (any cause)
  Autoagglutination (→ *artefactual* ↑ MCV)‡
5 Aplastic anemia
6 Paroxysmal nocturnal hemoglobinuria

* cf. congenital sideroblastosis: usually microcytic
‡ e.g. in cold hemagglutinin disease (CHAD; p. 192)

AUTOIMMUNE HEMOLYTIC ANEMIA

Investigation of suspected hemolysis
1 Etiologic clues on blood film
  — Spherocytes (hereditary or autoimmune hemolysis)
  — Schistocytes, helmet cells (microangiopathic hemolysis)
  — Sickled cells
2 Signs of marrow compensation
  — Polychromatophilic macrocytes
  — Reticulocytosis ('warm' > 'cold' hemolysis)
  — Occasional nucleated red cells
3 Confirmation of red cell lysis
  — Mild unconjugated (direct) hyperbilirubinemia
  — Urinalysis: urobilinogen +, bilirubin –
  — ↓ Haptoglobin*
  — ↓ Hemopexin
  — ↓ Folate (secondary, esp. in pregnancy)

4 Confirmation of marrow compensation
  — Erythroid hyperplasia on marrow aspirate
5 Signs of intravascular hemolysis
  — Hemoglobinemia, hemoglobinuria‡
  — Hemosiderinuria (implies chronicity; may → ↓ Fe^{2+})
  — Methemalbuminemia (Schumm's +; implies severity)
6 Further diagnostic investigations
  — Coombs' and Ham's tests
  — Cold agglutinins, Donath–Landsteiner antibody
  — Hb EPG; Heinz body prep; RBC G6PD levels
  — ^{51}Cr-RBC survival and sequestration study

* NB: False-negatives in acute phase reactions, false-positives in liver disease
‡ Associated with pink serum; cf. myoglobinuria

Coombs tests: what do they do?
1 Direct Coombs antiglobulin test (DAT)
  — Used to investigate *hemolysis*
  — i.e. Do the *patient's red cells* have antibody/C_3?
2 Indirect Coombs antiglobulin test (IAT)
  — Used in blood *crossmatching*
  — i.e. Does the intended *recipient's serum* contain antibodies to the planned red cell transfusion?

Autoimmune hemolysis: diagnostic aspects
1 'Warm' type
  — IgG-mediated extravascular (intrasplenic) hemolysis: +DAT, +IgG
  — Progressive anemia, mild jaundice, splenomegaly
  — Blood film: spherocytes, marked reticulocytosis
  — Often arises secondary to SLE, CLL, Hodgkin's, drugs
  — Often responds to steroids/azathioprine, splenectomy
  — Transfusion may be life-saving
2 'Cold' type
  — IgM-κ-mediated intravascular (intrahepatic) hemolysis: +DAT, +C_3
  — Autoagglutination on blood film
  — Symptom severity depends more on height of thermal amplitude than on absolute titer
  — May signify lymphoma, macroglobulinemia, infection
  — Treatment is best directed at the underlying condition
  — Transfusion should be avoided if possible; if absolutely necessary, warm blood and transfuse slowly

Features of drug-induced autoimmune hemolysis
1 'Methyldopa' (autoimmune) type
  — Mild (rarely significant) extravascular hemolysis
  — +DAT, +IAT (i.e. Coombs+ without drug), –C_3
  — May remain Coombs+ for years after drug ceased
2 'Penicillin' (hapten) type
  — IgG directed against drug (a hapten)
  — IgG adsorbs to red cell after prolonged high-dose R_x
  — Causes extravascular hemolysis
  — +DAT, –IAT (i.e. Coombs+ *only* in presence of drug)

3 'Quinine' (immune complex) type
— Intravascular hemolysis on second or subsequent exposures ('innocent bystander' mechanism)
— IgM-(or IgG-) mediated complement activation
— Drug-IgM complex dissociates from RBCs, leaving C_3
— +DAT, +C_3

6 Mutation in ankyrin/β-spectrin locus (not routine)
— Genetic heterogeneity reflects clinical picture

* Corrects with glucose; cf. 'autoimmune' spherocytosis

OTHER ANEMIAS

Significance of abnormal reticulocyte counts in anemia
1 Reticulocytosis
— Blood loss/hemorrhage
• Up to 15% reticulocytes
— Hemolysis
• Up to 30% reticulocytes
— Response phase of iron/B_{12}/folate deficiency
• Up to 50% reticulocytes
2 Reticulocytopenia (i.e. relative to degree of anemia)
— Aplastic anemia
— Chronic disease, e.g. uremia

Hypersplenism: diagnostic criteria
1 Cytopenia
2 Splenomegaly
3 Marrow hypercellularity
4 Cytopenia corrected by splenectomy

Anemia of chronic disease: laboratory features
1 Blood film
— Normocytic ± hypochromic; normal RDW
— Reticulocytopenia (for degree of anemia)
2 Iron studies
— ↓ Fe/TIBC/TF saturation
— ↑ Ferritin
3 Special studies
— ↓ Red cell survival
— ↓ Erythropoietin activity
— ↑ Red cell protoporphyrin
4 Bone marrow
— Absent sideroblasts (RBC precursors)
— ↑ Iron stores

Varieties of anemia in myxedema
1 Normochromic, normocytic
2 Macrocytic
— Suggests associated pernicious anemia
3 Microcytic (in female)
— Suggests menorrhagia

Diagnosis of hereditary spherocytosis
1 Family history (in 80%)
2 Clinical picture
— Recurrent mild unconjugated jaundice (DD$_x$ Gilbert's)
— ± Splenomegaly, anemia, gallstones
3 Numerous microspherocytes on blood film Negative Coombs test
4 ↑ MCHC (35–38 g%); normal MCV
5 Definitive diagnosis
— ↑ RBC osmotic fragility (high-salt lysis)
— Positive autohemolysis test*

Causes of a grossly abnormal ESR
1 > 100 mm/h
— Malignancy
• Myeloma
• Hodgkin's
• Carcinomatosis
— Sepsis, esp. active TB
— Active vasculitis, esp. giant-cell
— Uremia; profound anemia
2 < 3 mm/h*
— Polycythemia rubra vera
— Sickle-cell anemia
— Massive leukocytosis (e.g. in CLL)
— Hypofibrinogenemia (hereditary or DIC-induced)
— High-dose steroids or salicylates

* NB: 95% of these will be *normal*

NORMAL AND ABNORMAL HEMOGLOBINS

Factors improving tissue oxygenation by red blood cells*
1 Acidosis, hypercapnia
— Via Bohr effect
2 Hypoxia, anemia
Thyrotoxicosis; pregnancy
Renal failure
— Via ↑ red cell 2,3-DPG
3 Increased blood temperature
4 Low-affinity Hb (see below)

* i.e. reducing Hb affinity for oxygen; right shift of dissociation curve

Diagnostic value of hemoglobin electrophoresis
1 Hb S (sickle cell)
2 Hb A_2 (↑ in β-thal *trait* esp.)
3 Hb C, D, E

Hemoglobins with abnormal oxygen affinity
1 High-affinity hemoglobins
— e.g. Hb F; Hb Chesapeake, Hb Rainier, Hb Köln
— Detected as unexpected polycythemia on routine test
— Cause left shift of oxyhemoglobin dissociation curve*
— Usually asymptomatic with benign course
2 Low-affinity hemoglobins (rare)
— e.g. Hb Kansas, Hb Seattle, Hb Hammersmith
— Present with congenital cyanosis + 'pseudoanemia'
— DD$_x$: genetic methemoglobinemia ('Hb M')
3 Unstable hemoglobins
— 'Heinz-body anemias' (p. 157)
— Abnormal isopropanol/heat stability test
— Usually autosomal dominant transmission
— Respond to splenectomy

* Also occurs in smokers due to binding of carbon monoxide to Hb

HEMATOLOGIC MALIGNANCIES

Diagnostic priorities in bone marrow biopsy
1 Aspiration more important
  — Acute leukemias
  — Chronic myeloid leukemia ($\rightarrow$ karyotyping)
  — Myelodysplastic syndromes
  — Megaloblastosis, sideroblastosis
  — Thrombocytopenia, leukopenia
2 Trephine more important
  — Chronic lymphocytic leukemia*
  — Non-contributory aspirate: 'dry' or 'blood' tap

* NB: Can usually be diagnosed on blood film alone

Differential diagnosis of a dry tap
1 Operator inexperience
  — Needle tip in wrong place
  — Clot blocking needle lumen
2 Marrow fibrosis
  — Myelofibrosis
  — Myelodysplastic syndrome
  — Hairy cell leukemia
  — AIDS
3 Packed marrow
  — Leukemia, lymphoma
  — Metastatic carcinoma
  — Osteopetrosis
4 Empty marrow
  — Aplastic anemia
  — Aleukemic leukemia
  — Paroxysmal nocturnal hemoglobinuria (some)

Evaluation of the anemic patient with hypoplastic marrow
1 History
  — Toxin exposure (incl. drugs)
  — Previous transfusions*
2 Blood count: prognosis worse if
  — WCC < 500/mL
  — Platelets < 20,000/mL
  — Reticulocyte count < 1%
3 Marrow aspiration and trephine
  — Helps exclude
    • Myelofibrosis
    • Hypoplastic (aleukemic) leukemia
    • Metastatic carcinomatosis
  — Prognosis worse if cellularity < 25% normal
4 Ham's test
  — Excludes paroxysmal nocturnal hemoglobinuria
  — Prognosis better if positive
5 HLA-typing of siblings

* Higher success rate of marrow transplant if transfusions can be avoided altogether

Laboratory features of myelodysplastic syndromes
1 Film
  — Hypersegmented neutrophils, *or*
  — Hyposegmented neutrophils (Pelger–Huet-like)
2 NAP score
  — Low
3 Hb electrophoresis
  — Increased Hb F (often)

4 Marrow
  — Hypercellular
  — Scarcity of mature forms
  — Slight excess of blasts

Common cytogenetic aberrations in hematologic malignancies
1 Ph[1]
  — Reciprocal 9:22 translocation of *c-abl* oncogene and *bcr*
2 Blastic transformation of CML
  — Ph[2] (i.e. second Philadelphia chromosome)
  — Aneuploidy
  — Trisomy 8, isochromosome 17
3 8:14 translocation of c-*myc*
  — Lymphomas, esp. Burkitt's
4 15:17 translocation
  — Acute promyelocytic leukemia (M3)
5 8:21 translocation
  — M2 (AML with maturation; p. 163); good prognosis
  Chromosome 16 inversion
  — M4 (myelomonocytic AML); good prognosis
6 5q-
  — Refractory anemia (myelodysplastic, 'preleukemia')
  5q-/7q-
  — Iatrogenic leukemia (second malignancy)
  — Poor prognosis

MULTIPLE MYELOMA

Minimal diagnostic criteria for myeloma
1 Characteristic marrow aspirate
  — % Plasmacytosis (e.g. > 30%)
  — Morphology (plasmacytoma)
2 Monoclonal immunoglobulin spike, e.g.
  — IgG > 3.5 g/dL/24 h urine EPG
  — IgA > 2.0 g/dL/24 h urine EPG
  — κ/λ light chains > 1.0 g/dL/24 h urine EPG
3 Demonstration of *multiple* lesions
  — e.g. Repeated aspirations, skeletal survey

NB: Although the diagnosis will be supported by demonstration of a serum and/or urine paraprotein, such a finding is not sufficient for diagnosis, nor (given the occurrence of non-secretory myeloma) is it strictly necessary

Major prognostic variables in myeloma
1 Presence of renal impairment*
2 β_2-microglobulin levels‡
3 Plasma cell labelling index¶
4 Response to therapy

* NB: A minority of patients who present with renal failure recover function following rehydration; some others with irreversible failure may do quite well on dialysis
‡ Reflect disease bulk and/or renal function
¶ Measured using tritiated thymidine, thymidine kinase or BuDR

Paraprotein-related clinical patterns in myeloma
1 Hyperviscosity
  — IgG$_3$
2 Hypercalcemia; platelet dysfunction
  — IgA

3 Plasma cell leukemia
— IgE
4 Renal failure
— IgD
— Bence-Jones only
5 Hepatosplenomegaly
— μ heavy-chain disease

INVESTIGATING MYELOPROLIFERATIVE DISEASE

Thrombocytosis: factors favoring myeloproliferative disease
1 Physical examination
— Splenomegaly
2 Platelets
— Platelet count > 1000 x 10^9/L
— Giant platelets on film
— Abnormal aggregation → ↑ bleeding time
3 Blood film
— Basophilia
— Neutrophilia
4 Other laboratory studies
— ↑ NAP score
— ↑ B_{12}
— ↑ Uric acid
5 Clinical course
— Hemorrhage
— Thrombosis*

* Sudden increment in platelet count may indicate splenic vein thrombosis

Polycythemia? Laboratory features of polycythemia vera
1 Coexisting leukocytosis and/or thrombocytosis
2 Hb O_2 saturation > 92%*
3 ↑ NAP score
4 ↑ Plasma B_{12}
5 Low erythropoietin levels (limited assay availability)

* cf. chronic airways disease, smoking, altitude: Hb O_2 saturation < 90% (plus high erythropoietin levels)

CHRONIC MYELOID (GRANULOCYTIC) LEUKEMIA

Diagnosis of chronic myeloid leukemia (CML)
1 Clinical
— Splenomegaly ± pain/rub (infarct)
— Hemorrhagic or thrombotic phenomena (e.g. priapism)
— *No* predisposition to infection (normal WBC function)
2 Blood film
— WCC often > 100 x 10^9/L
— Predominant cells: neutrophils, myelocytes
— Left shift; basophilia ± eosinophilia
— Normochromic anemia ± thrombocytosis
3 Other laboratory studies
— ↓ NAP score (often zero)
— ↑ B_{12} (↑ TC-I; p. 158)
— ↑ Uric acid
4 Bone marrow
— < 10% myeloblasts (cf. blastic transformation)

— M:E ratio > 10:1 (usually)
— Rarely: Gaucher cells, sea-blue histiocytes
5 Philadelphia chromosome (Ph'; → > 90%)
— Generally unaffected by chemotherapy (i.e. may persist despite morphologic 'remission'*)
— Main reason for performing marrow examination

* cf. Philadelphia chromosome-positive ALL

Signs of acute (blastic) transformation of CML
1 Symptoms
— Fever
— Bone pain
2 Signs
— Increasing splenomegaly
— Lymphadenopathy
3 Laboratory
— ↑ WCC/platelets
— Rising NAP score
— Appearance of circulating TdT+ or CALLA+ blasts*
4 Bone marrow
— > 10% blasts
— New cytogenetic aberrations (p. 161)
5 Clinical course
— Refractoriness to busulfan

* Implies *lymphoblastic* transformation, better prognosis than myeloblastic

Differential diagnosis of normal or high NAP score in CML
1 Partial remission
2 Intercurrent infection (or other stress)
3 Pregnancy
4 Development of myelofibrosis
5 Blastic transformation
6 Leukemoid reaction (i.e. misdiagnosis)

Characteristics of Ph'-negative CML
1 'Juvenile' CML
— Age of onset typically < 5 years
— May be inherited
— A subacute form of chronic myelomonocytic leukemia and subset of malignant histiocytosis (p. 235)
— May be responsive to isotretinoin
2 Adult Ph'-negative CML
— Tends to be later onset than Ph+ CML
— Smaller spleen
— Lower WCC
— Higher lysozyme and Hb F
— Poorer prognosis

NB: 'Ph'-negative' CML may be clinically indistinguishable from Ph'-positive CML if chromosome 22 *bcr* rearrangement is subtle

CHRONIC LYMPHOCYTIC LEUKEMIA (CLL)

Significance of anemia in CLL
1 Marrow suppression ('chronic disease') in 95%
2 Autoimmune hemolysis (in 5%)
3 Hypersplenism (rare)

Immunologic considerations in CLL
1 Impaired humoral immunity
— 50% have hypogammaglobulinemia (esp. ↓ IgM)

2 Impaired cell-mediated immunity
— CD4:CD8 (helper–suppressor) ratio often inverted
3 Effect of therapy on immunity
— Steroids increase the risk of infectious complications
— Hypogammaglobulinemia may improve with chemo
— IV gammaglobulin reduces the incidence of bacterial infections in hypogammaglobulinemic patients
4 Paraproteins and hemolysis
— 5% of patients have a paraprotein
— 5–10% have a positive direct antiglobulin (Coombs) test
— Significant hemolysis/thrombocytopenia affects < 5%
— Thrombocytopenia *usually* indicates marrow failure (rather than autoimmune destruction)

OTHER LEUKEMIAS

Clinicopathologic hallmarks of selected leukemic subtypes
1 Acute promyelocytic leukemia (M3)
— Clinical: DIC-like coagulopathy* (in 90%)
— Film: Auer rods (see below)
— t(15:17) chromosomal translocation‡
2 Acute (myelo)monocytic leukemia (M4, M5)
— Clinical: gingival hyperplasia (± CNS/skin disease)
— Laboratory: lysozymuria (± hypokalemia)
3 B cell (Burkitt's-type) leukemia (L3)
— t(14:18) translocation (i.e. same as Burkitt's lymphoma)
4 T cell leukemia/lymphoma
— Mediastinal mass (poor prognosis)
5 Prolymphocytic leukemia (PLL)
— Massive splenomegaly; *absent* lymphadenopathy
— Marked anemia and leukocytosis
6 Chronic lymphocytic leukemia
— 'Smudge' cells and/or 'basket' cells on film
— Distinguished from well-differentiated lymphocytic lymphoma by degree of peripheral lymphocytosis
— May transform to PLL or diffuse lymphoma
7 Hairy cell leukemia
— Massive splenomegaly (DD$_x$: CML, myelofibrosis)
— Thrombocytopenia (due to hypersplenism)
— Anemia/leukopenia (due to marrow fibrosis/ failure)

* Fibrinolytic bleeding disorder with normal AT III and protein C levels (cf. DIC); *no* evidence for efficacy of heparin
‡ Affects α-retinoic acid receptor locus

Leukemias commoner in men than women
1 T cell leukemia/lymphoma
2 Chronic lymphocytic leukemia
3 Hairy cell leukemia
4 Prolymphocytic leukemia

Laboratory features of leukemias and lymphomas
1 Light microscopy
— Auer rods (in circulating blasts)
• AML (esp. M3)
— Reed–Sternberg cells
• Hodgkin's disease
— Pautrier microabscesses
• Mycosis fungoides
2 Electron microscopy
— Cerebriform nuclei
• Sézary syndrome
3 (Immuno)cytochemistry
— Anti-CALLA
• Good-prognosis ALL subtype
— Anti-CD4 (defines helper T cell phenotype)
• Sézary syndrome, mycosis fungoides
— Anti-CD8 (defines suppressor T cell phenotype)
• T cell CLL (some exceptions)
— Anti-light chains (κ, λ)
• Confirms monoclonality (malignant lineage) of immunocytes in effusions, CSF, marrow
— TdT
• ALL (except rare B cell subtype)
• Lymphoblastic transformation of CML
— Acid phosphatase (tartrate-resistant: TRAP)
• T cell ALL
• Hairy cell leukemia
— PAS
• ALL
— Peroxidase/Sudan black
• AML

LEUKEMIAS: CLASSIFICATION, STAGING AND PROGNOSIS

Acute non-lymphocytic leukemia: the FAB classification
1 M1 — Acute myeloblastic leukemia, undifferentiated
2 M2 — Acute myeloblastic leukemia with maturation
3 M3 — Acute promyelocytic leukemia
4 M4 — Acute myelomonocytic leukemia
5 M5 — Acute monocytic leukemia
6 M6 — Erythroleukemia

Poor prognostic signs in acute lymphoblastic leukemia
1 Adult onset
2 Male sex
— Associated with T cell leukemia and mediastinal mass
— Increased testicular relapse
3 CALLA negative (T cell, B cell, null cell)
4 Presentation with
— Initial WCC > 100 x 10^9/L
— Massive extramedullary disease
— CNS leukemia
5 Philadelphia chromosome-positive*‡

* cf. CML (p. 162): *better* prognosis
‡ cf. AML: poor prognosis indicated by 5q- or 7q- chromosomal deletion

CLL staging: modified Rai criteria
1 Stage 1 — Lymphocytosis + lymphadenopathy
2 Stage 2 — Lymphocytosis + hepato-/splenomegaly
3 Stage 3 — Lymphocytosis + anemia

4 Stage 4 — Lymphocytosis + anemia +
thrombocytopenia

NB: Lymphocytosis (> 15 x 10⁹/L; > 40% in marrow) alone is
sometimes referred to as stage 0

Life expectancy from diagnosis in CLL
1 Stage 1 disease — 12 years
2 Stage 2 disease — 8 years
3 Stage 3 disease — 4 years
4 Stage 4 disease — 2 years
5 Stage 5 disease — 1 year

LYMPHOMAS

Pros and cons of staging laparotomy in Hodgkin's disease
1 Pros
— Absent splenomegaly does not imply absent
splenic disease, nor must splenomegaly imply
splenic involvement; hence, of diagnostic value*
— Morbidity of radiotherapy may be reduced by
excluding splenic irradiation, thus preventing
irradiation of left kidney, left lung base and
cardiac apex
— Oophoropexy enables preservation of fertility in
young women requiring pelvic irradiation
— WBC/platelet counts may improve following
splenectomy, thus improving treatment tolerance
2 Cons
— Invasive, potentially morbid and hazardous
— Increased risk of infection post-splenectomy
(p. 198)
— Popularity of staging laparotomy in stage IA/IIA
patients (esp. those with lymphocyte-
predominant disease; p. 156) has declined, with
close follow-up post-radiotherapy now being
widely accepted

* Since 20% of patients with clinical stage II disease (normal
abdominal CT) actually have abdominal disease (incl. liver,
nodes), staging laparotomy remains the best way to confirm
such disease and hence to determine need for chemotherapy in
some cases

Staging of Hodgkin's disease: simplified Ann Arbor criteria
1 Stage 1 — Involvement of a single site (incl.
extranodal)
2 Stage 2 — Involvement of > 1 lymph node region
on the *same* side of the diaphragm
3 Stage 3 — Node involvement on *both* sides of
diaphragm
4 Stage 4 — Extranodal disease (esp. marrow or (liver)

Clinical staging of Hodgkin's disease: 'A' vs. 'B' criteria
1 'A' — Asymptomatic
2 'B' — Fevers > 38°C
— Sweats
— > 10% weight loss in last 6 months

Non-Hodgkin's lymphomas: Kiel histologic subtypes
1 Indolent
— Follicular (nodular)

• Centrocytic
• Centroblastic
— Diffuse small-cell
• Lymphocytic (WDLL, CLL-like)
• Centrocytic
• Immunocytic (lymphoplasmacytoid)
2 Aggressive
— Diffuse large cell
• Lymphoblastic (T cell or Burkitt-type)
• Centroblastic
• Immunoblastic

Assessing prognosis in lymphoma
1 Hodgkin's disease*
— Prognosis determined by disease *stage*, e.g.
• Stage IA/IIA disease → 90% cure
• Stage IIIB/IV disease → 30% cure
— Other poor prognosticators
• Advanced age
• Elevated ESR (> 30) following definitive R$_x$
2 Non-Hodgkin's lymphoma
— Prognosis mainly determined by *histology*, e.g.
• Indolent histology → median survival 5 years
• Aggressive histology → median survival 1 year‡

* Note that *older* patients with Hodgkin's disease have a
markedly worse prognosis than do young patients with the same
disease stage
‡ Paradoxically, *chemocurability* is greatest in 'aggressive'
histology

HYPERCOAGULABLE STATES

Indications for investigation of hypercoagulability
1 Family history of venous thrombosis
2 Recurrent venous thrombosis or pulmonary
embolism
3 Single episode of venous thrombosis in a young
patient
4 Unusual site of thrombosis
— Retinal vein thrombosis
— Renal vein thrombosis
— Hepatic vein thrombosis
— Arterial thrombosis

Laboratory characterization of suspected hypercoagulability
1 Exclude hyperviscosity
— Hb/PCV (polycythemia), platelets (thrombocytosis)
— Paraproteinemia
— Whole blood viscosity
2 Exclude defective fibrinolysis
— FDPs, hypofibrinogenemia (DIC)
— Schistocytes (TTP, DIC)
— Euglobulin clot lysis time (tPA deficiency/inhibitor)
— Factor XII deficiency
— Abnormal fibrinogen or plasminogen (activator)
3 Exclude primary deficiency of endogenous
anticoagulation
— Antithrombin III*
— Protein C*; protein S*
— Heparin cofactor II
4 Exclude inhibitors of endogenous anticoagulants
— Elevated levels of histidine-rich glycoprotein‡

— Elevated levels of platelet factor 4
— Factor V Leiden mutation¶
5 Exclude acquired inducers of hypercoagulability
— Lupus anticoagulant
— Acid hemolysis test (PNH)
— Fibrin monomers/fibrinopeptide A (malignancy)

* Deficiency *or* resistance states
‡ Binds and inactivates heparin
¶ Confers resistance to activated protein C, esp. in oral contraceptive users

Antithrombin III deficiency: causes
1 Hereditary
2 Estrogens (pregnancy, OCs, Ca prostate)
3 Liver disease
4 Nephrotic syndrome
5 Disseminated thrombosis*
6 Heparin therapy

* Since heparin acts via AT III, massive thrombosis (which depletes AT III levels) may be associated with relative heparin resistance

HEMOSTATIC DISORDERS

Investigation of thrombocytopenia
1 Check automated count by direct vision (exclude clotting)
2 Film
— Schistocytes (DIC, TTP)
— Blasts (acute leukemia)
3 Coagulation screen
— Helps further exclude DIC
4 Marrow aspirate
— Hypoplastic etiology
— Abundant megakaryocytes (ITP, hypersplenism)

Prolonged PT, APTT and thrombocytopenia?
1 Disseminated intravascular coagulation
2 Liver disease with hypersplenism
3 Heparin therapy* (p. 171)

* NB: The APTT is *not* prolonged by subcutaneous low-dose heparin therapy

Platelet function tests: clinical correlations
1 Von Willebrand's disease
— Normal aggregation in vitro
— Defective ristocetin aggregation
— Defective endothelial adhesion
  • Corrected by addition of normal plasma
2 Glanzmann's thrombasthenia
— Defective aggregation in vitro*
— Normal ristocetin aggregation
— Normal endothelial adhesion
3 Bernard–Soulier syndrome (glycoprotein IB deficiency)
— Giant platelets → 'thrombocytopenia'
— Normal aggregation in vitro
— Defective ristocetin aggregation
— Defective endothelial adhesion
  • *Not* corrected by addition of normal plasma
4 Aspirin ingestion
— Defective aggregation in vitro
  • Impaired release reaction to ADP

5 Dysproteinemia
  Myeloproliferative disease
  Uremia, liver disease
— Defective aggregation *and* adhesion

* i.e. to ADP, adrenaline, collagen

Hemophilia A: levels of severity
1 > 50% F VIII$_c$
— Normal hemostasis
2 20–40% F VIII$_c$
— Excess bleeding after major trauma
3 5–20% F VIII$_c$
— Excess bleeding after surgery or minor trauma
4 2–5% F VIII$_c$
— Moderate hemophilia; severe post-traumatic and occasional spontaneous bleeding
5 < 2% F VIII$_c$
— Severe hemophilia; frequent spontaneous bleeds into muscles and joints

Diagnosis of hemophilia
1 Low F VIII$_c$
2 Normal or increased F VIII$_{Ag}$
3 Normal F VIII$_{VWF}$ (cf. VWD: ↓)
4 Normal bleeding time (cf. VWD: ↑)
5 Carrier status? VIII$_c$: VIII$_{Ag}$ < 70%

Bleeding tendency with normal coagulation screen?
1 Vascular disorder
— Hereditary hemorrhagic telangiectasia
— Vasculitis, scurvy
2 Platelet dysfunction
— Aspirin ingestion
— Dysproteinemia (esp. IgA)
— Inherited platelet dysfunction
— Platelet factor III deficiency
3 Mild coagulopathy
— Von Willebrand's
— Mild hemophilia
— Factor XIII deficiency

THE PORPHYRIAS

The acute porphyrias*: what do they have in common?
1 All three are autosomal dominant
2 All three are often precipitated by drugs
3 All three are potentially life-threatening

* Acute intermittent or variegate porphyria; hereditary coproporphyria

Approach to investigation of suspected acute porphyria
1 Urinary PBG absent
— Excludes acute porphyrias
2 Urinary PBG absent
  Fecal screen negative
— Excludes both acute and latent porphyrias
3 Urinary PBG present
  Fecal screen negative
— Acute intermittent porphyria (acute or latent phase)

4 Urinary PBG present
  Fecal screen positive*
  — Variegate porphyria (acute phase)
5 Urinary PBG absent
  Fecal screen positive*
  — Variegate porphyria (latent phase)

NB: Urinary PBG and/or ALA are the hallmarks of porphyria-induced neurologic disease
* *Biliary* porphyrins may be positive in cases where fecal screen is negative

Investigation of suspected porphyria-induced photosensitivity

1 Urinary PBG absent
  Red cell screen negative } Excludes porphyric
  Fecal screen negative   } etiology
2 Urinary PBG present
  Fecal screen positive   } Variegate porphyria
  Biliary screen positive   }
3 Urinary PBG absent   } Porphyria cutanea
  Red cell screen negative } tarda
  Fecal screen positive   } Variegate porphyria
4 Urinary PBG absent   } Erythropoietic
  Red cell screen positive } coproporphyria
  Fecal screen negative   }
5 Urinary PBG absent   } Erythropoietic
  Red cell screen positive } uroporphyria/
  Fecal screen positive   } protoporphyria

'Safe' drugs in patients with porphyria

1 Aspirin, paracetamol, codeine
2 Penicillin; low-dose chloroquine*
3 Chlorpromazine, metoclopramide; sodium valproate
4 Propranolol, labetalol; digoxin
5 Insulin

* NB: *High-dose* chloroquine may precipitate porphyria cutanea tarda, whereas low-dose is therapeutic

Diagnostic significance of elevated RBC protoporphyrin

1 Porphyria
  — Erythropoietic protoporphyria
2 Ineffective erythropoiesis
  — Iron deficiency
  — Lead poisoning
  — Anemia of chronic disease

MANAGING HEMATOLOGIC DISEASE

PRINCIPLES OF BLOOD SUPPORT

The leukopenic patient: principles of management

1 Assume fever represents infection until proven otherwise
2 Take urine and blood cultures if febrile
3 If prolonged leukopenia anticipated*, perform
  — Baseline HSV/CMV/toxoplasma titers
  — Regular swabs of throat/axillae/nose/perineum
  — Removal of IUD
4 Monitor chest and perineum for sepsis

5 Avoid pelvic examinations unless indispensable

* e.g. bone marrow transplant

Granulocyte transfusions

1 Sole potential indication
  — Fever > 48 h in a severely neutropenic patient (< 500 cells/µL) receiving optimal antibiotics, esp. if
    • Positive blood cultures (esp. *Ps. aeruginosa*)
    • Imminent (< 1 week) marrow recovery unlikely
2 Problems
  — Questionable benefit*; expensive
  — Poor leukocyte function (esp. if obtained by filtration)
  — Transfusion reactions
  — Sensitization (alloimmunization)‡
  — Possible transmission of CMV
  — Pulmonary infiltrates (intravascular leukostasis)
  — Graft-versus-host disease if cells not irradiated

* Less important than prompt prescription of broad-spectrum antibiotics
‡ e.g. preventing increments to transfused platelets

Morbidity of massive stored blood transfusions

1 Infection
  — Hepatitis (HCV, HBV, CMV)
  — HIV seroconversion
2 Coagulopathy
  — Low in factors V, VIII and platelets*
3 Citrate toxicity (usually subclinical)
  — Metabolic alkalosis with hypocalcemia
4 Tissue hypoxia (reversible after 24 h)
  — Due to low 2,3-DPG of stored blood
5 Metabolic acidosis and/or K^+ (esp. if renal impairment)
  — Due to low pH of stored blood
6 Fever, fluid overload, hemolysis, DIC

* i.e. assuming packed cells (not whole blood) are used

Clinical utility of autologous blood transfusion

1 Advantages
  — No infective risk
  — No incompatibility risk
2 Indications
  — Elective surgery, esp.
    • Orthopedic surgery
    • Cardiac surgery
  — Pregnancy third trimester
3 Contraindications
  — Insufficient time prior to planned transfusion
  — Anemia, frailty, infection
  — Severe cardiac disease
    • Left main disease and/or unstable angina
    • Tight aortic stenosis

Therapeutic indications for phlebotomy

1 Polycythemia rubra vera
2 Idiopathic hemochromatosis
  Sideroblastosis with iron overload
3 Porphyria cutanea tarda
4 Polycythemia (Hb > 20 g/dL) due to chronic lung disease or cyanotic congenital heart disease; keep hematocrit ~ 65%

Constituents of fresh frozen plasma
1 Coagulation factors
2 Endogenous anticoagulants
3 C$_1$-esterase inhibitor
4 α_1-antitrypsin
5 Fibronectin
6 Immunoglobulins
7 Albumin

Indications for fresh frozen plasma
1 (Anti)coagulation factor deficiency *if* concentrate unavailable
2 Thrombotic thrombocytopenic purpura
3 Bleeding associated with thrombolytic therapy, warfarin overdosage or DIC

CLINICAL USE OF HEMOPOIETIC GROWTH FACTORS

Human recombinant colony-stimulating factors (CSFs)*
1 G-CSF (granulocyte colony-stimulating factor: filgrastim)
   — Increases granulocytes
2 GM-CSF (granulocyte-macrophage CSF: ecogramostim)
   — Increases granulocytes, monocytes, eosinophils
3 M-CSF (monocyte/macrophage CSF)
   — Increases monocytes
4 IL-3 ('multi-CSF')
   — Increases monocytes, granulocytes, eosinophils, basophils, erythrocytes
5 Erythropoietin
   — Increases erythrocytes
6 Thrombopoietin
   — Increases platelets

* cf. lymphoid growth factors (lymphokines, interleukins); p. 198

Potential indications for hemopoietic growth factor therapy
1 G-CSF
   — Kostmann's (inherited) neutropenia
   — Cyclic neutropenia
   — Marrow support in patients receiving conventional cancer chemotherapy, but at high risk of sepsis*
2 G-CSF *or* GM-CSF
   — Recruitment of peripheral blood stem cells (PBSC) for autologous marrow transplantation prior to high-dose cytotoxic therapy
3 Erythropoietin
   — Symptomatic anemia due to
     • Renal failure
     • Myeloma
   — Hypoproliferative anemias
   — Anemia prophylaxis in premature births
   — 'Priming' prior to autologous blood banking
4 Thrombopoietin
   — Thrombocytopenia (remains investigational)

* Survival benefit unproven

Toxicity of hemopoietic growth factor therapy
1 G-CSF
   — Bone pain following IV bolus injection

2 GM-CSF
   — Bone pain, fever, malaise, arthralgias
   — Skin rash at injection site
   — Capillary leak syndrome*: serous effusions/ ascites
   — Large-vessel venous thrombosis*
3 Erythropoietin
   — Thrombotic tendency if hematocrit rises too quickly

* Seen with high-dose treatment; may reflect secondary release of TNF or IL-1

SPLENECTOMY

Splenectomy: common indications in hematologic disease
1 Hereditary spherocytosis
2 Chronic ITP
3 Hairy cell leukemia
4 Occasional indications
   — Hodgkin's disease (staging laparotomy)
   — Idiopathic 'warm' autoimmune hemolytic anemia
   — Massive enlargement: pain, hypersplenism*

* e.g. in myelofibrosis or thalassemia

Management of the splenectomy patient
1 Patient selection
   — *Avoid* splenectomy if possible in children, esp. < 5 yrs (greatest risk of subsequent life-threatening sepsis)
2 Children requiring splenectomy
   — Prophylactic oral penicillin V until adulthood
3 All patients
   — Pneumococcal vaccination, *prior* to splenectomy if possible

HEMOLYTIC ANEMIAS

Management of warm autoimmune hemolytic anemia
1 Exclude drug-induced cause
2 Exclude B cell malignancy (bone marrow, EPG)
3 Treat underlying autoimmune disease if present
4 *Avoid* transfusion if possible
5 Trial of medical therapy
   — Steroids (prednisolone 60 mg/day)
   — Folate 5 mg/day
   — ± Azathioprine
6 Consider splenectomy if
   — Steroids ineffective or unacceptable
   — DAT $\rightarrow$ IgG only (no C$_3$)
   — ^{51}Cr-RBC studies confirm spleen as site of sequestration
7 Other therapies
   — Danazol
   — High-dose intravenous IgG
   — Cyclosporin A

Management of cold autoimmune hemolytic anemia
1 Keep patient warm
2 Exclude *M. pneumoniae*, infectious mononucleosis

3 Exclude B cell malignancy
4 Avoid steroids and splenectomy (they generally don't work)
5 If transfusion absolutely necessary
— Use washed packed cells (less complement)
— Infuse via blood warmer
6 Investigational therapy
— High-dose IV methylprednisolone
— Plasmapheresis/plasma exchange

Clinical significance of oxidant and antioxidant drugs
1 Oxidant drugs
— Precipitate favism (hemolysis in G6PD deficiency)
— Exacerbate methemoglobinemia
— Include*
• Nitrates (incl. nitroprusside)
• Phenacetin, paracetamol
• Sulfonamides, nitrofurantoin, primaquine
2 Antioxidant (reducing) drugs
— Used for treatment of severe methemoglobinemia (e.g. levels > 20%; may cause cerebral ischemia)
— Include
• Ascorbic acid
• Methylene blue (IV in emergencies)*

* NB: Notwithstanding its therapeutic role in methemoglobinemia, methylene blue may also stimulate hemolysis in G6PD deficiency

MANAGING HEMATOLOGIC MALIGNANCIES

Treatment options in acute lymphoblastic leukemia (ALL)
1 Induction/consolidation (95% → complete remission)
— Vincristine/prednisone
— Daunorubicin
— ± L-asparaginase, cytosine arabinoside
2 Maintenance (50% → cure) therapy
— Methotrexate/6-MP* (3 years)
3 Routine CNS prophylaxis‡
— Cranial irradiation
— Intrathecal methotrexate
4 Marrow transplant
— In second remission
— In first remission *if*
• Poor prognosis ALL, *or*
• Availability of HLA-identical donor

* Pharmacokinetics of 6-MP should be checked at beginning of maintenance to confirm adequate bioavailability for individual dosage schedule
‡ NB: Some centers also advocate prophylactic testicular irradiation, while others monitor this potential sanctuary site for relapse

Treatment options in acute myeloblastic leukemia (AML)
1 Induction/consolidation (70% → complete remission)
— Cytosine arabinoside + daunorubicin ± 6TG/VP-16
2 Marrow transplant*
— In first remission (or *early* relapse if age > 30)
3 Promyelocytic leukemia (M3)
— *all*-trans-retinoic acid (ATRA: 'differentiation' therapy)
— Platelets, FFP, tranexamic acid (for coagulopathy)

4 CNS prophylaxis
— Acute monocytic (M4, M5) leukemias only
5 Maintenance therapy, late intensification
— Doubtful value in AML

* Relatively more valuable for AML than ALL

Treatment of chronic lymphocytic leukemia (CLL)
1 Stage I/II disease
— Observe (unless *massive* adenopathy)
2 Stage III/IV disease
— Chlorambucil ± vincristine/prednisone (CVP)
— Second-line
• Fludarabine
• Deoxycoformycin
• 2-chlorodeoxyadenosine
3 Immune hemolysis/thrombocytopenia
— Steroids
— Splenectomy in selected patients
4 Recurrent infections
— Gammaglobulin (IV)

Indications for cytotoxic therapy in CLL
1 Symptomatic lymphadenopathy
2 Refractory constitutional symptoms
3 Non-immune cytopenia

Therapeutic approach to chronic myeloid leukemia (CML)
1 Chronic phase
— Busulfan (intermittent), hydroxyurea (daily)
— Bone marrow transplantation
2 Myeloblastic transformation (75%)
— No effective treatment known
3 Lymphoblastic transformation (25%)
— Vincristine/prednisone

Management modalities in hairy cell leukemia
1 Splenectomy
— For massive splenomegaly *or* hypersplenism
— Improves cytopenia; may improve survival
— Now becoming less popular
2 Deoxycoformycin, *or* 2-chlorodeoxyadenosine
— Impressive remission rates and durations
3 Interferon-α

Managing polycythemia vera
1 Mild disease, young patient (< 50), preoperative
— Phlebotomy
• May be technically difficult due to clotting
• Aim to keep hematocrit in normal range (≤ 0.45)*
2 Older patients (50–65) or associated thrombocytosis
— Hydroxyurea
• Alternatives: busulfan, chlorambucil (may cause leukemia)
3 Elderly or non-compliant patients
— ^{32}P
• Takes 6–12 weeks to work
• Risk of leukemia
4 Non-specific measures
— Allopurinol
— H_2-blockers

NB: *Pruritus* may or may not respond to normalization of hematocrit; if not, antihistamines may help
* cf. secondary polycythemia: do *not* venesect unless PCV > 0.54

Managing the dysproteinemias
1 Myeloma
 — Melphalan (or cyclophosphamide) ± prednisone
 — Doxorubicin/BCNU
 — Interferon-α
 — Apheresis for hyperviscosity
 — Erythropoietin for symptomatic anemia
 — IV immunoglobulin for infection prophylaxis*
 — Prophylactic long bone internal fixation as required
2 Macroglobulinemia
 — Chlorambucil, CVP
 — Plasmapheresis

* esp. for patients with poor IgG responses to pneumococcal vaccination

Management options in cutaneous lymphoma*
1 Topical nitrogen mustard
2 Whole skin electron beam therapy
3 PUVA (or home UVB)
4 Oral steroids
5 Combination cytotoxic therapy
6 Cyclosporin A; interferon-α; retinoids

* None is regularly effective

Management modalities in non-Hodgkin's lymphomas
1 Low-grade (indolent, usually nodular) lymphomas
 — CVP and/or local irradiation
 — Fludarabine
 — Treated with palliative intent
2 High-grade (aggressive, usually diffuse) lymphomas
 — CVP + doxorubicin (CHOP)
 — Treated with curative intent
3 Lymphoblastic lymphoma
 — Treated as for T cell ALL (incl. CNS prophylaxis)
4 Remission after first relapse
 — High-dose chemotherapy with marrow transplant
5 Refractory end-stage disease
 — Total body irradiation (palliative only)

Approach to the management of Hodgkin's disease
1 Pathologic stage IA
 — Local irradiation
2 Pathologic stage IIA (above diaphragm)
 — 'Mantle' irradiation*
3 Pathologic stage IIA (below diaphragm)
 — 'Inverted Y' irradiation‡
4 Pathologic stage III or IV
 Bulky disease (irrespective of stage)
 'B' symptoms (p. 164), irrespective of stage
 'E' (extranodal) disease
 — Combination chemotherapy (e.g. ABVD, MOPP)

* Supradiaphragmatic + upper paraaortic nodes
‡ All paraaortic, iliac and pelvic nodes

Toxicity of therapy for Hodgkin's disease
1 Induced by radiotherapy (e.g. mantle)
 — Hypothyroidism
 — Lhermitte's phenomenon (radiation myelitis)
 — Radiation pneumonitis/pericarditis
 — Reduced hemopoietic reserve
2 Induced by chemotherapy (e.g. MOPP)
 — Sterility (esp. in males)
 — Second malignancies (esp. if prior radiation)

Chemoresistance in Hodgkin's disease
1 Occurs in 25%
2 More common with
 — 'B' symptoms
 — Nodular sclerosing histology (→ frequent relapses)

Tumor lysis syndrome: features and clinical significance
1 Occurs after initial chemotherapy for sensitive tumors*, esp.
 — Burkitt's lymphoma
 — ALL
 — Germ-cell tumors
2 Metabolic effects
 — Hyperuricemia + urate nephropathy
 — Hyperphosphatemia + reciprocal hypocalcemia
 — Hyperkalemia (esp. if azotemic or acidotic)
3 Complications
 — Renal failure (typically irreversible: may be fatal)
 — Arrhythmias, cardiac arrest (due to hyperkalemia)
 — Tetany, weakness, paralytic ileus (hypocalcemia)
 — Severe metabolic acidosis
4 Prevention
 — Pretreatment allopurinol
 — Forced alkaline diuresis
5 Treatment of established syndrome
 — Hemodialysis

* NB: Can also occur following treatment of 'aleukemic' leukemias

BONE MARROW TRANSPLANTATION

Indications for bone marrow transplantation
1 Established indications
 — Aplastic anemia (preferably untransfused)
 — ALL (good prognosis) in second remission
 — ALL (poor prognosis: p. 163)
 — AML in first remission
 — Refractory lymphoma
 — CML in chronic phase
 — Severe combined immunodeficiency (SCID)
2 Occasional indications
 — Neuroblastoma
 — β-thalassemia major
 — Osteopetrosis
 — Hurler's syndrome
 — Chronic granulomatous disease
 — Wiskott–Aldrich syndrome
 — Paroxysmal nocturnal hemoglobinuria (severe)

Prerequisites for marrow transplantation
1 HLA- and MLC-compatible sibling
2 Recipient's age < 40 years (preferably < 20)

Advantages of peripheral stem cells over marrow reinfusion
1 Less traumatic than normal bone marrow harvest
2 Accelerated recovery of transplant hemopoiesis
3 Lower risk of disease relapse in neoplastic disorders

Complications of bone marrow transplantation
1   High-dose cyclophosphamide
   — Cystitis
   — Cardiomyopathy
2   Total body irradiation
   — Pancreatitis
   — Pneumonitis
   — Parotitis
   — Hepatic venoocclusive disease
   — Cataracts
3   Combined toxicity
   — Sterility
   — Second malignancy
4   Other
   — Infection
   — Cardiac tamponade (?due to infection)
   — Graft-versus-host disease
   — Disease relapse; graft failure

Differential diagnosis of CXR infiltrates in marrow transplant patients
1   Pneumonia, esp.
   — CMV
   — Parainfluenza virus
   — Respiratory syncytial virus (RSV)
2   Radiation pneumonitis
3   Graft-versus-host disease

GRAFT-VERSUS-HOST DISEASE (GVHD)

Prerequisites for developing GVHD
1   Graft must contain immunologically competent cells
2   Host must express antigens foreign to the graft
3   Host must be immunologically incapable of destroying the grafted immunocytes

Patients at high risk of GVHD
1   Older transplant recipients
2   Recipients of HLA-mismatched transplants
3   Recipients of grafts from allosensitized donors
4   Recipients of small-intestinal transplants
5   Recipients of unirradiated blood transfusions

Features and management of GVHD
1   Acute GVHD (occurs < 100 days post-transplant)
   — Mediated by cytotoxic T cells; affects ~ 50%
    • Dermatitis (bullous, morbilliform)
    • Hepatitis; abnormal LFTs → liver failure
    • Enterocolitis, diarrhea, nausea
2   Chronic GVHD (occurs > 100 days post-transplant)
   — Affects 30% long-term survivors, esp. if older
    • Dermatitis (scleroderma/lichen planus-like)
    • Conjunctivitis, stomatitis, esophagitis
    • Wasting, recurrent infections (bacterial, zoster)
3   Patients who have survived an episode of GVHD have a significantly lower risk of leukemic relapse
4   Prophylaxis
   — Cyclosporin (agent of choice in aplastic anemia)
   — ± Methotrexate
   — ± Autologous marrow purging with anti-T$_H$ antibodies

5   Established disease
   — Symptomatic treatment
   — Steroids, azathioprine
   — Thalidomide

Diagnostic criteria for hepatic venoocclusive disease*
1   Jaundice before day 30 post-transplant
2   Tender hepatomegaly
3   Ascites and weight gain

* Due to chemoradiotherapy-induced hepatic endothelial damage

THROMBOCYTOPENIA

Points to remember in managing the thrombocytopenic patient
1   Precautions on the ward
   — No aspirin
   — No intramuscular injections
   — No routine blood pressure measurements
2   Precautions at the bedside
   — Inspect skin and oral mucosa daily
   — Examine fundi daily
   — Remove IUD if prolonged cytopenia anticipated
3   Precautions in the laboratory
   — Check coagulation screen (esp. to exclude DIC)

What minimum platelet count mandates platelet transfusion?
1   For asymptomatic patients without bleeding or fever
   — 5×10^9/L
2   For patients with bleeding manifestations or fever
   — 10×10^9/L
3   For patients with coagulopathy, high-risk anatomical lesions or on heparin
   — 20×10^9/L

Predictors of response to splenectomy for ITP
1   Age < 60 years
2   Short history of ITP (i.e. not chronic)
3   Initial promising response to steroids
4   Post-operative platelet count > 500×10^9/L

Failed splenectomy for ITP?
1   Look at the blood film
   — Absent Howell–Jolly bodies suggest accessory spleen
2   Short-term control measures
   — IV gammaglobulin (esp. if recent onset ITP)
   — Vincristine or vinblastine
   — Plasmapheresis
3   Long-term control measures
   — Cyclophosphamide
   — Azathioprine
4   Experimental control measures
   — Colchicine
   — Danazol

Post-transfusion (thrombocytopenic) purpura
1   Occurs in susceptible 2–3% of population lacking Pl^{A1} antigen

2 Prior sensitization required (e.g. transfusion, pregnancy)
3 Usually occurs in older women 2–10 days post-transfusion
4 Widespread purpura and mucosal bleeding (10% mortality)
5 Diagnosis may be confirmed by direct detection of anti-Pl^{A1}
6 Management
— Pl^{A1}-negative transfusions
— High-dose IV IgG
— Steroids, plasmapheresis if necessary

Features of heparin-induced thrombocytopenia (HIT)
1 General
— Reports of overall average ~ 1–4%
— Incidence is not dose-dependent
— Commoner with bovine than porcine heparin
— Occurs rarely with low-dose sc heparin*
2 Type I: early-onset HIT
— Commoner type; occurs within 1 week
— Typically asymptomatic; bleeding *rare*
— Platelet count usually > 100 x 10^9/L
— Due to platelet-aggregating effect of heparin
— Treatment: continue heparin therapy
3 Type II: delayed-onset HIT
— Typically occurs 1–3 weeks after heparin commenced
— Can occur earlier if previous heparin exposures
— May cause
• Severe thrombocytopenia, bleeding
• Paradoxical arterial thromboembolism in 0.5% (due to platelet aggregation), possibly resulting in limb gangrene, stroke or death
— Caused by immune mechanism: heparin-IgG complexes bind platelets, causing
• Reduced survival and thrombocytopenia
• Aggregation and thrombosis
— Diagnosis: clinical picture (most important) *plus*
• Platelet aggregometry studies
• Two-point ^{14}C-serotonin release assay
— Treatment
• Cease heparin
• Commence warfarin ± dextran, *or*
• Switch to the heparinoid ORG 10172, *or*
• Add IV immunoglobulin, *or*
• Substitute hirudin (p. 172), esp, if paradoxical arterial thrombosis has supervened

* Low-dose heparin acts mainly at endothelial surfaces, rather than by direct peripheral anticoagulation
NB: Heparin may *increase* platelet counts in chronic ITP

HEMOPHILIA

Long-term complications of hemophilia A
1 AIDS
2 Chronic hepatitis (esp. non-A non-B)
3 Arthropathy
4 Narcotic addiction
5 F VIII antibodies (inhibitors: seen in 10%)

Replacement factor levels required in hemophilia
1 Minor hemarthrosis
— 10–20%
2 Dental extraction
Major joint/muscle bleed
— 20–50% (may need multiple transfusions)
3 Surgery, major trauma (esp. cranial)
— 50–100%

Management of bleeding in patients with factor VIII$_c$ inhibitors*
1 For *serious* hemorrhage or preoperatively
— Plasmapheresis
— Extracorporeal protein A adsorption of patient plasma
2 If inhibitor levels *low*
— Porcine factor VIII$_c$
— Alternate-day human factor VIII 'desensitization'
3 If inhibitor levels *high*
— Activated prothrombin complex concentrates (APCCs)
— Contain factor IX, II, X (but not VII) + proteins C and S
— These factor IX concentrates may be riskier for virus transmission
4 Other measures
— *Megadose* factor VIII plus APCCs
— Recombinant activated factor VII (factor VIIa)
— IV gammaglobulin + cyclophosphamide

* 25% of all hemophilia A patients (50% of severe cases) develop inhibitors

ANTICOAGULATION

Duration of anticoagulation: the rough guide
1 Prosthetic heart valve, *or*
Arterial emboli + mitral valve disease/atrial fibrillation, *or*
Recurrent thromboses or emboli
— Treat indefinitely
— Aim for INR 3–4
2 Life-threatening pulmonary embolism, *or*
Extensive proximal (ileofemoral) DVT
— Treat for 6–12 months
— Heparinize for 7 days prior to starting warfarin
— Aim for INR 2.5–3.5
3 Uncomplicated pulmonary embolus, *or*
Localized proximal DVT, *or*
Carotid TIA in a female
— Treat for 3–6 months
— Heparinize for 3 days prior to starting warfarin
— Aim for INR 2.5–3
4 Uncomplicated calf DVT
— Treat for 3 months
— Start heparin and warfarin together
— Aim for INR 2–2.5

Mechanisms of antithrombotic drugs
1 Heparin
— Binds to and activates AT III; this complex
• Inhibits thrombin-induced activation of factors V and VIII

- Inactivates factor Xa
- (Thus) prevents fibrin formation from fibrinogen
— Does *not* efficiently inactivate fibrin-bound thrombin (cf. hirudin)
— Is neutralized by other (non-AT III) heparin substrates, e.g. vitronectin, platelet factor IV; elevated plasma levels of these may cause heparin resistance

2 Warfarin
— Prevents activation of vitamin K, thereby inhibiting γ-carboxylation of factors II, VII, IX and X*

3 Streptokinase/urokinase
Tissue plasminogen activator (tPA)
— Activate plasminogen

4 Hirudin
— AT III-independent anticoagulant, formerly from leeches (*Hirudo medicinalis*); now recombinant
— Inactivates fibrin-bound thrombin; hence, more effective than heparin in preventing extension of preformed thrombi

* And also of the anticoagulant proteins C and S; hence, if deficiency of these proteins is suspected as a possible cause of thrombosis (p. 165), assay should be undertaken *prior* to commencing warfarin

Side-effects of heparin therapy
1 Bleeding ± thrombocytopenia (see above)
2 Osteoporosis (*if* full-dose treatment > 6 months)
3 Burning sensation of hands and feet
4 Alopecia

Indications for heparin therapy
1 Prophylaxis of thromboembolism
2 Treatment of established deep venous thrombosis
3 Unstable angina
4 Acute myocardial infarction
— Prevention of mural thrombus and/or reinfarction
5 Following thrombolytic therapy
— Maintenance of vessel patency

Mechanisms of antiplatelet drugs
1 Reduced thromboxane A_2 synthesis
— Aspirin (irreversibly acetylates cyclooxygenase)
— Sulfinpyrazone (reversibly acetylates cyclooxygenase)
2 Increased platelet cAMP
— Prostacyclin (PGI_2): activates adenyl cyclase
— Dipyridamole (inhibits phosphodiesterase)

Mechanisms of warfarin potentiation
1 ↑ Catabolism of coagulation factors
— Fever, thyrotoxicosis, post-operative
↓ Hepatic drug metabolism
— Liver disease, cardiac failure, acute alcoholic binge
↓ Renal excretion
— Renal failure, old age
2 ↑ Bleeding tendency (independent of coagulation)
— Aspirin, indomethacin, phenylbutazone
3 Potentiation of hypoprothrombinemia
— Aspirin; quin(id)ine

— Tetracycline, chloramphenicol
→ ↓ bacterial vitamin K synthesis
4 Drugs inhibiting hepatic metabolism
— Antibiotics (isoniazid, chloramphenicol, metronidazole, sulfonamides)
— Amiodarone; cimetidine; allopurinol; valproate
— Phenylbutazone (inhibits S-enantiomer metabolism)
5 Plasma protein displacement
— Clofibrate

Drugs inducing hepatic metabolism of warfarin
1 Phenytoin, phenobarbitone, carbamazepine
2 Chronic alcohol ingestion; cigarette smoking
3 Rifampicin; griseofulvin

'Safe' drugs in warfarinized patients
1 Analgesics
— Paracetamol
2 Sedatives, anticonvulsants
— Benzodiazepines
3 Antibiotics
— Penicillins, cephalosporins, aminoglycosides

NB: Caution must *always* be exercised when *changing* therapy of patients stabilized on warfarin

UNDERSTANDING HEMATOLOGIC DISEASE

Clinical varieties of B cell neoplasms
1 Dysproteinemias
— Benign monoclonal gammopathy
— Multiple myeloma, solitary plasmacytoma
— Waldenström's macroglobulinemia
— Heavy chain disease (α and γ)
— 'Primary' amyloidosis
2 Leukemias
— ALL (most cases)
— CLL (98% cases)
— Hairy cell leukemia
3 Lymphomas
— Most subtypes, incl. Burkitt's

Clinical varieties of T cell neoplasms
1 Mycosis fungoides
2 Sézary syndrome
3 T cell leukemia/lymphoma
4 Lymphoblastic lymphoma

The myelodysplastic syndromes ('preleukemias')
1 Classification
— Idiopathic refractory sideroblastic anemia (30%)
— Refractory anemia (40%)
— Refractory anemia with excess blasts (30%)
— Chronic myelomonocytic leukemia* (1%)
2 Acute leukemia (usually M4; p. 163) supervenes in 10%
3 Risk of leukemia is not reliably predicted by marrow features
4 Overall prognosis is inversely proportional to
— Transfusion requirement (i.e. ± leukemic transition)
— % Marrow blasts (→ ↑ AML transition, ↑ infection)

5 Low-dose cytosine arabinoside may help 'differentiate' dysplastic marrow precursors

* Consider diagnosis in Philadelphia-chromosome-negative CML

MULTIPLE MYELOMA

Relative incidence of myeloma subtypes
1 IgG — 50%
2 IgA — 30%
3 Light-chain (BJP) only — 10%
4 IgM — 5%
5 IgD — 2%
6 Biclonal — 2%
7 Non-secretory — 1%

Mechanisms of renal failure in myeloma
1 Intratubular precipitation of Bence-Jones protein
2 Prerenal (e.g. dehydration with IVP)
3 Sepsis (e.g. pyelonephritis) ± nephrotoxic antibiotics
4 Amyloid; plasma cell infiltration
5 Hypercalcemia, urate nephropathy
6 Hyperviscosity

Mechanisms of anemia in myeloma
1 Marrow failure (leukoerythroblastic)
2 Marrow failure (iatrogenic)
3 'Chronic disease' (± azotemia)
4 Dilutional
5 Bleeding (reduced platelet number and function)
6 Iatrogenic sideroblastosis (? preleukemic)

Spectrum of bony involvement in myeloma
1 Lytic lesions esp. (→ 60%)
 — Vertebral bodies (cf. carcinoma → pedicles)
 — Skull (usually painless; cf. carcinoma)
 — Mandible (classical)
2 Diffuse osteoporosis (→ 20%)
3 Skeletal survey more sensitive than isotope bone scan
 Osteosclerotic lesions are very rare; when present they may be associated with neuropathy (POEMS syndrome)
4 Serum alkaline phosphatase typically *normal*

Neurologic manifestations of myeloma
1 Spinal cord compression
 — Usually due to vertebral collapse
2 Confusion
 — Hyperviscosity
 — Hypercalcemia
 — Steroid-induced
3 Peripheral neuropathy
 — Amyloid
4 Cranial nerve palsies
 — Base of skull lesions

HEMOLYTIC ANEMIAS

Paroxysmal nocturnal hemoglobinuria: features
1 Pathogenesis

 — A clonal stem-cell defect
 — Red cell subpopulation develops with abnormal affinity and/or sensitivity to complement
 — May terminate in leukemia, aplasia, myelofibrosis
2 Clinical features
 — Episodic 'smoky' urine
 — Abdominal/back pain
 — Thrombotic events (e.g. Budd–Chiari syndrome)
3 Laboratory diagnosis
 — Anemia
  • Usually normochromic, but may be hypochromic
  • Macrocytes may be present
 — Hemoglobinuria, hemosiderinuria
 — Positive Ham's (acid hemolysis) test*
 — ↓ NAP; ↓ red cell acetylcholinesterase
 — Bone marrow hypoplastic in 25%
4 Management principles
 — Transfusion of washed packed red cells
 — Avoidance of whole blood or iron supplements
 — ± Androgens, folate, warfarin

* Sucrose lysis/sugar-water tests now outmoded

Causes of intravascular hemolysis
1 Paroxysmal nocturnal hemoglobinuria
 Paroxysmal cold hemoglobinuria (IgG-mediated)
 Cold hemagglutinin disease (IgM-mediated)
2 Intracardiac prostheses
 — Aortic valve replacements
 — Patch repair of ostium primum ASD
3 Incompatible blood transfusion
 Burns, snake venom, 'march' hemoglobinuria

Causes of microangiopathic hemolytic anemia
1 Thrombotic thrombocytopenic purpura (TTP)*
 Hemolytic uremic syndrome (HUS)*
2 Malignant hypertension
 Pregnancy-associated hypertension
3 Mucinous adenocarcinoma
4 Vasculitis
5 Transplant rejection

* Designates clinical syndrome which tends to be diagnosed TTP by hematologists and HUS by nephrologists; but read on

Identifiable precipitants of hemolytic uremic syndrome
1 Diarrheal infections
 — *E. coli* O157: H7 diarrhea
  • Produces *Shigella*-like toxins
  • Mainly affects children under 5
 — *Sh. dysenteriae* serotype I
  • Renal failure more likely if treated with ampicillin
2 Drugs
 — Mitomycin C
 — Cyclosporin
 — Ticlopidine, quinine
3 Other
 — SLE, scleroderma
 — Pregnancy
 — Transplantation

Thrombotic thrombocytopenic purpura
1 Diagnostic pentad
 — Thrombocytopenic purpura

— Microangiopathic hemolytic anemia
— Bizarre neurologic signs
— Fever
— Renal failure
2 Investigations
— Blood film: schistocytes, no spherocytes
— Coombs-negative
— PI, PTTK, FDPs, fibrinogen usually normal
— ANA negative in 80%
3 Management
— Plasma exchange ± FFP/antiplatelet therapy/ steroids
— Splenectomy

Features favoring TTP over hemolytic uremic syndrome
1 Usually affects adult *women* (may be autoimmune)
2 Usually *relapsing* clinical course
3 *Neurologic* involvement is more characteristic
4 Benefits from steroids or antiplatelet therapy

Differential diagnosis of HUS/TTP
1 Exotic infectious disease
— Malaria (± DIC)
— Viral hemorrhagic fever (e.g. dengue)
— Leptospirosis
2 Septicemia with DIC
— Gram-negative sepsis
— Pneumococcus, meningococcus
— *Staph. aureus*
— *M. pneumoniae*

Disseminated intravascular coagulation
1 Major causes
— Sepsis (Gram-negative septicemia, *P. falciparum*)
— Malignancy (e.g. disseminated prostate cancer)
— Obstetric disaster
2 Diagnosis
— Film: RBC fragments, thrombocytopenia
— ↑ PI, PTTK, TT
— ↑ FDPs (→ ↓ thrombin, ↓ platelet function)
— ↓ Fibrinogen, factors V and VIII, AT III
— + Ethanol gelation/soluble fibrin monomer complexes
3 Management
— Treat underlying condition
— Prevention (e.g. heparin prophylaxis in M3 AML)
— Symptomatic bleeding
• Platelets
• Transfusion
• Fresh frozen plasma
• Heparin (controversial): monitor AT III levels

HEMOGLOBINOPATHIES

Thalassemias: basic concepts
1 Thalassemias are a heterogeneous group of disorders due to abnormal production of globin chains
2 Anemia in (say) β-thalassemia results from
— Ineffective erythropoiesis (insufficient β-chains)
— Hemolysis (precipitation of relative α-chain excess)

3 Predominant genetic basis
— α-thalassemias
• Usually due to gene deletions (chromosome 16)
• Become symptomatic when α-globin production drops below ~ 25% normal
— β-thalassemias
• Usually due to complex (non-deletional) lesions on chromosome 11* (e.g. causing abnormal β-globin mRNA splicing/translation)
4 Incidence
— About 100,000 homozygotes worldwide
— Most of these are β-thalassemics

* In addition to β-globin, most of the other non-α-globin genes (γ — Hb F; δ, ε) are in this chromosome 11 cluster

Clinical categorization of thalassemias
1 Thalassemia trait
— Asymptomatic condition; may be detected on screening
2 Thalassemia minor
— Mild anemia with minimal symptoms
3 Thalassemia intermedia
— Moderate anemia and splenomegaly
— e.g. Hb C, Hb Lepore; Hb E plus β-thal trait
4 Thalassemia major
— Severe transfusion-dependent anemia

Features of α-thalassemia
1 αα/α-
— Asymptomatic carrier (α-thalassemia-2 trait)
— Occurs in 15–20% blacks
— Low normal MCV/MCHC, but rarely anemic
— Hb A_2, Hb F levels normal (cf. β-thal trait)
— 1–2% Hb Bart's (γ_4) in cord blood
2 α-/α-
— Homozygous α-thalassemia-2 trait
— Usually asymptomatic
— 5–10% Hb Bart's; normal Hb A_2; ± ↓ MCV
3 αα/– –
— Heterozygous α-thalassemia (α-thalassemia-1 trait)
— Low MCV, mild anemia; normal Hb A_2
— Blood film
• Target cells
• Some Hb H (β_4) inclusion bodies (Hb H < 1%)
4 α-/– –
— Hb H disease; offspring of α-thal-2 and α-thal-1 traits
— Moderate/severe anemia (similar to β-thal intermedia)
— Typical Hb H cells visible on cresyl violet stain
— Presentations in adult life: gallstones, splenomegaly
— 10–30% Hb H ± ↓ Hb A_2
— May improve with splenectomy
5 α° (– –/– –)
— Hydrops fetalis (→ stillbirth, perinatal death)
— 80% Hb Bart's, 20% Hb Portland (i.e. absent Hb A_2)

Features of β-thalassemia
1 β-thalassemia minor
— ↓ MCV (< 75 fL) but hematocrit > 30%*
— Basophilic stippling; targets, few teardrops

— ↓ Osmotic fragility (cf. spherocytosis, p. 160)
— ↑ Hb A$_2$ ± ↑ Hb F
— Definitive diagnosis by Hb EPG
2 Suspected thalassemia minor with normal Hb A$_2$
— α-thalassemia
— δβ-thalassemia (heterozygous; suspect if ↑ Hb F)
3 β-thalassemia major
— ↑ Hb F (>70%) ± ↑ Hb A$_2$ (cf. β-thal minor)
— β^0-thalassemia: no detectable Hb A
— β$^+$-thalassemia: up to 30% Hb A
— Blood film: teardrops, targets, nucleated red cells

* i.e. microcytosis excessive for degree of anemia, e.g. compared with iron deficiency anemia

Approach to the patient with thalassemia
1 Thalassemia trait
— Test partner (spouse-to-be) for trait; refer for genetic counselling if positive
— Educate patient against accepting oral iron on basis of ↓ MCV interpreted by doctors unaware of diagnosis
— Prescribe prophylactic folate and/or iron supplements during marrow stress, e.g. menorrhagia, pregnancy
2 Thalassemia intermedia
— Similar phenotype to thal major, but no need for chronic hypertransfusion
— Transfusion requirement may increase in infection, puberty; may benefit from splenectomy
3 Thalassemia major
— Hypertransfuse to maintain Hb > 10 g/dL
— Folate supplements; hepatitis B vaccination
— Splenectomy for hypersplenism or discomfort; pre-splenectomy pneumococcal vaccination
— Iron chelation regimen at earliest possible age*
— Genetic counselling, amniocentesis
— Hydroxyurea to increase Hb F (investigational)
— Monitor for siderosis-induced endocrine deficiency
— Bone marrow transplantation work-up

* Subcutaneous desferrioxamine *or* oral deferiprone/L1; organ damage otherwise begins after first 50–100 units (10–20 g Fe) transfused

---

SICKLE-CELL ANEMIA

Clinical spectrum of sickle-cell disease
1 Hb AS (sickle trait)
— 60% Hb A, 35% Hb S
— Normal life expectancy
— Hyposthenuria, nocturia, papillary necrosis
— Painless (micro)hematuria
— Bacteriuria in pregnancy; zinc wasting
— Hypoxia (e.g. unpressurized aircraft at high altitude) may precipitate splenic/retinal infarction

2 Hb SS (sickle-cell disease)*
— No Hb A; 85% Hb S, 10% Hb F
— Dactylitis, leg ulcers, cerebrovascular disease, gout, priapism (→ impotence), retinopathy
— Autosplenectomy usually supervenes before age 3
3 Hb SC (sickle-C disease)
— Sickle and target cells on film
— Thrombotic tendency
• Proliferative retinopathy
• Aseptic necrosis of femoral head or shoulder
• Hematuria
• Complications during pregnancy
4 Hb S + α-thal
— *Less* severe than Hb SS

* manifestations due to fibrous polymerization of Hb S ($\alpha_2\beta_2^{6Val \to Glu}$) on deoxygenation

Hepatic manifestations of sickle-cell anemia
1 Complications related to transfusion
— Hemochromatosis
— (Chronic) hepatitis B/C
2 Complications related to chronic hemolysis
— Gallstones
3 Complications related to repeated vascular occlusion
— Hepatic fibrosis or infarction
— Liver failure

Varieties of sickle-cell crises
1 Hemolytic crises
— May signify sepsis or associated G6PD deficiency
— Uncommon; transfusion not routinely indicated
2 Aplastic crises
— May signify parvovirus infection or folate deficiency
— Low reticulocyte count (cf. hemolytic crisis)
3 Thrombotic (vasoocclusive, painful) crises
— Commonest; may affect abdomen, lung, brain
— Infarcts precipitated by tissue hypoxia
— May be accompanied by fever, fits, dyspnea
— a HBD may be elevated
— Complications include
• Autosplenectomy (hyposplenism)
• Aseptic necrosis of bone
• Permanent brain damage
• Renal failure
4 Sequestration crises
— Most serious, esp. in infants (due to hypovolemia)
— Presents with rapid-onset hepato/splenomegaly
5 Therapy
— Hydroxyurea (→ ↑ Hb F levels*)

NB: Generally adequate to maintain Hb levels at 7–10 g/dL (since Hb S has a relatively low oxygen affinity)
* cf. Erythropoietin: therapeutically useless in this context

5.1 Gordon LI et al (1992) Comparison of a second generation combination chemotherapeutic regimen (m-BACOD) with a standard regimen (CHOP) for advanced diffuse non-Hodgkin's lymphoms. N Engl J Med 327: 1342–1349

Fisher RI et al (1993) Comparison of a standard regimen (CHOP) with three intensive chemotherapy regimens for advanced non-Hodgkin's lymphoma. N Engl J Med 328: 1002–1006

Two randomized ECOG and SWOG studies showing that CHOP still reigns supreme in the treatment of lymphoma.

5.2 Goldberg MA et al (1990) Treatment of sickle cell anemia with hydroxyurea and erythropoietin. N Engl J Med 323: 366–372

Small study indicating an increase in Hb F ('anti-sickling' Hb) and reduced hemolysis in sickle-cell patients receiving the antimetabolite hydroxyurea. Erythropoietin, on the other hand, yielded no benefit.

5.3 Lucarelli G et al (1993) Marrow transplantation in patients with thalassemia responsive to iron chelation therapy. N Engl J Med 329: 840–844

Brittenham GM et al (1994) Efficacy of deferoxamine in preventing complications of iron overload in patients with thalassemia major. N Engl J Med 331: 567–573

Two studies – the former retrospective and the latter prospective – assessing the efficacy of β-thalassemia intervention. Early adequate iron chelation is effective in preventing organ failure, but marrow transplantation also appears most useful in treating 'good-prognosis' patients with HLA-identical donors.

5.4 Lahtinen R et al (1992) Randomised, placebo-controlled multicentre trial of clodronate in multiple myeloma. Lancet 340: 1049–1052

Study of 350 patients in which biphosphonate-treated myeloma patients suffered less bone pain and less osteolytic progression.

5.5 Chapel HM et al (1994) Randomised trial of intravenous immunoglobulin as prophylaxis against infection in plateau-phase multiple myeloma. Lancet 343: 1059–1063

Study of 82 myeloma patients in which immunoglobulin-treated patients sustained no episodes of pneumonia or septicemia, whereas a matched placebo group incurred 10 such episodes. Benefit was maximal in patients with poor IgG response to Pneumovax inoculation.

5.6 Powles RL et al (1990) Bone-marrow transplant from father to son and subsequent graft from son to father. Lancet 335: 999–1000

One of those interesting little BMT anecdotes, this one about a dad who cured his son by donating marrow, but was subsequently cured himself by retrieving his original donation.

5.7 Swerdlow AJ et al (1992) Risk of second primary cancers after Hodgkin's disease by type of treatment: analysis of 2846 patients in the BNLI. BMJ 304: 1137–1143

Large analysis showing a 3-fold increased risk of cancer, esp. NHL (16-fold), leukemia (16-fold), bone sarcomas (15-fold), thyroid (9-fold), lung and colon (3-fold).

5.8 Vandenbroucke JP et al (1994) Increased risk of venous thrombosis in oral-contraceptive users who are carriers of factor V Leiden mutation. Lancet 344: 1453–1457

Case-control study of 155 thrombosis patients, showing a 4-fold increased apparent risk in OC takers and a further (multiplicative) 8-fold risk in patients with resistance to protein C-dependent fibrinolysis due to factor V Leiden mutation.

5.9 Gmür J et al (1991) Safety of stringent prophylactic platelet transfusion policy for patients with acute leukemia. Lancet 338: 1223–1226

Swiss study suggesting that platelet transfusions may not be necessarily indicated in leukemics with counts of 20,000 or more in the absence of bleeding signs. Indeed, for well patients, the 'danger level' may be more like 5000.

5.10 Ehrenforth S et al (1992) Incidence of development of factor VIII and factor IX inhibitors in haemophiliacs. Lancet 339: 594–598

Study of 80 hemophiliac children revealing 25% overall incidence of inhibitors (50% in severe cases) – a cumulative risk of 33% by age 6, much higher than previously believed.

Etchason J et al (1995) The cost-effectiveness of preoperative autologous blood donations. N Engl J Med 332: 719–724

Decision-analysis exercise suggesting that the low rates of transfusion infectivity now seen make autologous transfusion likely to be cost-ineffective.

CHAPTER 6

Immunology

Physical examination protocol 6.1   You are asked to examine a patient suspected of having a collagen-vascular disease

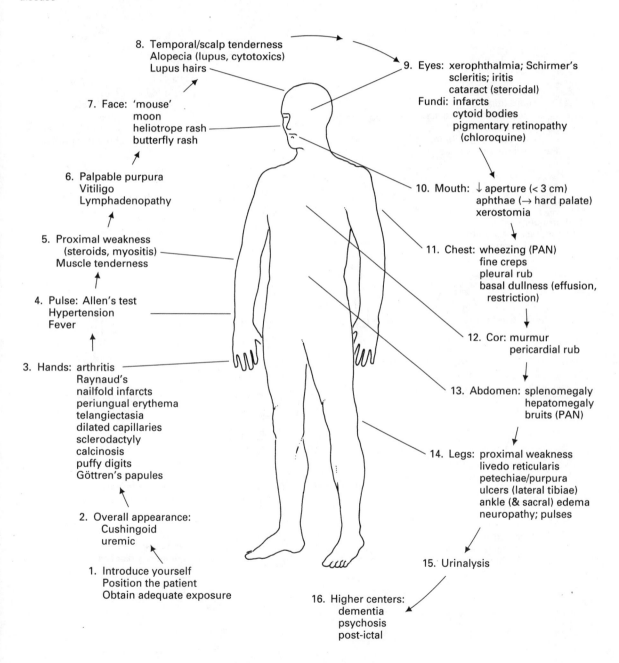

8. Temporal/scalp tenderness
   Alopecia (lupus, cytotoxics)
   Lupus hairs

7. Face: 'mouse'
   moon
   heliotrope rash
   butterfly rash

6. Palpable purpura
   Vitiligo
   Lymphadenopathy

5. Proximal weakness
   (steroids, myositis)
   Muscle tenderness

4. Pulse: Allen's test
   Hypertension
   Fever

3. Hands: arthritis
   Raynaud's
   nailfold infarcts
   periungual erythema
   telangiectasia
   dilated capillaries
   sclerodactyly
   calcinosis
   puffy digits
   Göttren's papules

2. Overall appearance:
   Cushingoid
   uremic

1. Introduce yourself
   Position the patient
   Obtain adequate exposure

9. Eyes: xerophthalmia; Schirmer's
   scleritis; iritis
   cataract (steroidal)
   Fundi: infarcts
   cytoid bodies
   pigmentary retinopathy
   (chloroquine)

10. Mouth: ↓ aperture (< 3 cm)
    aphthae (→ hard palate)
    xerostomia

11. Chest: wheezing (PAN)
    fine creps
    pleural rub
    basal dullness (effusion,
    restriction)

12. Cor: murmur
    pericardial rub

13. Abdomen: splenomegaly
    hepatomegaly
    bruits (PAN)

14. Legs: proximal weakness
    livedo reticularis
    petechiae/purpura
    ulcers (lateral tibiae)
    ankle (& sacral) edema
    neuropathy; pulses

15. Urinalysis

16. Higher centers:
    dementia
    psychosis
    post-ictal

Physical examination protocol 6.2 You are asked to examine a patient suspected of having Sjögren's syndrome

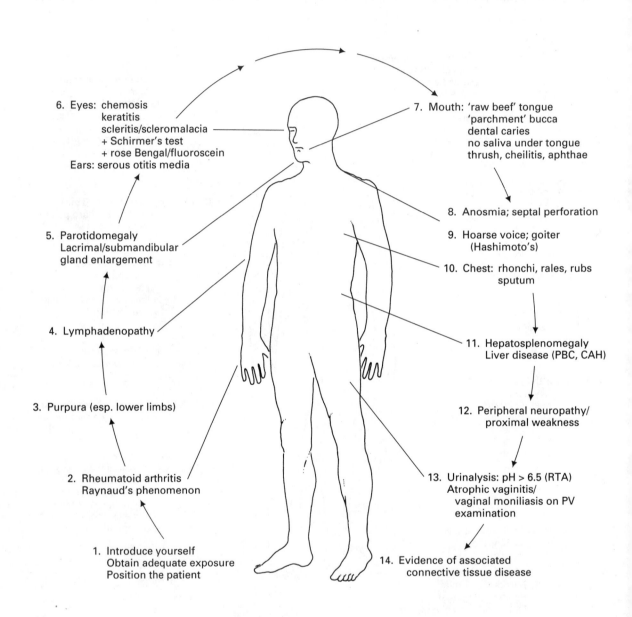

6. Eyes: chemosis
   keratitis
   scleritis/scleromalacia
   + Schirmer's test
   + rose Bengal/fluoroscein
   Ears: serous otitis media

5. Parotidomegaly
   Lacrimal/submandibular
   gland enlargement

4. Lymphadenopathy

3. Purpura (esp. lower limbs)

2. Rheumatoid arthritis
   Raynaud's phenomenon

1. Introduce yourself
   Obtain adequate exposure
   Position the patient

7. Mouth: 'raw beef' tongue
   'parchment' bucca
   dental caries
   no saliva under tongue
   thrush, cheilitis, aphthae

8. Anosmia; septal perforation

9. Hoarse voice; goiter
   (Hashimoto's)

10. Chest: rhonchi, rales, rubs
    sputum

11. Hepatosplenomegaly
    Liver disease (PBC, CAH)

12. Peripheral neuropathy/
    proximal weakness

13. Urinalysis: pH > 6.5 (RTA)
    Atrophic vaginitis/
    vaginal moniliasis on PV
    examination

14. Evidence of associated
    connective tissue disease

Physical examination protocol 6.3   You are asked to examine a patient with Raynaud's phenomenon and esophageal reflux

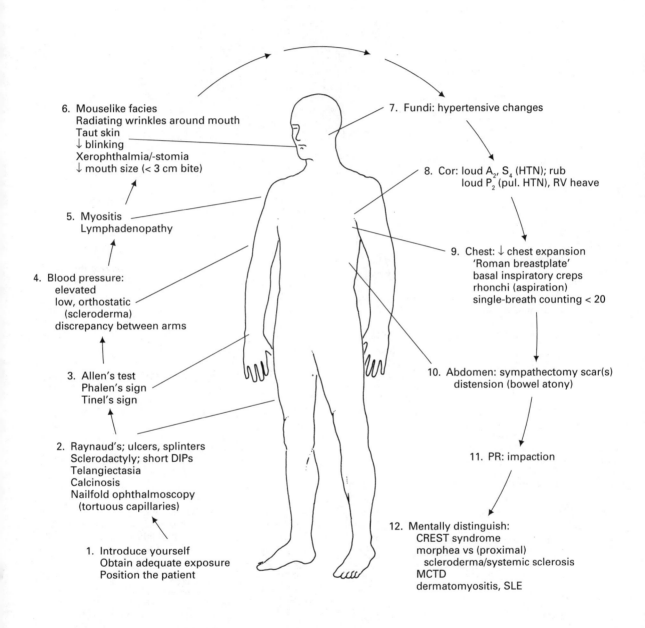

6. Mouselike facies
   Radiating wrinkles around mouth
   Taut skin
   ↓ blinking
   Xerophthalmia/-stomia
   ↓ mouth size (< 3 cm bite)

7. Fundi: hypertensive changes

8. Cor: loud A_2, S_4 (HTN); rub
   loud P_2 (pul. HTN), RV heave

5. Myositis
   Lymphadenopathy

9. Chest: ↓ chest expansion
   'Roman breastplate'
   basal inspiratory creps
   rhonchi (aspiration)
   single-breath counting < 20

4. Blood pressure:
   elevated
   low, orthostatic
     (scleroderma)
   discrepancy between arms

3. Allen's test
   Phalen's sign
   Tinel's sign

10. Abdomen: sympathectomy scar(s)
    distension (bowel atony)

2. Raynaud's; ulcers, splinters
   Sclerodactyly; short DIPs
   Telangiectasia
   Calcinosis
   Nailfold ophthalmoscopy
     (tortuous capillaries)

11. PR: impaction

1. Introduce yourself
   Obtain adequate exposure
   Position the patient

12. Mentally distinguish:
    CREST syndrome
    morphea vs (proximal)
      scleroderma/systemic sclerosis
    MCTD
    dermatomyositis, SLE

Physical examination protocol 6.4   You are asked to examine a patient for stigmata of amyloidosis

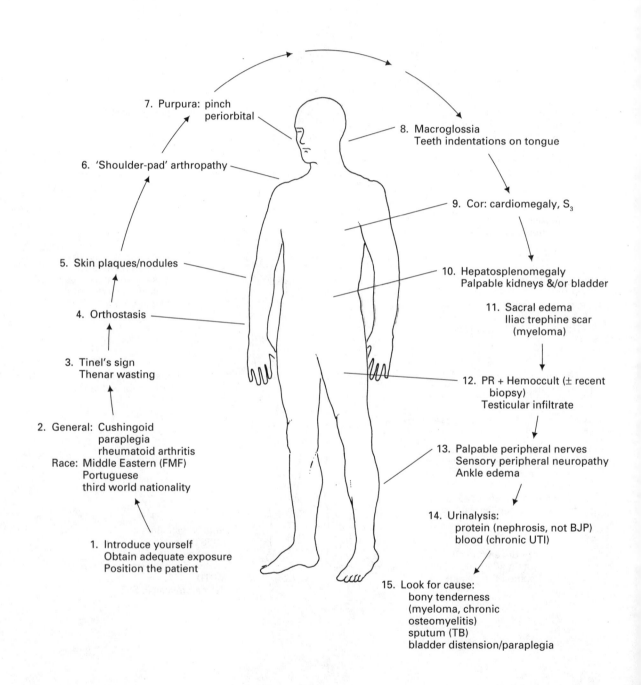

7. Purpura: pinch
   periorbital

6. 'Shoulder-pad' arthropathy

5. Skin plaques/nodules

4. Orthostasis

3. Tinel's sign
   Thenar wasting

2. General: Cushingoid
   paraplegia
   rheumatoid arthritis
   Race: Middle Eastern (FMF)
   Portuguese
   third world nationality

1. Introduce yourself
   Obtain adequate exposure
   Position the patient

8. Macroglossia
   Teeth indentations on tongue

9. Cor: cardiomegaly, S_3

10. Hepatosplenomegaly
    Palpable kidneys &/or bladder

11. Sacral edema
    Iliac trephine scar
    (myeloma)

12. PR + Hemoccult (± recent
    biopsy)
    Testicular infiltrate

13. Palpable peripheral nerves
    Sensory peripheral neuropathy
    Ankle edema

14. Urinalysis:
    protein (nephrosis, not BJP)
    blood (chronic UTI)

15. Look for cause:
    bony tenderness
    (myeloma, chronic
    osteomyelitis)
    sputum (TB)
    bladder distension/paraplegia

CLINICAL ASPECTS OF IMMUNOLOGIC DISEASE

Commonest immunologic short cases
1 Raynaud's (± SLE, MCTD, CREST, etc.)
2 Fibrosing alveolitis

Clinical classification of hypersensitivity reactions
1 Type I (immediate)
   — IgE-mediated → *eosinophil chemotaxis*, e.g.
   • Atopic asthma
   • Hay fever
2 Type II (membrane-bound antigen)
   — IgM/IgG-mediated → cell lysis (*cytotoxicity*) due to granulocyte/complement activation, e.g.
   • Transfusion reactions
   • AIHA, ITP, methyldopa hemolysis
   • Anti-GBM disease (Goodpasture's syndrome)
   — IgM/IgG-mediated → *receptor blocking* , e.g.
   • Pernicious anemia
   • Myasthenia gravis
   • Hashimoto's disease
   — IgM/IgG-mediated → *receptor activation*, e.g.
   • Graves' disease
3 Type III (circulating immune complexes)
   — IgA/IgG-mediated → *Arthus reaction* (antibody excess)
   • Hypersensitivity pneumonitis
   • Allergic bronchopulmonary aspergillosis
   — IgA/IgG-mediated → *serum sickness* (antigen excess)
   • Rheumatic fever
   • Post-infectious glomerulonephritis
   • Secondary syphilis
   • Lepromatous leprosy
   • Henoch–Schönlein purpura
4 Type IV (delayed)
   — T cell-mediated → *mononuclear chemotaxis*
   • Graft rejection, graft-versus-host disease
   • Contact dermatitis
   • Tuberculin reaction; TB gumma/caseation
   • Tuberculoid leprosy

VASCULITIS

Clinical stigmata of vasculitis
1 Leukocytoclastic vasculitis
   — Palpable purpura
2 Non-inflammatory obliterative endarteritis
   — Nailfold infarcts
   — Splinter hemorrhages
3 Necrotizing vasculitis
   — Purpura with skin ulceration
   — Mononeuritis multiplex
   — Motor neuropathy
   — Aneurysmal dilatations overlying arterial bifurcations
4 Cutaneous signs *sometimes* indicating vasculitis
   — Livedo reticularis
   — Atrophie blanche
   — Hemorrhagic bullae/vesicles/ulcers
   — Panniculitis; pustulonecrotic nodules
   — Scarring alopecia
   — Urticarial lesions > 24 h duration
5 Non-cutaneous signs *sometimes* indicating vasculitis
   — Hypertension
   — Microscopic hematuria
   — Retinal vasculopathy, cytoid bodies

Vasculitides with characteristic anatomic distributions
1 Cranial arteritis
   — Temporal, external carotid, other extracranial arteries
2 Takayasu's arteritis
   — Aortic arch
3 Behçet's syndrome
   — Ocular vessels, skin and mucosa, CNS
4 Degos disease
   — Gastrointestinal tract
5 Sneddon's syndrome
   — Skin, CNS

COLLAGEN-VASCULAR DISEASES

Differential diagnosis of purpura in collagen-vascular diseases
1 Vasculitis (see above)
2 Corticosteroid therapy
3 Thrombocytopenia
   — Immune (SLE) ± hypersplenism (Felty's)
   — Iatrogenic (penicillamine, gold)
   Platelet dysfunction
   — Iatrogenic (aspirin, other NSAIDs)
4 Amyloidosis
5 Cryoglobulinemia
6 Factor VIII antibodies (SLE, RA)

Raynaud's phenomenon: features suggesting secondary cause*
1 Symptoms
   — Abrupt onset
   — Digital edema, ulceration, gangrene
   — Thumb involvement
   — Dry eyes/mouth, dysphagia, breathlessness
   — Joint pain or swelling
2 Signs
   — Abnormal Allen's test
   — Telangiectasia
   — Puffy finger thickening
   — Tight skin around mouth
3 Nailfold capillaroscopy
   — *Avascular areas* with tortuous capillaries‡
4 Serology
   — Strongly positive autoantibody profile (esp. ANA)
   — Autoantibodies: topo I, dsDNA, centromere, nucleolar
   — Cryoglobulins; EPG and immunoglobulins
   — Hypocomplementemia (incl. C_7 deficiency)
   — Grossly elevated ESR ± elevated whole blood viscosity

5 Radiology
 — Digital artery occlusion on Doppler study/ arteriogram
 — Subcutaneous calcinosis on plain X-ray
 — Abnormal barium swallow

* Systemic diseases are responsible for ~ 20% of Raynaud's phenomenon; most cases are primary
‡ Highly specific for scleroderma or dermatomyositis

SCLERODERMA

Criteria for scleroderma diagnosis
1 Major criterion
 — Bilateral skin thickening proximal to MCP joints and associated with Raynaud's phenomenon
2 Supporting clinical findings
 — Sclerodactyly, pitted fingertip scars, finger pulp loss
 — Bibasilar pulmonary fibrosis
3 Supporting investigations
 — Nailfold capillaroscopy: enlarged and distorted capillary loops, reduced in number, plus hemorrhages
 — Positive ANA, esp. if nucleolar or centromeric pattern
 — Abnormal esophageal motility on barium swallow

Differential diagnosis of scleroderma
1 'Overlap' syndrome
 — Mixed connective tissue disease
 — CREST syndrome (strictly, a subtype of scleroderma)
 — Dermatomyositis, SLE
2 Eosinophilic fasciitis
 — Spares hands and feet (no Raynaud's)
 — No visceral complications
3 Morphea
 — Localized sclerodermatous plaques
 — No systemic features
4 Other sclerosing diseases
 — Carcinoid syndrome
 — Graft-versus-host disease
 — Amyloidosis
5 Sclerosant exposure, e.g.
 — Bleomycin
 — Silica; vinyl chloride monomer

Spectrum of pulmonary disease in scleroderma
1 Interstitial fibrosis ± (secondary) pulmonary hypertension
2 Primary pulmonary hypertension, esp. in CREST variant
3 Pleurisy
4 Aspiration pneumonitis
5 Restriction of chest wall expansion
6 Bronchioloalveolar cell carcinoma

Mechanisms of cardiac failure in scleroderma
1 Left ventricular failure
 — Severe hypertension
 — Myocardial fibrosis (scleroderma cardiomyopathy)

 — Reperfusion necrosis (?due to myocardial Raynaud's)
2 Right ventricular failure
 — Pulmonary hypertension (primary or secondary)
3 Pericarditis
 — Tamponade (acute)
 — Constriction (chronic)
4 Arrhythmias

Differential diagnosis of anemia in scleroderma
1 Normocytic
 — 'Chronic disease' ± uremia
2 Microcytic
 — Esophagitis, telangiectasia
3 Macrocytic
 — Bacterial overgrowth
4 Microangiopathic
 — Renal involvement with severe hypertension

Gastrointestinal presentations of scleroderma
1 Reflux esophagitis
 — Regurgitation
 — Epigastric pain; dysphagia
2 Post-prandial 'bloating'
 — Gastric dilatation, delayed emptying
 — Malabsorption
3 Steatorrhea
 — Bacterial overgrowth (due to gut hypomotility)
 — Lymphatic fibrosis
4 Anemia
 — Severe esophagitis ± peptic ulceration telangiectasia
 — Bacterial overgrowth
5 Constipation
 — Chronic intestinal pseudoobstruction
 — Fecal impaction; barium impaction

Esophageal abnormalities in the scleroderma patient
1 Distal hypoperistalsis (in 70%)
2 Reflux (in 60%)
3 Esophageal dilatation (in 50%)
4 Absent lower esophageal sphincter tone (in 40%)
5 Positive Bernstein (acid perfusion) test (in 30%)
6 Hiatus hernia (in 20%)
7 Stricture (in 10%)

Radiology of the lower gastrointestinal tract in scleroderma
1 Plain abdominal film
 — Fluid levels, dilated loops of bowel
 — Pneumoperitoneum*
2 Small bowel series
 — Flocculated barium ('moulage' sign)
 — Close-packed valvulae coniventes‡
 — Dilatation of second and third parts of duodenum
3 Barium enema
 — Megacolon; pneumatosis intestinalis
 — Wide-mouthed diverticula on antimesenteric border
 — Reduced motility, slow transit time

* = Pneumatosis intestinalis with cyst rupture
‡ 'Hidebound' or 'accordion' appearance

SYSTEMIC LUPUS ERYTHEMATOSUS

Clinical associations of SLE
1 IgA deficiency
2 C_2 deficiency (and other complement components)
3 α_1AT deficiency
4 Thymoma
5 Porphyria cutanea tarda
6 Klinefelter's syndrome

Adverse prognostic indicators in SLE
1 Associations of more aggressive disease
— Male sex; youth (esp. children)
— High-titer dsDNA Ab; ↓↓ complement (esp. C_3)*
— Sm Ab (predicts development of renal disease)
— IgG 'lupus band' on (uninvolved) skin biopsy‡
— Cryoglobulinemia; phospholipid antibody (p. 191)
2 Clinical evidence of established disease
— Renal involvement
• Heavy proteinuria
• Proliferative/membranous nephritis on biopsy
3 Development of infectious complications
— Gram-positive cocci, *Neisseria, Salmonella*, due to
• Autoimmune leukopenia/leukocyte dysfunction
• Hypocomplementemia, hyposplenism
— Opportunistic infections, due to:
• Steroid/immunosuppressive therapy

* Note that primary deficiencies of C_4 or other complement components (e.g. C_2) may cause a degree of hypocomplementemia unrelated to prognosis
‡ cf. IgM/A

Indicators of active disease in SLE
1 Clinical indicators
— Acute arthritis or vasculitis
— Worsening rash, mucosal ulceration, hair loss
— Pleurisy or pericarditis
— Hematuria, active urinary sediment (esp. red cell casts)
— Systolic hypertension
— Fits, psychosis, 'lupus headache'
2 Laboratory indicators
— Recent rise in dsDNA antibody titer
— ↓ C_3, ↓ THC (if recent)
— Leukopenia, lymphopenia, anemia, reticulocytosis, thrombocytopenia

Indications for renal biopsy in SLE
1 Exclusion of reversible renal failure in atypical disease
2 Confirmation of irreversible disease

Incidence, therapy and prognosis of lupus nephritis
1 40% of SLE patients develop clinical nephritis within 1 year
2 65% of SLE patients develop clinical nephritis within 5 years
3 90% of SLE patients have abnormal renal histology on biopsy
4 WHO type II or V (p. 307): 10–15% → renal failure in 5 years
5 WHO type III, IV: 20–30% → renal failure in 5 years

Pathophysiology of CNS lupus
1 Frank CNS vasculitis is *rare*; commonest pathology is a non-inflammatory vasculopathy with microinfarcts (i.e. bland thrombosis, often due to phospholipid antibodies; p. 191)
2 Vasculitis (± immune complexes) may cause
— *Extracerebral* disease, e.g. cranial nerve palsies, or
— *Focal cerebral* disease (e.g. chorea, stroke)*
3 CSF *antineuronal antibodies* are present in up to 80% of patients with 'diffuse' CNS lupus (fits, psychosis)
4 Antibodies to *ribosomal P antigen* in neuronal cytoplasm may be detectable in 90% of psychotic lupus patients
5 Such autoantibodies may prove to be useful in distinguishing primary CNS lupus from iatrogenic *steroid psychosis*

* NB: Phospholipid antibodies may also cause focal cerebral sequelae

Features of drug-induced SLE
1 Occurrence
— Older patients than primary SLE
— More frequently male (40% vs. 10% in primary SLE)
— Increases with dosage and duration of drug therapy
— Most cases are due to procainamide
— Primary SLE is not exacerbated by such drugs
2 Clinical patterns
— Lung, joint and serosal (esp. pleural) disease common
— Arthralgias, maculopapular rash, fever, cytopenias
— Renal disease *uncommon*; CNS disease *rare*
3 Serology
— ANA against histones (homogeneous pattern) in 95%
— Double-stranded DNA antibodies typically *absent*
— Complement levels *normal*
4 Slow acetylation status usual
— Incidence approaches 100% in hydralazine lupus
— Less marked association in primary SLE
5 HLA association
— DR4
— cf. Primary SLE: DR2, DR3
6 Course
— Symptoms persist for 1–3 months after drug ceased
— ANA can remain positive for 6–12 months

Features of neonatal SLE
1 Cutaneous type
— Commoner in female neonates (75%)
— Transient photosensitive skin eruptions, often discoid
— Associated thrombocytopenia, liver dysfunction
2 Cardiac type
— Commoner in male neonates
— Causes perinatal complete heart block in 95%
— Anti-Ro (SS-A) present in virtually 100%*
— La (SS-B), nRNP antibodies also often present

— 20% of affected neonates will need pacemaker insertion
— 15% will die of associated myocarditis
— Pathology: endomyocardial fibrosis → AV block
3 *Mothers* of affected neonates
— 70% asymptomatic at time of neonatal diagnosis
— 90% develop collagen disease (e.g. SLE) in 10 years
— Anti-Ro in a pregnant woman is an indication for fetal monitoring using echocardiography
— Fetal myocarditis is treated with dexamethasone (not inactivated by placenta) or plasmapheresis

* Of all anti-Ro-positive pregnant women (i.e. whether symptomatic or not), fewer than 3% have children with congenital heart block. Active maternal SLE causes far greater morbidity from intrauterine fetal death (± preeclampsia, phospholipid antibodies) or neonatal lupus

When to suspect primary complement deficiency in SLE
1 Early-onset disease
2 Absent total hemolytic complement (THC, CH_{50})*
3 Normal C_3, C_4 despite persistently active disease
4 Parental consanguinity

* DD_x: Blood sample left on bench in immunology laboratory over weekend

SJÖGREN'S SYNDROME

Clinical concomitants of Sjögren's syndrome
1 Dry mouth and eyes; also nose, throat, trachea, skin
2 Secondary otitis, bronchitis, pneumonitis
3 Dental caries
4 Vulvovaginitis → dyspareunia, pruritus vulvae
5 Atrophic gastritis
6 Recurrent parotidomegaly
7 Lymphadenopathy, splenomegaly; 'pseudolymphoma'
8 Lymphoma, thymoma
9 Cryoglobulinemia; Waldenström's macroglobulinemia
   Benign hyperglobulinemic purpura of Waldenström
10 Pulmonary atelectasis (esp. post-operative)
   Renal tubular acidosis (esp. post-partum)
11 Drug hypersensitivity
12 Autoimmune disease, esp. PBC, Raynaud's, Hashimoto's

Distinction of primary from secondary Sjögren's syndrome
1 No other evident connective tissue disease, esp.
— Rheumatoid arthritis
— SLE
— Scleroderma
2 Autoantibody profile
— ANA more commonly positive (90% vs 50%)
— Ro (SS-A) antibodies* more positive (80% vs 50%)
— La (SS-B) antibodies more positive (50% vs 10%)
— Antisalivary duct antibodies *less* positive (15% vs 60%)
3 Associated with HLA-DR3

— cf. Secondary type: HLA DR4

NB: Rheumatoid factor is positive in almost 100% of *both* primary and secondary Sjögren's syndrome
* Also commonly positive in SLE

Diagnosis of Sjögren's syndrome
1 Clinical sicca syndrome (± connective tissue disease, e.g. RA)
— Gritty eyes, dry mouth*
2 Ophthalmological examination
— Positive Schirmer's test
  • < 15 mm in 5 min
— Abnormal rose Bengal stain
  • Punctate uptake in conjunctival/corneal erosions
— Slit-lamp examination
  • Reduced tear film; erosions
3 Serology
— High-titer IgM rheumatoid factor
— High-titer ANA (± Ro, La)
4 Salivary/labial gland biopsy‡
— Lymphocytic infiltrate
— Acinar atrophy
— Myoepithelial islands

* Note that similar symptoms can occur due to other causes such as sarcoidosis, anticholinergic side-effects. Additional symptoms such as night sweats, adenopathy, weight loss may suggest lymphoma development
‡ Salivary gland scintigraphy may obviate the need for biopsy in centers where this expertise is available

OTHER CONNECTIVE TISSUE DISEASES

Diagnosis of polymyositis
1 Clinical
— Proximal weakness > wasting
— Muscle tenderness
— Heliotrope rash, Göttren's papules
2 Laboratory
— CPK
— EMG
— Muscle biopsy

Diagnosis of polyarteritis nodosa
1 Clinical
— Hypertension
— Mononeuritis multiplex
— Asthma (?Churg–Strauss variant)
2 Laboratory
— Neutrophilia, eosinophilia (?Churg–Strauss variant)
— ↑ESR
— Biopsy of clinically involved tissue
— Angiography (e.g. celiac axis) → aneurysms

Diagnosis of 'mixed connective tissue disease'
1 Clinical
— Raynaud's; puffy fingers/hands (scleroderma-like)
— Arthralgias/-itis; lymphadenopathy (SLE-like)
— Myositis, serositis, pneumonitis (polymyositis-like)
— Renal involvement rare

2 Laboratory
— High-titer (> 1:1024) speckled ANA
— High-titer (cf. SLE) anti-RNP Ab
— Negative dsDNA Ab; negative Sm Ab
— Normal complement levels
— Polyclonal hypergammaglobulinemia
— Abnormal upper (polymyositis-like) and/or lower (scleroderma-like) esophageal motility
— $\downarrow DL_{co}$
3 Therapy
— Steroid-responsive features
  • Myositis
  • Pleurisy
  • Depression
  • Interstitial lung fibrosis, pulmonary hypertension
  • Esophageal dysmotility
4 Clinical course
— 5–10% 10-year mortality
— Indiscriminate steroid use may cause osteoporosis

Clinical significance of mixed connective tissue disease (MCTD)
1 The diagnosis of MCTD is important because it implies the presence of *myositis*
2 Myositis is an indication for *steroids* even in cases with only *mild* symptoms
3 Even if only mild myositis symptoms, initial steroid therapy should be *aggressive* (e.g. prednisone 1 mg/kg)
4 Despite being traditionally regarded as 'mild' disease, complications such as fibrosing alveolitis may be *fatal* if undertreated

AMYLOIDOSIS

Clinical significance of amyloid components
1 AL
— Amyloid L-(light-chain) component
— Causes amyloid of monoclonal immunocytic origin
— Derived from light-chain (BJP) fragments, $\lambda > \kappa$*
— Occurs in
  • 10% myeloma cases (overall)
  • 25% BJP-only myeloma
  • 5% benign monoclonal gammopathy
2 AA
— Amyloid A-component
— Causes amyloidosis of reactive systemic origin
— Derived from the acute phase plasma protein SAA
— Occurs in
  • Familial Mediterranean fever‡
  • *Long-standing* (>10 yr) rheumatoid arthritis (10%), juvenile chronic arthritis (5%), Hodgkin's (5%), TB, leprosy, osteomyelitis
3 AP
— Amyloid P-component
— Pathogenetic significance unknown
— Resembles the acute phase reactant C-reactive protein

— Occurs with all amyloid subtypes *except* cerebral
— ^{123}I-AP scanning may be useful in diagnosis

* cf. most paraproteins and normal immunoglobulins: $\kappa > \lambda$
‡ May *present* with amyloid

Classification of clinical amyloidosis variants
1 Monoclonal immunocytic dyscrasia (AL-amyloidosis)
— Incl. myeloma-associated and 'primary' amyloidosis
2 Reactive systemic amyloidosis (AA-amyloidosis)
— 'Secondary' amyloidosis (similar to FMF type)
3 Endocrine amyloid (affects APUD cells), e.g. from
— Calcitonin-related fibrils in medullary thyroid Ca
— Amylin (amyloid islet polypeptide) in type II DM
4 Senile amyloid (affects heart, joints, seminal vesicles)
— Amyloid from plasma prealbumin ASc
5 Hemodialysis-associated (AH) amyloid ($\rightarrow$ bones, kidneys)
— Amyloid derived from plasma β_2-microglobulin*
6 Cerebral amyloid (Alzheimer's, Down's, senile dementia)
— Amyloid from β/A4-protein (APP derivative)
— Also $\rightarrow$ Dutch hereditary cerebral angiopathy
7 Hereditary (Icelandic) cerebral amyloid ($\rightarrow$ CVA)
— Amyloid from cystatin C (γ-trace protein)
8 Hereditary neuropathic amyloid (e.g. Portuguese amyloid)
— Amyloid from plasma transthyretin ('prealbumin')
9 Familial amyloid polyneuropathy (Iowa, USA)
— Amyloid from apolipoprotein A1
10 Hereditary nephropathic amyloid (FMF; similar to AA)
— Autosomal recessive; colchicine prophylaxis effective
11 Finnish hereditary amyloid
— Amyloid from abnormal gelsolin (binds actin)

* Not removed by dialysis; causes arthropathy, fracture

AL- ('primary') vs AA- ('secondary') amyloidosis
1 AL-amyloidosis $\rightarrow$ *mesenchymal* tissue deposition
— Macroglossia*
— Acquired factor X deficiency*
— Neuropathy
  • Peripheral (incl. carpal tunnel syndrome)
  • Autonomic
— Arthropathy
  • Large joints, e.g. 'shoulder-pads'
  • Carpal tunnel syndrome
— Purpura
  • 'Pinch' (non-thrombocytopenic) purpura
  • Post-proctoscopic periorbital purpura
— Cardiomyopathy (restrictive or HOCM)
  • Often associated with low-voltage ECG
— Hyposplenism
2 AA-amyloidosis $\rightarrow$ *parenchymal* tissue deposition
— Nephrotic syndrome‡
— Hepatosplenomegaly‡
— Goiter

* *Highly* specific for AL-amyloidosis
‡ Also occur in 'primary' amyloid

Diagnosis of amyloidosis
1 Paraproteinemia, *plus*

2 Biopsy (Congo red stain) of
   — Routinely biopsied site (e.g. marrow in myeloma)
   — Affected site* (e.g. sural nerve in neuropathy)
   — Deep rectal biopsy
   — Aspirated abdominal fat
3 Biopsy (polarized light microscopy)
   — 'Apple-green' birefringence
4 Electron microscopy
   — β-pleated sheets
5 Direct immunofluorescence of bone marrow plasma cells
   — Light-chain antibodies → monoclonal immunocytes
   — Polyclonality (e.g. in reactive systemic amyloidosis)

* NB: Due to increased risk of bleeding in amyloidosis, suspected renal amyloid is usually considered an indication for *rectal* biopsy

HIV AND AIDS

Clinical spectrum of HIV infection
1 Mononucleosis-like ('seroconversion') syndrome
   — Fever, rash, ± neuropathy, encephalitis
2 Asymptomatic phase (~ 7–10 years)*
   — CD4 count drops below 200/mm³
   — Active HIV replication continues, but largely confined to fixed lymphoid tissue (nodes, Kupffer cells)
3 AIDS-related complex (ARC)‡
   — e.g. Adenopathy¶, diarrhea, fever, weight loss, thrush
4 AIDS ('full-blown')
   — e.g. *P. carinii* pneumonia, cerebral toxoplasmosis, *Cryptosporidium* diarrhea

* Unless HIV acquired by *transfusion* → average latency ~ 4 years
‡ Persistent generalized lymphadenopathy + sweats, fever, weight loss = 'AIDS prodrome'
¶ i.e. ≥ two extrainguinal nodes > 1 cm diameter

INVESTIGATING IMMUNOLOGIC DISEASE

B lymphocytes: laboratory characteristics
1 Phenotype
   — Surface immunoglobulin (IgM, IgD) present
   — $\kappa:\lambda$ chains = 2:1
2 Function
   — IgG, A, M levels
   — Isohemagglutinins (IgM)
   — Antibodies to
     • Pneumococcus (IgM)
     • Tetanus/polio/diphtheria (IgG)
3 In vitro blastogenesis (T cell-dependent)
   — Inducible with pokeweed mitogen
4 Lymph node localization
   — Follicles, medullary cords

Phenotypic characterization of T cell subtypes
1 T cells (general)
   — Express CD3 (pan T cell*) cell-surface marker
2 Helper/inducer (T_H)
   — Normally comprise 70–80% T cells
   — Express CD4 (T cell receptor for HIV)
   — Lineage causing T cell leukemia (HTLV-1 +)
3 Suppressor/cytotoxic (T_S)
   — Normally comprise about 30% T cells
   — Express CD8

* cf. Ia antigen; expression excludes T cell origin

Characterization of T cell function in vitro and in vivo
1 Phenotype
   — Spontaneous E-rosette formation with sheep RBCs
2 Function
   — Primary response: DNCB sensitization
   — Lymphokine (MIF, LIF) production
   — 'Memory': DTH skin testing to tuberculin, *Candida*, mumps, trichophyton, tetanus, streptokinase
3 In vitro blastogenesis
   — Inducible with Con A, PHA
   — Specific antigen, e.g. herpes simplex type II
4 Lymph node localization
   — Paracortical

$T_H:T_S$ ratios in health and disease
1 *Normal* $T_H:T_S$
   — CD4:CD8 = 1.5–2.0
2 *Inverted* ratio ($T_H < T_S$)
   — With lymphopenia
     • AIDS*
   — With normal lymphocyte count
     • Common variable hypogammaglobulinemia
     • X-linked lymphoproliferative (Duncan's) disease
   — With lymphocytosis
     • CLL
3 *Exaggerated* ratio ($T_H \gg T_S$)
   — SLE
   — Sjögren's syndrome
   — Juvenile chronic arthritis
4 *Relative variations* of $T_H:T_S$ ratio
   — Leprosy
     • Tuberculoid: ↑ $T_H:T_S$
     • Lepromatous: ↓ $T_H:T_S$
   — Renal transplant
     • Acute rejection: ↑ $T_H:T_S$
     • Homograft infection (e.g. CMV): ↓ $T_H:T_S$
   — Graft-versus-host disease‡
     • Acute: ↑ $T_H:T_S$
     • Chronic: ↓ $T_H:T_S$
   — Active sarcoid¶
     • Bronchoalveolar lavage: ↑ $T_H:T_S$
     • Peripheral blood: ↓ $T_H:T_S$

* $T_H:T_S$ ratio normal in SCID, WAS, Nezelof's (i.e. despite lymphopenia)
‡ Acute GVHD is associated with hypergammaglobulinemia
Chronic GVHD with hypogammaglobulinemia
¶ Bronchoalveolar lavage fluid in active sarcoid is associated with lymphocytosis; cf. peripheral blood → lymphopenia

INVESTIGATION OF HYPERSENSITIVITY STATES

Drugs for which prick testing is reliable
1 β-lactams
2 Local anesthetics

Radioallergosorbent testing ('RAST'): indications*
1 Known high risk of anaphylaxis
   — e.g. Hypersensitivity to penicillin or insect sting
2 Preexisting skin hypersensitivity
   — Dermatitis, dermatographia, other skin disease
3 Recent (< 72 h) exposure to drugs inhibiting prick test
   — esp. Antihistamines, sympathomimetics
4 Highly suggestive history with negative prick test
   — e.g. Inhalant allergy (i.e. suspected false-negative)
5 Small children (< 5 years)

* = Relative contraindications to prick testing

Elevated IgE: differential diagnosis
1 Metazoan parasitic infestation
   — Trichinosis
   — Toxocariasis
   — Filariasis
   — Schistosomiasis
2 Pulmonary disease
   — Atopic asthma
   — Bronchopulmonary aspergillosis
   — Churg–Strauss syndrome
   — Löffler's syndrome
3 Skin disease
   — Pemphigus
   — Pemphigoid
4 Rare causes
   — Wiskott–Aldrich syndrome
   — Job's syndrome
   — Hodgkin's disease
   — Sézary syndrome
   — Selective IgA deficiency

NB: IgE is *not* elevated in the hypereosinophilic syndrome or in extrinsic allergic alveolitis (hypersensitivity pneumonitis)

IgA excess states
1 Elevated serum levels
   — Wiskott–Aldrich syndrome
   — Berger's (IgA nephropathy) disease
   — Henoch–Schönlein purpura
   — Alcoholic cirrhosis
   — Wegener's granulomatosis
2 Positive direct immunofluorescence
   — Extrarenal
     • Celiac disease
     • Dermatitis herpetiformis
     • Pyoderma gangrenosum
   — Renal
     • Berger's disease
     • SLE (IgA_1)
     • Henoch–Schönlein (IgA_2)
     • Alcoholic cirrhosis (IgA_2)

ABNORMALITIES OF PLASMA PROTEINS

Differential diagnosis of polyclonal hypergammaglobulinemia
1 Liver disease
2 Autoimmune disease, connective tissue disease
3 Sarcoidosis
4 Chronic infection
5 Hodgkin's disease, angioimmunoblastic lymphadenopathy
6 AIDS

Dominant polyclonal gammopathy in liver disease
1 Primary biliary cirrhosis — IgM
2 Chronic active hepatitis — IgG
3 Alcoholic cirrhosis — IgA (not invariably)

Secondary causes of hypogammaglobulinemia
1 Hematologic malignancy
   — Myeloma
   — Chronic lymphocytic leukemia
   — Non-Hodgkin's lymphoma
2 Some infections (e.g. EBV, rubella)
3 Nephrotic syndrome
4 Protein-losing enteropathy (e.g. intestinal lymphangiectasia)
5 Thymoma
6 Myotonic dystrophy

Paraproteinemia: differential diagnosis
1 Benign monoclonal gammopathy (diagnosis of exclusion)
2 Myeloma (IgG > A > BJP only > D > non-secretory > M > E)
3 Plasmacytoma
4 Macroglobulinemia
5 Heavy chain disease*†
6 Non-Hodgkin's lymphoma
7 Chronic lymphocytic leukemia
8 Essential cryoglobulinemia
9 Cold hemagglutinin disease (IgM)
10 Primary amyloidosis

* λ-heavy chain disease → lymphoma-like syndrome in elderly men
† α-heavy chain disease → malabsorption in young Mediterranean patients

Benign monoclonal gammopathy: diagnostic criteria
1 No increase with time
2 No immune paresis (i.e. other Ig levels normal)
3 Normal skeletal survey
4 Paraprotein level
   — < 20 g/L (IgG)
   — < 10 g/L (other)
   — Absent Bence-Jones protein
5 Marrow plasmacytosis < 10%

Components of normal serum protein electrophoresis
1 α_1 band
   — α_1AT; α_1 acid glycoprotein (orosomucoid)
   — αFP

2 α_2 band
— Haptoglobin
— Ceruloplasmin
— AT III
3 β_1 band
— Transferrin
β_2 band
— C_3

Abnormal electrophoretic patterns: clinical significance
1 α_1 pallor
— α_1AT deficiency
2 β pallor
— Frozen/stored specimen → in vitro C_3 activation
3 γ pallor
— Hypogammaglobulinemia (primary or secondary)
4 β-γ fusion
— IgA paraproteinemia
— FDPs (DIC)
— Alcoholic liver disease
— Hemoglobinemia (intravascular hemolysis)
5 ↓ Albumin
↑ Gammaglobulin
— Chronic liver disease (any etiology)
6 ↓ Albumin
↑ α_2 globulins
↓ Gammaglobulin
— Nephrosis
7 Discrete band cathodal to γ region in serum and urine
— Lysozyme (e.g. in AMOL, CGL)

Electrophoretic abnormalities of urine and CSF
1 In urine
— ↑ IgG: transferrin clearance
• Glomerular disease
— ↑ β_2 microglobulin: transferrin clearance
• Tubular disease
— Bizarre EPG
• Bladder cancer
• Factitious contamination
2 In CSF
— Strong prealbumin bands
↑ IgG: albumin ratio
Oligoclonal IgG bands
• Multiple sclerosis, neurosyphilis, SSPE

THE COMPLEMENT CASCADE

Complement abnormalities in disease
1 Acute phase reaction
— ↑ C_3 ↑ C_4 ↑ total hemolytic complement (THC)
2 Classical pathway activation
— ↓ C_3 ↓ C_4 ↓ THC
3 Alternate pathway activation
— ↓ C_3
— Normal C_4
— Normal or reduced THC
4 Fluid phase activation
— Normal C_3
— ↓↓ C_4 ↓ THC
— ↓ C_1-INH (see below)

5 Deficiency of classical pathway component
— ↓↓ THC
6 Poorly collected specimen
— ↓ THC ± ↓ $C_{3,4}$
Idiopathic angioneurotic edema
— *Normal* complement profile (cf. hereditary)

The alternate pathway: its pathogenetic significance
1 Function
— Antibody-independent resistance (e.g. via opsonization)
2 Activation
— Endotoxin (bacterial lipopolysaccharide)
3 Defectiveness
— Hyposplenism (p. 199)
4 Pathogenicity
— Post-infective glomerulonephritis
— Mesangiocapillary glomerulonephritis type II ('dense deposit disease') ± partial lipodystrophy
— Paroxysmal nocturnal hemoglobinuria

Phenotypes associated with primary complement deficiencies
1 C_1-esterase inhibitor (C_1-INH) deficiency
— Hereditary angioneurotic edema (see below)
2 C_2 deficiency (commonest deficiency; → 1 in 10,000)
— One-third → asymptomatic
— One-third → mild or atypical SLE
— One-third → recurrent pyogenic infections*
3 $C_{1q,r,s}$, C_2 or C_4 deficiency
— Mild SLE, glomerulonephritis, Henoch–Schönlein
4 C_3 deficiency (most serious deficiency)
— Life-threatening infections (encapsulated bacteria)
— May reflect deficiency of factor H/I or C_3b inactivator
5 Factor H deficiency
— Associated with hemolytic uremic syndrome
6 C_5 dysfunction (Leiner's syndrome; presents in infancy)
— Eczema, Gram-negative infections, diarrhea
7 C_7 deficiency
— Raynaud's phenomenon
8 C_{5-9} deficiency
— *Neisseria* (meningococcal/gonococcal) infections

NB: Total hemolytic complement may be undetectable in C_{1q} or C_2 deficiency (confusing in clinically mild SLE). All homozygous complement deficiencies are *rare* except for C_1-INH and C_2 deficiencies
* e.g. pneumococcal/*H. influenzae* sepsis, esp. meningitis

Features of hereditary angioneurotic edema (C_1-INH deficiency)
1 Presentations
— Non-pruritic skin swellings lasting at least 48–72 h
— Recurrent abdominal colic
— Upper respiratory tract obstruction
— Intestinal pseudoobstruction
— Family history of asphyxiation (glottal edema)
2 Diagnostic clues
— *No* inflammation, itching or urticaria with attacks
— Normal histamine levels during attacks
— Interictal low C_4

3 Acute management
— Purified C₁-esterase inhibitor (if available)
— Fresh plasma*
— Tracheostomy
4 Prophylaxis
— Danazol, stanozolol
— EACA, tranexamic acid
5 *Acquired* C_1-1NH deficiency may be associated with B cell malignancy or glomerulonephritis

* NB: Contains C_2/C_4 which may precipitate or worsen glottal edema

PATHOPHYSIOLOGY OF AUTOIMMUNE DISORDERS

Vasculitis: clinicopathological correlations
1 Large arteries
— Giant cell arteritis, Takayasu's
2 Medium-size arteries and veins
— Buerger's disease
3 Venules, veins, venae cavae, arteries
— Behçet's disease
4 Small-to-medium arteries and veins
— Churg–Strauss, Wegener's
5 Small-to-medium arteries
— PAN
6 Arterioles, capillaries, post-capillary venules
— Hypersensitivity (leukocytoclastic vasculitis → intradermal capillaries)
— Rheumatoid vasculitis
— Henoch–Schönlein purpura

Ultrastructural features of the vasculitides
1 Giant cell arteritis
— Absent fibrinoid necrosis
— Moderate giant cell infiltrate
— Mononuclear infiltration
2 Wegener's granulomatosis
— Marked fibrinoid necrosis
— Marked giant cell infiltrate
— Polymorph/mononuclear infiltration
3 Churg–Strauss syndrome
— Moderate fibrinoid necrosis
— Moderate giant cell infiltrate
— Eosinophil infiltration
4 Polyarteritis nodosa
— Marked fibrinoid necrosis
— Absent giant cells
— Polymorph/eosinophil infiltration
5 Hypersensitivity vasculitis
— Slight fibrinoid necrosis
— Absent giant cells
— Polymorph/lymphocyte infiltration

ANTINEUTROPHIL CYTOPLASMIC ANTIBODIES (ANCA)

Significance of antineutrophil cytoplasmic antibodies (ANCA)
1 Marker of systemic vasculitis
2 Positive in 80% cases of Wegener's
— Absence makes this diagnosis *unlikely*

3 Positive in 50% cases of microscopic polyarteritis (*not* PAN)
— Typically negative in leukocytoclastic vasculitis
4 Common immunofluorescent patterns
— Diffuse cytoplasmic (cANCA) staining
• Characteristic of Wegener's
• Finely granular in microscopic polyarteritis
• Antigen: neutrophil α-proteinase 3
— Perinuclear (pANCA) staining
• Non-specific (e.g. → severe infections)
• *Rarely* positive in Wegener's
• Antigen: myeloperoxidase (or elastase)
5 Variation with disease activity
— ANCA often (not always) parallels activity
— i.e. Can be used to monitor treatment
— Clinical relapses may be prevented by treating presumptively when ANCA rises
— Pathogenetic role of ANCA unproven
6 ANCA also positive in other vasculitides:
— Rapidly progressive glomerulonephritis*
— Churg–Strauss syndrome (p. 327), SLE
— Kawasaki syndrome (see below)

* Anti-GBM antibodies also seen in this context (p. 308)

Clinical significance of negative ANCA
1 Patient does not have vasculitis after all
2 Vasculitis is local – *not* systemic
3 Patient already commenced on therapy
4 Suboptimal assay system (in up to 30%)

Differential diagnosis of false-positive ANCA
1 Infection, esp.
— HIV
— Infective endocarditis
— Amebic abscess
2 Inflammatory bowel disease
— esp. With sclerosing cholangitis
3 Malignancy

KAWASAKI SYNDROME

Diagnosis of Kawasaki syndrome*
1 High fever > 5 days in a child aged < 5 years, *plus*
2 At least four of the following signs
— Conjunctival injection
— Cervical adenopathy
— Upper respiratory tract mucosal erythema
— Painful hand/foot erythema or edema
— Skin rash‡
3 Exclusion of
— Scarlet fever (gp A strep), rheumatic fever
— Severe staphylococcal infection with toxin
— Leptospirosis, Rocky Mountain spotted fever
— EBV infection
— Juvenile rheumatoid arthritis

* An epidemic systemic vasculitis of children
‡ Incl. 'reactivation' of previous BCG site

Management of Kawasaki syndrome
1 Monitor for potentially lethal vasculitic complications

— Echocardiographic detection of coronary aneurysms (usually detectable 2–4 weeks after symptom onset)
— Myocarditis, pancarditis; acute myocardial infarction
2 Therapy
— High-dose aspirin helps fever
— IV gammaglobulin

AUTOANTIBODIES

Pathogenetic autoantibodies*
1 Neuromuscular ion-channel disorders
— AChRAb (acetylcholine receptor antibody)
• Myasthenia gravis
— Antibody to voltage-gated calcium channels
• Eaton-Lambert (myasthenic) syndrome
— Antibody to membrane potassium channels
• Acquired neuromyotonia (Isaacs' syndrome)
Glutamic acid decarboxylase Ab
— 'Stiff-man' syndrome
2 Connective tissue pathologies
— Antibody to type II collagen
• Bilateral sensorineural hearing loss
• Relapsing polychondritis
— Anti-GBM (glomerular basement membrane)
• Goodpasture's syndrome
— Intercellular cement Ab
• Pemphigus
3 SLE-associated syndromes
— Anti-Ro (SS-A)
• Congenital heart block (maternal SLE)
— Antiphospholipid (p. 191)
• Thrombotic tendency in SLE
4 Endocrinopathies mediated by *agonistic* antibodies, e.g.
— TSH receptor Ab
• Graves' disease (→ goiter)
— β islet cell Ab
• Spontaneous hypoglycemia
5 Endocrinopathies mediated by *blocking* antibodies, e.g.
— TSH receptor‡ Ab
• 1° myxedema, Hashimoto's
— ACTH receptor Ab
• Addison's
— Gastrin receptor Ab
• Pernicious anemia
— FSH receptor Ab
• Premature menopause
— Insulin receptor Ab
• Type B insulin receptor abnormality
• Associated with acanthosis nigricans

* i.e. the autoantibody is thought to actually cause the phenotype, rather than being simply a diagnostic (epiphenomenal) marker
‡ *Mutations* affecting this receptor may also cause congenital hypothyroidism

Diagnostic patterns of antinuclear antibodies
1 Rim (peripheral)
— Associated with native (double-stranded) DNA antibodies to DNA sugar-phosphate backbone

— Titer parallels disease activity
2 Homogeneous (diffuse)
— Associated with histone* (or ssDNA) antibodies
— Rarely associated with dsDNA antibodies
3 Nucleolar
— Associated with antibodies to nucleolar RNA
4 Speckled
— Associated with antibodies to non-histone antigens
— Ribonucleoproteins
• U1 RNP (nRNP)
• rRNP
• Sm
• Ro (SS-A)
• La‡ (SS-B)
— Jo-1 (aminoacyl tRNA synthetase)
— Topoisomerase I (Scl-70)
— Centromere
— Ku¶

* Histones are DNA-binding chromatin proteins
‡ A nucleic acid-binding ATPase which terminates RNA transcription
¶ DNA-binding protein; associated with sclerodactyly

Features of ANA-negative SLE
1 Subacute presentation
2 Major skin involvement (e.g. photosensitive dermatitis)
3 Thrombocytopenia common
4 Renal and CNS disease unusual
5 Lupus band negative
6 Antibodies to Ro (SS-A) positive in ~ 50%*

NB: Only 5% of SLE cases are ANA-negative; hence, difficult to be sure of diagnosis in this situation. *Discoid* LE is usually ANA-negative
* Standard ANA immunofluorescence does *not* reliably detect anti-Ro (or antiphospholipid)

Serologic subsets of SLE
1 Most specific SLE markers
Predictive of renal disease, hypocomplementemia
— dsDNA antibodies (in 60% SLE patients)
— Sm antibodies (in 20%; → membranous G/N)
— PCNA antibodies (in 5%)
2 Drug-induced SLE (usually due to procainamide)
— Homogeneous ANA (in 95%)
3 Sjögren's, scleroderma, overlap syndromes
— Nucleolar ANA
4 Mixed connective tissue disease (pp. 184–185)
— Anti-U1
5 Scleroderma
— Antitopoisomerase I (Scl-70); Ku
6 CREST syndrome
— Anticentromere antibody*
7 Sicca syndrome
— La, Ro
8 Polymyositis (± pulmonary fibrosis)
— Jo-1‡

* Thus indicating good prognosis in scleroderma but *not* in Raynaud's (i.e. suggests progression to scleroderma)
‡ 25% of dermatomyositis patients will have anti-Jo-1; of these, 80% will have both myositis and lung fibrosis

Clinical associations of anti-Ro antibodies
1 Neonatal SLE
   — esp. Congenital heart block
2 Subacute cutaneous SLE (SCLE)
   — 'Polycyclic' lesions in photosensitive distribution
3 ANA-negative SLE
4 SLE due to homozygous C_2 deficiency
5 Sicca syndrome* ± arthritis
6 Pneumonitis, hyperglobulinemia

* 'Primary' Sjögren's syndrome

PHOSPHOLIPID ANTIBODIES

Detection of phospholipid antibodies
1 Anticardiolipin antibody tests
2 'Lupus anticoagulant' test
3 Reaginic tests for syphilis (biological false-positives)

What are phospholipid antibodies?
1 Anticardiolipin antibody
   — One of the family of antibodies which comprise antiphospholipid activity in plasma
   — Bind in solid-phase assays (e.g. ELISA)
2 The lupus anticoagulant (itself an antibody)
   — Detectable in ~ 30% SLE patients (incl. drug-induced)
   — Closely related to anticardiolipin antibody
   — Inhibits coagulation in vitro by antagonizing interaction between phospholipid moiety of prothrombin activator complex and prothrombin*
   — Antibody-phospholipid complex may activate factor XII and platelets by inhibiting β_2 glycoprotein 1 (β-GPI)
   — Paradoxical *thrombosis* in vivo‡; usually no bleeding
3 False-positive syphilis reagins
   — Distinct from lupus anticoagulant and anticardiolipin
   — Unrelated to antibodies found in 'true' syphilis
   — Distinguishable serologically from true syphilis reagins

* → Prolonged PTTK *uncorrected* by in vitro addition of normal plasma (i.e. a true 'anticoagulant')
‡ esp. with IgG phospholipid antibody; risk correlates with plasma level

Major features of antiphospholipid syndrome
1 Thrombosis (venous and/or arterial)
2 Thrombocytopenia
3 Recurrent miscarriages

Vascular complications of phospholipid antibodies*
1 Placental arterial insufficiency
   — Recurrent abortions (first and second trimester)
   — Intrauterine fetal death (second and third trimester)
2 CNS arterial insufficiency
   — TIAs, stroke, multiinfarct dementia
   — Vascular myelopathy (? ant. spinal artery thrombosis)
   — Migraine, amaurosis fugax, CRA occlusion

3 Cardiac insufficiency
   — Acute myocardial infarction
   — Coronary graft thrombosis
4 Pulmonary arterial insufficiency
   — Recurrent pulmonary emboli
5 Peripheral arterial insufficiency
   — Aortic arch syndrome
   — Axillary arterial thrombosis
   — Mesenteric arterial thrombosis
   — Peripheral vascular disease (incl. gangrene)
6 Venous thrombosis
   — Superficial thrombophlebitis
   — Deep venous thrombosis
   — Renal vein thrombosis (± bilateral)
   — Retinal vein thrombosis
   — Budd–Chiari syndrome
   — Portal vein thrombosis

* NB: Only 50% of cases have SLE; the others represent 'primary antiphospholipid syndrome'. Note also that arterial insufficiency in this context is *not* mediated by vasculitis, but by bland intimal thickening

Forms of hypertension associated with phospholipid antibodies
1 'Primary' pulmonary hypertension
2 Labile systemic hypertension
3 Portal venous hypertension

Additional manifestations of phospholipid antibodies
1 Thrombocytopenia, Coombs-positive hemolytic anemia
2 Chorea, epilepsy, psychiatric disturbance
3 Guillain–Barré syndrome
4 Libman–Sachs cardiac valve degeneration*
5 Splenomegaly
6 Livedo reticularis, splinter hemorrhages
7 Adrenal infarction, Addison's disease
8 Avascular necrosis of bone

* vegetations → regurgitation

Bleeding in patients with lupus anticoagulant? Exclude
1 Thrombocytopenia
2 Hypoprothrombinemia
3 Factor VIII antibodies

Long-term management of antiphospholipid syndrome
1 Low-dose aspirin (e.g. 75 mg/day)
2 History of venous thrombosis?
   — Warfarin (aim for INR ~ 2–2.5)
3 History of arterial thrombosis?
   — Warfarin (aim for INR ~ 3–4)
4 Steroids/immunosuppressives have not proven useful *except* in management of cytopenias

'COLD' AUTOANTIBODIES

The cryopathies: clinicopathological background
1 Cryoglobulinemia
   — May be monoclonal or polyclonal (usually IgM)
   — Clinical manifestations arise due to precipitation of immunoglobulins at low temperatures (i.e. < 37°C)

— Sequelae include
  • Raynaud's (may progress to gangrene)
  • Purpura (esp. legs)
  • Hepatosplenomegaly; abnormal LFTs
  • Arthralgias, fever
  • Confusion, weakness (hyperviscosity)
  • Renal failure, uremia (glomerulonephritis)
— Etiological associations
  • Connective tissue disease (e.g. SLE)
  • Myelo-/lymphoproliferative disease (e.g. CLL)
  • Infections: e.g. HBV, post-infectious nephritis
2 Cold agglutinins
  — Clinical manifestations due to IgM binding red cells at low temperatures → complement activation on rewarming to 37°C → hemolysis (p. 160)
  — Less often, red cell *autoagglutination* may supervene → vascular obstruction (Raynaud's, acrocyanosis)
  — Etiological associations
    • *M. pneumoniae* (anti-I; Rh specificity)
    • Infectious mononucleosis (anti-i)
    • Diffuse large-cell lymphoma
    • Waldenström's macroglobulinemia
3 Paroxysmal cold hemoglobinuria
  — Clinical manifestations due to low-temperature IgG (Donath–Landsteiner antibody) binding P antigen of red cell membrane → complement fixation → intravascular hemolysis on rewarming to 37°C
  — Hemoglobinemia/transient leukopenia may also occur
  — Etiological associations
    • Measles, mumps, varicella
    • Congenital syphilis
4 Cryofibrinogenemia
  — Manifestations may include cold urticaria (p. 368)
  — Etiological associations
    • Diabetes mellitus
    • Prostate cancer

TISSUE TYPING

Gene loci in the major histocompatibility complex (MHC)
1 HLA determinants (see below)
2 Complement components
  — e.g. C_2, C_4; C_3 convertase
3 Tumor necrosis factor
  — Proinflammatory cytokine implicated in rheumatoid arthritis and other autoimmune disorders
4 Heat-shock proteins (HSPs)
  — Molecular chaperones controlling protein folding
5 Genes affecting antigen processing and presentation
  — Located between DP and DQ loci
6 Unrelated ('class III') genes responsible for some 'HLA-linked' disorders, e.g.
  — Narcolepsy
  — 21-hydroxylase
  — Hemochromatosis

HLA antigens: patterns of expression and function
1 HLA A, B, and C antigens (*class I* antigens) are found on most nucleated cells (not RBCs) except trophoblast
  — Function: present foreign antigen (usually viral) to *cytotoxic T cells*
  — Mediate graft rejection
2 D-related (DR or *class II*) antigens are found on
  • B cells (basis of pretransplant MLC)
  • Activated T cells
  • Monocytes and macrophages
  • Sperm, epididymal cells
  — Function: present foreign antigen to *helper T cells*
  — Mediate immune responsiveness

Prevalence of HLA antigens in Caucasian populations
1 HLA-A3 — 25%
2 HLA-B8 — 10%
3 HLA-B27 — 5–10%
4 HLA-DR4 — 20–40%

HLA allele linkage disequilibrium: common haplotypes
1 A1, B8, DR3
  — Often occur together in Caucasians
  — May include deletion for C_4 complement component
2 A2, B35, DR4
  — Often occur together in American Indians
3 A30, B13, DR7
  — Often occur together in Chinese

HLA antigens: strongest disease associations
1 HLA-DQw6
  — Present in 20% controls
  — Present in > 95% *narcolepsy* cases (50-fold ↑ risk)
  — Also present in 80% Goodpasture's (anti-GBM disease)
2 HLA-B27
  — Present in 5–10% controls
  — Present in 90% *ankylosing spondylitis* (75-fold ↑ risk)
  — Also present in 80% *Reiter's syndrome* (25-fold ↑ risk)

Other disease associations with HLA antigens
1 A3
  — Idiopathic hemochromatosis (in 75%)
  — B7, B14 also linked to IHC
2 B5
  — Behçet's disease with ocular or colonic involvement
  — Takayasu's arteritis
3 B12
  — Behçet's disease
  — Minimal lesion nephrosis
4 B27
  — Psoriatic arthritis ± sacroiliitis
  — Juvenile chronic arthritis with sacroiliitis
  — Reactive arthritis
  — Acute anterior uveitis
  — Chronic balanitis; chronic prostatitis
  — 'Frozen shoulder'
  — Asbestosis
5 B35
  — Subacute (de Quervain's, viral) thyroiditis

Bw47
— 21-hydroxylase deficiency
Bw53
— Malarial resistance
6 Cw6
— Psoriasis vulgaris (20x ↑ risk)
Cw7
— Guillain–Barré syndrome (chronic relapsing subtype)
7 DP
— Beryllium hypersensitivity
8 DQ
— Pemphigus vulgaris
DQw3
— Ca cervix
9 DR2
— Multiple sclerosis (B7, DQw1)
— SLE (esp. with C_2 deficiency)
10 DR3 (and B8)
— Primary Sjögren's (sicca) syndrome
— Celiac disease/dermatitis herpetiformis (B8, DQw2)
— SLE (esp. neonatal or subacute cutaneous SLE)
— Addison's disease; Graves' disease
— Insulin-dependent diabetes (also DR4, B8, B15)
— HBsAg-negative chronic active hepatitis
— Myasthenia gravis
— Buerger's disease
— Membranous nephropathy
11 DR4
— Seropositive RA; secondary Sjögren's syndrome
— Polyarticular (RA-like) juvenile chronic arthritis
— Chronic (antibiotic-resistant) Lyme arthritis
— SLE (iatrogenic)
— Preeclampsia (familial)
12 DR5
— Pernicious anemia
— Hashimoto's thyroiditis
— Early-onset systemic (Still's) juvenile chronic arthritis
— HIV-associated sicca syndrome

DIAGNOSIS AND PROGNOSIS OF HIV INFECTION

Current status of HIV antibody testing
1 HIV ELISA is the best screen (cf. definitive test: Western blot)
2 ELISA may remain negative for 3–6 months post-infection (i.e. negative test does not exclude HIV infection)
3 ELISA is 99% sensitive if performed > 6 months post-infection
4 ELISA has a significant false-positive rate; hence, all positives need to be confirmed using Western blot
5 ELISA+ neonates of infected mothers may not have HIV
6 Some patients with AIDS do not have positive ELISA

HIV antibody tests: who should doctors screen?
1 Patients in whom HIV status is clinically relevant*

2 Patients whose blood has inadvertently contaminated a health professional (needlestick‡, mucosal exposure)
3 Donors of blood, semen, ova or transplant tissues
4 Regular clients of VD and drug detoxification clinics*
5 Prostitutes
6 Rapists

* Refusal of such patients to give informed consent for testing should be interpreted as signifying HIV positivity until proven otherwise
‡ Note that HBV is a far more frequent complication of needlestick; seroconversion occurs in only ~ 1% of needlestick injuries involving HIV-positive patients (cf. HIV blood *transfusion*: almost 100% seroconversion after one unit)

Predictors of poor prognosis in HIV infection
1 Advanced disease, late presentation, frail condition
2 Marked anemia
3 CD4+ lymphocyte count* < 100/mm^3
4 Loss of p24 antibody; p24 antigenemia
5 Female sex (prognosis generally worse than for males)

* NB: Rate of decline may predict likely long-term onset of AIDS

MANAGING IMMUNOLOGICAL DISEASE

INDICATIONS FOR IMMUNOMODULATORY THERAPY

Indications for plasmapheresis/plasma exchange
1 Hyperviscosity syndrome (acute or maintenance)
2 Non-oliguric anti-GBM disease (Goodpasture's)
3 Myasthenia gravis: crisis or prethymectomy
4 Essential mixed cryoglobulinemia
5 Acute Guillain–Barré syndrome
6 Thrombotic thrombocytopenic purpura

Potential indications for intravenous immunoglobulin
1 Immune thrombocytopenia
— Recent-onset ITP*
— Post-transfusion purpura
2 Symptomatic hypogammaglobulinemia
— Primary (incl. IgG subclass deficiencies)
— Secondary, e.g. in CLL (but see below)
3 Infection
— Neonatal sepsis‡
— Prophylaxis for marrow transplants, ICU patients
— CMV pneumonia (with ganciclovir)
— Pediatric AIDS
4 Autoimmune/vasculitis
— Kawasaki syndrome (with aspirin; p. 190)
— Acute Guillain–Barré syndrome
— Pure red cell aplasia
— Reduction of F VIII antibodies in hemophilia
— Severe allergic asthma in childhood

* Or autoimmune neutropenia/hemolysis; esp. pre-splenectomy
‡ Or prophylaxis for this in premature neonates
NB: High-dose IV IgG can cause transient hyperviscosity, aseptic meningitis and/or renal impairment but rarely transmits hepatitis or HIV. It does not appear *cost-effective* for chronic disorders such as CLL

Indications for hyposensitization
1 Bee/wasp sting anaphylaxis, *or*
   Severe reaction with strongly positive prick test
2 Severe allergic rhinitis if due to pollen/grass/
   housedust mite hypersensitivity (*not* in food
   allergy)
3 (Major) penicillin allergy *if essential* for management
   (e.g. life-threatening enterococcal endocarditis)

Therapeutic modalities in allergic rhinitis
1 Prophylaxis
   — Sodium cromoglycate (mast cell stabilizer)
   — Ketotifen* (antihistamine/mast cell stabilizer)
2 Antihistamines
   — Astemizole for prophylaxis
   — Terfenadine for symptoms
3 Associated nasal obstruction
   — Inhaled beclomethasone
4 Refractory symptoms
   — Hyposensitization

* Other actions include antianaphylactic, anti-PAF (platelet-
activating factor) and inhibition of SRS-A (i.e. leukotrienes C_4, D_4,
E_4)

Antihistamines: indications and toxicities
1 First-generation H_1-blockers
   — Diphenydramine
   — Chlorpheniramine
   — Hydroxyzine
2 Second-generation H_1-blockers
   — Terfenadine
   — Ketotifen
   — Astemizole
   — Cetirizine
3 Main indications
   — Allergic rhinoconjunctivitis
   — Chronic urticaria, pruritus, angioedema
4 Toxicities
   — CNS toxicity: somnolence (esp. first-generation)
   — Appetite stimulation, weight gain
   — Q-T_c prolongation (esp. terfenadine overdose)

DRUG-INDUCED IMMUNOLOGIC DISORDERS

Pathogenesis of drug fever
1 Hypersensitivity reactions
   — Penicillins, sulfonamides
   — Methyldopa; hydralazine (SLE)
   — D-penicillamine
2 Antituberculosis drugs
   — INH, PAS, rifampicin, streptomycin
3 Cytotoxics
   — Bleomycin, L-asparaginase
4 Dose-related pyrogens
   — Amphotericin B
5 Thermoregulatory dysfunction
   — Anticholinergics (impaired sweating)
   — Phenothiazines (hypothalamic effect)
6 Overdosage
   — Aspirin
   — Iodine (may → transient hyperthyroidism)

7 Drug abuse
   — Amphetamines, LSD, barbiturates, IV cocaine
   — Laxatives
8 Drug withdrawal
   — Corticosteroids
9 Malignant hyperthermia
   — Anesthetic agents, esp. inhalational
10 Rare (unlikely) causes
   — Digoxin
   — Chloramphenicol, tetracycline
   — Monocomponent insulin

Anaphylaxis: most frequent iatrogenic causes
1 Penicillins* (and other protein-binding haptens)
2 Insulin (and other human proteins)
3 Heterologous antisera (e.g. tetanus antitoxin)
4 Intravenous vitamin K
5 Iron dextran infusion
6 Streptokinase, protamine

* Frequency of penicillin-induced anaphylaxis is ~ 0.2%, with
approximately one-quarter of these proving fatal

Precipitants of anaphylactoid reactions*
1 Aspirin
2 Opiates: codeine, morphine
3 Gammaglobulin administration, blood transfusions
4 Anesthetic agents (e.g. thiopentone, curare)
5 Iodinated contrast agents (esp. in venography)
6 Hydrocortisone (very occasionally)

* i.e. *not* IgE-dependent and *not* requiring prior antigen
exposure; cf. anaphylaxis

Crossreactive drug sensitivity
1 p-Aminobenzoates
   — Sulfonamides
   — Sulfonylureas
   — Thiazides
   — Phenothiazines
   — Procainamide
   — Acetazolamide
2 Penicillins
   — Penicillin G
   — Semisynthetic penicillins
   — Penicillamine
   — Cephalosporins
3 Allopurinol-induced maculopapular rash is
   commoner if past history of ampicillin rash, esp. if
   renal dysfunction (ampicillin rash also commoner in
   allopurinol patients)

Clinical aspects of penicillin hypersensitivity
1 *Allergic* reactions most commonly occur with
   semisynthetic penicillins; such reactions represent
   major determinant (i.e. penicilloyl group of the
   cleaved β-lactam ring) hypersensitivity mediated by
   IgG/IgM antibodies
2 True IgE-dependent *anaphylactic* reactions are rare
   (incidence 0.05%, mortality 0.0002%); such reactions
   commoner with parenteral administration, esp. of
   benzylpenicillin, and represent *minor determinant*
   (penilloate, penicillin or penicilloic acid), or hapten,
   hypersensitivity

3 *Fatal* anaphylactic reactions usually occur in patients with *no* past history of penicillin allergy or atopy. To confirm a past history of anaphylaxis, prick testing is indicated

4 85% of patients with history of minor reactions can be re-exposed without toxicity, perhaps indicating transient sensitization; only major contraindication is anaphylaxis

5 Cephalosporin cross-sensitization occurs, but is uncommon

6 If penicillin is required for a serious bacterial infection in a patient with a history of penicillin-induced anaphylaxis, temporary desensitization may be undertaken and completed within 4 h*

* NB: Desensitization works by raising the cell threshold to IgE; it *cannot* be performed using steroid or antihistamine cover

IMMUNOSUPPRESSIVE THERAPY

Alternate-day steroids: guidelines for use
1 Benefits
   — Less growth retardation in children
   — Less HPA axis suppression
   — Fewer infective complications
   — Less aseptic necrosis, cataracts
2 Problems
   — Less likely to be effective in remission induction
3 Useful in
   — Polymyositis
   — Myasthenia gravis
4 Ineffective in
   — Giant cell arteritis
   — Severe rheumatoid arthritis
   — Chronic active hepatitis
   — Asthma

Therapeutic immunosuppression: which drug?
1 Azathioprine
   — Renal transplantation
   — HBsAg-negative chronic active hepatitis
   — SLE
   — Behçet's syndrome (esp. with uveitis)
2 Cyclophosphamide
   — Wegener's, lymphomatoid granulomatosis
   — PAN, systemic vasculitis, SLE with renal involvement
3 Methotrexate
   — Severe psoriasis (e.g. pustular)
   — Reiter's syndrome
   — Dermatomyositis, pemphigus (steroid-sparing)
4 Cyclosporin
   — Bone marrow transplantation (helps prevent graft rejection in aplasia, GVHD in leukemia)
   — Immunosuppression in renal transplantation
   — Anecdotal
     • Insulin-dependent diabetes (early stages)
     • Graves' ophthalmopathy
     • Sarcoidosis
     • Behçet's
5 Antilymphocyte (-thymocyte) globulin
   — Organ transplantation
   — Aplastic anemia

Mechanisms implicated in therapeutic immunosuppression
1 Corticosteroids
   — Polymorphs
     • ↓ Extravascular egress (impaired chemotaxis)
     • Post-phagocytic defect (↓ intracellular killing)
   — Mononuclears
     • Extravascular trapping (↓ T cell number/function)
     • Impaired antibody-antigen uptake
     • ↓ Immunoglobulin synthesis
   — Eosinopenia
   — ↓ Interleukin-2 levels
2 Azathioprine
   — Prodrug for 6MP (metabolized in liver)
   — Reduced lymphocyte proliferation
   — Impaired lymphokine release
   — Reduced antibody synthesis
3 Cyclosporin
   — Fungal cyclic polypeptide
   — Binds peptidyl prolyl isomerases*
   — No lympholytic action; no myelosuppression
   — ↓ IL-2 release (→ ↓ T cell activation)
   — ↓ IL-1 levels, ↓ helper T cell number
4 FK 506, rapamycin (investigational)
   — Macrolide (erythromycin-like) structure
   — Binds peptidyl prolyl isomerases (like cyclosporin)
   — 100 times more potent than cyclosporin
5 Antilymphocyte globulin
   — Reduction of circulating lymphocyte pool
   — Suppression of cell-mediated immunity

* Enzymes which mediate both protein folding and lymphocyte activation

General indications for cytotoxic immunosuppression
1 Uncontrolled disease despite non-cytotoxic therapy, esp. if major organ involvement (e.g. in vasculitis, sarcoid)
2 Unacceptable steroid side-effects
3 Organ transplantation
4 Wegener's granulomatosis, PAN

Comparative morbidity of immunosuppressive therapy
1 Azathioprine
   — Neutropenia; impaired cell-mediated immunity
   — Cholestasis, pancreatitis
   — Lymphomas; SCC (skin/cervix)
   — 4-fold ↑ bioavailability (hence, toxicity) if given with allopurinol (also true for oral 6MP)
2 Cyclophosphamide
   — Myelosuppression, sterility, alopecia
   — Cystitis, bladder fibrosis/cancer (avoided with mesna)
   — AML (less frequent than with chlorambucil)
3 Methotrexate
   — Hepatotoxicity (liver fibrosis) with long-term therapy
   — No demonstrated second malignancy rate
4 Cyclosporin*
   — Nephrotoxicity (esp. older patients)
     • Prolonged post-transplant oliguria
   — Lymphoma
     • May regress on dose reduction (?EBV-induced)
   — Hypertension
     • Despite normal renal function/renin levels

— CNS syndrome
  • Cortical blindness, confusion, pyramidal lesions
— Other: hepatotoxicity, hirsutism, gum
  hypertrophy‡, tremor, breast lumps, gout
5 Antilymphocyte globulin
— Transfusion reactions
— CMV viremia

* Ketoconazole delays cyclosporin metabolism, thus either increasing toxicity or reducing cyclosporin dose requirement by 60–80%
‡ NB: Some cases reported of gingival carcinoma arising on cyclosporin

Patient evaluation prior to glucocorticoid therapy
1 Urinalysis (glycosuria), urine culture
2 Blood pressure
3 Chest X-ray
4 Measurement of intraocular pressure in patients with diabetes, severe myopia or family history of glaucoma

INTERFERONS

Varieties of interferon
1 Interferon-α ('leukocyte')
— Derived originally from human monocytes
— Now mainly produced using recombinant techniques
2 Interferon-β (fibroblast)
— Derived from human fibroblasts
— 30% amino acid homology with interferon-α
3 Interferon-λ ('immune')*
— Derived from human T cells
— No homology with interferon-α or β

* May offer effective prophylaxis against infection in chronic granulomatous disease

Physiological actions of interferons
1 Inhibit viral replication (e.g. in chronic HBV infection)
2 Activate NK cells and macrophages
3 Increase HLA antigen expression
4 Increase plasma membrane rigidity

Indications for interferon-α immunotherapy
1 Established indications
— Hairy cell leukemia (90% response rate)
— Chronic active hepatitis B or C
— Juvenile laryngeal papillomatosis (HPV-induced)
— Kaposi's sarcoma in AIDS
2 Investigational indications
— Essential mixed cryoglobulinemia*
— CML (chronic phase)
— Lymphoma (cutaneous T cell, aggressive NHL)
— Islet cell tumors, esp. VIPoma
— Genital warts

* esp. if associated with anti-HCV

Toxicity of interferon
1 'Flu-like syndrome; lethargy, somnolence
2 Nausea, vomiting, anorexia, diarrhea
3 Thrombocytopenia and/or neutropenia
4 Dysgeusia, xerostomia
5 Abnormal liver function tests
6 Reversible cardiac dysfunction

TRANSPLANTATION

Renal transplantation: predictors of successful engraftment
1 Essential
— ABO compatibility
— Negative cytotoxic crossmatch (MLC)
2 Desirable
— HLA-B/DR matching (esp. DR)
— Prior transfusions

Marrow transplantation: predictors of successful engraftment
1 Negative cytotoxic crossmatch
2 HLA-B/DR matching
3 Satisfactory number of transplanted cells
4 No prior transfusions

Clinical hazards of bone marrow transplantation
1 For immunodeficiency (e.g. Wiskott–Aldrich)
— Graft-versus-host disease (GVHD) especially
2 For aplastic anemia
— Graft rejection especially
3 For acute leukemia
— GVHD, rejection and disease relapse constitute approximately equivalent risks to survival

Classification of transplant rejection
1 Hyperacute
— Complement-fixing antibodies in recipient serum prior to transplant → irreversible Ag-Ab reaction usually presenting as graft thrombosis
2 Acute
— Potentially reversible reaction due to cell-mediated immunity; occurs unpredictably and at any time
3 Chronic
— Irreversible process due to subendothelial antibody deposition and arteriolar narrowing

Post-transplant malignancies
1 Squamous cell carcinoma of skin
2 Squamous cell carcinoma of cervix (usually in situ)
3 Non-Hodgkin's lymphoma
— In azathioprine-treated patients → CNS
— In cyclosporin-treated patients → GIT/lung
4 Acute myeloblastic leukemia*

* NB: Only occurs after therapy with alkylators and/or irradiation

VASCULITIS THERAPY

Drug therapy in SLE: a rough guide
1 Minimally symptomatic disease
— Withhold medication
2 Tenosynovitis, arthralgias, pleurisy
— NSAIDs (except aspirin: potentially hepatotoxic)
3 Skin disease and/or joint symptoms resistant to NSAIDs
— Topical steroids (for rash)
— Hydroxychloroquine 200–400 mg/day
4 Refractory arthritis (sepsis excluded)
Immune leukopenia/thrombocytopenia

Fevers
— Prednisone 0.5 mg/kg/day
5 Immune hemolysis
Pneumonitis, peritonitis
Myositis
— Prednisone 0.75 mg/kg/day
6 Myopericarditis
Focal glomerulonephritis
Vasculitis, neuropathy
— Prednisone 1 mg/kg/day*
7 Diffuse proliferative glomerulonephritis
Membranous glomerulonephritis
— Acute phase (first 12 weeks)
• Pulse IV methylprednisolone 1 mg/kg/day, *plus*
• Cyclophosphamide* (2–3 mg/kg/day orally)
— Maintenance phase
• Azathioprine 1 mg/kg/day
8 Cerebral lupus
— Exclude infection, use anticonvulsants and tailor immunosuppression as above

NB: If prolonged therapy > 10 mg/day prednisone is required, azathioprine may be added as a steroid-sparing agent
* May prolong survival

General measures in Raynaud's phenomenon
1 Cold avoidance (effective in 50% of all patients)
— Thermal underwear
— Gloves, warm socks (may be electrically heated)
— Maintenance of *steady* ambient temperature
2 Other general measures
— Arm exercises, biofeedback
— Stop smoking (esp. in Buerger's disease)
— Cessation of β-blockers, ergotamine

Specific therapies for Raynaud's disease
1 Oral nifedipine 20–60 mg/day
— Drug of choice: reduces attack frequency and severity
— Inhibits both vasospasm and platelet aggregation
— Effective in 50% of patients requiring medication
Alternative calcium blockers
— Diltiazem 60 mg t.d.s.
— Nicardipine, felodipine, isradipine
2 Glyceryl trinitrate 2% ointment
— Useful for Raynaud's affecting odd sites, e.g. nipples
— Works only transiently; causes headaches
3 Iloprost (prostacyclin analog)
— Particularly useful in aborting prolonged severe attacks, e.g. to prevent digital ulceration/ necrosis
— Requires IV administration in hospital
4 Second-line approaches in mild disease
— ACE inhibitors
— α-blockers (thymoxamine, prazosin)
— Ketanserin, naftidrofuryl (serotonin antagonists)
— Sympathectomy (for Raynaud's of the feet)
5 Plasma exchange
— Cryoglobulinemia patients esp.
6 Unproven therapies popular with patients
— Evening primrose oil (linolenic/gamolenic acid)
— Fish oil (p. 77)

Approach to infective complications in the AIDS patient
1 Infections for which effective therapy exists
— *P. carinii* pneumonia (commonest infection)
• Prophylaxis: oral co-trimoxazole *or* nebulized pentamidine (less effective, better tolerated)
• Treatment: IV or oral co-trimoxazole depending on infection severity
• Adjunctive steroids may be of value in respiratory failure (PaO_2 < 9 kPa)
— Toxoplasmosis (e.g. cerebral mass lesions)
• R_x: sulfadiazine + pyrimethamine
— Cryptococcosis (e.g. meningitis or disseminated)
• R_x: (oral) fluconazole *or* (IV) amphotericin
— Candidiasis
• R_x: fluconazole
2 Infections for which promising therapy exists
— CMV
• Ganciclovir*, foscarnet
— *M. avium-intracellulare* (MAI)
• Azithromycin, clarithromycin
• Rifabutin, ciprofloxacin
3 Infections for which no effective therapy exists
— Cryptosporidiosis

* Efficacy now virtually established

Indications for *P. carinii* prophylaxis in HIV-infected patients
1 T_H (CD4 cell) count < 0.2×10^9/L
2 T_H:total lymphocyte ratio < 1.5
3 Oral thrush
4 Unexplained fever
5 Kaposi's sarcoma
6 Cerebral toxoplasmosis
7 Past history of *P. carinii* pneumonia

Mechanisms of zidovudine action
1 Structural analog of thymidine
2 Phosphorylated to zidovudine phosphates on entering cells
3 Zidovudine monophosphate inhibits production of important HIV metabolites, thymidine di- and triphosphate
4 Zidovudine triphosphate inhibits HIV reverse transcriptase

Subjective benefits of zidovudine therapy in AIDS
1 Improved functional capacity and quality of life
2 Reduced frequency of opportunistic infections
3 More rapid recovery from major infective complications*
4 Slowed disease progression‡
5 Improved survival from HIV encephalopathy

* May also hasten neuropathy resolution during initial seroconversion phase
‡ Also in ARC, but not in asymptomatic phase

Quantitative indices of zidovudine benefit
1 ↑ Weight
2 ↑ CD4+ lymphocyte number
3 ↓ HIV p24 antigenemia
4 ↑ Platelets (if thrombocytopenic)

Limitations of zidovudine therapy
1 Limited efficacy
   — *Inhibits* HIV reverse transcriptase* but does not *eradicate* intracellular HIV
   — Transient effect (resistance develops)
2 Toxicity
   — Nausea
   — Macrocytic anemia/neutropenia
   — Mitochondrial myopathy‡
3 Short half-life (~ 1 h)
   — Frequent (e.g. 4-hourly) dosage may be required¶
4 Expense

* Thus preventing infection of new CD4+ cells
‡ DD_x: polymyositis, primary HIV myopathy. Hence, proceed to biopsy if no improvement after 2 weeks' zidovudine cessation; inflammatory infiltrates may indicate steroids plus zidovudine reintroduction
¶ Optimal dosage schedule is *not* yet empirically established

UNDERSTANDING IMMUNOLOGICAL DISEASE

Isotypes, idiotypes and antiidiotypic antibodies
1 The class of an antibody (IgG, IgM, etc.) is its *isotype*
2 Highly variable heavy and light chain regions (where antigen and antibody combine, i.e. in the Fab fragment) constitute a unique antibody specificity termed *idiotype*
3 Particular structural antigenic determinants comprising a given idiotype are termed *idiotopes*
4 An immunoglobulin contains many idiotopes which can generate a large number of *antiidiotypic antibodies* raised against these antigens (cf. rheumatoid factors: antibodies raised against the constant Fc portion of the antibody)
5 Circulating idiotype/antiidiotype immune complexes have been demonstrated, e.g. in cryoglobulinemia, SLE

Regulatory functions of some interleukins
1 Interleukin 1 (IL-1)
   — Following antigen recognition, IL-1 is released by activated macrophages, leading to stimulation of helper (CD4+) T cells with release of IL-2
   — Also induces proliferation of activated B cells
2 Interleukin-2 (IL-2), 'T cell growth factor'
   — Mitogenic for T cells and natural killer (NK) cells
   — Released by CD4+ (helper) T cells*
   — Stimulates IFN-γ production
3 Interleukin-3 (IL-3, multi-CSF)
   — Released by T cells and other cells
   — Stimulates growth of most hemopoietic stem cells

* cf. IL-1; released by monocytes/macrophages

Lymphocytes: functional aspects
1 B cells
   — Defense against extracellular bacteria, protozoa

   — Prevention of viral reinfection in immune host
2 T cells
   — Defense against intracellular bacteria
   — Defense against viruses (esp. herpes), fungi, protozoa
3 K ('killer') cells
   — Mediate antibody-dependent cell-mediated cytotoxicity (ADCC), e.g. against measles
4 NK ('natural killer') cells
   — Non-antigen specific action
   — Postulated but unproven role in 'tumor surveillance'

CLINICAL IMMUNE DEFECTS

Clinical patterns of lymphocyte dysfunction
1 Ataxia-telangiectasia (Louis–Bar syndrome)
   — ↓ IgA
   — ↓ Cell-mediated immunity
   — Causes recurrent sinopulmonary infections
   — May terminate as lymphoma
2 Wiskott–Aldrich syndrome (WAS)
   — ↓ IgM; ↑ IgA/E
   — ↓ Cell-mediated immunity
   — ↓ Platelets
   — Causes eczema, abscesses, bleeding
   — May terminate as lymphoma

Infective complications of compromised immunity
1 Defective cell-mediated immunity (incl. Hodgkin's, sarcoid)
   — Intracellular bacteria (TB, *Listeria* spp.)
   — Candidiasis, cryptococcosis
   — CMV, HZ; toxoplasmosis
   — *Pneumocystis*, atypical mycobacteria
2 Hypogammaglobulinemia (incl. CLL, myeloma)
   — Extracellular bacteria (e.g. pneumococcus, *Staph. aureus*)
   — *Mycoplasma* (septic arthritis, pneumonia)
   — CNS enteroviruses (e.g. ECHO in Bruton's)
   — Warts (↓ IgM); giardiasis, *Campylobacter* enteritis
3 Hyposplenism/post-splenectomy
   — Encapsulated bacteria (pneumococci, *H. influenzae*, *Salmonella* spp., *Neisseria* spp.); babesiosis*
4 Hypocomplementemia
   — ↓ $C_{2,3}$ → recurrent pyogenic infections, esp.
     • *Staph. aureus*
     • Streptococci
     • *H. influenzae*
   — ↓ $C_{6,7,8}$ → *Neisseria* spp. esp.
5 Combined B and T cell defects (CLL, SCID, WAS, Louis–Bar)
   — Recurrent sinopulmonary infections (CMV, Gram-negatives, anerobes, *Staph. aureus*)
6 Steroid therapy
   — Aspergillosis
   — *P. carinii*

* In endemic areas, e.g. Massachusetts

PROBLEMS WITH POLYMORPHS

Clinical patterns of leukocyte dysfunction
1 Chédiak–Higashi syndrome
  — ↓ Neutrophil function (↓ intracellular killing)
  — Associated with partial oculocutaneous albinism
  — Due to myeloperoxidase deficiency
  — Treatable with vitamin C
2 Chronic granulomatous disease of childhood (CGDC)
  — ↓ Intracellular killing (post-phagocytic defect)
  — ↓ H_2O_2 generation
  — + NBT test (diagnostic)
  — *Staph. aureus*/Gram-negatives/*Nocardia* spp./ *Serratia*
3 Job's/hyper-IgE syndrome
  — ↓ Intracellular killing
  — ↓ T cell number
  — ↑ IgE
  — Recurrent staphylococcal abscesses; herpes
4 'Lazy leukocyte' syndrome
  — ↓ Chemotaxis
5 Leukocyte adhesion deficiency (LAD)
  — Defective β-chain of LFA-1 integrin
  — Associated with neutrophilia, but absent pus formation
  — Severe bacterial childhood infections (e.g. pneumonia)

Infective complications of neutrophil dysfunction
1 Neutropenia
  — Pneumonia (enterococci, Gram-negatives, *Staph. aureus*)
  — Perirectal suppuration
  — Pharyngostomatitis (esp. candidal)
  — Recurrent bacteremias
2 Defective neutrophil chemotaxis (steroids, diabetes, alcohol)
  — Abscesses, cellulitis (*Staph. aureus*, strep, *Ps. aeruginosa*)
3 Defective intracellular killing (CGDC, Job's, Chédiak–Higashi)
  — Abscesses (*E. coli, Staph. aureus*)
  — Septic arthritis/osteomyelitis (*Salmonella, Serratia*)

PRIMARY IMMUNE-DEFICIENT STATES

Varieties of primary immunoglobulin deficiency
1 X-linked (Bruton's) agammaglobulinemia*
2 IgG subclass deficiencies
3 Selective IgA deficiency
4 Common variable immunodeficiency

* Prone to enteroviral (esp. echovirus) infections; antibody-deficient patients are otherwise not usually troubled by viral infections

Selective IgA deficiency*: clinical features
1 Sinopulmonary infections (± otitis media)
2 Giardiasis (severe and prolonged)
3 Autoimmune diathesis (e.g. thrombocytopenia), atopy

4 Anaphylactic reactions triggered by small amounts of IgA in transfusions (blood or plasma) or gammaglobulin

* Surface IgA present *but* B cells fail to differentiate to plasma cells; may be associated with ↓ IgG_2. Often asymptomatic; affects one in 700

Common variable hypogammaglobulinemia*: complications
1 Allergies; autoimmune diathesis
2 Gastrointestinal complications
  — Giardiasis
  — Gluten-sensitive enteropathy/dermatitis herpetiformis
  — Nodular lymphoid hyperplasia
  — Achlorhydria/atrophic gastritis; 50 x ↑ gastric cancer
3 Splenomegaly; lung/liver granulomata
4 Polyarthritis
5 Thymoma esp. in late-onset disease (i.e. onset after 40 years)

* *Normal* B cell number – cf. Bruton's – but fail to differentiate into plasma cells and secrete immunoglobulins; hence, low serum IgG and IgA

SECONDARY IMMUNE DEFECTS

Etiology of acquired hyposplenism
1 Splenectomy
  — Trauma (incl. operative)
  — Hypersplenism, esp.
    • ITP
    • Hereditary spherocytosis
    • Thalassemia
  — Hodgkin's staging (now uncommon)
2 Autosplenectomy
  — Repeated infarction in sickle-cell disease
3 Celiac disease
4 Rare
  — SLE
  — Ulcerative colitis
  — Amyloidosis
  — Sarcoidosis
  — Thyrotoxicosis
  — Lymphoma, CML

Recommended vaccinations for the hyposplenic patient
1 Pneumococcal*
2 Hib (*H. influenzae* type b)
3 Meningococcal groups A and C

* Best evidence for efficacy is in patients vaccinated *prior* to elective splenectomy; doubtful value post-splenectomy

Features of overwhelming post-splenectomy infection (OPSI)
1 Incidence of OPSI is 1% in children, 0.1% in adults
2 Incidence is greatest in first 3 years post-splenectomy
  Ten-year OPSI incidence is ~ 7%
3 Pneumococcal OPSI is a particular risk if age < 20

4 Incidence of OPSI varies with indication for splenectomy
5 10–20% of OPSI cases are polymicrobial

Effective antibiotic prophylaxis regimens post-splenectomy
1 Phenoxymethylpenicillin
   • 125 mg b.d. (age < 6)
   • 250 mg b.d. (age 6–12)
   • 500 mg b.d. (age > 12)
2 Amoxycillin
   — Covers *H. influenzae* as well as pneumococcus
   • 250 mg b.d. (age < 10)
   • 500 mg b.d. (age > 10)
3 Erythromycin
   — If penicillin-allergic
   • 125 mg b.d. (age < 3)
   • 250 mg b.d. (age > 3)

Clinical associations of thymoma
1 Myasthenia gravis (40%)
2 Pure red cell aplasia (*not* corrected by thymectomy)
3 Common variable hypogammaglobulinemia
4 Chronic mucocutaneous candidiasis
5 Autoimmune disease
   — Sjögren's syndrome
   — SLE
   — Dermatomyositis
   — Hashimoto's/Graves' disease
   — Pemphigus

Predispositions to recurrent localized infections
1 Recurrent candidiasis
   — Steroids (incl. estrogens, pregnancy)
   — Broad-spectrum antibiotic therapy
   — T cell defects
2 Recurrent boils (furunculosis)*
   — Hypogammaglobulinemia
   — Hypocomplementemia
   — Job's/hyper-IgE syndrome
3 Recurrent candidiasis *or* boils
   — Diabetes mellitus
   — Iron deficiency‡
   — HIV infection

* Usually idiopathic
‡ Often subclinical; no anemia

Skin infections in immunosuppressed patients
1 'Transplant elbow'
   — *Staph. aureus*
2 Cellulitis
   — Streptococci
3 Opportunistic bacteria
   — *Nocardia*, atypical mycobacteria
4 Fungi
   — *Aspergillus, Cryptococcus*
5 Viruses
   — Herpes simplex, varicella-zoster; HPV

HIV AND ACQUIRED IMMUNODEFICIENCY

Immunological abnormalities in the AIDS patient
1 T cells

   — ↓ Helper (CD4+) T cell number*
   — ↓ T cell function (↓ IL-2/IFN-α response to Ag)
   — ↓ Cytotoxic (CD8+) T cell response to HIV-infected cells
   — Cutaneous anergy
2 B cells
   — ↓ Function (↓ humoral response to vaccination)
   — Activation → polyclonal hypergammaglobulinemia
3 NK cells
   — ↓ Number and function
4 Monocytes/macrophages
   — ↓ Function (↓ IL-1, chemotaxis, antigen presentation)

* Normally > 0.7 x 10^9/L; falls to < 0.2 x 10^9/L

Some molecular biological aspects of HIV
1 Structurally related to animal lentiviruses and contains
   — Core protein (p24)
   — Reverse transcriptase
   — Envelope (*env*) glycoproteins (gp120, gp41)
2 HIV-2 (West Africa) expresses different *env* region Hence, may be associated with 'false-negative' serology
3 The *env* protein gp120 resembles the T_H marker CD4 HIV binds and enters T_H cells via CD4 Most AIDS manifestations reflect consequent T_H dysfunction

High-risk transmission modes for HIV infection
1 Bloodborne transmission
   — Needle sharing, e.g. heroin addicts
   — Multiple transfusions, esp. hemophiliacs
   — Transplacental/peripartum neonatal infection
2 Venereal transmission
   — Homosexuals
   — Prostitutes (female or male)
   — Promiscuous heterosexuals, esp. uncircumcised

Occurrence of Kaposi's sarcoma in HIV-infected cohorts
1 Seen commonly in homosexuals with AIDS*
2 Seen occasionally in intravenous drug abusers with AIDS
3 Seen rarely in hemophiliacs with AIDS

* Fecal–oral contact appears to predispose

Infective complications of early HIV infection
1 Oral candidiasis
2 Herpesviruses (zoster, recurrent herpes simplex, CMV)
3 Staphylococcal infections
4 Oral hairy leukoplakia* (EBV)
5 Antibiotic hypersensitivity reactions

* Virtually pathognomonic of HIV infection

Infective complications of advanced HIV infection
1 *Pneumocystis carinii* pneumonia*
2 CMV infection, esp. pneumonitis/retinitis/colitis‡
3 Invasive mucosal candidiasis, esp. esophageal
4 Cryptococcosis, aspergillosis, histoplasmosis
5 Intestinal cryptosporidiosis, isosporiasis (esp. in Haitians)

6 Disseminated (extraintestinal) strongyloidiasis
7 Toxoplasmosis, esp. CNS
8 Mycobacterial infections, esp. *avium-intracellulare*¶
9 Recurrent *Salmonella* bacteremias
10 Disseminated zoster

* Presentation of AIDS in 50%; affects 80% of patients at least once; 10% die with first infection; 50% relapse within 12 months
‡ Treat with ganciclovir; cf. CMV adrenalitis, treat with steroid replacement
¶ May cause marrow depression; infection confirmed in 50% of AIDS autopsies

Indirect sequelae of HIV infection*

1 Progressive multifocal leukoencephalopathy (JC virus)
2 Cerebral lymphoma (EBV)
3 Kaposi's sarcoma (but see ref. 6.9)

4 Hairy leukoplakia
5 Cardiomyopathy‡

* i.e. believed to be precipitated by immunodeficiency (e.g. via a second viral infection) rather than directly by HIV
‡ Infective basis unproven; also may occur with interferon-α therapy

Neurologic complications of HIV infection

1 Subacute diffuse encephalitis
2 Meningitis (incl. cryptococcal)
3 Progressive multifocal leukoencephalopathy
4 Space-occupying lesion(s)
   — Cerebral toxoplasmosis*
   — Non-Hodgkin's lymphoma
5 Myelitis (CMV, HSV type 2)
6 Neuropathies

* Negative serology makes diagnosis unlikely

REVIEWING THE LITERATURE: IMMUNOLOGY

6.1 Valentine MD et al (1990) The value of immunotherapy with venom in children with allergy to insect stings. N Engl J Med 323: 1601–1603

Venom immunotherapy effectively prevented further systemic reactions to insect stings in this semi-randomized study of 242 once-bitten children. However, since only 9% of non-immunized children had a second 'reaction' to stings, the authors conclude that immunization is unnecessary for most 'insect-sting-allergic' children.

6.2 International Rheumatic Fever Study Group (1991) Allergic reactions to long-term benzathine penicillin prophylaxis for rheumatic fever. Lancet 337: 1308–1310

Study of 1790 patients receiving monthly penicillin injections to prevent recrudescence of rheumatic fever. Prophylaxis was effective, while anaphylaxis occurred in only 0.2% per year (3% had an allergic reaction). One fatality was due to anaphylaxis, but overall this regimen seems well worthwhile.

6.3 Weeks JC et al (1991) Cost effectiveness of prophylactic intravenous immune globulin in chronic lymphocytic leukemia. N Engl J Med 325: 81–86

Study estimating cost-benefit of IV gammaglobulin prophylaxis in CLL patients: works out as ~ $6 million per quality-adjusted life year saved.

6.4 Galli M et al (1990) Anticardiolipin antibodies (ACA) directed not to cardiolipin but to a plasma protein cofactor. Lancet 335: 1544–1547

Khamashta MA et al (1990) Association of antibodies against phospholipids with heart valve disease in systemic lupus erythematosus. Lancet 335: 1541–1544

The first study showed that antiphospholipid antibodies could also be directed against β_2-glycoprotein I (apolipoprotein H) as well as against cardiolipin, consistent with the recognized thrombotic association (see text). The second paper confirms the association of mitral valve vegetations (in 16%) and mitral regurgitation (38%) – so-called Libman–Sacks endocarditis – with phospholipid antibodies.

6.5 Boumpas DT et al (1992) Controlled trial of pulse methylprednisolone versus two regimens of pulse cyclophosphamide in severe lupus nephritis. Lancet 340: 741–745

Lewis EJ et al (1992) A controlled trial of plasmapheresis therapy in severe lupus nephritis. N Engl J Med 326: 1373–1379

The first study suggested that prolonged courses of pulse cyclophosphamide are superior to pulse steroids in preserving renal function in SLE, while the second indicated that addition of plasmapheresis to such regimens is generally useless.

6.6 Miller FW et al (1992) Controlled trial of plasma exchange and leukapheresis in polymyositis and dermatomyositis. N Engl J Med 326: 1380–1384

Study indicating lack of significant benefit in patients receiving either plasma exchange or apheresis.

6.7 Anderson RM et al (1991) The spread of HIV-1 in Africa: sexual contact patterns and the predicted demographic impact of AIDS. Nature 352: 581–586

Analysis suggesting that African AIDS may decimate much of the continent's population over the next few decades.

6.8 Goedert JJ et al (1991) High risk of HIV-1 infection for first-born twins. Lancet 338: 1471–1475

Clark SJ et al (1991) High titers of cytopathic virus in plasma of patients with symptomatic primary HIV-1 infection. N Engl J Med 324: 954–960

Ou C et al (1992) Molecular epidemiology of HIV transmission in a dental practice. Science 256: 1165–1169

Three papers attesting to the infectivity of bloodborne HIV. The first indicated a 50% risk of 'first-born' HIV transmission, compared with 19% of second-born twins, suggesting that intrapartum trauma associated with initial delivery could be responsible; Caesarean section (only) partially reduced this differential. The second paper shows that within 2 weeks of symptom onset, primary HIV patients have up to 1000 tissue culture-infective HIV doses per ml of their plasma. The final paper summarizes the infamous case of the dentist who transmitted HIV to five of his patients.

Bryson YJ et al (1995) Clearance of HIV infection in a perinatally infected infant. N Engl J Med 332: 833–838

Controversial study in which a putatively HIV-positive infant appeared to develop secondary immunity to the virus, which disappeared.

6.9 Simonds RJ et al (1992) Transmission of human immunodeficiency virus type I from a seronegative organ and tissue donor. N Engl J Med 326: 726–732

Urnovitz HB et al (1993) HIV-1 antibody serum negativity with urine positivity. Lancet 342: 1458–1459

Two papers showing that all which is seronegative is not gold. In the first case report, viral culture and PCR detected (in retrospect) HIV in the blood and tissues of an organ donor who had died prior to developing antibodies. In the second study of 12 patients, false-negative results from serum ELISA and/or Western blot were ultimately straightened out by doing urine ELISA in conjunction with cell-mediated immune responses.

Huang YQ et al (1995) Human herpesvirus-like nucleic acid in various forms of Kaposi's sarcoma. Lancet 345: 759–761

One of several PCR studies spotting the expression of herpes-like DNA sequences in Kaposi's – now characterised as HHV-8.

6.10 Hamilton JD et al for the Veterans Affairs Cooperative Study (1992) A controlled trial of early versus late treatment with zidovudine in symptomatic human immunodeficiency virus infection. N Engl J Med 326: 437–443

Concorde Coordinating Committee (1994) Concorde: MRC/ANRS randomised double-blind controlled trial of immediate and deferred zidovudine in symptom-free HIV infection. Lancet 343: 871–881

Lenderking WR et al for the AIDS Clinical Trials Group (1994) Evaluation of the quality of life associated with zidovudine treatment in asymptomatic human immunodeficiency virus infection. N Engl J Med 330: 738–743

Three studies hinting at limited benefit for zidovudine therapy. The Veterans' study of 338 patients indicated no improvement in survival and significant side-effects; but there did appear to be some delay in progression for patients treated early. In contrast, the large Concorde study looked at 1749 patients and detected no statistically significant difference in outcome attributable to the timing of zidovudine intervention; treatment of asymptomatic patients was therefore discouraged. The other American study of 1338 asymptomatic HIV patients concluded that zidovudine side-effects cancelled out any net benefit of early intervention, notwithstanding apparently delayed progression.

CHAPTER 7

Infectious disease

Physical examination protocol 7.1   You are asked to examine a patient with fever of unknown origin

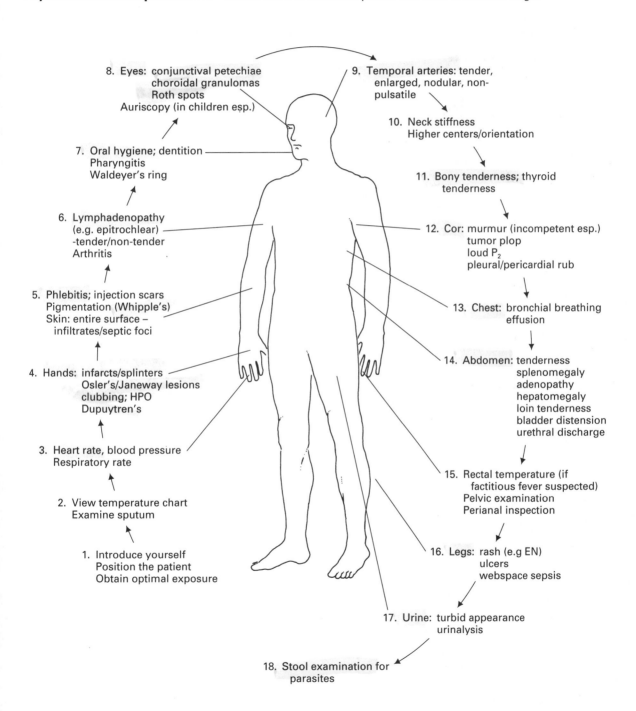

8. Eyes: conjunctival petechiae
   choroidal granulomas
   Roth spots
   Auriscopy (in children esp.)

7. Oral hygiene; dentition
   Pharyngitis
   Waldeyer's ring

6. Lymphadenopathy
   (e.g. epitrochlear)
   -tender/non-tender
   Arthritis

5. Phlebitis; injection scars
   Pigmentation (Whipple's)
   Skin: entire surface –
   infiltrates/septic foci

4. Hands: infarcts/splinters
   Osler's/Janeway lesions
   clubbing; HPO
   Dupuytren's

3. Heart rate, blood pressure
   Respiratory rate

2. View temperature chart
   Examine sputum

1. Introduce yourself
   Position the patient
   Obtain optimal exposure

9. Temporal arteries: tender,
   enlarged, nodular, non-
   pulsatile

10. Neck stiffness
    Higher centers/orientation

11. Bony tenderness; thyroid
    tenderness

12. Cor: murmur (incompetent esp.)
    tumor plop
    loud P_2
    pleural/pericardial rub

13. Chest: bronchial breathing
    effusion

14. Abdomen: tenderness
    splenomegaly
    adenopathy
    hepatomegaly
    loin tenderness
    bladder distension
    urethral discharge

15. Rectal temperature (if
    factitious fever suspected)
    Pelvic examination
    Perianal inspection

16. Legs: rash (e.g EN)
    ulcers
    webspace sepsis

17. Urine: turbid appearance
    urinalysis

18. Stool examination for
    parasites

Diagnostic pathway 7.1   The patient has an enlarged spleen. Which etiologies would you suspect most strongly?

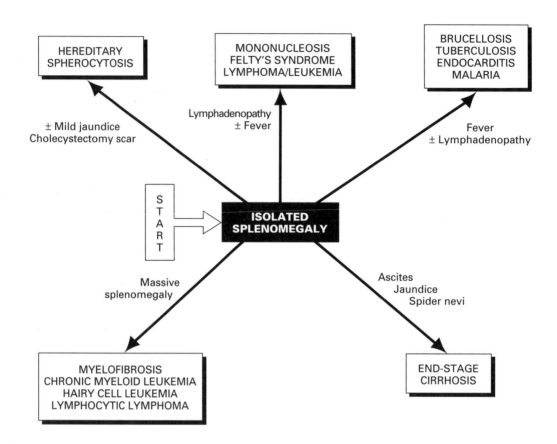

CLINICAL ASPECTS OF INFECTIOUS DISEASE

Commonest infectious disease short cases
1 Pneumonia
2 Infective endocarditis

Fever of unknown origin*: direct questions
1 Past medical history
   — Rheumatic fever
   — Tuberculosis
   — Splenectomy
2 Recent drug use
   — Antibiotics
   — Alcohol
   — Intravenous narcotics
3 Recent foreign travel
4 Recent sexual contacts and practices
5 Animal exposure (occupational or domestic)
6 Recent insect or tick bites (been camping?)
7 Recent ingestion of unusual or exotic food (incl. water, raw milk)
8 Family history and racial background

* defined here as fever with negative signs, CXR, MSU and blood cultures

Common fevers in patients returning from tropical countries
1 Malaria
2 Dengue (and Lassa, Ebola, etc.; p. 213)
3 Typhoid
4 Tick typhus
5 Amebic liver abscess
6 Schistosomiasis; visceral leishmaniasis
7 Tuberculosis
8 Brucellosis

Factitious fever: clinical clues
1 Patient's apparent well-being
2 Normal physical examination, cool skin, no sweating
3 No correlation between fever spikes and heart rate
4 Consistently normal rectal temperature
5 Dramatic fluctuations of temperature, often > 41°C
6 Absence of normal diurnal variation
7 Normal WCC, ESR
8 Recovery of multiple and/or unusual organisms
9 Typical patient profile: young, female, (para)medical

Classic fever patterns
1 Fevers recurring every 48 h
   — 'Tertian' malaria
     • *P. vivax* (± *ovale*): 'benign tertian'
     • *P. falciparum*: 'malignant tertian'
2 Fevers recurring every 72 h
   — 'Quartan' malaria
     • *P. malariae*
3 Fevers lasting 1–2 weeks, alternating with afebrile periods of similar duration
   — Hodgkin's disease (Pel–Ebstein fever; rare)
4 Fevers recurring every 3 weeks
   — Cyclic neutropenia

Differential diagnosis of night sweats
1 Pulmonary tuberculosis
2 Lymphoma
3 Brucellosis; abscess; endocarditis
4 Alcoholic withdrawal
5 Nocturnal hypoglycemia
   Nocturnal dyspnea
   Nightmares

Diagnostic significance of localized lymphadenopathy
1 Inguinal adenopathy
   — Venereal diseases* (pp. 206, 216)
   — Perianal sepsis or malignancy
   — Lymphoma
2 Occipital adenopathy
   — Scalp infection (e.g. fungal) or neoplasm
   — Viral infection (e.g. rubella)
3 Cervical adenopathy
   — Mononucleosis; other viral infection
   — Streptococcal infection
   — TB (scrofula)
   — Lymphoma
   — Kikuchi's histiocytic necrotizing lymphadenitis
4 Axillary adenopathy
   — Catscratch disease; dogbite
   — Lymphoma; lung or breast cancer
5 Epitrochlear adenopathy
   — Miliary TB
   — Local pyogenic infection
   — Lymphoma

* 'Groove sign' (adenopathy above and below inguinal ligament) is said to be classic of LGV

TUBERCULOSIS: CLINICAL

Skin manifestations of TB
1 Primary skin inoculation
   — Ulcer with regional adenopathy
2 Lupus vulgaris
   — Nodules, scarring, face and neck
3 Scrofuloderma
   — Cervical adenopathy, skin fixation
4 Erythema nodosum
   — Signifies onset of Mantoux reactivity
5 Erythema induratum (Bazin's disease)
   — Cyanotic nodules on calves with central necrosis

Manifestations commoner in primary TB infections
1 Chest
   — Pleurisy and/or large pleural effusion*
   — Lower zone infiltrate + ipsilateral hilar adenopathy
2 Cervical adenopathy
3 Erythema nodosum
4 Phlyctenular conjunctivitis
5 Acute miliary dissemination

* May follow rupture of peripheral caseous foci

Time-course of sequelae following untreated primary TB
1 First 3–4 weeks post-inoculation
   — Positive tuberculin test

— Erythema nodosum, fevers
— Phlyctenular conjunctivitis
  • esp. In children
2 After 4–8 weeks
— Appearance of primary focus on CXR
3 After 2–6 months
— Pleural effusion
4 After 3–12 months
— Bronchial rupture (erosion by caseating nodes)
— Tuberculous meningitis
— Miliary TB
5 After 1–3 years
— Bone and joint involvement
6 After 5 years
— Skin involvement
— Renal involvement

Misleading clinical presentations of TB
1 Night sweats, hilar adenopathy
  Misdiagnosis: lymphoma
2 PUO, granulomas, splenomegaly, erythema nodosum
  Misdiagnosis: sarcoidosis*
3 Right iliac fossa mass and/or ileitis on barium studies
  Misdiagnoses: Crohn's disease, yersiniosis, actinomycosis
4 Ureteric stricture(s)
  Misdiagnosis: idiopathic retroperitoneal fibrosis*
5 Headache, meningism, CSF lymphocytosis, neg. Gram-stain
  Misdiagnosis: viral meningitis
6 Constrictive pericarditis
  Misdiagnosis: restrictive cardiomyopathy‡
7 Bloodstained ascites
  Misdiagnosis: abdominal malignancy
8 Scrotal (epididymal) mass
  Misdiagnoses: tumor, syphilitic (testicular) gumma

* NB: Treated with steroids
‡ Attributable to (for example) endomyocardial fibrosis in African migrant

Clinical features of tuberculous meningitis
1 Significance
— Potentially life-threatening
2 Onset
— Subacute (days – weeks)
3 Symptoms and signs
— Fever
— Headache, meningism
— Impaired consciousness
4 Complications
— Hydrocephalus, cerebral edema, convulsions
— Cranial nerve palsies
— Arachnoiditis; hemiparesis
— SIADH

NON-TUBERCULOUS MYCOBACTERIA

Clinical significance of non-tuberculous mycobacteria
1 Rarely transmitted between humans
2 Clinical pattern of involvement similar to that of TB
3 Positive culture does not necessarily indicate pathogenicity in non-immunosuppressed patients
4 Clinical infection may indicate need for HIV serologic testing

Clinical spectrum of non-tuberculous mycobacterial disease
1 Pulmonary
— *M. avium-intracellulare*
  • Commonest and most serious pathogen
  • Predilection for diseased lungs or AIDS
  • Resistant to therapy (> 20% die)
— *M. fortuitum/chelonei*
  • Predilection for diseased lungs
  • Responds poorly to therapy
— *M. kansasii*
  • Responds well to therapy
— *M. xenopi, M. szulgai, M. simiae* (rare)
2 Skin/soft tissue
— *M. marinum*
  • Swimming-pool granuloma
  • Responds poorly to drug therapy
  • Usually resolves spontaneously
— *M. ulcerans*
  • Responds poorly to drug therapy
  • Treat by excision
— *M. fortuitum/chelonei*
  • Occurs following trauma or surgery
  • Best treated by initial debridement
3 Lymphadenitis (esp. cervical)
— *M. scrofulaceum*
  • Occurs in healthy children
  • Best treated by excision
  • Responds poorly to drug therapy
— *M. avium-intracellulare*
  • Treat by excision (see also p. 218)

SEXUALLY TRANSMITTED DISEASES

Post-exposure time-course of syphilitic presentations
1 Primary chancre
— 3–6 weeks
2 Secondary (skin) lesions
— 6 weeks–4 months
3 Meningitis
— 2–12 months
4 Meningovascular syphilis
— 4–8 years
5 General paresis of the insane (GPI)
— 5–25 years
6 Tabes dorsalis
— 10–50 years

Skin signs of secondary syphilis
1 Symmetric papulosquamous psoriasiform rash involving palms and soles; ± paronychia
2 Condylomata lata
3 Mucous patches (buccal)
  Mucosal erosions ('snail track' ulcers)
  Split papules
4 Leukoderma ('necklace of Venus')
5 Erythema nodosum
6 'Moth-eaten' alopecia

Clinical features of disseminated gonococcal infection
1 Typically occurs in young women or male homosexuals
   Symptoms of (primary) gonococcal infection may be absent
   Complicates approximately 2% of gonorrhea cases
2 Symptoms and signs include
   — Fever
   — Arthralgias/arthritis ± tenosynovitis
     • Asymmetrical; polyarticular, predilection for small joints of hands/wrists (cf. Reiter's)
   — Pustular hemorrhagic skin lesions, esp. on limbs
   — Myocarditis (may simulate rheumatic fever)
   — Hepatitis (may simulate hepatitis B, cholecystitis)
   — Perihepatitis (Fitz-Hugh Curtis syndrome*); if laparotomy is carried out in error, 'violin-string' adhesions are classically seen between the liver and abdominal wall (spread from fallopian tubes)
3 Laboratory investigations
   — Cultures of urethra, endocervix, rectum, pharynx
   — Blood and synovial fluid cultures: positivity of one tends to exclude the other; only 25% of clinically involved joints will yield gonococci
   — Culture of skin lesions (positive only occasionally)
4 Pathogen characteristics
   — Auxotype requires hypoxanthine/uracil for culture
   — Serum-resistant (resists serum antibody/C_3)
   — Penicillin-sensitive (exquisitely and regularly so)

* Also seen in chlamydial infection; rarely, occurs in bacteremic males

Vaginal discharges: typical presentations
1 *Candida albicans*
   — Predispositions
     • Oral contraceptives
     • Antibiotics (esp. tetracyclines)
     • Diabetes mellitus
   — Presentation
     • Marked pruritus vulvae
     • Perineal erythema
   — Discharge
     • Scanty, cheesy, little odor
   — Diagnosis
     • Gram-stain
2 *Trichomonas vaginalis*
   — Venereally transmitted
   — Presentation
     • Foul-smelling discharge
     • Pruritus often absent
     • Variable skin irritation
   — Discharge
     • Yellow, foamy, offensive; often profuse
   — Diagnosis
     • Direct microscopy: dark-field illumination
3 *Gardnerella vaginalis*
   — Venereally transmitted
   — Presentation
     • Malodorous discharge
     • No skin irritation
   — Discharge
     • Greyish, foul-smelling ('fishy' odor)
   — Diagnosis
     • Positive amine test
     • 'Clue cells' on microscopy

4 Gp B streptococci
   — Uterine discharge post-partum
   — Discharge
     • Foul-smelling lochia

ANAEROBIC INFECTION

Common anaerobic infections
1 Dental infections
2 Gynecological sepsis (e.g. septic abortion)
3 Abscesses: cerebral, lung, liver
4 Aspiration pneumonia
5 Biliary tract sepsis
6 Bite wounds

Factors predisposing to anaerobic infection
1 Mucosal injury
2 Microvascular disease
3 Tissue necrosis
4 Foreign bodies

ZOONOSES

Zoonoses: diseases transmitted to humans by animals
1 Anthrax (*B. anthracis*)
   — From goats, sheep
2 Leptospirosis/Weil's disease (*L. icterohemorrhagicae*)
   'Plague' (*Y. pestis*)
   — From rats
3 Brucellosis (esp. *B. melitensis*)
   Q fever (*C. burneti*)
   Leptospirosis (*L. hardjo*)
   — From cattle
4 Salmonellosis (esp. *S. enteritidis*)
   — From cattle, poultry (esp. hens' eggs)*
5 Toxocariasis (*T. canis*)
   Bite wounds (*Pasteurella multocida*)
   Canicola fever (*L. canicola*)
   Blastomycosis, leptospirosis
   Hydatids (*E. granulosus*)
   Capnocytophagia canimorsus (DF-2)
   — From dogs
6 Toxoplasmosis (*T. gondii*)
   Tularemia; catscratch disease
   — From cats
7 Campylobacter enteritis (*C. jejuni, C. coli*)
   — *C. jejuni* is the common human pathogen
   Yersiniosis (*Y. enterocolitica*)
   — From birds, poultry, pigs, dogs, cats
8 Rabies (rabiesvirus; a rhabdovirus)
   — From foxes, bats, small carnivores
   — From infected domestic dogs (or cats) in urban centers

* cf. *Shigella* spp.: man is the natural host

Clinical features of specific zoonoses
1 *Toxocara canis* ('visceral larva migrans')
   — Transmitted to children by dogs
   — Systemic presentation (→ age 1–4): rash, fever, cough, failure to thrive, eosinophilia

— Retinal presentation ($\rightarrow$ older children): strabismus, unilateral loss of visual acuity, no eosinophilia
— Diagnosis: ELISA or biopsy
— R_x: thiabendazole* (if symptomatic), plus steroids for allergic manifestations

2 *Toxoplasma gondii*
— Presentation: usually subclinical; may present with isolated non-tender adenopathy (DD_x: lymphoma)
— Systemic presentation: malaise, fever, headache, mononucleosis-like syndrome
— Ocular presentation: posterior uveitis (usually due to reactivation of in utero infection)
— Severe congenital presentation (maternal infection in first/second trimester) may cause thrombocytopenia, hepatosplenomegaly, hydrocephalus
— Other presentations: CNS toxoplasmosis (e.g. in AIDS)
— Diagnosis
  • Sabin–Feldman dye test (if available)
  • IgM antibody (for acute infections only)
— R_x: sulfadiazine/pyrimethamine and folinic acid

3 *Echinococcus granulosus* (hydatid disease)
— Transmitted to humans by dogs (definitive host) from sheep and cattle (intermediate hosts)
— Presentation: enlarging cyst(s), esp. in liver and lung
— Diagnosis: serology, biopsy (Casoni test non-specific)
— Indications for surgery
  • Lung cyst
  • Liver cyst > 5 cm } unless calcified
— Needle aspiration contraindicated

4 Brucellosis
— Presentation: back pain, arthralgias, epididy-moorchitis, scrotal pain, cough, splenomegaly, endocarditis, weight loss, chronic fatigue, depression
— Diagnosis: blood cultures, marrow culture, serology
— R_x: doxycycline *plus* streptomycin (or rifampicin)

5 Leptospirosis
— Septicemic phase: fever, aches and pains, conjunctival infection; renal involvement (pyuria, hematuria); diagnose by finding leptospires in blood or CSF
— 'Immune phase': meningism, uveitis, rash; diagnose by demonstrating leptospiruria
— Weil's disease (i.e. severe leptospirosis): jaundice, renal failure, cardiovascular collapse; with any serotype
— Diagnosis (general): serology
— R_x: parenteral penicillin or doxycycline‡

6 Yersiniosis
— Organisms multiply in Peyer's patches
— Ileitis/enterocolitis (esp. in children)
— Mesenteric adenitis (may mimic appendicitis)
— Reactive polyarthritis, erythema nodosum
— Diagnosis: stool culture, paired sera
— R_x: symptomatic ± co-trimoxazole

7 *C. canimorsus* (DF-2)
— Immotile Gram-negative bacillus; normal in dogs

— Predispositions: dogbite (75%), alcoholism (25%), splenectomy (25%), chronic airways disease or immunosuppression (25%)
— Sepsis $\rightarrow$ meningitis/pneumonia/endocarditis
— R_x: penicillin G (resistant to aminoglycosides)

* cf. 'cutaneous larva migrans' – caused by *Ancylostoma caninum/braziliense* – is treated with *topical* thiabendazole
‡ NB: Efficacy uncertain; may precipitate Herxheimer reaction (p. 221)

Organisms transmitted by human bite injuries
1 Streptococci, staphylococci
2 *Bacteroides* spp.
3 *Eikenella corrodens*
4 *Fusobacterium* spp.
5 *Peptostreptococcus* spp.

FOOD POISONING

Clinical spectrum of food poisoning
1 *Salmonella* (esp. *enteritidis, typhimurium*)
— Incubation period 12–48 h (toxin and infection)
— Source: raw meat/chicken/eggs/mayonnaise
— Fever, pain, diarrhea; may last several days (cf. typhoid)
— Incubation period 1–3 weeks
— Source: human fecal-oral transmission, polluted water
— Causes headache, initial constipation, fever (cf. cholera), cough, orchitis

2 *Staphylococcus aureus*
— Short incubation period 1–6 h (preformed toxin)
— Source: cold food (dairy products, sliced meats, salads), esp. if handled
— Vomiting prominent, no fever

3 Shigellosis
— Source: houseflies

4 *Listeria monocytogenes* ('Vacherin cheese disease')
— Incubation period 1 week
— Source: hot dogs/chicken, soft cheese, coleslaw, paté, salads
— Pregnancy infection $\rightarrow$ intrauterine fetal death
— Meningitis (30% die)
— Septicemia (esp. in T cell defects)

5 *Bacillus cereus*
— Incubation period 1–6 h (preformed toxin)
— Source: fried rice ($\rightarrow$ vomiting; incubation 1–5 h)
— Diarrheal form $\rightarrow$ incubation 10–12 h

6 *Clostridium botulinum*
— Incubation period 12–36 h (preformed toxin)
— Source: canned food
— Vomiting, paralysis, apnea; constipation; nerve palsies

7 *Clostridium perfringens* (formerly *welchii*) – type A strain
— Incubation period 12–24 h (preformed toxin)
— Source: undercooked meat, poultry, vegetables, stews, gravy, pies
— Abdominal pain, diarrhea

8 Cryptosporidiosis
— Source: water, milk, raw sausages/offal
— Predispositions: travel, livestock exposure

— Causes watery diarrhea
— Common in AIDS (± isosporiasis)
9 Yersiniosis (see above)
— Source: pigs, raw pork

Seafood poisoning: specific pathogens and syndromes
1 *Vibrio parahemolyticus*
— Incubation period 24 h (toxin and infection)
— Source: seafood/shellfish (esp. shrimp)
— Vomiting, diarrhea; may last up to 5 days
2 *Vibrio vulnificus*
— Source: oysters, other raw shellfish
— Septicemic illness, shock, hepatitis, osteomyelitis, DIC
— Sensitive to ciprofloxacin
3 Domoic acid poisoning
— Source: mussels
— Excitotoxic encephalopathy
4 Eustrongyloidiasis; gastric anisakiasis
— Source: eating sushi
5 *Diphyllobothrium latum*
— Finnish infestation
— Secondary B_{12} deficiency
6 Ciguatera fish poisoning
— Toxin from flagellate *G. toxicus*
— Causes nausea, abdominal cramps, oropharyngeal paresthesiae, shooting pains in legs, pain in teeth
7 Scombroid fish poisoning (with mackerel, tuna, anchovies)
— Scombrotoxin = histamine (from fish histidine)
— Nausea, flushing, diarrhea, dizziness
— Treatable with cimetidine
8 Norwalk virus, hepatitis A (p. 144)
— Source: raw shellfish, cold foods prepared by handlers

INFECTIVE DIARRHEAS

Common pathogens implicated in traveller's diarrhea*
1 Gram-negative bacilli
— Enterotoxigenic *E. coli*
— *Salmonella* spp.
— *Shigella* spp.
2 Curved motile Gram-negative bacilli
— *Vibrio* spp.
— *Campylobacter* spp.
— *Plesiomonas shigelloides*‡
— *Aeromonas hydrophila*
3 Protozoa
— *Giardia lamblia*
— Amebiasis
— Cryptosporidiosis
4 Viruses
— Norwalk (parvovirus)

* Therapy/prophylaxis: (1) ciprofloxacin, (2) doxycycline
‡ From eating oysters

Clinical spectrum of *E. coli* diarrhea
1 Enterotoxigenic *E. coli* (ETEC)
— Clinically resembles cholera
— Commonest cause of traveller's diarrhea

— Organisms adhere to small bowel mucosa and release toxins
2 Enterohemorrhagic *E. coli* (EHEC)
— *E. coli* O157:H7 releases verotoxins, causing
  • Hemorrhagic colitis (mimics IBD)
  • Hemolytic uremic syndrome, TTP (p. 173)
3 Enteroinvasive *E. coli* (EIEC)
— Clinically resembles shigellosis (dysentery)
— Colonic invasion → mucosal ulceration
4 Enteropathogenic *E. coli* (EPEC)
— Adhere to gut mucosa, destroy microvilli
— Common cause of infantile diarrhea

Features of *Campylobacter** enteritis
1 Source: chickens (esp. fast-food), unpasteurised milk (or bird-pecked bottles)
— Illness resembles salmonellosis, shigellosis
— Affects older children and young adults
2 Rapid onset; duration less than 1 week
— Relapses in 25%
3 Severe abdominal pain, fever, myalgia, backache
— May simulate acute abdomen
— Bloody diarrhea in 60% ± toxic megacolon
4 Reactive arthritis (esp. if HLA B27+)
— May simulate inflammatory bowel disease
5 Culture requires special conditions ($\uparrow CO_2$, $\downarrow O_2$)
6 Antibiotics usually *not* indicated
— Erythromycin in severe disease
— Asymptomatic carriers *rare*

* *C. jejuni, C. coli*

Features of viral gastroenteritis
1 Rotavirus, esp. group A (DD_x = *Pestivirus*)
— Affects infants, young children (6 months – 2 years)
— Incubation period 1–3 days; illness duration 1 week
— Mucosal IgA production confers lifelong immunity
— Vomiting prominent, dehydration common
2 Parvoviruses (esp. Norwalk virus)
— Affects all ages (esp. older children and adults)
— Produces winter epidemics ('winter vomiting disease')
— Fever, vomiting, abdominal pain common
— Illness duration ~ 48 h; incubation period 1–2 days
— No predictable development of immunity
— Asymptomatic carriage may occur (cf. *Campylobacter*)
— Frequently transmitted via shellfish ingestion
3 Astroviruses
— Usually affect children; may coinfect with rotavirus
— Cause mild, rotavirus-like diarrheal illness
4 Enteric adenoviruses
— Affect children (~ 3% of infantile gastroenteritis)

PRESENTATIONS OF INFECTIOUS DISEASE

'Spot' diagnosis of infectious diseases
1 Horder's spots
— Facial macules in psittacosis

2 Forschheimer's spots
— Soft palate lesions in rubella
3 Koplik's spots
— Bluish-grey buccal nodules in measles
4 Roth spots
— Pale-centered retinal infarcts in SBE*
5 Rose spots
— Truncal rash in 20% typhoid patients
6 Target lesions (erythema multiforme)
— *M. pneumoniae*, herpes simplex (esp.)

* Due to either septic microemboli or vasculitis

Clinical features of toxic shock syndrome
1 Toxic (fever > 39°C)
2 Shock (systolic BP < 90 mmHg)
3 Rash
— Initially a diffuse 'sunburn-like' macular erythroderma
— About 10 days post-onset generalized desquamation supervenes, particularly affecting palms and soles
4 At least three of
— Vomiting or diarrhea
— Mucosal (conjunctival/pharyngeal/vaginal) hyperemia
— Myalgias ± rhabdomyolysis (↑ CPK)
— Sterile pyuria and/or azotemia
— Abnormal liver function tests
— Thrombocytopenia
— Confusion (in absence of shock or high fever)
5 Vaginal/endocervix cultures for *Staph. aureus* (phage gp 1) are positive in about 98% of untreated patients*
Cultures of blood, throat and CSF are generally negative (very occasionally blood cultures may grow *Staph. aureus*). Staphylococcal exotoxin may be identified
6 Treatment consists of supportive measures (since symptoms are primarily toxin-mediated) ± flucloxacillin

* Not all cases occur in tampon users, e.g. nasal surgery may also predispose

UNUSUAL MICROORGANISMS

The rickettsioses: clinical syndromes
1 *R. rickettsii*
— Rocky Mountain spotted fever
2 *R. tsutsugamushi*
— Scrub typhus
3 *R. prowazekii*
— Epidemic typhus (louseborne; human reservoir)
— Brill–Zinser disease (recrudesence of latent disease)
4 *R. typhi*
— Endemic typhus (fleaborne; rodent reservoir)

Lyme disease (*Borrelia burgdorferi*): signs
1 Skin lesions
— Erythema chronicum migrans
2 Neurological
— Meningism, cranial nerve palsies, neuropathy

3 Cardiac
— AV block, myopericarditis
4 Arthritis
— Recurrent, asymmetric, often affects knee

Clinical spectrum of *M. pneumoniae* infection
1 Community-acquired pneumonia, esp. in young patients
2 Cold agglutinin production ± hemolytic anemia
3 Erythema multiforme, Stevens–Johnson syndrome
4 Non-specific musculoskeletal and/or gastrointestinal upset
5 Neurologic effects: Guillain–Barré, aseptic meningitis
6 D_x: rising CFT, *M. pneumoniae* IgM/IgA, sputum ELISA

Catscratch disease
1 Transmitted by cats
— Caused by *Afipia felis*, a Gram-negative bacillus
2 Presentation
— Red papule with regional adenopathy
— Adenopathy suppurative in 30%
3 Differential diagnosis
— Mycobacterial lymphadenitis
4 Diagnosis
— Biopsy with Warthin–Starry stain
5 Treatment
— Symptomatic

MALARIA AND OTHER PARASITES

Malarial subtypes: the clinical distinction
1 *P. falciparum*
— Causes 75% malaria in Africa (+ almost all deaths)
— Presents within 3 months of exposure (cf. *vivax*)
— High mortality; dense parasitemia; often drug-resistant
— Presentations
  • 'Cerebral malaria' (RBCs aggregate) ± hypoglycemia
  • 'Blackwater fever'*
  • Acute renal failure, DIC; pulmonary edema
— Does *not* relapse following effective treatment
2 *P. vivax*
— Responsible for 90% malaria in Asia
— Difficult to eradicate (due to exoerythrocytic phase)
— 10% of cases present over a year after exposure
— Manifests with persistent splenomegaly and/or anemia
— Prone to splenic rupture (may be spontaneous)
— Blood film: Schüffner's dots within parasitized red cell
— Symptoms may recur every few months for 10 years
3 *P. ovale*
— Contracted only in Africa
— Also exhibits exoerythrocytic phase and Schüffner's dots (hence primaquine treatment required; p. 219)
4 *P. malariae*
— Long incubation; prodromal symptoms common

— Red cell parasitization may persist for decades
— Late recrudescences may occur for up to 50 years; splenomegaly persists; symptoms usually mild
— Hematuria, nephrotic syndrome may occur

* Intravascular hemolysis → hemoglobinuria
NB: *Quinine* R$_x$ has been linked to both hypoglycemia and hemoglobinuria

Endogenous protective factors in malarial regions
1 Acquired immunity (partial)
2 HLA Bw53*
3 Hemoglobinopathy
— Hb S heterozygosity‡
— Ovalocytosis
— G6PD deficiency
— Increased Hb F levels¶
4 ?Malnutrition
— ?Due to accompanying iron deficiency

* Allelic frequency in Africa is 40-fold greater than Europe
‡ Confers 80% protection
¶ e.g. in thalassemia minor

Predispositions to severe malaria
1 Extremes of age
2 Pregnancy
3 Hyposplenism* (p. 199)

* incl. autosplenectomy in sickle-cell disease; cf. Hb S heterozygotes

Laboratory markers of severe malaria
1 Hypoglycemia
2 Renal failure
3 Neutrophilia*
4 Markedly deranged LFTs
5 Elevated CSF protein (+ lactate)

* WCC more commonly low or normal in mild disease; anemia, thrombocytopenia may also be associated

Classical presentations of parasitic disease
1 'Duodenal ulcer' type pain
— *Strongyloides stercoralis*
2 Iron-deficiency anemia ± hypoalbuminemia
— Hookworm (*Ancylostoma*/*Necator*)
3 Intestinal/biliary obstruction
— *Ascaris lumbricoides*
4 Rectal prolapse (+ bloody diarrhea, anemia)
— *Trichostrongylus;Trichura* (whipworm)
5 Malabsorption
— *Giardiasis* (a protozoon), capillariasis
6 Pruritus ani
— *Enterobius* (pinworm, threadworm)
7 Hemoptysis (lung abscesses)
— Paragonomiasis (may simulate TB)
'Anchovy sauce' expectoration
— Amebiasis (a protozoon) (hepatic)
8 'Grape skin' expectoration
— Echinococcosis (hydatid disease)
9 Terminal hematuria
— *Schistosoma hematobium*
10 Portal hypertension
— *Schistosoma japonicum*
11 Pulmonary hypertension
— *Schistosoma mansoni*

12 'Swimmer's itch'
— Non-human schistosome cerceriae*
13 Cholangitis, pancreatitis, cholangiocarcinoma
— *Clonorchis sinensis*
14 Lymphedema, elephantiasis
— Filariasis
15 Vitamin B$_{12}$ deficiency
— *Diphyllobothrium latum*
16 Megaesophagus/-colon, cardiomyopathy
— Chagas' disease (*Trypanosoma cruzi*)

* cf. 'swimming pool granuloma': from *Mycobacterium marinum* (p. 206)

VIRAL DISEASES

Lymphotropic viruses
1 EBV
2 CMV
3 HHV-6 (human herpesvirus-6)*
4 Adenoviruses

* Also known as human B cell lymphotropic virus (HBLV); resembles CMV

Distinguishing features of mononucleosis-like syndromes
1 EBV
— Affects mainly adolescents (12–25 years)
— Pharyngitis/tonsillitis prominent, may be exudative
— Palatine petechiae characteristic, fever common
— Tender cervical lymphadenopathy usual
— Splenomegaly frequent
— Lymphocytosis in 90% of cases
  • Relative lymphocytosis > 50%
  • Atypical lymphocytosis > 10%
— Liver function tests abnormal in 90% (jaundice 5–10%)
— Ampicillin rash in 90% of exposed cases
2 CMV
— Affects mainly young adults (25–35 years)
— Pharyngitis absent; fever prominent
— Lymphadenopathy/splenomegaly unusual
— Hepatomegaly usual (granulomatous hepatitis on biopsy); liver function tests often abnormal (esp. alkaline phosphatase); jaundice rare
— Implicated in Rasmussen's encephalitis (refractory partial epilepsy + focal neurologic defects)
— Atypical lymphocytosis less common than with EBV
— Virus isolable from urine long after infection
— Virus also isolable from secretions (e.g. saliva) or from buffy coat (i.e. leukocyte) blood fraction (best test)
— Ampicillin rashes occur with same frequency as EBV
3 Toxoplasmosis (a protozoon)
— Affects all age groups
— Systemic symptoms unusual (usually subclinical)
— Pharyngitis absent
— Non-tender 'rubbery' lymphadenopathy common, may persist for up to 12 months

— Splenomegaly unusual
— Liver dysfunction, atypical lymphocytosis absent
— Ampicillin rash not associated
— May respond to antibiotics (spiramycin; co-trimoxazole, pyrimethamine/sulfadimidine)
4 HHV-6 (human herpesvirus-6)
— Mononucleosis-like syndrome affects adults
— Children → exanthem subitum (roseola infantum)
— Fever unusual; non-specific viral syndrome
— Non-tender cervical adenopathy
— Virus persists in salivary glands
— Atypical lymphocytosis usual
— May cause pneumonia/encephalitis in immunosuppressed
5 Early HIV infection
— Affects mainly homosexuals (> IV drug abusers)
— Occurs within 2–6 weeeks of primary HIV infection
— Sudden onset (cf. EBV: insidious)
— Short duration (about 2 weeks)
— Prominent *rash* (± fever/pharyngitis/adenopathy)
— Often associated with oral/genital/anal *ulcers* ?reflecting portal of virus entry
— Cough and/or watery diarrhea also common
— No atypical lymphocytosis
— No hepatosplenomegaly or abnormal liver function
— Neurologic abnormalities unusual (cf. later HIV)
— Patients usually well for 2–3 years subsequently

Parvovirus B19: the clinical spectrum
1 Erythema infectiosum
— 'Fifth disease', 'slapped-cheek' syndrome
— Often misdiagnosed as rubella; peak age 4–11
2 Anemia
— Aplastic crises, e.g. in sickle-cell‡, spherocytosis
— In AIDS, ALL, Nezelof's syndrome*
3 Symmetric polyarthropathy (esp. in adult women)
— Rubella-like; rheumatoid factor negative
4 Fetal abnormalities
— e.g. Hydrops

* Treatable with IV gammaglobulin
‡ May be followed by nephrotic syndrome

Human papillomavirus (HPV): clinical associations
1 Type 1
— Plantar warts
2 Type 3
— Flat warts
3 Type 5/8
— Skin SCCs in transplant patients
4 Type 7
— Common warts in food handlers
5 Types 6 and 11
— Condylomata acuminata (genital warts)
— Juvenile laryngeal papillomatosis
6 Type 13
— Oral leukoplakia
7 Type 16 (and others, esp. 18)
— SCC cervix
— SCC penis
— SCC vulva
8 Type 30
— SCC larynx

9 Type 31
— Genital warts*

* Usually subclinical

Complications of viral infections
1 Influenza A
— Staphylococcal/pneumococcal pneumonia
— Meningococcal disease
2 Measles
— Reactivation of pulmonary TB
— Bacterial pneumonia
— Encephalomyelitis, SSPE
3 Mumps
— Meningitis, deafness, thyroiditis, pancreatitis
— Paroxysmal cold hemoglobinuria
— Orchitis (common), sterility (rare)
4 Varicella-zoster
— Miliary calcification on CXR
— DIC
5 CMV
— Guillain–Barré syndrome
— Myopericarditis
— Necrotizing pneumonitis in transplant patients
6 Coxsackie A
— Aseptic meningitis, paralysis
— Herpangina
— 'Hand, foot and mouth' disease (esp. A16)
— Acute hemorrhagic conjunctivitis (esp. A24)*
7 Coxsackie B
— Pleurodynia; myopericarditis
— Pancreatitis, orchitis
— ? Diabetes mellitus
8 JC virus (a papovavirus)
— Progressive multifocal leukoencephalo-pathy
9 Parvovirus
— Fifth disease ('slapped cheek' syndrome)
— Aplastic crisis in sickle-cell disease
10 Creutzfeldt–Jakob
— Myoclonic jerks; dementia
— Transmissible by corneal transplantation

* Also caused by enterovirus 70

VIRAL HEMORRHAGIC FEVERS

Classification of the viral hemorrhagic fevers
1 Togaviruses
— Alphaviruses (mosquitoborne)
  • Chikungunya fever (Asia)
  • O'nyong nyong (Africa)
— Flaviviruses (mosquito- and tickborne)
  • Dengue fever (Asia, Africa, Pacific, Caribbean)
  • Yellow fever (Africa, S. America)
  • Kyasanur Forest disease (Asia)
  • Omsk hemorrhagic fever (Central Asia)
2 Bunyaviruses (mosquito- and tickborne)
— Congo-Crimean fever (Africa, Asia)
— Rift Valley fever (Africa)
— Korean hemorrhagic fever (Hantaan virus: Asia)
3 Arenaviruses (rodentborne)
— Lassa fever (Africa)

— Argentinian hemorrhagic fever (Junin virus)
— Bolivian hemorrhagic fever (Machupo virus)
— Venezuelan hemorrhagic fever
4 Filoviruses (nosocomial transmission)
— Marburg virus disease (Europe, Asia, Africa)
— Ebola virus disease (Africa)

The viral hemorrhagic fevers: differential diagnostic features

1 Marburg/Ebola viruses
— Filoviruses; African endemicity
— Nosocomial spread (transmissible by blood products)
— Different incubations, similar manifestations
— Presentation (abrupt onset)
  • Headache, conjunctivitis, back pain, arthralgias
  • Diarrhea ± melena
  • Pleurisy, psychosis, proteinuria
  • DIC; characteristic hemorrhagic rash
2 Lassa fever
— An arenavirus*; African endemicity
— Rodentborne; transmission similar to filoviruses
— Presentation (insidious onset; may be subclinical)
  • Pharyngitis, lymphadenopathy, nephrosis
  • Hypoxic death, esp. in pregnancy
— Management: barrier nursing, ribavirin‡
3 Dengue fever
— A flavivirus (four serotypes); South Pacific endemicity
— Presentation
  • Rash, DIC
  • Shock (esp. in infants with previous infection)
4 Korean hemorrhagic fever with renal syndrome
— Due to Hantaan virus; rodentborne¶
— Presentation
  • Nephrosis, acute renal failure
  • *Mild* hemorrhagic signs in Korean variant
Hantavirus pulmonary syndrome (a distinct hantavirus)
  • Fulminant non-cardiogenic pulmonary edema
5 Congo-Crimean fever
— Tickborne
— Similar to Kyasanur Forest disease (India)
— Presentation
  • Severe hemorrhagic sequelae
  • Chest pains, oropharyngitis
6 Yellow fever
— Mosquitoborne
— Similar to Rift Valley fever (also in Africa)
— Presentation
  • Arthritis
  • Retinal damage
  • Jaundice (hence 'yellow') in convalescent phase
  • Black vomitus (+ other hemorrhagic signs)

* Similar syndromes seen with other arenaviruses, notably Junin (Argentinian) and Machupo (Bolivian) fevers
‡ NB: For Junin-type disease, give 500 mL high-titer immune plasma
¶ Same virus probably responsible for nephropathica epidemica in Scandinavia (a related bunyavirus may cause Balkan nephropathy)

Diagnoses suggested by direct microscopy

1 Acid-fast bacteria to Ziehl–Neelsen staining
— *Mycobacteria* spp.
Catalase-positive, niacin-negative, INH-resistant
— Atypical (non-tuberculous) mycobacteriosis
2 Weakly acid-fast organisms
— *Nocardia* (aerobic) spp.
— *Actinomyces* (anaerobic) spp.
3 Dark-field examination
— *Treponema pallidum*
4 Silver methenamine stain
— *P. carinii*
5 Indian ink stain (CSF)
— *Cryptococcus neoformans*
6 Romanowsky-type stain, thick and thin films
— *Plasmodia* spp.
7 Gram-negative diplococci in WBCs (cervical/urethral swab)
— *Neisseria gonorrheae*
8 Inclusion bodies within urethral epithelial cells
— *Chlamydia trachomatis*
9 Pyogenic meningitis in adults: Gram-positives in CSF
— Pneumococcal meningitis*
Pyogenic meningitis in adults: Gram-negatives in CSF
— Meningococcal meningitis*

* Presumptive diagnosis

Diagnostic value of throat swabs

1 Gp A β-hemolytic strep (see below)
2 Gonococcal pharyngitis
3 *Mycoplasma pneumoniae*
4 Diphtheria, pertussis
5 Some viral infections: polio, rubella

Diagnosis of streptococcal pharyngitis

1 Throat swab (culture)
— Heavy growth confirms diagnosis
— Diagnosis excluded by negative swab
— 'Light growth' unhelpful
2 Throat swab (rapid antigen test)
— ELISA directly confirms strep antigen presence
— 90% specificity and sensitivity
3 Supportive tests
— C-reactive protein (p. 350)
  • Levels higher in bacterial than viral infections
— ASO titer
  • Rising titer useful if retrospective D_x needed
— Heterophile antibody ('Mono spot')
  • Useful in excluding EBV
4 Therapeutic trial of antibiotics
— Little *diagnostic* value
— May be more *cost-effective* than investigation*

* Though delaying treatment to await test results does not appear to increase incidence of complications

Diagnostic utility of bone marrow culture

1 Miliary tuberculosis
2 Brucellosis
3 Typhoid
4 Kala-azar

TUBERCULOSIS: INVESTIGATIONS

Diagnostic criteria in pulmonary tuberculosis
1 Suggestive
   — Clinical context
   — Radiographic appearance*
   — Positive tuberculin test, esp. if converts
   — Positive antibody to 38-kDa TB antigen
2 Presumptive
   — Acid-fast bacilli in sputum/gastric washings
   — Caseating granulomata on biopsy
3 Definitive
   — *Mycobacterium tuberculosis* isolated on culture

* NB: *Activity* of TB *cannot* be assessed from CXR

Diagnosis of tuberculous meningitis
1 Routine CSF examination
   — ↑ Mononuclears
   — ↑ Protein
   — ↓ Glucose
2 Special CSF examination
   — ↓ Chloride
   — ↓ Serum/CSF bromide partition ratio
   — Positive tryptophan assay
3 Diagnostic CSF examination
   — Acid-fast bacilli on Ziehl–Neelsen staining, confirmed as tuberculous on culture (NB: usually negative)
4 CXR, tuberculin test
   — Useless (negative in up to 50%)

The false-negative tuberculin test: differential diagnosis
1 Extremes of age
2 Very recent infection (< 10 weeks since inoculation)
3 Viremia (e.g. measles, influenza)
   Following live vaccination (e.g. rubella)
4 Severe systemic disease
   — Septicemia (incl. miliary tuberculosis)
   — Carcinomatosis and/or cytotoxic therapy
   — Uremia, malnutrition
   — Tuberculous meningitis
5 Defective T cell function
   — Hodgkin's disease and/or thymic irradiation
   — Sarcoidosis
   — Wiskott–Aldrich, di George, SCID
   — AIDS (NB: test hazardous to perform)
6 Drugs
   — Steroids, other immunosuppressives
7 Technical problems
   — Inadvertent subcutaneous injection
   — Adsorption of antigen to syringe
   — Substandard potency of preparation

SYPHILIS SEROLOGY

What tests are available for diagnosing syphilis?
1 Dark-field examination
   — For direct spirochetal identification
2 Reaginic (flocculation) tests
   — VDRL (best test; quantitative)
   — WR (little used now)
   — RPR (used in outlying areas)
3 Specific treponemal serologic tests*
   — FTA-ABS
   — TPI
   — TPHA

* Positive for life after initial infection; hence, *not* appropriate for monitoring therapeutic adequacy

Positive dark-field examination: differential diagnosis
1 Primary syphilitic chancre
2 Secondary syphilis (mucosal lesions)
3 Congenital syphilis (mucosal lesions)
4 Non-pathogenic oral or rectal treponemes

Sensitivity of reaginic tests (e.g. VDRL) in established syphilis
1 Primary syphilis
   — Positive in 80% (reliably negative within 2 years of R_x)
2 Secondary syphilis
   — Positive in 99%
3 Late/latent syphilis
   — Positive in 70% (may remain positive long after R_x)
4 Neurosyphilis
   — CSF positive in 50% (i.e. 50% false-negative rate*)

* cf. CSF VDRL: false-positives *rare* unless 'bloody tap' contaminates sample

Causes of chronic reaginic false-positives
1 Non-treponemal bacterial infections
   — Leprosy*, leptospirosis*, malaria*
   — Venereal: LGV, chancroid (p. 216)
   — Tuberculosis, psittacosis, rickettsial disease
2 Viral infections
   — Infectious mononucleosis*
   — Viral hepatitis
   — HIV
3 Autoimmune disease
   — SLE*
4 Narcotic abuse
5 Chronic liver disease
6 Pregnancy
7 Neoplasia
   — Carcinomatosis
   — Myeloma, lymphoma
8 Multiple blood transfusions

* May also cause false-positive treponemal serology (e.g. FTA-ABS)

Choosing the most appropriate test in suspected syphilis
1 Primary (recent) exposure
   — Dark-field examination of primary chancre
   — FTA-ABS is the first test to become positive
2 Secondary syphilis
   — Dark-field examination if skin/mucosal lesions present
   — VDRL
3 Screening (pregnant women, prostitutes, contacts of cases)
   — VDRL
   — If positive, do FTA-ABS

4 Follow-up (of primary/secondary/late syphilis) after therapy
   — VDRL at 3, 6, 12 months*
   — If titer unchanged after 12 months, re-treat
5 Exclusion of neurosyphilis
   — CSF FTA-ABS (negativity reliably excludes diagnosis)

* Titer should decline 4-fold by 3 months and 8-fold by 6 months

Diagnostic significance of syphilis serology
1 Positive VDRL
   Positive FTA-ABS
   — Syphilis (yaws, pinta, bejel)
2 Positive VDRL
   Negative FTA-ABS
   — Biological false-positive
3 Negative VDRL
   Positive FTA-ABS
   — Early, latent, late or treated syphilis
4 Positive FTA-ABS (IgM)
   — Congenital syphilis*

* cf. IgG only: implies passive transfer of maternal antibody

Neurosyphilis: CSF monitors during treatment
1 Total protein
2 Mononuclear cell count
3 Quantitative VDRL titer *if* positive prior to treatment*

* CSF VDRL is 100% specific but only 50% sensitive

FEVER OF UNKNOWN ORIGIN

Considerations in the investigation of unexplained fever
1 Exclude
   — Drug allergy
   — Surreptitious drug abuse
   — Factitious fever
2 Bone marrow examination
   — Aspiration/trephine (lymphoma)
   — Bone marrow culture (p. 213)
3 Unusual organism suspected
   — Acid-fast stains, etc. (pp. 213, 226)
   — Thick and thin blood films
   — Plasma immunoassays
     • *Candida* enolase antigenemia
     • *Aspergillus* antigenemia
4 Abscess suspected
   — CT/ultrasound
   — Scintigraphy
     • ^{67}Gallium-scanning
     • ^{111}Indium-leukocyte (or -IgG) scanning
5 Invasive fungal infection suspected (e.g. post-transplant)
   — Plasma (1→3) β-D-glucan
   — *Candida* enolase antigenemia
6 HIV serology or PCR (p. 193)

Fever of unknown origin: diagnoses localized by gallium scan
1 Abscess (e.g. subphrenic)
2 Lymphoma
3 Hepatoma
4 Sarcoidosis

Infections causing profound peripheral eosinophilia
1 Trichinosis (diagnosis by serology or muscle biopsy)
2 Visceral larva migrans (*Toxocara canis*) esp. in children
3 Tropical pulmonary eosinophilia (filariasis)

DIAGNOSTIC STUDIES IN OTHER INFECTIONS

Infectious mononucleosis: making sense of the serology
1 VCA (viral capsid antibody; IgG)
   — Positivity indicates past or present infection
2 EA (antibody to EBV 'early antigen')
   — Appears within 2–3 weeks of symptom onset
   — 'D' (diffuse) component disappears within months; useful marker of current infection if positive
   — 'R' (restricted) component may persist for years, esp. in relapsing disease
3 EBV-specific IgM (i.e. to viral capsid antigen)
   — Tends to parallel heterophile antibody rise (see below)
   — Usually becomes negative within 3 months of onset
   — Extremely useful in heterophile-negative cases; the best test for confirming acute disease
4 EBNA (EBV-associated nuclear antigen)
   — Viral antigen detected by immunofluorescence
   — Indicates infected cells harboring viral genome
5 EBNA antibody (IgG)
   — Appears late
   — Indicates previous infection; persists lifelong
6 Heterophile antibody (IgM)
   — i.e. Heterophile agglutinins for sheep erythrocytes
   — Basis of Paul–Bunnell test (diagnostic); present in 90%
   — Similar (Forssman-type) agglutinins seen in hepatitis, lymphomas, etc; adsorbed out by guinea pig kidney*
   — May be misleadingly negative for up to a month after symptom onset; tedious and expensive to perform

* cf. positive Paul–Bunnell: antibodies adsorbed out by ox (beef) erythrocytes

Weil–Felix reactions: diagnostic significance
1 Epidemic (*R. prowazekii*) typhus
   — OX-19 positive
     Brill–Zinsser disease (recurrent epidemic typhus)
   — All negative
2 Scrub (*R. tsutsugamushi*) typhus
   — OX-K positive
3 Rocky Mountain (*R. rickettsii*) spotted fever
   — OX-I9 and OX-2 positive
4 Q (*Coxiella burneti*) fever
   — All negative (see below)
5 *Proteus* spp. infections, brucellosis, typhoid, leptospirosis
   — False-positives

Diagnosis of Q fever
1 Complement fixation test (CFT)
2 Acute disease → 4 x ↑ phase II antibody titer
3 Chronic disease → persistent ↑ phase I and II Ab titer
4 Endocarditis → > 1: 200 phase I Ab titer

Diagnosis of genital ulcers ± inguinal adenopathy
1 Positive dark-field examination
— Primary syphilis
2 *H. ducreyi* on microscopy/culture
— Chancroid
3 Donovan bodies on microscopy
— Granuloma inguinale*
4 *Chlamydia* on culture/serology
— Lymphogranuloma venereum
5 *H. simplex* on viral culture
— Genital herpes
6 Negative microbiology
— Consider Behçet's/Reiter's syndrome

* Bipolar staining bacilli visible within monocytes, reflecting presence of *Calymmatobacterium inguinale*

Laboratory diagnosis of specific infections
1 Gonorrhea
— Immediate plating and Gram-stain
— Urethral culture in chocolate (blood) agar
— Endocervical/anorectal/pharyngeal culture in Thayer–Martin (antibiotic-enriched) medium
2 Typhoid
— Blood cultures; stool and urine cultures
— Widal test: > 4 x ↑ antibody titer to 'O' (cell wall) antigen
3 Cryptococcal meningitis
— Cryptococcal antigen in CSF (most sensitive test)
— CSF culture (most specific test)
— Indian ink stain (quickest test)

MANAGING INFECTIOUS DISEASE

PRINCIPLES OF ANTIBIOTIC CHEMOTHERAPY

Mechanisms underlying antibiotic activity
1 Interference with bacterial cell wall synthesis
— β-lactams (penicillins, cephalosporins)
• Prevent proteoglycan crosslinking
— Vancomycin
• Inhibits proteoglycan formation
2 Interference with fungal cell wall synthesis
— Imidazoles (ketoconazole, miconazole, clotrimazole)
• Inhibit ergosterol synthesis (making cells 'leaky')
3 Interference with bacterial protein synthesis
— Aminoglycosides
• Distort bacterial 30S ribosomal subunit → ↓ mRNA attachment and translation
— Tetracycline
• Blocks aminoacyl-tRNA binding to 30S ribosome
— Chloramphenicol
• Blocks 50S ribosome transpeptidation
— Erythromycin
• Blocks bacterial 50S ribosomal translocation
— Fusidic acid
• Inhibits ribosomal GTPase (= elongation factor)

4 Interference with folate metabolism
— Sulfonamides (PABA analogs → ↓ dihydropteroate)
— Trimethoprim (inhibits bacterial DHFR)
— 5-flucytosine (fungal antimetabolite)
5 Interference with bacterial DNA gyrase (topoisomerase II)
— Nalidixic acid
— Ciprofloxacin, norfloxacin*
6 Other mechanisms
— Metronidazole: inhibits anaerobic electron transfer
— Nitrofurantoin: interferes with bacterial acetyl CoA
— Rifampicin: inactivates bacterial RNA polymerase
— Acyclovir: inhibits viral DNA polymerase‡

* Both contraindicated in children
‡ Drug is selectively activated by viral thymidine kinase

Bioavailability of antibiotics at specific sites of infection
1 CSF
— Cefotaxime, cefuroxime, ceftriaxone*
— Penicillins (during meningitis only)
— Chloramphenicol; erythromycin; metronidazole
— Isoniazid/rifampicin/pyrazinamide
— 5-flucytosine, fluconazole
2 Bile
— Penicillins (e.g. mezlocillin)
— Cephalosporins
— Erythromycin
3 Urine
— Penicillins, cephalosporins
— Sulfonamides, trimethoprim
— Aminoglycosides
— Nitrofurantoin, nalidixic acid
— Ethambutol
— Fluoroquinolones
— Fluconazole, flucytosine

* i.e. *unlike* other cephalosporins

Non-absorbable antibiotics
1 Nystatin
2 Neomycin
3 Colistin
4 Framycetin
5 Vancomycin

Bactericidal antibiotics
1 β-lactams*
— Penicillins
— Cephalosporins
— Imipenem (a carbapenem)
— Aztreonam (a monobactam)
2 Aminoglycosides
3 Rifampicin
4 Metronidazole
5 Fluoroquinolones

* cf. β-lactamase *inhibitors* (p. 222): negligible antibacterial activity

Relative indications for bactericidal antibiotic therapy
1 Infective endocarditis
2 Bacterial meningitis
3 Febrile neutropenia

TREATMENT OF ANAEROBIC INFECTIONS

Antibiotics with anaerobic specificity
1 Metronidazole
  Imipenem } Good activity against
  Chloramphenicol } *Bacteroides fragilis*
  Co-amoxiclav*
2 Clindamycin
  Cefoxitin } Moderate activity against
  Piperacillin } *Bacteroides fragilis*
3 Penicillin G
  Tetracycline } Poor activity against
  Erythromycin } *Bacteroides fragilis*

* Amoxicillin + clavulanic acid

Metronidazole: indications for parenteral administration
1 Prior to urgent surgery if anaerobic sepsis suspected
2 Proven anaerobic infections resistant to oral or rectal therapy
3 Patients with vomiting, diarrhea and known anaerobic sepsis
4 Life-threatening sepsis in patients with anaerobic source

PROPHYLACTIC ANTIBIOTICS

Antibiotic prophylaxis regimens
1 Rheumatic fever (maintenance prophylaxis)
  — 1.2×10^6 U penicillin G IM monthly, *or*
  — 250 mg penicillin V orally b.d. until adulthood; lifelong prophylaxis if significant valve disease
2 Infective endocarditis (*intermittent* prophylaxis)
  — Dental work
    • Amoxycillin 3 g p.o. 1 h pre, 6 h post, *or*
    • Clindamycin 300 mg IV pre, 150 mg p.o. 6 h post
  — Genitourinary/colonic instrumentation
    • Ampicillin 1 g IV + gentamicin 2 mg/kg IV 30 min pre, then amoxycillin 1 g orally q 6 h
  — Penicillin allergy
    • Clindamycin 600 mg p.o. 1 h before, *or*
    • Vancomycin 1 g slow IV + gentamicin, *or*
    • Teicoplanin 400 mg IV + gentamicin
3 Tuberculosis
  — Isoniazid 300 mg daily p.o. for 12 months, *plus*
  — Pyridoxine 25 mg daily p.o. for 12 months
4 *Pneumocystis carinii* (in marrow transplant recipients)
  — Trimethoprim/sulfamethoxazole (best)
  — Aerosolized pentamidine (expensive, less effect)
5 Infant contacts of epiglottitis (*H. influenzae* type B)
  — Rifampicin 20 mg/kg daily for 4 days

Malarial prophylaxis: general measures
1 Minimize or avoid travel to endemic regions
2 Avoid mosquito bites
  — Cover exposed skin with clothing, esp. at night
  — Use repellents and (within bedrooms/tents) insecticide
  — Use bednets if mosquitos cannot be excluded

Prophylactic antimalarial chemotherapy regimens*
  — Non-resistant area, *or* during pregnancy‡
    • Chloroquine
  — Endemic non-falciparum chloroquine resistance
    • Chloroquine + pyrimethamine/dapsone
  — Falciparum area
    • Mefloquine (in highly resistant areas), *or*
    • Chloroquine + proguanil
    • Doxycycline (investigational)

* NB: Recommendations change often
‡ Ideally, pregnant women should *avoid* elective travel to malarious areas

MANAGING MYCOBACTERIAL DISEASE

Relative indications for BCG vaccination
1 Medical or laboratory workers exposed to tubercle bacilli
2 Neonates exposed to active TB
3 Tuberculin-negative children/adolescents in endemic areas

Therapeutic indications for tuberculin skin testing
1 To assess need for isoniazid prophylaxis in non-BCG-treated contacts (esp. children) of active tuberculosis cases
2 To assess need for BCG immunization in children
3 To assess TB prevalence in different communities
4 To investigate individuals suspected of having active TB

Indications for prophylactic isoniazid therapy
1 A tuberculin-positive patient younger than 50 (esp. a child) who
  — Is a member of a household in which a recent diagnosis of TB has been made
  — Has a chest X-ray suggesting TB
2 A tuberculin-positive individual who
  — Is about to commence immunosuppressive treatment
  — Has a predisposition to TB
    • Hodgkin's disease, leukemia (e.g. CLL, hairy cell)
    • Silicosis, sarcoidosis, alcoholism
    • Poorly controlled insulin-dependent diabetes
    • Post-gastrectomy
3 Recent tuberculin conversion in absence of BCG vaccination

Chemotherapy of established tuberculosis
1 Standard (presensitivity) regimen for pulmonary TB
  — 6 months* INH + rifampicin (strongly bactericidal), *plus*
  — 2 months pyrazinamide (weakly bactericidal), *plus*
  — 2 months ethambutol (bacteriostatic), *or*
  — 2 months streptomycin (weakly bactericidal)
2 Sputum cultures still positive after 4 months of above?
  — Reculture and check for acquired resistance
  — If no resistance, recommence R_x for 9 months
  — If resistance demonstrated, use second-line drug(s)

3 Pulmonary TB in pregnancy or during lactation
   — Isoniazid (plus pyridoxine supplements) for 9 months
   — Add ethambutol for 2 months if resistance suspected
   — Rifampicin probably safe in second and third trimesters
   — Avoid streptomycin at all stages
4 Pulmonary TB in child < 16 years old
   — Isoniazid and rifampicin for 9 months
   — Third drug not mandatory unless resistance suspected
5 Immunosuppressed patients
   — Isoniazid and rifampicin for 12 months
   — Ethambutol and pyrazinamide for 2 months
6 Renal TB
   — Avoid streptomycin and ethambutol if azotemic

* NB: If *cavities* on initial CXR, continue isoniazid and rifampicin for 9 months

Indications for corticosteroids in tuberculosis*
1 Absolute indication
   — Acute hypoadrenalism due to tuberculous ablation of adrenal glands
2 Life-threatening tuberculous meningitis
3 Controversial indications
   — Spinal or ureteric stenosis
   — Pericarditis
   — Acute miliary dissemination with septic shock
   — Refractory large pleural effusion(s)

* NB: Steroids absolutely contraindicated *unless* the patient is receiving antituberculous chemotherapy

Therapies useful for drug-resistant TB*
1 Amikacin (or capreomycin)
2 Ciprofloxacin
3 Cycloserine, ethionamide, PAS
4 Clofazimine, co-amoxiclav
5 Surgical excision of tuberculous foci

* Assuming resistance to INH, rifampicin, pyrazinamide, ethambutol and streptomycin

Toxicity of antituberculous chemotherapy
1 Isoniazid
   — Hepatitis (see below)
   — SLE (pp. 183, 190)
   — Pyridoxine deficiency (rare)
     • Pellagra-like rash
     • Neuropathy; optic neuritis ($\downarrow$ green vision)
     • Sideroblastosis*
   — *Potentiation* of phenytoin, warfarin
2 Rifampicin
   — Daily administration
     • *Antagonism* of oral contraceptives, warfarin, steroids, digoxin and sulfonylureas
     • Asymptomatic elevation of transaminases
   — Intermittent administration
     • Flu-like illness: affects Caucasians receiving R_x < 3 times/week for 3–6 months (20% mortality)
     • Hepatitis‡
     • Venous thrombosis
     • Hemolysis, thrombocytopenia; azotemia

3 Streptomycin
   — Hypersensitivity reactions
     • Rash, malaise, PUO; eosinophilia
   — Vestibular damage (esp. if renal impairment)
   — Teratogenicity
4 Ethambutol
   — Optic neuritis, esp. in renal impairment
5 Pyrazinamide
   — Hepatotoxicity in ~ 10%
6 Less commonly used antituberculous drugs
   — Cycloserine
     • Fits, psychoses, pyridoxine deficiency
   — Ethionamide
     • Hepatotoxicity
   — Prothionamide
     • Neuropathy; nausea; psychoses

* Commoner in (i) high dosage schedule (> 15 mg/kg/day), (ii) slow acetylation status, (iii) alcoholism and (iv) pregnancy
‡ NB: Also colors urine orange

Features of isoniazid-associated hepatotoxicity
1 Occurs in about 1%; usually within 3 months (may be fatal)
2 *Not* dose-related
   Not consistently related to acetylator phenotype*
3 Risk factors
   — Male sex
   — Age > 35 years (8-fold increase if > 65 years)
   — Alcoholism
   — Other hepatotoxic R_x (e.g. rifampicin, pyrazinamide)
4 Clinically indistinguishable from viral hepatitis
5 Liver function tests should only be *routinely* performed in the latter 'at-risk' group or in symptomatic patients
6 Cease R_x if ALT/AST exceed three times upper limit of normal

* Though an association with rapid acetylation has been reported

Problems in managing the alcoholic with TB
1 Poor compliance necessitating supervised (intermittent) treatment schedule; predisposes to rifampicin toxicity
2 Increased risk of hepatotoxicity
3 Increased risk of toxic amblyopia
4 Increased risk of pyridoxine deficiency
5 Neuropathy/optic neuritis, rash and sideroblastosis may arise due to other (non-iatrogenic) alcohol-related causes

Therapy of non-tuberculous mycobacteria
1 *Mycobacterium avium-intracellulare*
   — Indolent disease
     • Standard anti-TB regimens (up to 2 years)
     • Azithromycin, clarithromycin
     • Rifabutin, ciprofloxacin
   — Aggressive local disease
     • Surgery (lobectomy)
   — Aggressive widespread disease
     • Multidrug combinations, e.g. clofazimine, ansamycin, ciprofloxacin and ethambutol
2 *Mycobacterium marinum*
   — Expectant (conservative) management

— Excision of involved skin
— Rifampicin, ethambutol, doxycycline
3 *Mycobacterium scrofulaceum*
— Lymphadenectomy
4 *Mycobacterium fortuitum-chelonei*
— Excision of soft-tissue abscesses
— Doxycycline; amikacin, sulfonamides, erythromycin
5 *Mycobacterium kansasii*
— Isoniazid ⎫
— Rifampicin ⎬ For 2 years
— Ethambutol ⎭
6 *Mycobacterium xenopi*
— Standard anti-TB therapy

Leprosy: therapeutic options
1 Dapsone + rifampicin + clofazimine
2 Sparfloxacin + clarithromycin
3 Fusidic acid (or rifampicin) + ciprofloxacin
4 Thalidomide (for reactions following antibiotics in males)

Diseases which may respond to dapsone
1 Leprosy
2 Dermatitis herpetiformis
3 Pyoderma gangrenosum
4 Relapsing polychondritis

ANTIBIOTIC PRESCRIBING STRATEGIES

Antibiotic therapy of venereal disease
1 Genital gonorrhea
— Ceftriaxone 250 mg IM *or* (oral) cefixime 800 mg stat
— Tetracycline 500 mg q.i.d. for 5 days, *or*
— Single-dose oral amoxicillin 3 g (*if* sensitive)
— Single-dose ciprofloxacin 100 mg (*if* penicillin-resistant)
— Spectinomycin (*if* ciprofloxacin-resistant)
2 Gonococcal pharyngitis*
— Trimethoprim/sulfamethoxazole for 5 days
3 Gonococcal proctitis‡
— Single-dose ciprofloxacin 100 mg, *or*
— Spectinomycin 4 g IM
Gonococcal proctitis with positive VDRL
— Procaine penicillin (see below)
4 Syphilis¶
— Procaine penicillin 600,000 U IM daily
— Primary/secondary: for 10 days
— Latent/gummatous: for 15 days
— Neurological/aortitic: for 20 days
5 Chlamydial urethritis
— Azithromycin 1 g stat, *or*
— Doxycycline 100 mg b.d. for 7 days, *or*
— Tetracycline 500 mg q.i.d. for 14 days

* Usually unresponsive to amoxycillin or spectinomycin
‡ Unresponsive to tetracycline in males and, usually, to amoxycillin
¶ *Resistant* to spectinomycin; cf. gonorrhea

Treatment strategies in malaria
1 *P. falciparum* (sensitive)

— Chloroquine (base) 600 mg stat orally, then 300 mg 6 hours later, then 300 mg daily for 2 days
2 *P. falciparum* (resistant, fulminant or cerebral)
— Exchange transfusion (5–10 units) if parasitemia > 10%*
— IV quinine dihydrochloride 20 mg/kg (= 15 mg/kg quinine base) over 4 h, then 10 mg/kg q 8 h; 5% dextrose to obviate risk of hypoglycemia, *or*
— Artemether (oral or IM)
— Amodiaquine‡ 600 mg/day ± tetracycline, *or*
— Mefloquine 20 mg/kg for two doses, *or*
— Oral artesunate followed by mefloquine
— *No* steroids
3 *P. vivax/ovale*
— Due to exoerythrocytic (cryptobiotic) phase, add primaquine (base) 7.5 mg orally b.d. for 2 weeks to the chloroquine-based regimen
— Inadequate treatment may lead to late relapse
4 *P. malariae*
— Relapse *not* prevented by primaquine; relapses may occur decades later and must be fully re-treated

* NB: *Iron chelation* has also been reported to hasten resolution of parasitemia and coma in cerebral malaria
‡ Risk of agranulocytosis; no longer used for prophylaxis

Antibiotic chemotherapy of infection in the AIDS patient
1 *P. carinii*
— Co-trimoxazole; pentamidine
2 *C. albicans* (mucosal)
— Topical clotrimazole
— Oral ketoconazole
C. albicans (esophageal, invasive or disseminated)
— IV amphotericin B ± 5-FC
3 *T. gondii*
— Pyrimethamine/sulfadiazine
4 *C. neoformans*
— Amphotericin B* *plus* 5-FC
— Maintenance fluconazole
5 *Salmonella/Shigella* spp.
— IV ampicillin
6 Herpes simplex, varicella-zoster
— Acyclovir (nucleoside analog of guanosine, a herpesvirus thymidine kinase substrate)
CMV
— Ganciclovir (dihydroxypropoxymethylguanine)
— Foscarnet (phosphonoformic acid)

* Oral fluconazole may also be effective in acute management of non-life-threatening cryptococcal meningitis

OPTIMIZING ANTIBIOTIC THERAPY

Indications for fluoroquinolone therapy
1 Serious Gram-negative infections
— Acute Gram-negative osteomyelitis (IV ciprofloxacin)
— Severe necrotizing otitis externa (oral ciprofloxacin)
— Infective exacerbations of cystic fibrosis
2 Bacterial gastroenteritis
— Traveller's diarrhea
— Invasive salmonellosis

3 Complicated urinary tract infections, e.g.
  — Pyelonephritis
  — Trimethoprim-resistant cystitis
  — Indwelling catheter in situ
  — Chronic or relapsing prostatitis
  — Penicillinase-producing *N. gonorrheae* urethritis
4 Prophylaxis
  — Eradication of *Salmonella* carrier state
  — Asymptomatic contacts of meningococcal infection

Which macrolide?
1 Clarithromycin*
  — Undiagnosed community-acquired pneumonia, e.g.
    • Legionnaire's disease
    • *Mycoplasma* pneumonia
    • Psittacosis
2 Azithromycin
  — *C. trachomatis* keratitis
  — Toxoplasmal encephalitis
  — *M. avium-intracellulare* infections (500 mg/day)
  — Single-dose (1 g) therapy of chlamydial NSU‡
3 Erythromycin
  — Penicillin-allergy + Gram-positive cocci, e.g.
    • Strep throat
    • Pneumococcal pneumonia
  — Prophylactic or cautionary use
    • *C. diphtheriae* carrier state
    • *B. pertussis* (pre-paroxysmal)
    • Severe *Campylobacter* enterocolitis¶

* Improved activity against *H. influenzae* and high serum levels; hence, preferred for undiagnosed respiratory illnesses (if *severe*; if not, an aminopenicillin may be preferable)
‡ NB: Far more expensive than doxycycline or erythromycin
¶ *If* treatment indicated; ciprofloxacin is also effective

Drug of choice: tetracycline
1 Chlamydial disease (doxycycline)
  — Urethritis ('NSU')
  — Lymphogranuloma venereum
  — Non-gonococcal pelvic inflammatory disease
  — Epididymo-orchitis
  — TWAR pneumonia
2 Zoonoses
  — Brucellosis (doxycycline*)
  — Lyme disease (doxycycline)
  — Rickettsioses
3 Small intestinal infections‡
  — Whipple's disease (due to *Tropheryma whippelii*)
  — Severe *Yersinia* enteritis¶
  — Bacterial overgrowth
4 Mild-to-moderate acne vulgaris/rosacea
5 Broad-spectrum cover in renal failure (doxycycline)

* As part of combination therapy (p. 207)
‡ Efficacy due to poor gastrointestinal absorption; hence, high fecal levels
¶ Extraintestinal manifestations may be better treated with co-trimoxazole

Drug of choice: chloramphenicol
1 Pyogenic meningitis/encephalitis (children < 5)
2 Cerebral abscess
3 Severe (para)typhoid fever*
4 Acute epiglottitis

5 High oral bioavailability required‡

* Resistant strains now recognized; ciprofloxacin may be better
‡ e.g. refractory chest infections due to cystic fibrosis

Drug of choice: co-trimoxazole*
1 Major indications
  — *Pneumocystis carinii* (treatment or prophylaxis)
  — Nocardiosis (treatment or prophylaxis)
2 Other susceptible pathogens
  — Toxoplasmosis
  — *Klebsiella Serratia/Enterobacter* spp.
  — Yersiniosis, cyclosporiasis, melioidosis
  — Chancroid, granuloma inguinale
3 Refractory bronchitis/UTI/otitis media

* Trimethoprim/sulfamethoxazole

Drug of choice: co-amoxiclav*
1 Bite wounds (human or animal)
  — *P. multocida*
  — *Eikenella corrodens*
  — Streptococci, anaerobes
2 Resistant respiratory tract infections
  — Staphylococcal
  — *Moraxella catarrhalis*
  — *H. influenzae*
3 Complicated urinary tract or pelvic infections
  — *Proteus* spp.
  — *Klebsiella* spp.
  — Anaerobes, *E. coli*

* Amoxicillin plus clavulanic acid

Drug of choice: vancomycin
1 Pseudomembranous colitis (oral)
2 Methicillin-resistant staphylococci (MRSA)
3 Bacterial endocarditis
  — (Major) penicillin allergy
  — Prosthetic valve involvement
4 Shunt infections in dialysis patients*

* Vancomycin *not* dialysable

Drug of choice: metronidazole (or tinidazole)
1 Giardiasis
2 Trichomoniasis, *Gardnerella* vaginitis
3 Amebic dysentery
4 Anaerobic infections
5 Abscesses (incl. hepatic, cerebral)*

* NB: Many liver abscesses are due to *microaerophilic* strep – *Str. milleri* – and may therefore be resistant

CEPHALOSPORINS

A rough guide to the cephalosporins
1 First generation: strong Gram-positive activity
  — Cephalothin, cephazolin (IV), cephalexin (oral)
    • Active against β-lactamases, incl. *Staph aureus*
    • Weak Gram-negative activity
2 Second generation: intermediate activity spectrum
  — Cefoxitin
    • Moderate Gram-positive and Gram-negative activity (but not to *Staph aureus*, *Ps. aeruginosa*)

— Cefuroxime
   • Penetrates CSF; active against *H. influenzae*
3 Third generation: strong Gram-negative activity
  — Cefotaxime
   • Weak Gram-positive activity*
   • Does not cover anerobes or *Ps. aeruginosa*
   • Good CSF penetration‡
  — Ceftazidime (and, to some extent, cefoperazone)
   • Gram-negative cover includes *Ps. aeruginosa*

* Fails to cover *Str. fecalis* or *Staph aureus*
‡ Currently the drug of choice for undiagnosed childhood bacterial meningitis

Common problems with cephalosporin therapy
1 Poor penetration of sputum and CSF
2 Development of Gram-negative resistance
3 Significant incidence of cross-sensitivity in penicillin allergy
4 Expense

PENICILLINS

Microorganisms highly sensitive to penicillin G
1 Non-enterococcal (gp A and B) streptococci
2 *Clostridia* spp. (except *Cl. difficile*)
3 *Actinomyces* spp., *Corynebacteria* spp., *L. monocytogenes*
4 *Neisseria meningitidis*
5 Leptospira
6 *Borrelia burgdorferi**
7 *Treponema pallidum*
8 *C. canimorsus* ('DF-2'), *P. multocida*

* In *complicated* Lyme borreliosis; rash alone can be treated with tetracycline

Ampicillin/amoxicillin as first-line therapy?
1 Non-life-threatening community-acquired pneumonia
2 Acute bacterial exacerbations of chronic bronchitis
3 Meningitis due to *L. monocytogenes*
4 Urinary tract infections in pregnancy
5 Dental/surgical prophylaxis of bacterial endocarditis

Penicillin allergy or resistance: which antibiotic?
1 Pyogenic meningitis
  Aspiration pneumonia
  — Cefotaxime
  — Chloramphenicol
2 Typhoid
  — Ciprofloxacin
  — Chloramphenicol
3 Lobar pneumonia
  — Clarithromycin
  Rheumatic fever prophylaxis
  — Erythromycin
4 Acute bronchitis
  Sinusitis, otitis
  — Ciprofloxacin
5 Osteomyelitis
  — Ciprofloxacin
  — Clindamycin
6 Gonorrhea

  — Ciprofloxacin or ceftriaxone
  — Azithromycin (also covers *C. trachomatis*)
  — Spectinomycin
7 Syphilis
  — Erythromycin
8 Life-threatening staph infections
  — Vancomycin ± aztreonam

Antibiotics for endocarditis in penicillin allergy
1 Prophylaxis
  — Vancomycin
2 Staphylococcal or non-enterococcal streptococcal endocarditis
  — Vancomycin
  — Oral ciprofloxacin* + rifampicin
3 Enterococcal endocarditis
  — Penicillin desensitization → ampi- + aminoglycoside, *or*
  — Vancomycin (pending MIC, MBC) + aminoglycoside
4 Right-sided *Staph aureus* endocarditis
  — Flucloxacillin + tobramycin
  — Oral ciprofloxacin + rifampicin (on discharge)

* NB: Pneumococci also usually resistant

Pneumococcal infections: approximate duration of therapy
1 Otitis media — 5 days
2 Pneumonia — 10 days
3 Meningitis — 2 weeks
4 Septic arthritis — 4 weeks
5 Empyema — 6 weeks

Clinical features of Jarisch–Herxheimer reaction
1 Occurs due to rapid release of microbial endotoxin
2 Typically occurs within 1–6 h of bactericidal antibiotic therapy, esp. penicillins
3 Manifests with abrupt onset of fever, chills, myalgias, hyperventilation, tachycardia (± hypotension)
4 Classically occurs following initial treatment of *secondary syphilis*, but also occurs in other infections (esp. penicillin-treated spirochetal diseases, e.g. leptospirosis)

ANTIBIOTIC SENSITIVITY AND RESISTANCE

Characteristic patterns of antibiotic resistance
1 *Klebsiella* spp.
  — Penicillins (incl. ampicillin, ticarcillin)
2 *H. influenzae*
  — Penicillin G, cephalosporins; ampicillin (5%)
  — Erythromycin
3 Streptococci, anaerobes
  — Aminoglycosides*
4 *Proteus* spp., gp B streptococci
  — Tetracyclines
5 Listeriosis
  — Cephalosporins

* NB: Enterococcal strep are only 'sensitive' to aminoglycosides when used with a penicillin

Patterns of bacterial susceptibility to antibiotics
1 *Ps. aeruginosa*
   — Combination therapy (for serious infections)
     • Aminoglycoside + antipseudomonal penicillin
   — Extended-spectrum penicillins
     • Piperacillin (most potent)
     • Azlocillin
   — Other β-lactams
     • Imipenem/cilastatin
     • Ceftazidime
     • Aztreonam
2 *Staph aureus*
   — Drug of choice
     • Flucloxacillin
     • Nafcillin (for staphylococcal meningitis)
   — Second-line regimens
     • Clindamycin, erythromycin
     • Amoxicillin/clavulanic acid (co-amoxiclav)
   — Multiresistant ('methicillin-resistant': MRSA)
     • Vancomycin
     • Fusidic acid, rifampicin
3 *H. influenzae**
   — Cefotaxime (drug of choice for invasive disease)
   — Ampicillin/amoxicillin ± clavulanic acid
   — Chloramphenicol; clarithromycin; ciprofloxacin

* Note that *corticosteroids* confer additional therapeutic benefit in comatose children with *H. influenzae* meningitis (ref. 7.3)

Established synergy of antibiotic combinations
1 *Pseudomonas* infections
   — Aminoglycoside + antipseudomonal penicillin
2 *Str. fecalis* endocarditis
   — Ampicillin + gentamicin
3 Cryptococcal meningitis
   — Amphotericin B + 5-FC

Microorganisms commonly expressing β-lactamases
1 Staphylococci (95%)
2 Gonococci
3 Enterococci
4 Enterobacteriaceae, incl. *E. coli*
5 *H. influenzae*

β-lactamase inhibitors
1 Clavulanic acid
2 Sulbactam
3 Tazobactam

Antibiotics rapidly engendering resistance if used alone
1 *M. tuberculosis*
   — Rifampicin, streptomycin, pyrazinamide
2 *Staph aureus*
   — Fusidic acid, rifampicin, erythromycin
   — second and third-generation cephalosporins*
3 *Ps. aeruginosa*
   — Piperacillin, azlocillin, imipenem‡, aztreonam
4 Gram-negatives
   — Nalidixic acid, ciprofloxacin (esp. IV)
5 Fungi (e.g. *C. neoformans*)
   — Flucytosine (5-FC), fluconazole

6 Viruses
   — Ganciclovir

* e.g. cefoxitin (induces β-lactamase)
‡ Usually combined with cilastatin, a renal dipeptidase inhibitor (→ ↑ urinary imipenem levels, ↓ nephrotoxicity); has the broadest activity spectrum of any antibiotic

Mechanisms of antibiotic resistance to *Staph aureus*
1 'Plasmid resistance'
   — Express β-lactamases (e.g. TEM-1)
     → cleave antibiotic (β-lactam) ring
   — Certain bacteria (e.g. *Klebsiella, Ps. aeruginosa, Serratia, Enterobacter*) induce β-lactamases only in response to antibiotic exposure; these inducible enzymes are *resistant* to clavulanic acid
2 Reduced bacterial cell wall permeability
   — e.g. pen B mutation → ↓ porin expression (porins permit antibiotic entry)
   — Similar mechanism underlies resistance to vancomycin
   — β-lactamase-resistant drugs (or inhibitors) do *not* help
3 'Methicillin resistance' (MRSA)‡
   — Chromosomally-dependent ('intrinsic') resistance due to expression of penicillin-binding proteins
   — e.g. pen A mutation → ↓ PBP2
4 'Tolerance'
   — Development of MBC:MIC ratio > 32 (reflecting failure of autolytic bacterial enzyme activation by β-lactam)
5 Staphylococcal DNA gyrase mutations
   — Confer ciprofloxacin resistance

‡ Resist not only methicillin but also all other penicillins, cephalosporins, aminoglycosides, quinolones, erythromycin and clindamycin

Major indications for specific aminoglycosides
1 Gentamicin
   — Suspected Gram-negative sepsis
   — Adjunctive to β-lactams as broad-spectrum cover
2 Amikacin
   — Gentamicin resistance
3 Tobramycin
   — Suspected *Ps. aeruginosa*
4 Streptomycin
   — TB, brucellosis
5 Netilmicin
   — Concern over nephrotoxicity

Drug therapy of miscellaneous infections and infestations
1 Giardiasis
   — Metronidazole 2 g daily for 3 days, *or*
   — Tinidazole 2 g stat (single oral dose)
2 Hepatic amebiasis
   — Metronidazole 400 mg t.d.s. for 5 days
   Cecal amebiasis
   — Metronidazole 800 mg t.d.s. for 5 days* (or emetine)
3 Toxoplasmosis
   — Pyrimethamine/sulfadiazine; spiramycin
4 Scabies

— Topical gammabenzene hexachloride 1%
— Single-dose oral ivermectin
Lice
— Permethrin (topical)
5 Hookworm, whipworm, echinococcus
— Mebendazole
6 *Strongyloides, Toxocara*
— Thiabendazole
7 *Ascaris*, pinworm
— Pyrantel pamoate (or albendazole)
8 *Schistosoma japonicum* (plus other schistosomes), paragonomiasis, clonorchiasis, neurocysticerosis
— Praziquantel
9 Onchocerciasis ('river blindness'), bancroftian filariasis
— Ivermectin (single oral dose)
Other filariases
— Diethylcarbamazine (single-dose)
10 *Trypanosoma brucei gambiense*
— Eflornithine (IV)
Trypanosoma brucei rhodesiense
— Suramin

* Colonic amebiasis requires higher doses than hepatic, because metronidazole is very efficiently absorbed in the small intestine

ANTIBIOTIC TOXICITY

Potential morbidity of antibiotic use
1 Nitrofurantoin
— Neuropathy (esp. with renal impairment)
— Pulmonary fibrosis
— Hemolytic anemia; megaloblastosis
— Cholestasis → chronic active hepatitis
2 Chloramphenicol
— Idiosyncratic aplastic anemia (→ 1:25,000)
— Dose-related myelosuppression
— Neuropathy, optic atrophy
— Depression of antibody synthesis
3 Erythromycin
— Abdominal pain*
— Phlebitis (with IV use)
4 Ticarcillin
— Fluid (sodium) overload; hypokalemia
— Impaired platelet function, seizures
— Inactivation of gentamicin/tobramycin if admixed
5 Metronidazole
— Dysgeusia
— Disulfiram-type reactions
— Painful neuropathy
6 Amphotericin B
— Fever, rigors; vomiting; phlebitis
— Azotemia (75%); hypokalemia, renal tubular acidosis
— Anemia
7 Ciprofloxacin
— May precipitate theophylline toxicity
— Arthralgias in children
— Photosensitivity, psychosis, transaminitis, crystalluria
8 Vancomycin
— Rapid infusion → 'red-man' syndrome (histamine release); hydroxyzine prophylaxis may help

— Phlebitis, ototoxicity, nephrotoxicity

* Via activation of GI tract motilin receptors (p. 141)

Antibiotics which may precipitate seizures
1 High-dose β-lactams
— e.g. Ticarcillin, piperacillin
2 Imipenem
3 Fluconazole
4 Fluoroquinolones

Tetracyclines: toxic manifestations
1 Common
— Diarrhea
— Esophagitis
— Moniliasis
2 Benign intracranial hypertension
3 Photosensitization (demeclocycline)
Vertigo (minocycline)
4 Worsening of renal failure
5 Hepatotoxicity, esp.
— Intravenous use
— In pregnant women
— With preexisting renal impairment
6 Teeth staining when administered to children aged < 8 years*

* Or to pregnant women; ingestion during the third trimester may result in staining of the child's secondary (permanent) dentition

Aminoglycoside toxicity: variations between drugs
1 Deafness (cochlear VIII toxicity)
— Amikacin (most)
— Neomycin, gentamicin, tobramycin (moderate)
2 Ataxia (vestibular VIII toxicity)
— Streptomycin, gentamicin, tobramycin (most)
— Amikacin (moderate)
— Netilmicin (least)
3 Nephrotoxicity*
— Gentamicin, tobramycin (most)
— Amikacin (moderate)
— Netilmicin, streptomycin (least)

* Worsened by concurrent frusemide or cephalothin

Disadvantages of aminoglycosides
1 Narrow therapeutic range (must monitor levels)
2 Ineffective against anaerobes and strep/staph*
3 Failure to penetrate CSF, bile, abscesses
4 Must be given IV

* But synergistic with concomitant β-lactams

IATROGENIC INFECTIONS

Infections occurring in prosthetic appliances
1 Prosthetic valves, arterial grafts
— *Staph albus*
— *Staph aureus*
— *Str. viridans*
— Gram-negative bacilli
2 Prosthetic joints
— *Staph albus*

— *Staph aureus*
— Gram-negative bacilli
3 CSF shunts
— *Staph albus* (75%)
— *Staph aureus*
— Gram-negative bacilli
4 Intraocular lens implant
— *Staph albus*
— *Staph aureus*

Microorganisms transmissible by blood transfusion
1 Hepatitis viruses
— HCV, HBV, δ agent (p. 145)
2 HIV
3 CMV
4 Syphilis
5 Malaria, babesiosis
6 *Trypanosoma cruzi* (Chagas' disease)
7 Rare
— Brucellosis, yersiniosis
— EBV, HAV

Approach to the febrile neutropenic patient
1 Culture blood, urine and other relevant sites
2 Commence presumptive treatment with either
— Antipseudomonal β-lactam (e.g. piperacillin) *plus* an aminoglycoside (e.g. gentamicin), *or*
— Oral ciprofloxacin *if* neutropenic duration expected to be short (investigational)
3 If penicillin-allergic or uremic, substitute
— Ceftazidime, *or*
— Imipenem/cilastatin
4 Add amphotericin B if
— Fever and neutropenia persist > 1 week, *or*
— Fever persists > 3 days and condition deteriorating, *or*
— Fever persists despite resolution of neutropenia, *or*
— Sinus tenderness, nasal ulcers, CXR focal lesion, *or*
— Central line cultures are positive for *Candida*
5 Add vancomycin if
— *Staph albus* identified on blood culture, *or*
— Endemic MRSA and persistent fever
6 Add metronidazole (or clindamycin) if
— Perianal tenderness, *or*
— Necrotizing gingivitis
7 Add acyclovir if
— Ulcerative or vesicular mouth lesions

ANTIFUNGAL DRUGS

Principles of antifungal chemotherapy
1 For *any* disseminated or life-threatening fungal infection, e.g. invasive aspergillosis, rhinocerebral mucormycosis
— Intravenous amphotericin B ± 5-FC
— AIDS patients: maintenance oral fluconazole
For visceral leishmaniasis
— Liposomal amphotericin B
— Pentavalent antimony; aminosidine

2 Candiduria with indwelling catheter in situ
— Oral 5-FC ± amphotericin B bladder washouts
3 Chronic mucocutaneous candidiasis
Paracoccidioidomycosis
— (Oral) ketoconazole
4 Less serious infections
— Oropharyngeal candidiasis
• Amphotericin lozenges ± nystatin/clotrimazole
— Esophageal candidiasis
• Fluconazole
— Petriellidosis; *Pseudallescheria boydii*
• Miconazole (IV)
— Tinea capitis
• Oral griseofulvin (or ketoconazole)
— Tinea corporis
• Topical clotrimazole/tolnaftate
— Pityriasis ('tinea') versicolor
• Selenium sulfide (topical) shampoo
5 Cryptococcal meningitis
— IV (or intraventricular) amphotericin B, *plus*
— Oral (or intravenous) 5-FC (at least 6 weeks)
— *Maintenance* fluconazole in HIV patients

Indications for itraconazole
1 Invasive mycoses
— Histoplasmosis, blastomycosis
— Sporotrichosis, chromomycosis
— Non-life-threatening invasive aspergillosis
2 Dermatophyte infections
— Onychomycosis (toenail tinea)

Indications for fluconazole
1 Mucosal candidiasis *or* systemic candidemia
— In non-neutropenic patients
2 Coccidioidomycosis
3 CNS cryptococcosis
— Definitive therapy for non-life-threatening infections
— Maintenance therapy for HIV-infected patients

Disadvantages of ketoconazole therapy
1 Toxicity
— Nausea, hepatotoxicity
— Inhibition of steroid hormone synthesis*
• Impotence (antiandrogenic; useful in Ca prostate)
• Dysfunctional uterine bleeding
• Hypoadrenalism (useful in Cushing's)
2 Drug interactions (also common with itraconazole)
— Antagonism of ketoconazole by coadministered drug
• Absorption ↓ by antacids, H_2-blockers
• Mutual antagonism by rifampicin (↑ liver metabolism), isoniazid, phenytoin
— Potentiation of coadministered drug
• Cyclosporin A toxicity (esp. in renal transplants), but also permits cyclosporin dose reduction
• Phenytoin toxicity (?warfarin, tolbutamide)
— Disulfiram-like effect with alcohol

* cf. triazoles (fluconazole, itraconazole): specific for fungal cytochrome P_{450}, *no* effect on steroid metabolism

ANTIVIRAL CHEMOTHERAPY

Antibiotic regimens for viral infections
1 Herpes simplex
   — Keratitis: 3% acyclovir ointment five times daily
   — Genital (acute attack): 1 g/day acyclovir p.o.
   — Genital (prophylaxis): 800 mg/day acyclovir p.o.
   — Encephalitis: IV acyclovir (10 mg/kg q 8 h)
   — Acyclovir resistant disease in AIDS? Foscarnet
2 Varicella-zoster
   — Disseminated: IV acyclovir (10 mg/kg q 8 h)*
   — Ophthalmic: 3% ointment *plus* oral acyclovir
     4 g/day
3 HIV
   — Zidovudine (AZT) 250 mg q 4 h orally
4 Influenza A (prophylaxis or therapy)
   — Amantadine/rimantidine, 200 mg/day
5 Influenza B, RSV
   — Ribavirin aerosol
6 Lassa fever
   — Ribavirin orally
7 HPV (in juvenile laryngeal papillomatosis)
   — Interferon (IV)
8 Rhinovirus (for the common cold)
   — Interferon (intranasally)‡
9 CMV in the immunosuppressed patient
   — Ganciclovir (prevents retinitis, pneumonitis,
     colitis)
10 Hepatitis viruses (see p. 145)

* NB: Acyclovir therapy *not* yet proven to affect incidence or severity of post-herpetic neuralgia
‡ Doesn't work for RSV, adenovirus or (para)influenza

VACCINES

Active immunization: mechanisms of vaccine action
1 Toxoids
   — Tetanus, diphtheria, botulinum
2 Recombinant vaccines
   — Hepatitis B (HBsAg)
3 Pooled surface proteins
   — Pneumococcus
   — *H. influenzae* type B ('Hib')
   — Typhoid (parenteral Vi vaccine)
4 Attenuated (live) organisms*
   — Viruses: polio, measles, rubella, mumps
   — BCG
   — Hepatitis A
   — Cholera (CVD 103-HgR)¶
   — Typhoid (oral Ty21a vaccine)¶
5 Killed organisms‡
   — Influenza A
   — Rabies

* *Hazardous* (hence, contraindicated) in immunosuppressed patients
‡ *Ineffective* (hence, contraindicated) in immunosuppressed patients
¶ NB: Efficacy of cholera and typhoid vaccines for travellers remains modest

Indications for pneumococcal vaccine
1 Patients aged 2–70
   — Hyposplenism (p. 199)
   — Chronic renal failure
2 Patients aged 55–70
   — Diabetes mellitus
   — Chronic liver disease
   — Cardiac and/or pulmonary disease
   — CSF leaks

Indications for passive immunization
1 Pooled gammaglobulin
   — Hepatitis A
     • Family contacts
     • Institutional outbreaks
     • Travellers in tropical/developing countries*
   — Measles
     • Immunosuppressed contacts of acute cases‡
2 Hyperimmune globulin
   — Hepatitis B
     • Percutaneous/mucosal exposure to positive sera
     • Sexual contacts of acute cases (optional)
     • Newborns of HBsAg+ mothers (at 0, 3, 6 months)
   — Rh isoimmunization (→ Rh(D)-negative mother)
     • After delivery of Rh+ infant
     • On abortion of pregnancy with Rh+ father
     • Following inadvertent transfusion of Rh+ blood
   — Varicella-zoster
     • Immunosuppressed contacts of acute case
     • Newborn contacts of acute case
   — Rabies
     • Subjects exposed to rabid animals
   — Tetanus
     • Prophylaxis (exposure of non-immune subject)
     • Therapeutic (on diagnosis of disease: urgent)

* Repeat passive immunization every 4 months
‡ If exposed less than a week previously

Efficacy of active immunization
1 Pneumococcal vaccination
   — Prevents 60% infections
2 Influenza vaccination
   — Prevents 70% infections
3 Hepatitis B vaccination
   — Prevents 90% infections
4 MMR (measles, mumps, rubella) vaccination
   — Prevents 95% infections
5 DPT (diphtheria, pertussis, tetanus) vaccination
   — Prevents 99% infections

UNDERSTANDING INFECTIOUS DISEASE

A simplified classification of microorganisms
1 Viruses
   — RNA
     • Myxoviruses (e.g. influenza)
     • Paramyxoviruses (e.g. measles, mumps, RSV)
     • Picornaviruses (e.g. enteroviruses*, hepatitis A)
     • Reoviruses (e.g. rotavirus)
     • Rhabdoviruses (e.g. rabies)
     • Arenaviruses (e.g. Lassa fever)

- Togaviruses (e.g. rubella, dengue)
- Retroviruses (e.g. HIV, HTLV)
— DNA
  - Herpesviruses (HSV, VZ, CMV, EBV, HHV-6/8)
  - Adenoviruses
  - Parvoviruses
  - Papovaviruses (e.g. HPV, JC virus)
  - Hepadnaviruses (e.g. hepatitis B)
2 Bacteria
  — Cell-wall-deficient
    - *Mycoplasma* spp.
  — Obligate intracellular
    - *Chlamydiae, Rickettsiae*
  — Helically coiled
    - Spirochetes (*Treponema, Leptospira, Borrelia*)
    - *Helicobacter pylori*
    - *Campylobacter* spp.
    - *Aeromonas* spp., *Plesiomonas* spp.
  — 'Higher' bacteria
    - *Mycobacteria* spp.
    - *Corynebacteria* spp.
    - *Actinomyces, Nocardia*
  — Eubacteria (the rest)
3 Fungi
  — Yeasts (grow as hyphae, increase by budding), e.g.
    - *Candida albicans*
    - *Cryptococcus neoformans*
  — Molds (grow as mycelia, increase by branching), e.g.
    - *Aspergillus fumigatus*
    - Dermatophytes (e.g. tinea)
  — Dimorphic, e.g.
    - *Histoplasma capsulatum*
4 Parasites
  — Protozoa
    - *Plasmodium* spp.
    - *Toxoplasma gondii*
    - *Entameba histolytica*
    - *Giardia lamblia*
    - *Pneumocystis carinii*‡
    - *Trichomonas vaginalis*
  — Multicellular (worms)
    - *Schistosoma* spp.
    - *Strongyloides stercoralis*
    - *Echinococcus granulosus*
    - *Toxocara canis*
    - Filariasis

* Includes ECHO, polio, Coxsackie viruses
‡ *Pneumocystis* may be genetically closer to *fungi* than protozoa

Gram-staining: clinically relevant organisms
1 Gram-positive cocci
  — *Staphylococcus* spp.
  — *Streptococcus* spp.
2 Gram-negative cocci
  — *Neisseria* spp. (gonococcus, meningococcus)
3 Gram-positive bacilli
  — *Clostridium* spp.
  — *Bacillus* spp.
  — *Corynebacterium diphtheriae*
  — *Actinomyces israeli*
  — *Gardnerella vaginalis*
  — *Listeria monocytogenes*

4 Gram-negative bacilli
  — Enterobacteriaceae*
  — *Pseudomonas aeruginosa*
  — *Hemophilus influenzae*
  — *Campylobacter jejuni/coli*
  — *Brucella* spp.
5 Acid-fast bacilli
  — *Mycobacteria* spp.
  — *Nocardia* spp., *Actinomyces* spp. (weakly acid-fast)

* Includes *E. coli, Proteus, Klebsiella, Salmonella/Shigella* spp.

EPIDEMIOLOGY OF INFECTIOUS DISEASE

Seasonality of infectious disease
1 Summer/autumn
  — Legionnaire's disease
  — Leptospirosis
  — Polio; enteroviruses
  — Arboviruses (e.g. Ross River virus)
2 Autumn/winter
  — Hepatitis A
  — Coxsackie B
  — Coronaviruses; RSV
3 Winter/spring
  — Mumps
  — Infectious mononucleosis
  — Lymphocytic choriomeningitis
  — Rotavirus; Norwalk (parvovirus)
4 Spring or autumn
  — Rhinoviruses

Insect vectors of infectious disease
1 Malaria
  — *Anopheles* mosquito (female)*
2 Yellow fever
  — *Aëdes* mosquito
3 Leishmaniasis
  — *Phlebotomus* sandfly
4 *Trypanosoma cruzi*
  — *Reduviid* arthropod
5 *Trypanosoma gambiense*
  — *Tsetse* fly
6 *Shigella* spp.
  — Housefly (*Musca domestica*)
7 Babesiosis
  — *Ixodes* tick

* Bite only between dusk and dawn

Incubation periods of various infective agents
1 Rapid-onset (incubation period often < 1 week)
  — Viruses
    - Herpes simplex (esp. type I)
    - Yellow fever
  — Bacterial
    - Cholera (*V. cholerae*)
    - Bacillary dysentery (*Shigella*)
    - Scarlet fever (*Str. pyogenes*; p. 229)
    - Diphtheria (*C. diphtheriae*)
    - *Neisseria* spp. (gonococcus, meningococcus)
    - *H. influenzae*
    - Anthrax (*B. anthracis*)

2 Delayed-onset (incubation period often > 3 weeks)
   — Viruses
     • Hepatitis A/B
     • Epstein–Barr virus
     • Rabies
   — Bacteria
     • Syphilis (*T. pallidum*)
     • Leprosy (*M. leprae*)
   — Protozoa
     • Amebiasis (*E. histolytica*)
     • Chagas' disease (*T. cruzi*)
   — Worms
     • Filariasis
     • Schistosomiasis

Infectious disease: periods of infectivity
1 Hepatitis A
   — Prior to icteric phase
2 Measles
   — From prodrome until 4 days after onset of rash
3 Mumps
   — Three days preparotitis until 1 week after
4 Rubella, chickenpox
   — One week prior to onset of rash until 1 week after
5 Scarlet fever, diphtheria
   — Onset until 3 weeks after (↓ by antibiotic therapy)

The childhood exanthemata
1 Measles (rubeola)
2 German measles (rubella)
3 Scarlet fever
   — Due to toxin-producing streptococci
4 Filatov–Dukes disease
   — Variant of scarlet fever, *or*
   — Due to toxin-producing staph infections
5 Erythema infectiosum ('fifth disease')
   — Due to parvovirus B19 infection
6 Exanthem subitum (roseola, 'sixth disease')
   — Due to HHV-6 infection (p. 212)

Pathogen or contaminant? A guide to normal flora
1 Mouth
   — Anaerobes
   — *Str. viridans*
   — Pneumococcus
   — *H. influenzae*
2 Skin
   — *Propionibacterium acnes*
   — *Staphylococcus* spp.
3 Colon
   — Anaerobes
   — Enterobacteriaceae, esp. *E. coli*
4 Vagina
   — Lactobacilli
   — Anaerobes
   — Gp B streptococcus

Infections which commonly persist in the host
1 Herpesviruses (p. 226)
2 Hepatitis B and C viruses
3 Toxoplasmosis
4 Malaria (esp. *P. malariae*)
5 *Strongyloides stercoralis*
6 TB

Dental caries: the most prevalent infectious disease of humans
1 *Str. mutans* is the most cariogenic bacterium in plaque (an accretion on tooth enamel in which acid accumulates)
2 Dietary sucrose reduces plaque pH thus inducing demineralization of hydroxyapatite enamel
3 Immunization against *Str. mutans* reduces plaque load and caries by stimulating production of secretory IgA (± IgG)
4 Fluoride also reduces caries
5 Necrotizing ulcerative gingivitis or chronic periodontal disease may occur due to treponemal spirochetes, esp. *T. denticola* and *T. socranskii*

OCCUPATIONAL EXPOSURE TO INFECTIOUS DISEASE

Nosocomial sources of infection
1 Air conditioners
   — Aspergilli, staphylococci
2 Humidifiers
   — *Acinetobacter* spp.
   — *Pseudomonas* spp.
3 Water reservoirs
   — *Legionella pneumophila*, *Pseudomonas* spp.
4 Foods (e.g. salads)
   — Gram-negatives, staphylococci, streptococci
5 Endogenous flora
   — Enterobacteriaceae, staphylococci (incl. MRSA)
6 Reactivation
   — TB, herpesviruses, mycoses
7 Parenteral nutrition
   — Candidiasis, staphylococci
8 Blood transfusions
   — Hepatitis B and C, CMV, HIV, HTLV
   — Malaria, Chagas' disease (developing countries)
9 Hydrotherapy pools, whirlpool baths
   — *Ps. aeruginosa* folliculitis
10 Other patients and staff
   — Herpesviruses (esp. zoster)
   — *Listeria* spp.
   — *Cl. difficile*

Seroconversion risk after needlestick from viral index case
1 HIV
   — 0.5%
2 HCV
   — 5%
3 HBV
   — 25%*

* Risk varies widely depending on virion titer and HBeAg status

MECHANISMS OF INFECTIOUS DISEASE

Microorganisms which form spores
1 Fungi
2 *Clostridium* spp. (e.g. → botulism)
3 *Bacillus* spp. (e.g. → anthrax)

Diseases mediated by exotoxins
1 Clostridial disease
   — Tetanus (*Cl. tetani*)
   — Botulism (*Cl. botulinum*)
   — Gas gangrene (*Cl. perfringens*)
   — Antibiotic-associated colitis (*Cl. difficile*)
2 Diphtheria
3 Cholera
   Enterotoxigenic *E. coli* diarrhea
4 Staphylococcal food poisoning
   Toxic shock syndrome

Diseases in which prion proteins are implicated
1 Scrapie
2 Kuru
3 Creutzfeldt–Jakob
4 Gerstmann–Sträussler–Schenker syndrome
5 Familial fatal insomnia

Microbiological determinants of the 'gay bowel' syndrome
1 Pruritus ani
   — *Enterobius vermicularis* (pinworm)
   — *Pthirus pubis* (pubic lice)
   — *Sarcoptes scabiei* (scabies)
2 Perianal lesions
   — Condylomata acuminata (HPV 6, 11)
   — Condylomata lata (secondary syphilis)
   — Primary syphilitic chancre (simulates fissure)
   — Granuloma inguinale (*H. ducreyi*: donovanosis)
   — Herpetic vesicles
3 Proctitis
   — *C. trachomatis* (non-LGV serotypes)
   — *N. gonorrheae*
   — *T. pallidum*
   — Herpes simplex
4 Proctocolitis
   — *C. trachomatis* (LGV serotypes)
   — *Sh. flexneri*
   — *Campylobacter* spp.
   — *E. histolytica**
5 Enteritis
   — *G. lamblia*
6 AIDS-associated gastrointestinal infections
   — Cryptosporidiosis (small intestine)
   — Candidiasis (esophageal)
   — *M. avium-intracellulare* (may mimic Whipple's)
   — *S. typhimurium*
   — *Isospora belli, Cyclospora* spp.
   — CMV

* NB: May be non-pathogenic commensal

Predispositions to mucormycosis (invasive zygomycosis)
1 Diabetes (→ rhinocerebral)
2 Malnutrition (→ gastrointestinal)
3 Burns (→ cutaneous)
4 Leukemia (→ pulmonary)
5 Immunosuppression (→ disseminated)

Predispositions to osteomyelitis
1 'Standard-risk' individuals
   — *Staph aureus* in 60%

2 Sickle-cell disease
   — *Salmonella* spp.
3 Drug addiction
   — *Ps. aeruginosa* (→ pelvis, vertebrae)

Clinical manifestations of *H. influenzae* (HI) infection
1 Capsulated HI → children
   — Acute epiglottitis*
   — Meningitis
   — Septic arthritis
2 Non-capsulated HI → children
   — Otitis media
   — Conjunctivitis
3 Non-capsulated HI → adults
   — Exacerbation of chronic bronchitis

* Caused by type B *H. influenzae* which is often resistant to ampicillin

Varieties and features of chlamydial infection
1 Non-specific urethritis (NSU)
   — Caused by *C. trachomatis* serotypes D-K
   — Commonest sexually transmitted disease
   — Presentations
     • Seropurulent urethral discharge
     • Persistent symptoms after gonorrhea therapy
     • Failure of presumptive β-lactam therapy
     • Reiter's syndrome; Fitz-Hugh Curtis syndrome
     • Pelvic inflammatory disease, infertility
   — Diagnosis: chlamydial isolation
2 Lymphogranuloma venereum (LGV)
   — Caused by *C. trachomatis* serotypes L1–L3
   — Systemic venereal disease endemic in tropics
   — Commonest in males (5:1), esp. homosexuals
   — Presentations
     • Painful inguinal adenopathy (may suppurate)
     • 'Groove sign' (nodes indented by inguinal lig.)
     • Ulcerative proctitis; rectal stricture
     • Rectovaginal or rectovesical fistula
     • Genital elephantiasis (esp. in women)
   — Diagnosis: serology
3 Trachoma inclusion conjunctivitis (TRIC)
   — Caused by *C. trachomatis* serotypes A-C (hyperendemic)
   — Estimated to affect 500 million people
   — Commonest avoidable cause of blindness (→ keratitis)
   — Diagnosis: chlamydial isolation
4 Psittacosis
   — Caused by *C. psittaci*
   — Occupational hazard of bird-fanciers
   — Presentations
     • Atypical pneumonia
     • Myocarditis, endocarditis (rarely)
   — Diagnosis: serology
5 Epidemic pneumonia (TWAR)
   — Caused by *C. pneumoniae**
   — Causes 10–30% of pneumonia in Finland
   — Presentations
     • Prolonged, often relapsing illness

- Prominent pharyngitis, laryngitis
- Atypical pneumonia (mimics psittacosis)
— Resistant to erythromycin‡, responds to tetracycline
— Diagnosis: serology (distinguishable from *C. psittaci*)

* Named TWAR after first two isolates, TW-183 and AR-39; morphologically resembles *C. psittaci*
‡ cf. other atypical pneumonias (p. 337)

STREPTOCOCCI

Pathogenicity of streptococci

1 *Str. pyogenes* (= Gp A β-hemolytic strep; see below)
   — Acute invasive suppurative effects
   - Impetigo
   - Cellulitis, pyoderma
   - Pharyngitis
   — Other acute sequelae
   - Scarlet fever
   - Erysipelas
   - Puerperal sepsis
   - Wound infection
   — Late non-suppurative sequelae
   - Rheumatic fever
   - Post-infective nephritis
2 *Str. pneumoniae* (pneumococci)
   - Pneumonia, esp. community-acquired lobar
   - Meningitis
   - Otitis media
3 *Str. viridans*: a broad term including
   — *Str. sanguis*
   - Infective endocarditis (commonest strep cause)
   — *Str. fecalis* (enterococci)
   - Urinary tract infection
   - Infective endocarditis (penicillin-resistant)
   — *Str. bovis* (enterococci)
   - Infective endocarditis (penicillin-sensitive)
   — *Str. milleri*
   - Liver and/or brain abscess
   — *Str. mutans*
   - Dental plaque/caries

Characterization of streptococci

1 Diagnostically relevant Lancefield antigen groups

   — Gp A
   - *Str. pyogenes*
   — Gp B
   - *Str. agalactiae* (e.g. post-partum)
   — Gp D
   - Enterococci
2 Diagnostically relevant in vitro hemolysis
   — α-hemolytic*
   - *Str. viridans*
   - Pneumococci
   — β-hemolytic‡
   - *Str. pyogenes*

* α-hemolytic organisms convert unlysed red cell hemoglobin in 5% blood agar to greenish (hence, 'viridans') compounds
‡ β-hemolytic organisms lyse red cells in 5% blood agar

Pyogenic streptococci

1 *Str. pyogenes*
   — i.e. Gp A β-hemolytic strep
   — Nephritogenic, skin and invasive (esp. M1) strains (incl. 'flesh-eating' bacteria)
2 Pneumococci
   — Gram-positive diplococci on microscopy
3 *Str. milleri*
   — Anaerobic strep

NB: *Str. pyogenes* and pneumococci *rarely* cause streptococcal endocarditis

Streptococcal infections: clinical correlations

1 Untreated Gp A streptococcal pharyngitis predisposes to rheumatic fever (cf. primary skin infections)
2 *Both* pharyngeal and cutaneous Gp A streptococcal infections predispose to post-strep glomerulonephritis
3 Prompt antibiotic therapy does *not* prevent post-strep glomerulonephritis (cf. rheumatic fever)
4 Latent periods between initial infection and complications
   - 4 weeks for rheumatic fever
   - 2 weeks for nephritis following impetigo
   - 1 week for synpharyngitic nephritis
5 ASO titers are strongly positive in strep pharyngitis, but only weak in impetigo (streptolysin O inactivated by skin lipids)
6 Elevated or changing ASO titers may also be associated with erythema nodosum or Henoch–Schönlein purpura

7.1 Cohen S et al (1991) Psychological stress and susceptibility to the common cold. N Engl J Med 325: 606–612

'Stress' questionnaire preceded intranasal administration of virus to 394 volunteers. Both infection (viral isolation and/or rising titers) and symptoms were commoner in the 'stressed-out' cohort.

7.2 van der Meer J et al (1992) Efficacy of antibiotic prophylaxis for prevention of native-valve endocarditis. Lancet 339: 135–139

Controversial study suggesting that prophylactic antibiotics prevent (at best) 'only' 49% of native-valve endocarditis cases, making national prophylaxis programs likely to be cost-ineffective.

7.3 Schaad UB et al (1993) Dexamethasone therapy for bacterial meningitis in children. Lancet 342: 457–461

Double-blind study of 115 children in which adjunctive dex (0.4 mg/kg IV q 12 h for 48 h, prior to ceftriaxone) was shown to improve outcome, thus supporting the results of earlier studies. Hence, host response may be at least as important as microbial virulence in mediating morbidity of such infections.

7.4 Russel JA et al (1992) Allogeneic bone-marrow transplantation without protective isolation in adults with malignant disease. Lancet 339: 38–40

Hammond J et al (1992) Double-blind study of selective decontamination of the digestive tract in intensive care. Lancet 340: 5–9

Two more studies casting doubt on the efficacy of prophylactic antimicrobial measures. In the first, handwashing alone in a single room compared well with strict (gown-and-glove) protocols from other institutions. In the second study, enteral antibiotics (colistin, amphotericin and tobramycin) conferred no additive benefit in ICU patients receiving 72 h IV cefotaxime.

7.5 Wilkins E, Ivanyi J (1990) Potential value of serology for diagnosis of extrapulmonary tuberculosis. Lancet 336: 641–644

First report of serologic response to a putative 38-kDa *Myco. tuberculosis* antibody, enabling earlier diagnosis and therapy.

7.6 Goodrich JM et al (1991) Early treatment with ganciclovir to prevent cytomegalovirus disease after allogeneic bone marrow transplantation. N Engl J Med 325: 1601–1607

Merigan TC et al (1992) A controlled trial of ganciclovir to prevent cytomegalovirus disease after heart transplantation. N Engl J Med 326: 1182–1186

Two transplant studies indicating improved outcomes following use of the antiherpetic drug ganciclovir to prevent CMV infections.

7.7 Malik IA et al (1992) Randomised comparison of oral ofloxacin alone with combination of parenteral antibiotics in neutropenic febrile patients. Lancet 339: 1092–1096

Provocative randomized study comparing the in-hospital course of 60 febrile neutropenic patients receiving either the oral fluoroquinolone alone or conventional parenteral β-lactam/aminoglycoside therapy. No significant differences in efficacy were identified.

7.8 Saag MS et al (1992) Comparison of amphotericin B with fluconazole in the treatment of acute AIDS-associated cryptococcal meningitis. N Engl J Med 326: 83–89

Powderly WG et al (1992) A controlled trial of fluconazole or amphotericin B to prevent relapse of cryptococcal meningitis in patients with the acquired immunodeficiency syndrome. N Engl J Med 326: 793–798

Two prospective randomized studies confirming the value of fluconazole in AIDS-associated cryptococcal meningitis, either in primary treatment or subsequent maintenance.

Wingard JR et al (1991) Increase in *Candida krusei* infection among patients with bone marrow transplant-ation and neutropenia treated prophylactically with fluconazole. N Engl J Med 325: 1274–1277

The downside of prophylactic antibiotic therapy.

7.9 Summerfield JA et al (1995) Mannose binding protein gene mutations associated with unusual and severe infections in adults. Lancet 345: 886–889

Opsonic and complement activation defects due to mutations of mannose binding protein have previously been recognized to predispose to childhood infections, but this is the first report of such an association in adults.

7.10 Niruthisard S et al (1992) Use of nonoxynol-9 and reduction in rate of gonococcal and chlamydial cervical infections. Lancet 339: 1371–1375

Potentially important public health study indicating that vaginal spermicide (N-9) usage was associated with a major reduction of bacterial sexually transmitted infections.

CHAPTER 8

Metabolism, nutrition and genetics

Physical examination protocol 8.1   You are asked to assess the nutritional status of a patient with diarrhea

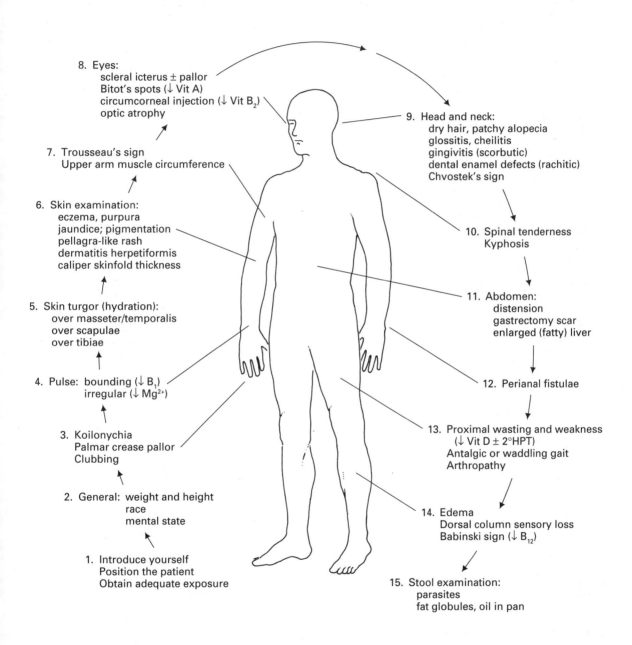

8. Eyes:
   scleral icterus ± pallor
   Bitot's spots (↓ Vit A)
   circumcorneal injection (↓ Vit B$_2$)
   optic atrophy

7. Trousseau's sign
   Upper arm muscle circumference

6. Skin examination:
   eczema, purpura
   jaundice; pigmentation
   pellagra-like rash
   dermatitis herpetiformis
   caliper skinfold thickness

5. Skin turgor (hydration):
   over masseter/temporalis
   over scapulae
   over tibiae

4. Pulse: bounding (↓ B$_1$)
   irregular (↓ Mg^{2+})

3. Koilonychia
   Palmar crease pallor
   Clubbing

2. General: weight and height
   race
   mental state

1. Introduce yourself
   Position the patient
   Obtain adequate exposure

9. Head and neck:
   dry hair, patchy alopecia
   glossitis, cheilitis
   gingivitis (scorbutic)
   dental enamel defects (rachitic)
   Chvostek's sign

10. Spinal tenderness
    Kyphosis

11. Abdomen:
    distension
    gastrectomy scar
    enlarged (fatty) liver

12. Perianal fistulae

13. Proximal wasting and weakness
    (↓ Vit D ± 2°HPT)
    Antalgic or waddling gait
    Arthropathy

14. Edema
    Dorsal column sensory loss
    Babinski sign (↓ B$_{12}$)

15. Stool examination:
    parasites
    fat globules, oil in pan

CLINICAL ASPECTS OF METABOLIC AND NUTRITIONAL DISORDERS

Commonest metabolic/nutritional short cases
1 Paget's disease
2 Marfan's syndrome
3 Wernicke–Korsakoff syndrome

WILSON'S DISEASE

Potential misdiagnoses in Wilson's disease
1 Coombs-negative hemolytic anemia due to hypersplenism
2 Idiopathic ('lupoid', HBsAg-negative) chronic active hepatitis
3 'Juvenile cirrhosis'
4 Schizophrenia, manic-depressive psychosis
5 Demyelination; primary cerebellar degeneration; Hallervorden–Spatz disease; idiopathic epilepsy

Other complications of Wilson's disease
1 Renal tubular acidosis (proximal type)
2 Amenorrhea, recurrent abortions
3 Chondrocalcinosis; pathological fractures
4 'Sunflower' cataracts
5 Pigmentation, blue lunules
6 Penicillamine toxicity

Diagnosis of Wilson's disease
1 Clinical signs
   — Hepato/splenomegaly
   — Kayser–Fleischer rings*
   — Slurred speech, 'batswing' tremor, rigidity, chorea
2 Copper metabolism
   — ↑ *Free* serum copper
   — ↓ *Total* serum copper
   — ↓↓ Serum ceruloplasmin (false-negatives in hepatitis)
   — ↑ 24-h urinary copper (usually > 100 μg; *not* pathognomonic), esp. post-penicillamine
   — Delayed rate of radiocopper incorporation into ceruloplasmin (definitive but rarely performed)
3 Liver biopsy (prone to sampling error)
   — ↑ Liver copper (> 60 μg/g dry weight)‡
   — Histology: fatty infiltration, hepatitis, cirrhosis
4 CT brainscan
   — Cortical atrophy, basal ganglia hypodensities

* Exclusion may require slit-lamp examination; absence excludes Wilson's as cause of neurological signs, but presence is *not* pathognomonic
‡ Most diagnostic test, though positives also may be seen in PBC

Drugs preventing clinical manifestations of Wilson's disease
1 Oral zinc (blocks gastrointestinal copper uptake)
2 Trientine (triethylene dihydrochloride)*
3 D-penicillamine

* An alternative to D-penicillamine in Wilson's, but *not* in cystinuria or rheumatoid arthritis

SKELETAL DISORDERS

Diagnostic criteria for Marfan's syndrome
1 Major criteria
   — Mitral valve prolapse with regurgitation
   — Dilated aortic root with regurgitation
   — Dissecting ascending aortic aneurysm
   — Lens dislocation with iridodonesis (shaky iris)
2 Minor criteria
   — Isolated mitral valve prolapse
   — Severe myopia (> 4 diopters)
   — High arched palate
   — Scoliosis, 'funnel' chest, asthenic build
   — Spontaneous pneumothorax
   — Arachnodactyly; flat feet
   — Joint hypermobility (esp. ankle)
   — Positive family history

The patient with Paget's*: clinical examination
1 Deformity of long bone(s), e.g. tibia
2 Bruit over deformity
3 Skull enlargement; associated bruit
4 Cervical spondylosis (p. 264)
5 Deafness (usually nerve)
6 Hyperdynamic circulation ± congestive cardiac failure

* see also p. 357

Presentations of primary hyperparathyroidism
1 Asymptomatic (in 30%)
   — Hypercalcemia detected on 'routine' biochemical test
2 Renal calculi (in 50%)
3 'Acute' presentations
   — Polydipsia/polyuria/dehydration
   — Nausea, vomiting, anorexia, constipation
   — Lethargy, dementia, psychosis
4 'Chronic' presentations
   — Nephrocalcinosis
   — Band keratopathy
5 Rare presentations
   — **P**eptic ulcer
   — **P**ancreatitis
   — **P**roximal myopathy
   — **P**athological fracture (of 'brown tumor')
   — **P**seudogout
   — **P**ituitary tumors ⎫
   — **P**ancreatic tumors ⎬ MEN1 (p. 115)
   — **P**heochromocytoma ⎭

NUTRITIONAL DISORDERS

Clinical presentations of vitamin deficiency
1 Vitamin A deficiency
   — Xerophthalmia, night blindness, Bitot's spots
   — Hyperkeratosis
2 Thiamine deficiency
   — Beri-beri (esp. in Asians)
     • Muscle weakness
     • Tachycardia, heart failure

— Wernicke–Korsakoff syndrome*, esp. in
  • Alcoholics ($\downarrow$ erythrocyte transketolase activity)
  • Also → hemodialysis/renal transplant patients
  • May be precipitated by IV glucose
  • May be mimicked by niacin deficiency
3 Pellagra (niacin deficiency)
  — Dermatitis (and glossitis)
  — Diarrhea
  — Dementia
4 Strachan's syndrome (? vitamin B-complex deficiency)
  — Orogenital dermatitis
  — Amblyopia
  — Painful peripheral neuropathy
5 Scurvy (vitamin C deficiency)
  — Weakness, fatigue, arthralgias
  — Ulcers, poor wound healing
  — Gingivitis, purpura
  — Subperiosteal hemorrhages (may be palpable)
6 Osteomalacia/rickets (vitamin D deficiency)
  — Tetany (in children)
  — Bone disease
  — Proximal myopathy
7 Vitamin E deficiency (e.g. cystic fibrosis, ileal resection)
  — Peripheral neuropathy, areflexia
  — Spinocerebellar degeneration, ataxia
  — Hemolysis

* NB: IV thiamine treatment usually reverses coma and ocular palsies, but nystagmus or ataxia often persist

Clinical presentations of trace element deficiency
1 Zinc deficiency (genetic, short bowel, diarrhea, alcoholism or TPN)
  — Acrodermatitis enteropathica; alopecia
  — Poor wound healing
  — Impaired taste (hypogeusia); photophobia
2 Selenium deficiency (may occur in TPN)
  — Muscle pain, hemolytic anemia
  — Keshan disease → childhood cardiomyopathy in China
3 Copper deficiency
  — Hypochromic microcytic anemia
4 Chromium deficiency
  — Glucose intolerance
  — Peripheral neuropathy; encephalopathy
5 Manganese deficiency
  — Nausea, dermatitis

Differential diagnosis of a pellagra-like rash
1 Pellagra (dietary niacin deficiency)
  — esp. With high-maize (leucine-rich, tryptophan-poor) diet; leucine inhibits tryptophan → niacin
2 Hartnup disease (inherited aminoaciduria)
  — Tryptophan malabsorption → nicotinamide deficiency
3 Carcinoid syndrome
  — $\uparrow\uparrow$ 5-hydroxytryptamine → $\downarrow\downarrow$ tryptophan (precursor)
4 Isoniazid toxicity
  — Prevents pyridoxine activation → $\downarrow\downarrow$ niacin precursors

Sorting out vitamin B_6 metabolism
1 'Niacin' = vitamin B_3 = nicotinic acid = pyridine 2-carboxylic acid
2 Nicotinic acid is a precursor of *nicotinamide* which is in turn a precursor of NAD (nicotinamide adenine dinucleotide) and NADP (NAD phosphate), both of which participate in cellular oxidation/reduction reactions
3 'Pyridoxine' (vitamin B_6) = one of three pyridine (niacin precursor) moieties in the diet; it is converted to the active coenzyme pyridoxal phosphate
4 Pyridoxal phosphate is involved in intermediary amino acid metabolism and binds to muscle glycogen phosphorylase

Predispositions to acquired folate deficiency
1 Alcoholism
2 Blind loop syndrome
3 Celiac disease

Differential diagnosis of B_{12} deficiency and a laparotomy scar
1 Post-gastrectomy
2 Ileal resection for Crohn's

HYPOTHERMIA

Predispositions to hypothermia
1 Environmental
  — Any severe or immobilizing illness
  — Poverty, poor housing, advanced age
  — Exposure
2 Reduced heat production
  — Hypothyroidism, adrenal failure
  — Malnutrition
  — Exhaustion (decreased shivering)
3 Increased heat loss
  — Erythroderma
  — Extensive burns
  — Vasodilatation, esp. if alcohol-induced
4 Impaired heat regulation/poikilothermia
  — Stroke
  — Autonomic neuropathy
5 Drug overdose, esp.
  — Phenothiazines
  — Barbiturates

Systemic complications of profound hypothermia
1 Metabolic
  — Acidosis, hyperkalemia
  — Hypoglycemia
2 Cardiovascular
  — Reduced cardiac output, BP, heart rate
  — ECG: 'J' waves, ventricular dysrhythmias, asystole
  — Myocardial infarction*
3 Renal
  — Initial diuresis → hypovolemia → oliguria
4 Respiratory
  — Reduced oxygen consumption *and/or* tissue hypoxia
  — Pulmonary edema, pneumonia; apnea

5 Gastrointestinal
— Erosive gastritis, pancreatitis
— Drug toxicity (↑ hepatic metabolism on rewarming)
6 CNS
— Amnesia, mydriasis
— Hallucinations, paradoxical undressing
— Reduced cerebral blood flow, coma

* e.g. if externally rewarmed without IV fluid replacement (p. 241)

Metabolic considerations in near-drowned patients
1 Fresh-water (hypotonic, hypervolemia) drowning
— Often leads to *mild* hypoxia only, due to surfactant inactivation and/or intravascular hemolysis
2 Salt-water (hypertonic) drowning
— Often causes *severe* hypoxia due to pulmonary edema
3 'Dry drowning'
— Death due to reflex laryngospasm without aspiration
4 Post-resuscitative course may be complicated by
— Aspiration pneumonia
— Acute tubular necrosis
— Disseminated intravascular coagulation
5 Prognosis post-resuscitation
— Hypothermia → better prognosis
— Neurologic signs → poor prognosis

Medical problems affecting underwater divers
1 Decompression sickness ('the bends')
— Symptom onset varies: 10 min → days
— Arteriovenous/lymphatic obstruction
— Tissue rupture
— Muscle fascial compartmental syndrome
2 Nitrogen narcosis ('rapture of the depths')
— Mimics drunkenness
— Occurs with air diving below 40 meters
3 Barotrauma
— Face squeeze; facial nerve baroparesis
— Dental or skin barotrauma
— Gastric rupture

HYPERTHERMIA

Differential diagnosis of hyperthermia
1 Fever (due to infection)
2 Heat stroke (exacerbated by anticholinergic therapy)
3 Iatrogenic (general)
— Bleomycin, L-asparaginase, interferon
— MAOI or sympathomimetic overdose ± tricyclics
4 Malignant hyperthermia
5 Neuroleptic malignant syndrome

Malignant hyperthermia or neuroleptic malignant syndrome?
1 Malignant hyperthermia (MH)
— Autosomal dominant etiology
— Caused by *many* inhalational anesthetics, e.g. halothane, suxamethonium*
— *Peripheral* origin (post-synaptic muscle contraction)

— High fever develops within minutes; may be fatal
— Often complicated by metabolic acidosis/hyperkalemia
— Muscle necrosis → myoglobinuria, renal failure, ↑ Ca^{2+}
— Associations: central core disease, myotonic dystrophy
— Prophylaxis or therapy: dantrolene sodium
2 Neuroleptic malignant syndrome (NMS)
— Idiosyncratic etiology (impossible to predict)
— Precipitated by phenothiazines/butyrophenones‡
— *Central* origin (CNS dopaminergic inhibition)
— Develops insidiously over 1–3 days: fluctuating consciousness, dystonias, autonomic instability
— 20% mortality due to aspiration pneumonitis, acute myoglobinuric renal failure, arrhythmias
— Neuromuscular blockers (e.g. pancuronium) may cause flaccid paralysis (cf. MH: no effect)
— Therapy: dantrolene or bromocriptine (takes days)

* cf. Pseudocholinesterase deficiency: specific for suxamethonium
‡ Also seen in L-DOPA 'drug holidays' in Parkinson's disease

AROMATIC ABNORMALITIES

Gustatory/olfactory clues to diagnosis of metabolic disorders
1 Skin
— Salty (cystic fibrosis)
— Caramel (maple syrup urine disease)
— Sweaty feet (isovaleric acidemia)
2 Urine
— Rotting fish (trimethylaminuria)*
— Mouse-like (phenylketonuria)

* Fish odor also detectable in breath, sweat, saliva, vaginal secretions

Anosmia: differential diagnosis
1 Post-traumatic
— e.g. Skull fracture (commonest cause)
2 Frontal/olfactory groove meningioma
→ Asymptomatic unilateral loss
3 Inherited disease
— Kallman's syndrome, Refsum's disease
4 Post-coryzal or chronic rhinitis; cadmium poisoning
5 Sjögren's syndrome, Paget's disease
6 CNS disease: Alzheimer's, Parkinson's

UNUSUAL DISORDERS

Diagnoses worth considering in obscure clinical presentations
1 Occult malignancy, esp. Ca lung/liver/kidney, lymphoma
2 Occult infection: tuberculosis, syphilis, infective endocarditis
3 Sarcoidosis
4 Polyarteritis nodosa
5 Iatrogenic

6 Functional
 — Alcoholism/narcotic addiction
 — Depression
 — Hysteria
 — Self-inflicted disease

Fibrosing syndromes in clinical medicine
1 Retroperitoneal fibrosis
2 Constrictive pericarditis
3 Sclerosing cholangitis
4 Riedel's thyroiditis
5 Peyronie's disease
6 Fibrosing alveolitis
7 Systemic sclerosis (scleroderma)

Clinical varieties of histiocytosis
1 Class I (Langerhans cell) histiocytosis*
 — Letterer–Siwe disease (→ infants)
 • Hepatosplenomegaly/lymphadenopathy
 • Cytopenias (marrow infiltration by H-X cells)
 • Lung infiltrates, recurrent pneumothoraces
 — Hand–Schüller–Christian disease (→ adolescents)
 • Skull lesions
 • Exophthalmos; ear discharge
 • Diabetes insipidus (in 30%)
 — Eosinophilic granuloma (→ adults)
 • Multiple lytic bony deposits (esp. in skull)
 • Malaise, weight loss, fever
 • Lung fibrosis
2 Class II histiocytosis
 — Hemophagocytic (non-Langerhans) syndromes
 • Sinus histiocytosis + massive adenopathy
3 Class III histiocytosis
 — Malignant histiocytosis
 • 'True histiocytic' lymphoma (celiac disease)
 • Histiocytic medullary reticulosis
 • Leukemias: AML (M4/M5), CMML (p. 172)

* = 'Histiocytosis X', a group of histologically benign conditions (though clinical course may be lethal). Treatable with etoposide

CLINICAL PRESENTATIONS OF INHERITED DISEASE

Gaucher's (adult non-neuronopathic) disease: features
1 Occurs due to deficiency of β-glucosidase
2 Presents with
 — Hypersplenism ± massive splenomegaly
 — Bone pain due to
 • Infarcts/aseptic necrosis
 • Bone cysts (→ distal femur)
 • Vertebral collapse
 • Pathological fracture
 — Pingueculae; pigmentation
 — Pneumonia
3 Normal life expectancy
 — i.e. In adult (type III) disease
4 Best screening test
 — Serum acid phosphatase (tartrate-resistant)
5 Definitive diagnosis
 — Demonstration of Gaucher cells in marrow, liver or node (= PAS +ve cells, 'crumpled silk' cytoplasm*)

* NB: Gaucher cells may also be seen in CGL, myeloma, ITP

Clinical spectrum of mitochondrial disease
1 Progressive external ophthalmoplegia, incl. Kearns–Sayre
 — Ophthalmoplegia + retinitis pigmentosa + complete heart block + increased CSF protein
2 Hypermetabolic proximal myopathy
 — e.g. Luft's: heat intolerance, fever, weakness
 — May mimic thyrotoxicosis
3 'Ragged red fiber' syndrome
 — Myopathy resembles facioscapulohumeral dystrophy
 — Associated with myoclonic epilepsy, lactic acidosis
4 Cytochrome deficiencies
 — e.g. Menke's ('kinky hair') syndrome

NB: Diseases of mitochondrial DNA are inherited via the maternal genome

Inborn abnormalities of connective tissue: features
1 Marfan's syndrome
 — Autosomal dominant, variable penetrance
 — Increasing frequency with paternal age
 — 30% sporadic mutation rate
 — Occurs due to fibrillin gene mutations
 — Signs
 • Armspan > height; scoliosis
 • Joint hypermobility
 • Arachnodactyly, 'wrist', 'thumb' signs
 • High palate, iridodonesis
 • Pectus deformity; MVP, AI
2 Osteogenesis imperfecta
 — Occurs due to qualitatively abnormal type I collagen
3 Homocystinuria (autosomal recessive)
 — Some phenotypic similarity to Marfan's, but
 • Atherothrombotic tendency
 • Subclinical osteoporosis
 • Downward lens dislocation
 • 30% incidence of mental retardation
 — Responds to
 • Dietary methionine restriction
 • Cystine supplements
 • Pyridoxine (in 50%)
 • Betaine
4 Pseudoxanthoma elasticum (dominant or recessive)
 — Characterized by
 • Flexural xanthoma-like lesions, lax skin
 • Fundal angioid streaks
 • Premature atherosclerosis (→ hypothyroidism)
 • Diagnostic calcium deposition on skin biopsy
 — Occurs due to production of abnormal elastin
5 Ehlers–Danlos syndromes (dominant or recessive)
 — Characterized by
 • Joint hypermobility, recurrent dislocations
 • Purpura
 • 'Fish-mouth' scarring
 • Diverticulosis, pneumothoraces
 — Type IV
 • GI bleeding, perforation, aneurysm rupture
 • Occurs due to ↓ type III collagen
 — Type VI
 • Retinal detachment, corneal perforation
 • Occurs due to ↓ lysyl hydroxylase

— Type VII
  • Velvety skin, short stature
  • Occurs due to ↓ procollagen protease
— Type VIII manifests as periodontitis
6 Disorders due to reduced lysyl oxidase activity
— Ehlers–Danlos type V (X-linked)
— Cutis laxa (X-linked)
  • Emphysema, pulmonary hypertension
— Menke's 'kinky hair' syndrome
  • Defective copper absorption

Laurence–Moon or Bardet–Biedl syndrome?
1 Features in common
— Mental retardation
— Hypogonadism
— Obesity
— Retinopathy
2 Additional features of Laurence–Moon syndrome
— Ataxia
— Spastic paraparesis
3 Additional features of Bardet–Biedl syndrome
— Polydactyly
— Renal abnormalities
  • Persistent fetal lobulation
  • Cystic dysplasia, clubbed calices
  • Nephrogenic diabetes insipidus
  • Aminoaciduria

INVESTIGATING METABOLIC DISORDERS

Causes of misleading results
1 (Pseudo)hyponatremia
— Dilutional
  • High-grade paraproteinemia
  • Chylomicronemia (ketoacidosis, hyperlipidemia)
  • IV therapy: mannitol or parenteral fat emulsions
2 Spurious hyperkalemia
— Sample hemolysis
  • (Leukemic) white cell count > 200,000/mL
  • Difficult venepuncture
  • Delay in processing specimen
3 Spurious hyperchloremia
— Bromism
4 Spurious hyperglycemia
— Venepuncture adjacent to dextrose infusion site
5 Spurious hypercalcemia
— Prolonged venous stasis
— Calcium binding by myeloma paraprotein (rare)
Spurious normocalcemia
— Hypoalbuminemia (esp. in cancer patients)
6 ↑ Triglycerides, ↑ gastrin, ↓ growth hormone
— Patient not fasted
7 Elevated CPK
— Recent intramuscular injection
8 Elevated acid phosphatase
— Recent rectal examination
9 Negative urinalysis for ketones
— Alcoholic ketoacidosis (leads to high β-hydroxybutyrate but normal acetone)

ELECTROLYTE DISORDERS AND THE ANION GAP

High anion gap metabolic acidosis*: common precipitants
1 Uremia
2 Ketoacidosis (diabetic or alcoholic)
3 Lactic acidosis (± dehydration, alcohol intoxication)
4 Overdose
— Aspirin
— Methanol, ethylene glycol
— Paraldehyde

* Anion gap = $Na^+ - Cl^- - HCO_3^-$; normal range = 8–12 mEq/L

Differential diagnosis of a low anion gap*
1 Hypoalbuminemia
2 Paraproteinemia
3 Electrolyte imbalance
— Hypercalcemia
— Hypermagnesemia
— Lithium intoxication

* May mask biochemical recognition of metabolic acidosis

Hyperchloremic (normal anion gap) acidosis: pathogeneses
1 Renal tubular acidosis
2 Gastrointestinal
— Diarrhea, esp. in neonates
— Pancreatic/biliary fistula
— Ureteroenterostomy ± obstructed ileal bladder/vesicocolic fistula
3 Iatrogenic
— Acetazolamide
— Cholestyramine
— Parenteral nutrition with fructose, sorbitol

Normal anion gap acidosis with hyperkalemia*: causes
1 Treated diabetic ketoacidosis
2 Obstructive uropathy
3 Early uremic acidosis, esp. if due to medullary disease
4 Mineralocorticoid deficiency or insensitivity

* a.k.a. type 4 renal tubular acidosis

Lactic acidosis: antecedents and diagnosis
1 Type A
— Precipitated by *any* cause of severe tissue hypoxia
2 Type B
— Idiopathic onset in elderly debilitated patients
— Alcohol abuse and/or liver disease
— Uremia
— Some leukemias, myeloproliferative disorders
— Diabetes mellitus ± metformin ± ketoacidosis
3 Clinical
— Hyperventilation without dehydration*
4 Diagnosis requires exclusion of other causes of high anion gap acidosis ± demonstration of elevated plasma lactate

* cf. hyperosmolar coma (p. 101): vice versa

Clinical features of D-lactic acidosis

1 Occurs in
  — Short-bowel syndrome
  — Jejunoileal bypass
2 Increased frequency if
  — Thiamine deficiency
  — Renal tubular acidosis
  — Large oral sugar load
3 Due to
  — Increased colonic lactate load leading to hyperabsorption
  — Selective failure to metabolize D-lactate isomer
4 Features
  — Confusion, ataxia, nystagmus, stupor
  — Mimics alcoholic inebriation
5 Treatment
  — Bicarbonate infusion
  — Thiamine (if deficient)
  — Reduce colonic flora (and ?alkalinize gut)
    • Oral vancomycin, neomycin, metronidazole

Examples of mixed metabolic acidosis

1 Normal plus high anion gap acidoses
  — Renal tubular acidosis leading to nephrocalcinosis
  — Diabetic with hyporeninemic hypoaldosteronism developing ketoacidosis
2 Mixed normal anion gap acidoses
  — Acetazolamide therapy in patients with preexisting renal tubular acidosis
3 Mixed high anion gap acidoses
  — Alcoholic ketoacidosis complicated by lactic acidosis
  — Methanol intoxication and lactic acidosis

Diagnostic significance of urinary chloride in metabolic alkalosis

1 *All* forms of metabolic alkalosis have low *serum* chloride
2 *Urinary* chloride is *normal* in some (*normovolemic*) metabolic alkaloses, e.g.
  — Primary hyperaldosteronism
3 Urinary chloride *absent* in *hypovolemic* metabolic alkaloses
  — Gastric losses (prolonged vomiting, suction)
  — Following excessive use of diuretics
4 This is because the hypovolemic stimulus for ADH secretion *overrides* hypoosmolar stimulus for ADH suppression
  — i.e. Renal Na+ (and Cl−) are *conserved*
5 This leads to a *paradoxical aciduria* which persists until NaCl (volume) *and* KCl (electrolyte) replenishment is achieved
  — i.e. Resolution of the alkalosis is *chloride-dependent*

Some causes of hypouricemia

1 Proximal renal tubular disease (e.g. Wilson's disease)
2 SIADH (e.g. acute interminent porphyria, Guillain–Barré)
3 Chronic liver disease
4 Carcinomatosis
5 Hereditary xanthinuria (xanthine oxidase deficiency)
6 Drug-induced: allopurinol, high-dose aspirin, NSAIDs, sulfinpyrazone, diflunisal, probenecid

Indications for serum magnesium estimation

1 Severe or intractable diarrhea and/or malabsorption, e.g.
  — Short bowel syndrome
  — Inflammatory bowel disease
2 Life-threatening alcohol withdrawal
3 Refractory cardiac arrhythmias (esp. ventricular) Unexplained digoxin toxicity
4 Apathetic thyrotoxicosis
5 Hypocalcemia and/or tetany unresponsive to calcium
6 Neuromuscular symptoms after cisplatin or mannitol
7 Investigation of chronic fatigue

Clinically important causes of hypophosphatemia

1 Insulin treatment of diabetic ketoacidosis
2 Alcoholic withdrawal supported with dextrose infusions
3 Proximal renal tubular dysfunction
4 Following starvation or severe burns
5 Osteomalacia (unless associated with renal failure)
6 Iatrogenic
  — Hyperalimentation
  — Phosphate-binding antacids, hemodialysis
  — Paracetamol overdose ($\rightarrow \uparrow$ renal losses)

Manifestations of hypophosphatemia

1 Due to reduced erythrocyte 2,3-DPG (esp. in ketoacidosis)
  — Tissue hypoxia $\rightarrow$ ataxia, confusion, convulsions
2 Due to reduced intracellular ATP
  — Platelet dysfunction $\rightarrow$ bleeding
  — Hemolytic anemia, leukocyte dysfunction
3 Due to rhabdomyolysis (esp. in alcoholics)
  — Renal failure
  — Delayed hypercalcemia
  — Cardiomyopathy

HYPERCALCEMIA

Common causes of hypercalcemia

1 Hyperparathyroidism
2 Malignancy
  — Via production of PTHrP
  — Osteolytic bone metastases ± 'flare'

Steroid-suppressible hypercalcemia: differential diagnosis

1 Granulomatous diseases
  — Sarcoidosis
  — TB, histoplasmosis, leprosy
2 Vitamin D intoxication
3 Multiple myeloma

Differential diagnosis of hypercalcemia with detectable iPTH*

1 Hyperparathyroidism
  — Primary
  — Tertiary (p. 318)
  — Secondary, *if* overzealous phosphate-binding R_x
2 Immobilization
  — Urinary cAMP normal

3 Malignancy
   — Urinary cAMP often increased
   — iPTH normal; PTHrP* often increased
4 Pheochromocytoma
   — Part of MEN2 (Sipple's syndrome; p. 115)
   — Catecholamine-stimulated PTH release‡

* iPTH = immunoreactive PTH; PTHrP = parathyroid hormone-related protein
‡ Hence, hyperparathyroidism may reflect hyperplasia *or* adenoma

Steps in the diagnosis of primary hyperparathyroidism
1 $\uparrow Ca^{2+}$; ± $\downarrow PO_4^{2-}$ (normalization may presage renal failure)
2 $\uparrow$ iPTH
   — Normal levels do not exclude the diagnosis*
   — The C-terminal fragment is generally assayed, though the N-terminal fragment confers activity
3 Elevated nephrogenous cAMP‡
4 Supportive (but not diagnostic) evidence
   — Phosphaturia (> hypercalciuria)
   — *Mild* $\uparrow$ serum alkaline phosphatase
   — Hyperchloremic acidosis (p. 236) with alkaline urine
   — No evidence of malignancy
5 Definitive diagnosis
   — Hyperplasia/adenoma confirmed at neck exploration
   — Resection followed by normalization of serum · calcium

* Undetectable levels do
‡ Not suppressible with oral calcium tolerance test

Differential diagnosis of normocalcemic hypercalciuria
1 Idiopathic
2 Medullary sponge kidneys
3 Immobilization (esp. in Paget's disease)
4 Sarcoidosis
5 Acromegaly; Cushing's syndrome
6 (Mild) primary hyperparathyroidism*
7 Renal tubular acidosis
8 Iatrogenic
   — Corticosteroids
   — Frusemide

* Definitively diagnosed by elevated serum iPTH and/or urinary cAMP

Hypercalcemia: selected clinical aspects
1 Dehydration may arise due to any combination of
   — Vomiting
   — Reduced fluid intake (anorexia, obtundation)
   — Nephrogenic diabetes insipidus
2 Azotemia may supervene due to
   — Prerenal failure (i.e. secondary to dehydration)
   — (Acute) vasoconstriction, $\downarrow$ glomerular permeability
   — (Chronic) tubule vacuolization or nephrocalcinosis
3 Immobilization hypercalcemia (and hypercalciuria)
   — More frequent in patients with Paget's disease
   — Corticosteroids or phosphate R_x are contraindicated
4 Gut hyperabsorption contributes to hypercalcemia in
   — Sarcoidosis

   — 'Milk-alkali' syndrome
   — Primary hyperparathyroidism
5 Familial hypocalciuric ('benign familial') hypercalcemia
   — Classically presents as failed neck exploration for hyperparathyroidism
   — Commonest hypercalcemia in patients < 10 years
6 Rhabdomyolysis hypercalcemia
   — May lead to initial hypocalcemia with azotemia
   — Hypercalcemia ensues during early renal recovery

Metabolic consequences of traumatic rhabdomyolysis*
1 Hyperkalemia; hypercalcemia (see above)
2 Hypovolemic shock
3 Myoglobinuric renal failure (p. 306)
4 Cardiomyopathy
5 Disseminated intravascular coagulation

* 'muscle crush syndrome'

VITAMIN D

Differential diagnosis of hypervitaminosis D
1 Intoxication with exogenous vitamin D
   — Renal failure
   — Hypoparathyroidism
   — Megadose ingestion
2 Granulomatous diseases
   — $\uparrow$ Extrarenal conversion of 25-OH-D to 1,25–$(OH)_2D$
   — Causes include sarcoidosis and lymphoma

Abnormal patterns of vitamin D metabolism in disease
1 Vitamin D intoxication
   — $\uparrow$ 25-Hydroxycholecalciferol ($25-D_3$)
   — Normal $1,25-D_3$
2 Sarcoidosis
   — Normal $25-D_3$
   — $\uparrow 1,25-D_3$ (even in *anephric* patients)
3 Chronic renal failure
   — Normal $25-D_3$
   — $\downarrow 1,25-D_3$
   — $\uparrow 24,25-D_3$
4 Rickets
   — Normal $1,25-D_3$ (vitamin D-resistant rickets)
   — $\downarrow 1,25-D_3$ (type I vitamin D-dependent rickets)
   — $\uparrow 1,25-D_3$ (type II vitamin D-dependent rickets)

Differential diagnosis of abnormal vitamin D metabolism
1 $\uparrow 1,25-D_3$
   — Primary hyperparathyroidism
   — Pregnancy
   — Sarcoidosis
2 $\downarrow 1,25-D_3$
   — Malignancy-induced hypercalcemia
   — Post-menopausal osteoporosis
   — Chronic renal failure
3 $\uparrow 25-D_3$
   — Vitamin D intoxication
   $\downarrow 25-D_3$
   — Osteomalacia
   — Hypomagnesemia

— Chronic liver disease (e.g. PBC)
— Chronic peritoneal dialysis
— Nephrotic syndrome
— Phenytoin use*

* Stimulates vitamin D catabolism

DIAGNOSTIC ASPECTS OF METABOLIC BONE DISEASE

Clinical significance of elevated urinary hydroxyproline*
1 Paget's disease (often > 50 x ↑)
2 Hereditary hyperphosphatasia (often > 50 x ↑)
3 Hyperparathyroidism
4 Osteomalacia (*except* renal tubular type)
5 Thyrotoxicosis

* Indicates collagen breakdown; correlates with serum alkaline phosphatase

Features of pseudohypoparathyroidism
1 Features *not* found in 'idiopathic' hypoparathyroidism
— Familial occurrence
• X-linked dominant (maternal) transmission*
— Physical examination
• Short fourth and fifth metacarpals‡
• No enamel hypoplasia or candidiasis
— Laboratory
• Normal or elevated serum iPTH
• Subnormal increment of urinary phosphate and nephrogenous cAMP after PTH infusion
2 Features *not* found in pseudopseudohypopara-thyroidism¶
— Clinical
• Associated endocrine abnormalities, e.g. hypothyroidism, amenorrhea
— Laboratory
• Hypocalcemia, hypocalciuria, hyperphosphaturia
• Normal or elevated serum iPTH
• Subnormal increment of urinary phosphate and nephrogenous cAMP after PTH infusion
3 Signs more typical of pseudopseudohypopara-thyroidism
— Mental retardation, dwarfism, obesity
— Subcutaneous calcification
4 Common features of pseudo- and pseudopseudo-variants
— Both may have Albright's osteodystrophy
— Both associated with G-protein (G$_s$) mutations
5 *All* may respond to pharmacological doses of calcitriol

* cf. Idiopathic: familial (autoimmune) variety is autosomal recessive
‡ Part of Albright's osteodystrophy (cf. Turner's syndrome → short fourth metacarpal; Down's syndrome → short, curved middle phalanx of fifth finger, 'clinodactyly')
¶ Now classified as a pathogenetic subset of pseudohypoparathyroidism

Diagnostic considerations in osteomalacia
1 Pathogenetic factors
— Main source of vitamin D for most people is sunlight

— Elderly people with little sun exposure may become vitamin D deficient due to dietary malabsorption induced (say) by gastrectomy
2 Proximal myopathy
— May be a prominent presenting symptom
— Arises in part due to hypophosphatemia
— Arises in part due to vitamin D deficiency per se
3 Diagnosis
— Characteristic radiographic features (p. 240)
— Biochemical triad
• Hypocalcemia
• Hypophosphatemia
• Serum alkaline phosphatase
— Definitive
• Bone biopsy

RADIOGRAPHIC FEATURES OF BONE DISEASE

Radiologic stigmata of hyperparathyroidism
1 General
— Widespread osteopenia
2 Most specific sign
— Subperiosteal resorption of radial aspects of middle phalanges of second and third fingers
3 Other erosive/resorptive changes
— Resorption of distal phalangeal tufts
— 'Brown tumors'*
— 'Fleabitten' mandible
— 'Salt-and-pepper' skull
— Loss of (dental) lamina dura
— Distal clavicular erosions
4 Metastatic calcification
— Nephrocalcinosis, renal calculi
— Chondrocalcinosis
— Vascular calcification (secondary hyperparathyroidism)

* bone cysts → phalanges, metacarpals, long bones

Classical spinal X-rays in metabolic bone disease
1 'Rugger-jersey' spine
— Renal osteodystrophy
— Osteopetrosis ('bone-within-bone')
2 'Ivory vertebrae'
— Paget's disease
— Hodgkin's disease
3 'Codfish' vertebrae
— Osteoporosis
— Osteomalacia
— Sickle-cell disease

Classical skull X-rays in bone disease
1 Osteoporosis circumscripta
— Paget's disease
2 'Raindrops' (many lytic lesions, no osteoblastic reaction)
— Myeloma
3 'Salt-and-pepper' skull
— Hyperparathyroidism
4 Wormian bones
— Osteogenesis imperfecta
5 'Hair-on-end' appearance
— Inherited anemias

6 'Punched-out' skull lesions
   — Histiocytosis X
7 Enlarged frontal sinuses
   — Acromegaly
8 Absent frontal sinuses
   — Kartagener's syndrome
9 Hyperostosis frontalis interna
   — Normal variant (esp. in women)

Other radiographic anomalies in bone disease
1 Rickets
   — Widened epiphyseal plate with indistinct borders
   — Splaying of bone ends (esp. wrists, knees)
   — Deformities: tibial bowing, frontal bossing
2 Osteomalacia
   — Pseudo-('Milkman's') fractures, Looser's zones*
3 Scurvy
   — Sclerotic bone edge ('dense white line') at epiphysis
   — No widening of epiphyseal plate (cf. rickets)
   — Periosteal elevation due to hemorrhage (seen post-R_x)
4 Heavy metal poisoning
   — Dense 'white line' at metaphysis (cf. scurvy)
5 Osteoid osteoma
   — Densely sclerotic lesion surrounded by radiolucency
   — Causes aspirin-sensitive bone pain in young patient
6 Osteopetrosis
   — 'Erlenmeyer flask' deformity of metaphyses

* Affect pubic rami, proximal femurs, lateral scapulae, rib

ISOTOPE BONE SCANNING

Possible indications for isotope bone scans
1 Suspected metastatic bone disease
2 Suspected (X-ray negative) fracture, esp.
   — ? Stress fracture
   — ? Sternal fracture
   — ? Scaphoid fracture
3 Suspected aseptic necrosis
   — Efficacy limited by non-specificity
4 Suspected sacroiliitis with non-diagnostic X-ray findings
   — Value in this context is controversial
5 Suspected periprosthetic infection (→ gallium scanning)
6 Paget's disease

Increased uptake on isotope bone scan?
1 New bone formation
   — Focal increase
     • Fracture*
     • Metastasis‡
   — Diffuse increase
     • Paget's disease
     • Hyperparathyroidism
     • Osteomalacia
2 Hyperemia
   — Infection¶
   — Trauma

3 Some primary tumors
   — Ewing's sarcoma
   — Osteosarcoma, neuroblastoma

* NB: Sacral and sternal lesions are often difficult to assess
‡ Solitary lesions and/or skull lesions can be difficult to interpret
¶ Osteomyelitis best diagnosed by bone scan ± ^{67}Ga or ^{111}In scan (esp. if prosthetic joint infection suspected)

Reduced uptake on isotope bone scan?
1 Avascular necrosis (incl. radiation osteonecrosis)
2 Multiple myeloma
3 'Eosinophilic granuloma' (p. 235)

NB: In patients with *pain*, normal uptake virtually excludes a bony origin

---

INVESTIGATION OF BONE METABOLISM

Diagnostic tests of bone density
1 X-ray
   — Singh index
2 Photodensitometry
   — e.g. Radial (or hip) bone mass
3 Iliac crest bone biopsy
   — Invasive; sampling error is a problem

Markers of osteoblastic activity (new bone formation)
1 Isotope (^{99m}Tc-phosphate) bone scan
2 Serum alkaline phosphatase (esp. bone isoform)
3 Serum osteocalcin

Markers of osteoclastic activity (bone resorption)
1 Acid phosphatase (tartrate-resistant)
2 Urinary hydroxyproline*
3 Urinary pyridinium crosslinks (of collagen)

* Utility reduced by non-specificity and insensitivity

INVESTIGATION OF GENETIC DISEASE

Biochemical screens available for inborn errors of metabolism
1 Benedict's test (copper reduction)
   — Galactosemia
2 DNP (dinitrophenylhydrazine) test
   — Maple syrup urine disease
3 Nitroprusside test
   — Homocystinuria
4 Alkaline silver reduction
   — Alkaptonuria (ochronosis)
5 Urinary colorimetry
   — Orotic aciduria

Presymptomatic disease identifiable by genetic linkage analysis
1 Huntington's chorea
2 Myotonic dystrophy
3 Duchenne muscular dystrophy
4 Neurofibromatosis (incl. acoustic variant)
5 Cystic fibrosis
6 α/β-thalassemias
7 Polycystic kidney disease

8 Familial adenomatous polyposis
9 Multiple endocrine neoplasia

Familial Mediterranean fever (recurrent polyserositis): diagnosis
1 History
   — Ethnic origin, positive family history
   — Previous attacks ± failed exploratory laparotomy
2 Acute episodes
   — Mild leukocytosis, ↑ ESR, ↑ fibrinogen during attacks
   — Rapid defervescence following attacks
3 Signs of chronicity
   — Proteinuria (if amyloidosis has supervened)
4 Important diagnostic exclusions
   — Normal amylase
   — Normal microbiology (incl. joint fluid)
   — Negative ANA and rheumatoid factor
5 Therapeutic normalization with colchicine
   — Effective symptom prophylaxis
   — Plasma dopamine β-hydroxylase (best test)

MANAGING METABOLIC DISEASE

Therapeutic priorities in metabolic derangements
1 Lactic acidosis
   — Removal of underlying cause (e.g. alcohol)
   — IV bicarbonate
2 Alcoholic ketoacidosis
   — Intravenous glucose, *plus*
   — Intravenous thiamine
3 Diabetic ketoacidosis
   — Insulin
   — Fluid and electrolyte balance
4 Hyperosmolar (non-ketotic diabetic) coma
   — IV fluids (use hypotonic saline unless hypotensive)
   — Insulin (usually unnecessary long-term; cf. DKA)
5 Hypoglycemic coma
   — Prevention
   — Immediate therapeutic trial of IV dextrose (± naloxone) in any undiagnosed unconscious patient*
6 Myxedema coma
   — Exclude hypothermia/-glycemia/-natremia/ -adrenal
   — Low-dose IV T_3 with hydrocortisone

* If Wernicke–Korsakoff syndrome possible, give IV thiamine as well

Management approach to the hypothermic patient
1 Sinus rhythm, core temperature > 32°C
   — Passive external rewarming
2 Sinus rhythm, core temperature < 32°C, *or* Arrhythmia, core temperature > 32°C
   — Active core rewarming:
     • Heated humidified air via endotracheal tube
     • Pleural or peritoneal lavage with heated (40–45°C) crystalloid or colloid fluid
3 Arrhythmia, core temperature < 32°C
   — Extracorporeal core rewarming
     • Cardiopulmonary bypass loop

   • Extracorporeal venovenous rewarming
   • Hemodialysis
   — Bretylium 10 mg/kg for ventricular fibrillation

MANAGEMENT OF ELECTROLYTE ABNORMALITIES

Hypokalemia: when is prophylactic supplementation indicated?
1 Patients clinically hypovolemic due to gastrointestinal losses who are commencing resuscitation with IV fluids
2 Patients undergoing insulin and fluid replacement for diabetic ketoacidosis *unless* hyperkalemic *and*
   — ECG changes of hyperkalemia, *or*
   — Biochemical evidence of prerenal failure, *or*
   — Known coexisting hyporeninemic hypoaldosteronism
3 Patients with anticipated large renal losses, e.g.
   — Post-obstructive diuresis
   — Sjögren's syndrome → post-partum
   — Wilson's disease → renal tubular disease + cirrhosis
4 Patients commencing therapy with
   — Loop diuretics
   — Ticarcillin
   — Amphotericin B
5 Patients stabilized on digoxin and commencing therapy with
   — Thiazides
   — Corticosteroids

An approach to acute hyperkalemia
1 Exclude diabetic ketoacidosis as a cause*
2 Check result on fresh specimen to exclude hemolysis artefact
3 Identify and remove precipitating cause if possible
4 Give 50 mL 50% dextrose IV, then soluble insulin (8–12 units)
5 Give 50 mL 8.4% sodium bicarbonate IV
6 Give 20 mL 10% calcium gluconate IV *if* ECG changes present
7 Give 15 g cation-exchange resin orally q 6 h and 30 g PR q 12 h
8 Dialysis (esp. peritoneal) may be indicated

* Since hyperkalemia of insulin deficiency may be associated with total body potassium deficit (and hence require K^+ *supplements* with insulin)

Approach to management of severe hyponatremia*
1 Asymptomatic patient (e.g. on diuretics; normotensive; low plasma sodium found on routine testing)
   — Discontinue diuretic
   — Restrict water intake
   — Encourage dietary salt intake until Na^+ normal
2 Minimally symptomatic patient, hypotensive, no CNS signs
   — Restrict water intake
   — IV normal saline to reexpand plasma volume
3 Symptomatic patient, CNS signs present (e.g. post-op)
   — Restrict water intake

— Slow hypertonic (3%) saline infusion
— Calibrate rate to increase plasma Na^+ by a *maximum* of 1 mmol/h (25 mmol/48 h) until Na^+ > 125 mmol/L
— Too rapid infusion → central pontine myelinolysis
— Hypervolemic SIADH patients may require frusemide

* plasma Na^+ < 110 mmol/L

Hazards of bicarbonate administration in metabolic acidosis
1 High sodium/osmotic load
2 Aggravation of tissue hypoxia (↑ Hb affinity for oxygen)
3 Paradoxical fall in CSF pH, leading to hypoventilation

MEDICAL TECHNOLOGY

Potential indications for hyperbaric oxygen therapy
1 Decompression sickness ('the bends')
2 Air embolism
3 Inhalational poisoning
— Carbon monoxide
— Smoke inhalation
— Hydrogen cyanide (adjunctive only)
4 Infections
— Gas gangrene
— Anaerobic sepsis with tissue necrosis
— Mucormycosis, actinomycosis
— Refractory chronic osteomyelitis
5 Impaired wound healing
— Radiation necrosis (esp. of bone)
— Severe thermal burns
— Diabetic wounds (if large vessels OK)
— Ischemic crush injury/compartment syndrome*
— Jeopardized skin flaps
— Hemorrhagic radiation cystitis

* Must be treated immediately to be effective

Iatrogenic consequences of synthetic implantable devices
1 Infection, commonly affecting
— Prosthetic hip
— Cardiac valve replacement
— CSF shunts
— Soft contact lenses; lens implants
— Long-term vascular access catheters
— Indwelling urinary catheters
2 Thromboembolism, commonly affecting
— Vascular grafts
— Valve replacements
3 Specific valve problems
— Valve failure (acute incompetence)
— Valve thrombosis (acute stenosis)
— Hemolysis
4 Specific IUD problems
— Pelvic inflammatory disease, infertility
— Ectopic pregnancy; septic abortion
— Uterine perforation, peritonitis
— *Actinomyces*/fungal infections (plastic IUDs)

NUTRITIONAL SUPPLEMENTATION

'Essential' amino acids*
1 Neutral (non-polar, uncharged)
— Valine, leucine, isoleucine
2 Polar uncharged
— Threonine
3 Strongly basic
— Lysine
4 Aromatic
— Histidine, phenylalanine, tryptophan
5 Sulfur-containing
— Methionine

* i.e. unable to be endogenously synthesized from precursors

Treatment approaches to morbid obesity
1 Dietary caloric restriction
— ± Psychotherapy, behavior modification, exercise
2 Anorexia-inducing drugs (controversial)
— Dexfenfluramine (for maximum of 12 weeks)
— Also improves peripheral insulin sensitivity
3 Surgery
— Jaw wiring
— Gastric stapling

Indications for hyperalimentation (parenteral nutrition)
1 Short bowel syndrome
2 Crohn's disease with severe malabsorption
3 Prolonged ileus
4 Pancreatic/intestinal fistula
5 Hypermetabolism (e.g. severe sepsis or burns)
6 Hyperemesis gravidarum (or other feeding difficulty)

Metabolic complications of total parenteral nutrition (TPN)
1 Hyperglycemia (may be aggravated by occult chromium deficiency) if insufficient insulin added to infusion
Hypoglycemia (most commonly due to kinking of dextrose infusion containing insulin, which continues to act)
Hyperosmolar coma (may be precipitated by sepsis)
2 Hypercalcemia (e.g. due to hypervitaminosis A or D)
Osteomalacia (in long-term TPN)
3 Hyperchloremic acidosis (prevent with acetate supplement)
Lactic acidosis (→ fructose infusions in neonates)
4 Hypophosphatemia (esp. during dextrose infusions)
Pseudohyponatremia (during infusion of fat emulsions)
Hypokalemia, hypomagnesemia, copper/zinc deficiency
5 Exfoliative dermatitis
— Due to ↑ vitamin A, ↓ zinc/fatty acids
6 Muscle wasting
— May be avoidable by glutamine supplementation
7 Liver disease
— Fatty infiltration
— Lymphocytic infiltration (+ transaminitis)
— Jaundice (± cholestasis, sepsis)
— Hyperammonemia (± encephalopathy)

VITAMIN THERAPY

Indications for high-dose vitamin supplements
1 Vitamins A,D,E,K
  — Hereditary abetalipoproteinemia (Bassen–Kornzweig)
  — Biliary atresia, ileal atresia
  — Cystic fibrosis
2 Vitamin B_6
  — Homocystinuria
  — Idiopathic refractory sideroblastic anemia
  — Renal oxalate stones
  — Unexplained infantile convulsions
3 Vitamin B_{12}
  — Transcobalamin II deficiency
  — Juvenile pernicious anemia
  — Homocystinuria
4 Folate
  — Congenital megaloblastosis
5 Vitamin K
  — Coagulopathy due to liver disease (esp. post-partum)

Toxicity of vitamin overdosage
1 Vitamin A
  — Skin dryness, fissuring, hair loss
  — Bone pain, hypercalcemia
  — Raised intracranial pressure ('pseudotumor')
  — Hepatic fibrosis
2 Vitamin B_3 (niacin)
  — Pruritus, hair loss
  — Peptic ulcer
  — Abnormal liver function tests
3 Vitamin B_6 (pyridoxine)
  — Sensory neuropathy
  — Antagonism of L-DOPA
4 Vitamin C
  — Renal oxalate stones
5 Vitamin D
  — Hypercalcemia
  — Hypertension
6 Vitamin E
  — Warfarin potentiation ($\downarrow$ vitamin K absorption)
7 Vitamin K
  — Hemolysis

Drug-induced vitamin deficiencies
1 Pyridoxine (B_6)
  — Isoniazid (in slow acetylators)
  — D-penicillamine
  — Hydralazine; cycloserine; chloramphenicol; L-DOPA
  — ?Oral contraceptives
2 Folate
  — Cholestyramine
  — Phenytoin
  — 'Antifolates', e.g. methotrexate, pyrimethamine
  — Sulfasalazine (may 'unmask' mild deficiency)
3 B_{12}
  — Chloramphenicol; long-term metformin, neomycin
4 B_1 (thiamine)
  — Nitrofurantoin

B_2 (riboflavin)
  — Thalidomide
5 Vitamin D
  — *Long-term* phenytoin/phenobarbitone (?hepatic induction $\rightarrow$ inactivation of 1,25-DHCC)
  — Cadmium poisoning ('ouch-ouch' disease = malacia)
6 Vitamin K
  — Warfarin
  — Aspirin
  — Megadose vitamin E

Disorders which may respond to pyridoxine
1 Homocystinuria
2 Primary hyperoxaluria
3 Idiopathic refractory sideroblastic anemia
4 Alcoholics developing neuropathy while taking isoniazid
5 Depression in women taking contraceptive pill
6 Vomiting in pregnant women
7 Convulsions of obscure cause in neonates

MANAGEMENT OF METABOLIC BONE DISEASE

Hyperparathyroidism: indications for surgical management
1 Renal calculi
  Progressive renal impairment due to nephrocalcinosis
2 Recurrent peptic ulceration (exclude gastrinoma)
3 Progressive reduction in height (vertebral osteopenia)
  Recurrent pancreatitis
  Recent onset of psychiatric symptoms
4 Severe or progressive radiological abnormalities*
5 High calcium (> 3.0 mmol/L) in patient from remote location

NB: Provided that surgical expertise is available, it may be best to operate if there is *any* doubt about the significance of symptoms
* e.g. osteitis fibrosa cystica with 2°/3° hyperparathyroidism in renal failure

Therapeutic modalities in post-menopausal osteoporosis
1 Hormone replacement therapy, esp. estrogens
2 Biphosphonates (etidronate, tiludronate)
3 Exercise*
4 Calcium citrate supplements (800 mg/day)
5 Subcutaneous or intranasal calcitonin
6 Vitamin D supplements (400–800 IU/day)

* Significance may relate to ovulatory effects rather than to activity alone

Biphosphonates: mechanisms and indications
1 Drugs
  — Etidronate
  — Pamidronate
  — Clodronate
  — Tiludronate
2 Mechanism of action
  — Pyrophosphate analogs; bind hydroxyapatite
  — Inhibit osteoclast-mediated bone resorption

3 Indications
  — Paget's disease (etidronate)
  — Hypercalcemia of malignancy (pamidronate)
  — Painful bone mets: myeloma, Ca breast (clodronate)
  — Vertebral osteoporosis (etidronate)
4 Unlicensed indications
  — Hyperparathyroidism (1°, 2°, 3°)
  — Prevention of heterotopic ossification
5 Toxicity
  — Malacia, fractures (etidronate; inhibits mineralization)

Rationâle for vitamin D supplements in osteoporosis
1 Relative indications
  — Lack of sun exposure
  — Little physical activity } esp. in winter
  — Low dietary vitamin D*
2 Oral vitamin D supplements suppress winter rise of PTH (→ ↓ bone density) due to reduced skin vitamin D synthesis
3 Antimyopathic effect of vitamin D supplements *may* also reduce falls in elderly independent of effects on bone density (unproven)

* Fatty fish/oils, liver, eggs, milk are the only substantive dietary sources

UNDERSTANDING METABOLIC DISEASE

Racial predispositions to disease
1 Ashkenazy Jews
  — Gaucher's
  — Tay–Sachs
  — Riley–Day
  — Niemann–Pick
  — Bassen–Kornzweig
  — Bloom's
  Non-Ashkenazy (Sephardic) Jews
  — Familial Mediterranean fever (recurrent polyserositis)
2 African Negro, Mediterranean littoral
  — Sickle-cell anemia
  — Thalassemias
  — Hb C
3 Lebanese
  — Hypercholesterolemia
  — Behçet's
4 Chinese
  — α-thalassemia
  — Alactasia
5 Northern European Caucasians
  — Idiopathic hemochromatosis
  — Phenylketonuria
  — Acute intermittent porphyria
  Swedes
  — Cystic fibrosis
  — Giant-cell arteritis
  — α_1-antitrypsin deficiency
  — LCAT deficiency
  Finns
  — Imerslund's disease
  — *Diphyllobothrium latum* infestations
  — Mulibrey nanism (→ pericarditis)

  — Congenital nephrosis
6 Eskimos (esp. Yupik)
  — Congenital adrenal hyperplasia
  — Pseudocholinesterase deficiency
  — Rapid acetylation status (close to 100%)
7 Other races
  Thais
  — Hb H disease (Hb Constant Spring → 2–5%)
  Pima Indians/Micronesians/Yemenite Jews
  — Type II (non-insulin-dependent) diabetes mellitus
  South Africans
  — Variegate porphyria
  Scots
  — Peptic ulceration (acid hypersecretion)
  Quebecois
  — Tyrosinemia (→ cirrhosis, renal tubular acidosis)

INHERITED DISEASES

Factors maintaining heterozygote mutation frequency
1 Duchenne muscular dystrophy
  — New mutations
2 Hemoglobinopathies (e.g. sickle-cell anemia, thalassemias)
  — Resistance to malaria
3 Cystic fibrosis
  — Resistance to cholera toxin
4 Peptic ulcer diathesis, lipid storage diseases
  — Resistance to TB
5 Congenital adrenal hyperplasia
  — Resistance to *H. influenzae* #B
6 Idiopathic hemochromatosis
  — Resistance to iron-deficiency anemia (in women)
7 Type I (insulin-dependent) diabetes mellitus
  — Reduced miscarriages
8 Type II (non-insulin-dependent) diabetes mellitus
  — Protects against starvation

Single-gene defects exhibiting autosomal dominant transmission
1 Familial hypercholesterolemia
2 Multiple polyposis
3 Neurofibromatosis
4 Tuberous sclerosis
5 Myotonic dystrophy
6 Huntington's chorea
7 Marfan's syndrome
8 Acute intermittent porphyria
9 Adult polycystic kidney disease

Single-gene defects exhibiting autosomal recessive transmission
1 Cystic fibrosis
2 β-thalassemia
3 Sickle-cell anemia
4 Phenylketonuria
5 Galactosemia
6 Tay–Sachs disease
7 Infantile polycystic kidney disease

Single-gene defects exhibiting X-linked recessive transmission

1 Hemophilias A and B
2 Duchenne muscular dystrophy
3 Alport's syndrome
4 Lesch–Nyhan syndrome
5 Nephrogenic diabetes insipidus
6 Testicular feminization syndrome
7 G6PD deficiency

GENETIC COUNSELLING

Referral for genetic counselling: potential indications

1 Suspected chromosomal abnormality
2 Diagnosed congenital and/or heritable abnormality
3 Abnormal mental or physical development
4 Abnormal sexual development
5 Unexplained infertility
6 Repeated abortions

Risk assessment in genetic counselling (general)

1 Risk of spontaneous abortion in established pregnancy
— 15%
2 Risk of married couple's infertility
— 10%
3 Risk of baby being born with physical or mental defect
— 2%

4 Risk of perinatal death or stillbirth
— 1%
5 Risk of death in infancy
— 0.5%

GENETIC DIAGNOSIS

Methods of localizing abnormal genes to specific chromosomes

1 Gene linkage (of a disease locus with a marker), e.g.
— Narcolepsy with HLA gene cluster
— Ataxia telangiectasia with polymorphic markers
2 Mutation-specific gene probes, e.g.
— Sickle-cell anemia
— α_1-antitrypsin deficiency
— β-thalassemias
— Phenylketonuria
— Cystic fibrosis

Dermatoglyphic stigmata of Down's syndrome

1 Distal axial triradius
— In 85%
2 Simian crease (single transverse palmar flexion crease)
— In 50%
3 Supernumerary ulnar loops

REVIEWING THE LITERATURE: METABOLISM, NUTRITION AND GENETICS

8.1 Fiatarone MA et al (1994) Exercise training and nutritional supplementation for physical frailty in very elderly people. N Engl J Med 330: 1769–1775

High-intensity resistance exercises prevented frailty and weakness in this prospective comparison with multinutrient supplementation.

Cummings SR et al (1995) Risk factors for hip fracture in white women. N Engl J Med 332: 767–773

Numerous risk factors (other than osteoporosis) were identified for hip fracture in this study of 9516 women, including previous hyperthyroidism, benzodiazepine and caffeine intake, sedentary lifestyle and impaired vision.

8.2 Belongia EA et al (1990) An investigation of the cause of the eosinophilia-myalgia syndrome associated with tryptophan use. N Engl J Med 323: 357–365

Cox IM et al (1991) Red blood cell magnesium and chronic fatigue syndrome. Lancet 337: 757–760

Two studies purporting to illuminate the pathogenesis of this perplexing condition – but it remains as mysterious as ever.

8.3 Khin-Maung U et al (1990) Effect of short-term inter-mittent antibiotic treatment on growth of Burmese (Myanmar) village children. Lancet 336: 1090–1093

Children aged 3–4 treated with antibiotics (to eliminate malabsorption due to bacterial overgrowth) grew more, but no other age group did. Overall, a disappointingly negative result.

8.4 Grantham-McGregor SM et al (1991) Nutritional supplementation, psychosocial stimulation, and mental development of stunted children: the Jamaican study. Lancet 338: 1–5

Independent benefits on cognitive function were apparent with either stimulation or milk-based nutritional supplements, indicating that malnutrition underlies at least some developmental stunting in deprived communities.

8.5 Silverman K et al (1992) Withdrawal syndrome after the double-blind cessation of caffeine consumption. N Engl J Med 327: 1109–1114

Even subjects drinking as few as 2–3 cups of coffee a day experience significant withdrawal symptoms (fatigue, headache, loss of concentration) when caffeine intake is reduced.

8.6 Mills JL et al (1995) Homocysteine metabolism in pregnancies complicated by neural tube defects. Lancet 345: 149–151

Case-control study of 81 infants with neural tube defects, indicating an abnormality in maternal homocysteine metabolism (?due to methionine synthase defect). This suggests that periconceptional supplementation with B_{12} as well as folate may help avoid neural tube defects.

8.7 Stacpoole PW et al (1992) A controlled clinical trial of dichloroacetate for treatment of lactic acidosis in adults. N Engl J Med 327: 1564–1569

Randomized study of 252 lactic acidosis patients, showing that DCA was of absolutely no clinical use.

8.8 Cross SJ et al (1992) Safety of subaqua diving with a patent foramen ovale. Br Med J 304: 481–482

Unlike previous studies from the US, this study did not document any excess risk of decompression sickness in individuals with a patent foramen ovale.

Reul J et al (1995) Central nervous system lesions and cervical disc herniations in amateur divers. Lancet 345: 1403–1405

MRI study of scuba diving veterans showing subcortical brain damage and cartilage degeneration

8.9 Tilyard MW et al (1992) Treatment of postmenopausal osteoporosis with calcitriol or calcium. N Engl J Med 326: 357–362

Chapuy MC et al (1992) Vitamin D_3 and calcium to prevent hip fractures in elderly women. N Engl J Med 327: 1637–1642

Reid IR et al (1993) Effect of calcium supplementation on bone loss in postmenopausal women. N Engl J Med 328: 460–464

Riggs BL et al (1990) Effect of fluoride treatment on the fracture rate in postmenopausal women with osteoporosis. N Engl J Med 322: 802–809

Watts NB et al (1990) Intermittent cyclical etidronate treatment of postmenopausal osteoporosis. N Engl J Med 323: 73–79

The second study showed that the combination of D_3 and calcium was effective; the first suggested that D_3 may be the more important component. The third, however, confirmed that calcium alone is indeed effective in its own right. Unfortunately, the fourth study suggested that fluoride is not useful, since it increases skeletal fragility by decreasing bone mineralization. The last confirmed that etidronate increases vertebral bone mass as well as (in this study) reducing fracture incidence.

Finkelstein JS et al (1994) Parathyroid hormone for the prevention of bone loss induced by estrogen deficiency. N Engl J Med 331: 1618–1623

Small study of 40 endometriosis patients, apparently showing that PTH prevents LHRH-induced bone loss in premenopausal women.

8.10 Leibel RL et al (1995) Changes in energy expenditure resulting from altered body weight. N Engl J Med 332: 621–628

Important study of 40 obese and non-obese subjects, showing that changes in body weight were translated into compensatory alterations of metabolic energy expenditure which tended to oppose or minimize weight change – thus providing some explanation for the failure rate of most dietary approaches to obesity.

Manson JE et al (1995) Body weight and mortality among women. N Engl J Med 333: 677–685

All-cause mortality was higher in overweight individuals.

Prentice AM, Jebb SA Obesity in Britain: gluttony or sloth? Br Med J 311: 437–439

Sloth.

CHAPTER 9

Neurology

Physical examination protocol 9.1   You are asked to examine the cranial nerves

6. **CN V:** muscles of mastication, trigeminal sensation
    Motor: clench teeth (masseter, temporalis);
      open mouth against resistance (pterygoids;
      jaw deviates to weak side)
    Sensory: ophthalmic/maxillary/mandibular sensation/
      corneal reflex (distinguish efferent VII limb)
      jaw jerk (?hyperactive)

7. **CN VII:** muscles of facial expression
    facial asymmetry or general wasting
    show teeth (if weak, ask to 'smile')
    puff out cheeks; screw up eyes
    frown; lift eyebrows
    Ask to test taste
    Ask to test lacrimation (Schirmer's test) if face weak

5. **CN III, IV, VI:** pupils and extraocular
    movements; exophthalmos;
    enophthalmos (Horner's); ptosis;
    lid retraction, lid lag
    Pupils (CN III): turn out lights
      equal? regular?
      direct and consensual light reflex?
      accommodation?
    Extraocular movements:
      diplopia? strabismus?
      nystagmus?
      fatiguability?

8. **CN VIII:** auditory and vestibular function
    Auditory: ticking watch,
      whispered numbers (other ear
      occluded)
      Weber's and Rinne's test
    Vestibular: Hallpike maneuver, etc.,
      if indicated

4. **CN II:** acuity, fields, fundi
    Test acuity with glasses on:
      Snellen's chart, newspaper,
      count fingers; hand threat
    Fields to confrontation:
      visual inattention
      map central scotoma
      map enlarged blind spot
    Fundi: ask to dilate pupils; turn
      out lights; red reflex, cataract;
      rubeosis iridis; optic disc
      retinal vessels; venous
      pulsations; macula
      ('look straight at the
      light now')

9. **CN IX, X:** pharyngeal function and
    sensation
    Test palate elevates in midline
      ('Aaah': CN X); moves away
      from paretic side
    Ask to test gag reflex bilaterally
      (CN IX)
    Speech: nasal (bulbar palsy),
      'Donald Duck' (pseudobulbar)
    Bovine cough (recurrent laryngeal
      branch of CN X)

10. **CN XI:** trapezius and sternomastoids
    shrug shoulders upwards against
    resistance; rotate jaw against
    resistance (rotating to right tests
    left sternomastoid)

11. **CN XII:** tongue
    wasting, fibrillation (lower motor neuron lesion)
    stick tongue out (deviates to weak side)
    rapid movements: side-to-side quickly
      'la-la-la-la-la-la-la'
    percussion myotonia (if myotonic dystrophy suspected)

3. Ask to examine olfaction
    If request granted, test bilaterally
      (cortical representation is ipsilateral)

2. General inspection:
    craniotomy scar
    ptosis, proptosis
    facial weakness, hemiplegia
    catheter

12. If appropriate, ask to proceed further, e.g.:
    auscultate carotids/orbits/skull/heart for bruit
    take blood pressure; assess pulse regularity
    look for absent abdominal reflexes (demyelination)
      absent ankle jerks (tabes dorsalis)
      extensor plantar responses
      glycosuria

1. Introduce yourself (note speech in reply)
    Position yourself opposite patient

Physical examination protocol 9.2   You are asked to assess a patient who has had difficulty walking

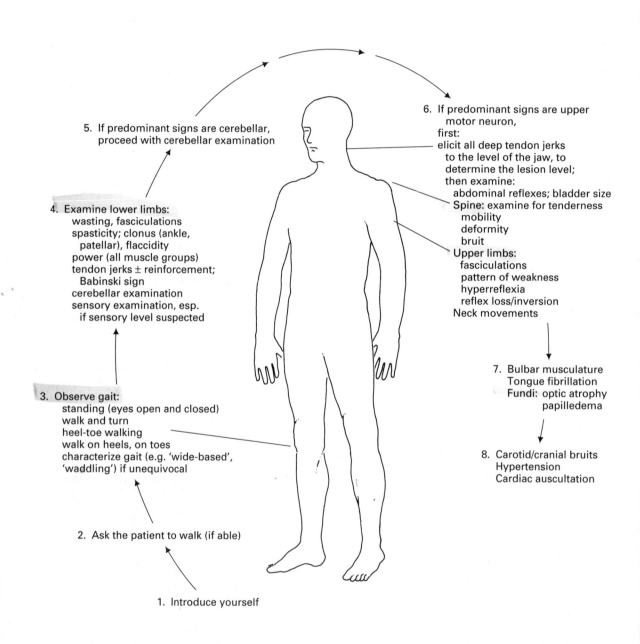

5. If predominant signs are cerebellar,
    proceed with cerebellar examination

6. If predominant signs are upper
    motor neuron,
    first:
    elicit all deep tendon jerks
    to the level of the jaw, to
    determine the lesion level;
    then examine:
      abdominal reflexes; bladder size
    Spine: examine for tenderness
      mobility
      deformity
      bruit
    Upper limbs:
      fasciculations
      pattern of weakness
      hyperreflexia
      reflex loss/inversion
    Neck movements

4. Examine lower limbs:
      wasting, fasciculations
      spasticity; clonus (ankle,
        patellar), flaccidity
      power (all muscle groups)
      tendon jerks ± reinforcement;
      Babinski sign
      cerebellar examination
      sensory examination, esp.
        if sensory level suspected

7. Bulbar musculature
    Tongue fibrillation
    Fundi: optic atrophy
      papilledema

3. Observe gait:
      standing (eyes open and closed)
      walk and turn
      heel-toe walking
      walk on heels, on toes
      characterize gait (e.g. 'wide-based',
      'waddling') if unequivocal

8. Carotid/cranial bruits
    Hypertension
    Cardiac auscultation

2. Ask the patient to walk (if able)

1. Introduce yourself

Physical examination protocol 9.3 You are asked to examine a patient who has noticed wasting of the hand muscles

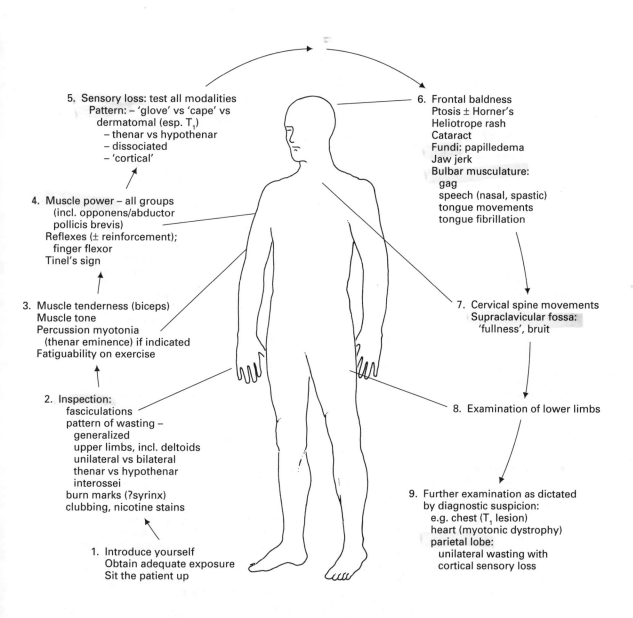

5. Sensory loss: test all modalities
   Pattern: – 'glove' vs 'cape' vs
   dermatomal (esp. T_1)
   – thenar vs hypothenar
   – dissociated
   – 'cortical'

4. Muscle power – all groups
   (incl. opponens/abductor
   pollicis brevis)
   Reflexes (± reinforcement);
   finger flexor
   Tinel's sign

3. Muscle tenderness (biceps)
   Muscle tone
   Percussion myotonia
   (thenar eminence) if indicated
   Fatiguability on exercise

2. Inspection:
   fasciculations
   pattern of wasting –
   generalized
   upper limbs, incl. deltoids
   unilateral vs bilateral
   thenar vs hypothenar
   interossei
   burn marks (?syrinx)
   clubbing, nicotine stains

1. Introduce yourself
   Obtain adequate exposure
   Sit the patient up

6. Frontal baldness
   Ptosis ± Horner's
   Heliotrope rash
   Cataract
   Fundi: papilledema
   Jaw jerk
   Bulbar musculature:
   gag
   speech (nasal, spastic)
   tongue movements
   tongue fibrillation

7. Cervical spine movements
   Supraclavicular fossa:
   'fullness', bruit

8. Examination of lower limbs

9. Further examination as dictated
   by diagnostic suspicion:
   e.g. chest (T_1 lesion)
   heart (myotonic dystrophy)
   parietal lobe:
   unilateral wasting with
   cortical sensory loss

Physical examination protocol 9.4   You are asked to examine the patient's cerebellar function

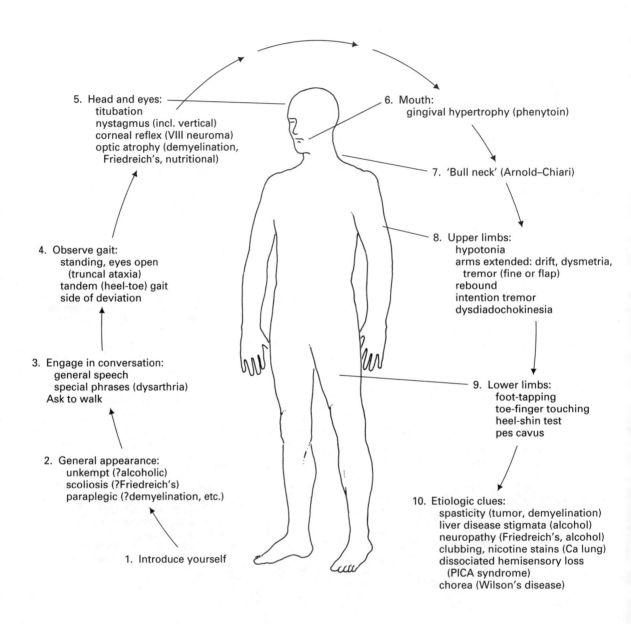

5. Head and eyes:
   titubation
   nystagmus (incl. vertical)
   corneal reflex (VIII neuroma)
   optic atrophy (demyelination,
    Friedreich's, nutritional)

6. Mouth:
   gingival hypertrophy (phenytoin)

7. 'Bull neck' (Arnold–Chiari)

4. Observe gait:
   standing, eyes open
    (truncal ataxia)
   tandem (heel-toe) gait
   side of deviation

8. Upper limbs:
   hypotonia
   arms extended: drift, dysmetria,
    tremor (fine or flap)
   rebound
   intention tremor
   dysdiadochokinesia

3. Engage in conversation:
   general speech
   special phrases (dysarthria)
  Ask to walk

9. Lower limbs:
   foot-tapping
   toe-finger touching
   heel-shin test
   pes cavus

2. General appearance:
   unkempt (?alcoholic)
   scoliosis (?Friedreich's)
   paraplegic (?demyelination, etc.)

1. Introduce yourself

10. Etiologic clues:
   spasticity (tumor, demyelination)
   liver disease stigmata (alcohol)
   neuropathy (Friedreich's, alcohol)
   clubbing, nicotine stains (Ca lung)
   dissociated hemisensory loss
    (PICA syndrome)
   chorea (Wilson's disease)

Physical examination protocol 9.5   You are asked to examine a patient for signs of parkinsonism

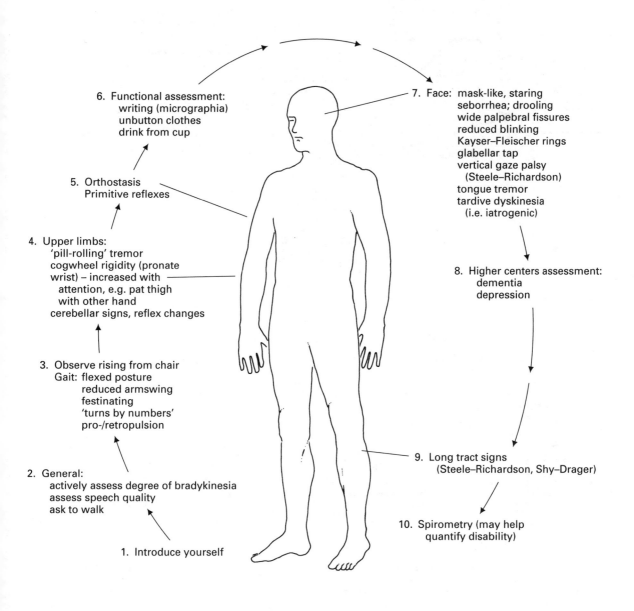

6. Functional assessment:
   writing (micrographia)
   unbutton clothes
   drink from cup

7. Face: mask-like, staring
   seborrhea; drooling
   wide palpebral fissures
   reduced blinking
   Kayser–Fleischer rings
   glabellar tap
   vertical gaze palsy
     (Steele–Richardson)
   tongue tremor
   tardive dyskinesia
     (i.e. iatrogenic)

5. Orthostasis
   Primitive reflexes

4. Upper limbs:
   'pill-rolling' tremor
   cogwheel rigidity (pronate
   wrist) – increased with
     attention, e.g. pat thigh
     with other hand
   cerebellar signs, reflex changes

8. Higher centers assessment:
   dementia
   depression

3. Observe rising from chair
   Gait: flexed posture
     reduced armswing
     festinating
     'turns by numbers'
     pro-/retropulsion

9. Long tract signs
   (Steele–Richardson, Shy–Drager)

2. General:
   actively assess degree of bradykinesia
   assess speech quality
   ask to walk

10. Spirometry (may help
    quantify disability)

1. Introduce yourself

Diagnostic pathway 9.1 This patient has a speech defect. What do you make of it?

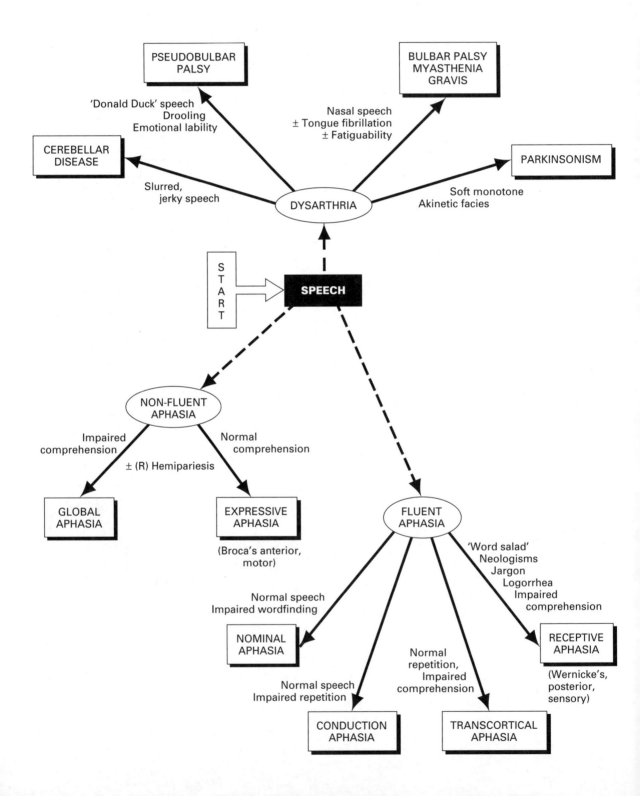

Diagnostic pathway 9.2   This patient is troubled by ptosis. Can you shed any light on the pathophysiology?

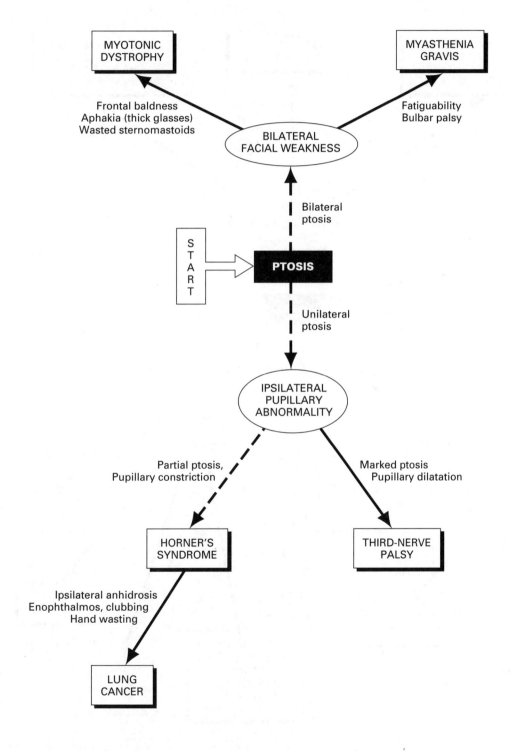

Diagnostic pathway 9.3   The patient is concerned about his legs. What do you think is the problem?

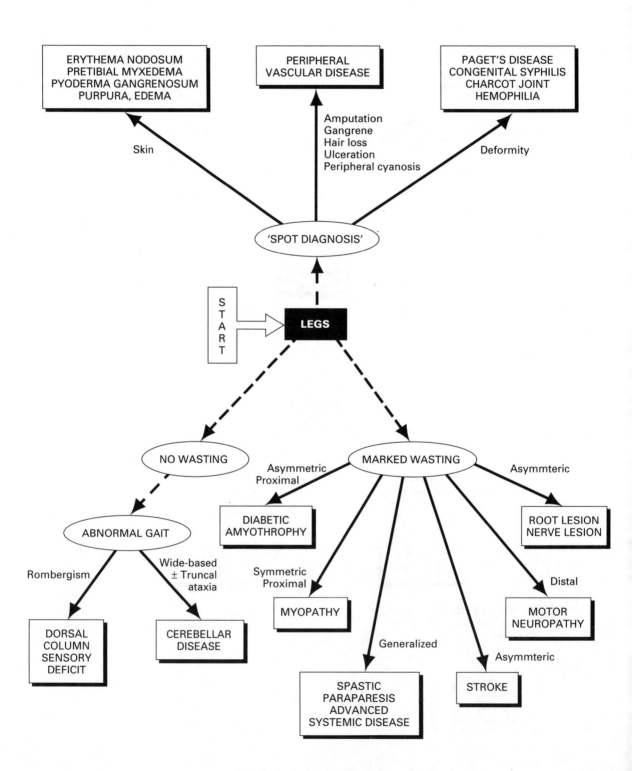

CLINICAL ASPECTS OF NEUROLOGIC DISEASE

Commonest neurologic short cases
1 Spastic paraparesis
2 Peripheral neuropathy
3 Ocular palsy

Clinical assessment of muscle weakness (MRC criteria)
1 Grade 1 — flicker of voluntary muscle activity*
2 Grade 2 — able to move with gravity eliminated
3 Grade 3 — able to move against gravity
4 Grade 4 — able to move against resistance
5 Grade 5 — normal power

* Paralysis = grade 0

Multiple CNS deficits: causes
1 Multiple sclerosis
  Multifocal leukoencephalopathy
2 Multiple infarcts
3 Multiple metastases
  Meningeal carcinomatosis
4 Meningovascular syphilis
5 Vasculitis (e.g. PAN)

Multiple cranial nerve palsies?
1 Malignancy
  — Brainstem tumor (e.g. nasopharyngeal Ca → VI)
  — Meningeal carcinomatosis
  — Perineural tumor infiltration
2 Infection
  — Basal meningitis (e.g. cryptococcal, tuberculous)
  — Meningovascular syphilis (now rare)
  — Herpes zoster
3 Sarcoidosis
  — esp. VII; ± VIII, II
4 Vasculitis
  — esp. Wegener's (→ VIII)
5 Paget's disease
  — Usually causes hearing loss only
6 Hyperostosis cranialis interna (familial)
  — Recurrent VII palsies ± I, II, VIII
7 Idiopathic
  — Tolosa–Hunt syndrome (p. 262)
  — Orbital pseudotumor
  — Idiopathic cranial polyneuropathy

Signs suggesting brainstem pathology
1 Conjugate gaze palsy/internuclear ophthalmoplegia
2 Vertical nystagmus
3 Opisthotonos and/or cerebellar signs
4 Crossed (cranial nerves vs long tract) signs
5 Deviation of eyes and head to paralysed side (cf. cortical)
6 Bilateral extensive deficit

Signs suggesting extracapsular (cortical) disease
1 Localized deficit
2 Dysphasia (cf. capsular lesion → pure dysarthria)
3 Hemianopia
4 Decreased proprioception/two-point discrimination
5 Apraxia
6 Obtundation

Clinical distinction between meningitis and encephalitis
1 Meningitis
  — Conscious state unimpaired
  — Meningism (including headache)
  — Prominent fever
  — ± Cranial nerve lesions (lower motor neuron)
2 Encephalitis
  — Early impairment of consciousness (drowsiness, coma)
  — Focal neurologic signs (upper motor neuron)
  — Convulsions
  — Associated hydrophobia (rabies)
  — Associated temporal lobe epilepsy (HSV)

Assessment of neurologic function in the unconscious patient
1 Pupils
  — Midbrain lesions
    • Light reflex may be lost
    • Hippus (fluctuation in pupil size)
    • Ciliospinal reflex (dilatation on pinching neck)
  — Pontine lesions
    • Pinpoint pupils
  — Lateral medullary lesions
    • Horner's syndrome
  — Diffuse cerebral damage
    • Fixed dilated pupils (*not* diagnostic)
  — Metabolic depression (e.g. overdose)
    • All brainstem reflexes lost *except* pupil light reflex
2 Reflexes
  — Corneal
    • Depressed in bilateral cerebral damage
  — Jaw jerk
    • Hyperactive in bilateral UMN lesions
  — Gag reflex
3 Conjugate gaze deviation (p. 262)
4 Caloric and oculocephalic testing (p. 263)
5 Spontaneous respiratory movements

EPILEPSY

Features of fits
1 Absence (< 30 sec)
  — Staring, blinking ± automatisms*
  — Immediate return of consciousness
  — Characteristic EEG (p. 269)
2 Tonic-clonic (1–5 min)
  — Fall ± cry; cyanosis
  — ± Tongue-bite, incontinence
3 Myoclonic (1–5 sec)
  — Brief limb jerks
4 Complex partial ('psychomotor'; last minutes)
  — Déjà vu, jamais vu
  — Hallucinations (esp. olfactory, gustatory)
  — *Prominent* post-ictal confusion‡
5 Simple partial (focal; seconds – minutes)
  — EEG may be normal¶
  — *No* post-ictal confusion
  — Examples: an 'aura', Rolandic epilepsy

— May generalize via Jacksonian march
— ± *Painful* sensations (in *parietal lobe* origin)

* Chewing, lip smacking, finger twiddling, etc.
‡ If *temporal lobe* in origin; *not* in frontal lobe variety
¶ Or there may be contralateral epileptiform discharges

Disorders mimicking epileptic seizures
1 Hyperventilation, agoraphobia, panic disorders
2 Cardiac arrhythmias
3 Migraine
4 Vasovagal syncope
5 Breath-holding episodes (infants)
6 Non-epileptic myoclonus, tics, habit spasms

Common precipitants of status epilepticus
1 Subtherapeutic anticonvulsant levels
— Poor compliance
— Recent dose reduction
2 Metabolic derangement
— Severe hyponatremia
— Hepatic encephalopathy
— Alcohol withdrawal
3 Inflammatory
— Encephalitis
— Cerebral vasculitis (e.g. SLE)
4 Head injury
5 Drug overdose
— e.g. Theophylline, cocaine

CEREBROVASCULAR DISEASE: BACKGROUND

Clinical characterization of stroke
1 Mechanism
— (Athero)thrombotic
— (Cardio)embolic
— Lacunar/hypertensive
— Vasculitis
— Aneurysmal
2 Site
— Internal carotid
— Middle cerebral
— Anterior or posterior cerebral
— Vertebrobasilar

Symptoms suggesting carotid insufficiency
1 Amaurosis fugax
— Complete or partial visual loss in *one* eye
2 Dysphasia
3 Unilateral limb weakness/paresthesiae *without* other (brainstem) features

Symptoms suggesting vertebrobasilar ischemia
1 Bilateral blindness
2 Other *bilateral* motor/sensory symptoms
3 Focal symptoms *plus* vertigo or diplopia

Clinical significance of transient ischemic attacks
1 30% of patients will have only one episode
2 30% will continue to have TIAs alone
3 30% will have a completed stroke within 3 years
4 30% of the latter will do so within 3 months of presentation

5 30% of asymptomatic carotid bruits go on to TIA and/or CVA
6 30% of carotid-type TIAs will have normal arteriography

Carotid-type TIAs: factors predictive of angiographic disease
1 Ipsilateral retinal emboli
2 Reduced superficial temporal and/or carotid artery pulse
3 Presence of forehead/scleral collaterals
4 Ipsilateral central retinal artery diastolic pressure < 20 mmHg
5 Ipsilateral carotid bruit, esp. if diastolic extension present; severe stenosis may → high-pitched, low-intensity bruit

Neurologic syndromes associated with hypertension
1 Lacunar infarcts
2 Intracranial hemorrhage
3 Hypertensive encephalopathy

Intracranial hemorrhage: classic site involvement
1 Aneurysms, amyloid angiopathy
— Subarachnoid
2 Arteriovenous malformations
— (Peri)ventricular, pons
3 Hypertension
— Basal ganglia (putamen/caudate), thalamus
4 Warfarin
— Cerebellar

PRESENTATIONS OF CEREBROVASCULAR DISEASE

Features suggestive of intracerebral hemorrhage
1 Gradual onset, smooth progression
2 Obtunded sensorium
3 Vomiting (95%), headache (50%)
4 Hypertension ± fundal stigmata/cardiomegaly
5 Diagnostic confirmation by CT

Signs suggestive of basal pontine hemorrhage
1 Rapid onset of decerebrate rigidity progressing to coma
2 Ophthalmoplegia with (classically) small reactive pupils
3 Abnormal oculocephalic and oculovestibular reflexes
4 Cheyne–Stokes/ataxic respiration
5 Sweating

Signs and symptoms of cerebellar hemorrhage
1 Subacute onset of occipital headache, vertigo and vomiting
2 Skew deviation of eyes; ocular bobbing (nystagmus unusual)
3 Paresis of gaze to affected side
4 Hemiparesis unusual (cf. putaminal/thalamic type)
5 Good recovery after prompt surgical evacuation

Clinical patterns of lacunar infarction
1 Pure motor hemiplegia
— Pontine

— Posterior limb of internal capsule
- Associated with dysarthria
- Typically affects upper limb > lower
2 Dysarthria – clumsy hand syndrome
— Caused by pontine infarction
— Associated with homolateral facial weakness
3 Pure hemisensory loss
— Due to thalamic infarction (posterolateral nucleus)
4 Ipsilateral ataxia/crossed hemiparesis
— Due to midbrain infarction
5 Dementia/incontinence/affective lability
— Due to bipyramidal (pseudobulbar) palsy*

* Differential diagnosis = normal pressure hydrocephalus

Clinical deterioration following an apparently completed stroke?
1 Infarct extension
2 Hemorrhage into infarct
3 Further emboli
4 Worsening cerebral edema/vasospasm
5 Misdiagnosis (e.g. tumor/vasculitis)

Presentations of arteriovenous malformations
1 Epilepsy (45%)
2 Hemorrhage (40%; may mimic aseptic meningitis)
3 Headache (often migrainous: 15%)
4 Pseudotumor (neurologic deficit due to vascular 'steal')
5 Apparent 'spontaneous' stroke
— Age under 20
— During third trimester

Diagnostic considerations in the young patient with 'stroke'
1 Disseminated sclerosis
2 Cardiac disease
— Arrhythmias (esp. atrial fibrillation)
— Valvular disease (esp. mitral valve stenosis/prolapse)
— Infective endocarditis
3 Vascular
— Classic migraine
— Arteriovenous malformation/aneurysm
— Vasculitis (e.g. SLE)
— Severe hypertension
— Hypercoagulable state
4 Intracranial tumor
5 Infection
— Encephalitis (e.g. HSV type 1)
— Neurosyphilis
6 Post-ictal
7 Functional
— Hyperventilation (may simulate TIA)
— Hysteria

Clinical features of lateral medullary (PICA*) syndrome
1 Abrupt onset of vertigo and hiccups
2 Bilateral nystagmus
— Maximal to side of lesion
— Often varies with posture
3 *Contralateral* body anesthesia for pain and temperature

4 *Ipsilateral*
— Facial anesthesia for pain and temperature
— Palatal paresis
— Taste loss
— Horner's syndrome
— Ataxia

* Posterior inferior cerebellar artery

LOCALIZING PATTERNS IN CEREBRAL DISEASE

Clinical manifestations of frontal lobe lesions
1 **A**nosmia — homolateral
Ataxia — Brun's
Aphasia — Broca's
Apathy
Amnesia
Atrophy (optic)
2 Mass effects (papilledema, field defects, Foster–Kennedy)
3 Incontinence
4 Spastic paraparesis or contralateral UMN signs
5 Primitive reflexes (palmar-mental/grasp/snout/ pout/suck)

The aphasias: how to distinguish them
1 Broca's
— Affected region: left frontal (inferoposterior)
— Associated features: nil
— Fluency: strained, 'effortful'
— Repetition: impaired
— Comprehension: intact
2 Wernicke's
— Affected region: left temporal (supero-posterior)
— Associated features: euphoria, agitation
— Fluency: abundant, melodic
— Repetition: impaired
— Comprehension: impaired
3 Global
— Affected region: left perisylvian (large area)
— Associated features: hemiplegia*
— Fluency: absent
— Repetition: impaired
— Comprehension: impaired
4 Conduction
— Affected region: left supramarginal gyrus‡
— Associated features: ± right facial/arm weakness
— Fluency: grossly normal
— Repetition: impaired
— Comprehension: intact
5 Transcortical (motor)
— Affected region: left frontal¶
— Associated features: nil
— Fluency: non-fluent, 'explosive'
— Repetition: intact
— Comprehension: intact
6 Thalamic (atypical)
— Affected region: anterolateral thalamus
— Associated features: ± amnesia
— Fluency: abundant, ± logorrhea

— Repetition: intact
— Comprehension: impaired

* Assuming single lesion; separate frontal and temporoparietal lesions can cause global aphasia without hemiplegia
‡ Or left auditory cortex plus insula
¶ Anterosuperior to Broca's area

Clinical manifestations of temporal lobe lesions
1 Superior quadrantanopia
2 Fluent aphasia (lesion in Wernicke's area)
3 Uncinate fits, depersonalization, micro-/macropsia
4 Bilateral disease (rare)
   — Deafness
   — Severe amnesia
   — Kluver–Bucy syndrome

Clinical manifestations of parietal lobe lesions
1 Non-dominant lobe lesions
   — Dressing apraxia
   — Constructional apraxia (draw clock, house, 5-point star)
   — Anosognosia
2 Dominant lobe lesions
   — Ideomotor apraxia ('brush teeth, use saw, drink a cup')
   — Receptive dysphasia (in inferior lesions)
   — Gerstmann's
     • Alexia + acalculia
     • Finger agnosia
     • Left–right confusion
   — Agraphia (in posterior lesions)
3 Anterior lobe lesions
   — Astereognosis/graphesthesia
   — Sensory inattention
   — ↓ Proprioception/two-point discrimination
   — Focal sensory deficits
4 Posterior lobe lesions
   — Visual inattention, sensory inattention
   — Homonymous (albeit incongruous) hemianopia*
   — ↓ Optikokinetic nystagmus
5 Wasting (→ 'parietal lobe weakness')

* Or inferior quadrantanopia

Clinical manifestations of occipital lobe lesions
1 'Cortical' blindness, or
   Altitudinal hemianopia, or
   Congruous crossed hemianopia
2 Smooth pursuit defects, impaired opticokinetic nystagmus
3 Visual agnosia; visual hallucinations
4 Achromatopsia; prosopagnosia; topographical amnesia

Predominant lateralization of some cortical functions
1 Left cerebral cortex
   — Language
   — Mathematical ability
2 Right cerebral cortex
   — Spatioperceptual ability
   — Music appreciation

Classic localization of some CNS deficits
1 Mammillary bodies
   — Wernicke's

2 Amygdaloid bodies
   — Aggressive behavior
3 Hippocampus
   Ventromedial temporal lobe
   — Memory loss
4 Butterfly glioma of corpus callosum
   — Typically asymptomatic until advanced

EXAMINING THE EYES

Clinical criteria for characterizing blindness
1 Complete blindness
   — Absent pupillary reactions
   — Absent opticokinetic nystagmus
2 Cortical blindness
   — Normal pupillary reactions (i.e. to light)
   — Absent opticokinetic nystagmus
3 Anton's syndrome
   — Cortical blindness (as above)
   — Blindness denied by patient*
4 Hysterical blindness
   — Normal pupillary reactions
   — Normal opticokinetic nystagmus
   — Blindness claimed by patient

* ? Due to destruction of visual association areas ± hallucinations, amnesia

Causes of painful visual loss
1 Optic neuritis
2 Acute glaucoma
3 Giant cell arteritis
4 Central retinal artery (CRA) occlusion*
5 Migraine

* Cause *par excellence* of amaurosis fugax

Classic patterns of visual field defect
1 Central field defects
   — Central scotoma
     • Macular pathology, e.g. demyelination
   — Central arcuate scotoma
     • Early glaucoma
   — Pericentral scotoma (normal acuity)
     • Retinitis pigmentosa
     • Chloroquine retinopathy
   — Centrocecal scotoma (extends to involve blind spot)
     • Toxic optic neuritis, e.g. methanol, 'nutritional'
   — Congruous homonymous scotoma
     • Localized lesions of occipital cortex
2 Hemianopias
   — Bitemporal hemianopia
     • Central chiasmal lesion, esp. pituitary tumor
   — Incongruous homonymous hemianopia
     • Optic tract lesion (rare)
   — Congruous homonymous hemianopia
     • Lesion of occipital lobe optic radiation
   — Homonymous hemianopia with macular sparing
     • Lesion of occipital cortex (usually vascular)
   — Bilateral homonymous hemianopia*
     • Small island of central vision

3 Quadrantanopias (usually due to tumors)
— Superior
• Lesion of temporal lobe optic radiation
— Inferior
• Lesion of parietal lobe optic radiation
4 Field defects in one eye only
— Retinal detachment
— Branch retinal vein occlusion
— Ischemic optic neuropathy ($\rightarrow$ inferior defect)
— Vasculitis
5 Concentric visual field constriction
— Hysteria ('tubular' vision)
— Advanced glaucoma or papilledema
— 'Panretinal' laser photocoagulation‡
6 Other patterns of field defect
— Enlarged blind spot
• Early papilledema
— Visual inattention
• Lesion of posterior parietal lobe

* Due to bilateral posterior cerebral artery occlusion
‡ Causes peripheral field loss with normal acuity; cf. diabetic maculopathy impairs acuity with peripheral field sparing

Chiasmal lesions: clinical signs aiding localization
1 Posterior chiasm lesions
— Due to suprasellar or third ventricle tumors
— Typically involve macular fibers only
— Manifest with central scotoma only
2 Anterosuperior chiasm lesions
— Due to meningiomas (sphenoid ridge, frontal lobe) or aneurysms (anterior cerebral/ communicating)
— Manifest with inferior temporal quadrant loss
3 Anteroinferior chiasm lesions
— Due to pituitary tumor, meningitis
— Involve maculopapillary bundle as well as chiasm
— Cause bitemporal hemianopia plus central scotoma
4 Posteroinferior chiasm lesions
— Due to pituitary tumors
— Initially cause bitemporal superior quadrantanopia
— May $\rightarrow$ optic atrophy, inferotemporal or nasal field loss

'Examine the eyes': important details
1 Position the patient in front of you (e.g. in chair, side of bed)
2 Inspection checklist
— Glasses (e.g. thick lenses, for aphakic patients)
— Ptosis (unilateral or bilateral)
— Proptosis (view orbits from all angles); ± pulsating
— Enophthalmos (esp. if pupil constricted), dry skin
— Rubeosis iridis; arcus senilis; band keratopathy
3 Visual acuity
— Test with patient's glasses on (newsprint, eye chart)
— Unilateral blindness? Exclude glass eye
4 Visual fields
— Test for visual inattention
— Map blind spot (and central scotoma, if present)
5 Fundoscopy
— Look for red reflex

— Characterize opacities (e.g. cataract)
— Indicate that you would like to dilate the pupils
— Comment on retinal vessels, venous pulsations, disc
— Inspect macula last ('look straight at the light now')
6 Extraocular movements
— Ask re diplopia in any direction
— Cover eyes sequentially when double image maximal (peripheral image is from the diseased eye)
— Is nystagmus present? Look for optic atrophy, dysarthria, bulbar palsy, cerebellar signs, etc.
— Is there fatiguability?
7 Pupils
— Check for regularity and circularity
— Turn off lights if possible to examine reactivity
— Test direct *and* consensual response to light in each eye
— Horner's syndrome? Check for ipsilateral facial anhidrosis (signifies lesion proximal to carotid bifurcation, e.g. in brachial plexus)
8 Palpate globes and temporal arteries for tenderness
9 Auscultate orbits (and skull if indicated)
10 Auscultate carotids if CVA suspected; ask to take BP, etc.

THE ABNORMAL FUNDUS

Papilledema: fundoscopic criteria
1 Loss of physiologic cup
2 Elevation of disc head (quantifiable in diopters)
3 Blurring of disc margins
4 Distended non-pulsatile veins
5 Subhyaloid hemorrhages at disc margins

Differential diagnosis of optic disc swelling
1 Pseudopapilledema: benign congenital anomalies, e.g.
— Drüsen of the disc (may $\rightarrow$ field defect)
— Hypermetropia
2 Papilledema
— Visual acuity: normal (unless long-standing disease)
— Visual field testing: enlarged blind spot
— Disc swelling usually bilateral (cf. papillitis)
3 Papillitis
— Subjective loss of brightness and color
— Pain on eye movement; tenderness on globe palpation
— Visual acuity: early, marked reduction
— Visual field testing: central scotoma (macular disease)
— Disc swelling usually unilateral (cf. papilledema)
— May progress to optic atrophy if long-standing
— Marcus–Gunn phenomenon (p. 261)
4 Retrobulbar neuritis
— Similar to papillitis, but
• *No* visible disc swelling
• Temporal disc pallor may be the only fundal sign
• Commonest presentation of demyelination

5 Posterior uveitis
 — Visual acuity only reduced if macular edema present
 — Visual field testing usually normal
 — Disc swelling may be unilateral or bilateral
 — Cellular infiltrate visible in vitreous
6 Ischemic optic neuropathy
 — Visual field testing → inferior altitudinal defect
 — Disc swelling: pale, asymmetric
 — Hypertensive vascular signs, else resembles papillitis

Disorders causing retinal arteriolar constriction
1 Malignant hypertension
2 Central retinal artery occlusion
3 Retinitis pigmentosa
4 Cinchonism

Disorders causing dilated retinal veins
1 Polycythemia, hyperviscosity
2 Central retinal vein (CRV) thrombosis
3 Increased intracranial pressure
4 CO_2 retention
5 Caroticocavernous fistula

Causes of angioid streaks (breaks in Bruch's membrane)
1 Paget's disease
2 Acromegaly
3 Pseudoxanthoma elasticum
4 Ehlers–Danlos syndrome
5 Hereditary hyperphosphatasia
6 Sickle-cell anemia

RETINOPATHY

Retinal hemorrhages: their morphologic significance
1 'Dot' hemorrhages
 — Microaneurysms in the posterior pole of the retina
 — Fundoscopic hallmark of diabetic retinopathy
2 'Blot' hemorrhages
 — Small hemorrhages deep in the posterior retinal pole
 — Vertical course of nerve fibers restricts spread here
 — Also characteristic of diabetic retinopathy
3 'Flame' hemorrhages
 — Rupture of superficial retinal capillary plexus
 — Track horizontally along superficial nerve fiber layer
 — Characteristic of grade III/IV hypertensive retinopathy
4 Preretinal ('subhyaloid') hemorrhages
 — Fluid level visible between retina and vitreous
 — Caused by new vessel rupture (e.g. proliferative diabetic retinopathy) or rapid rise in intracranial pressure (e.g. subarachnoid/intracerebral hemorrhage)
5 Subretinal hemorrhages
 — Greenish/brown appearance
 — Indicate choroidal pathology

6 Full-thickness hemorrhages
 — Widespread, dark, irregular appearance
 — Indicate retinal ischemia; predispose to new vessels

Retinopathy: hypertensive or diabetic?
1 Hypertensive
 — AV (arteriovenous) nipping*
 — Flame hemorrhages
 — Papilledema
2 Diabetic
 — Microaneurysms
 — Dot and blot hemorrhages
 — New vessel formation

* Not useful in assessing *severity* of hypertension

CLINICAL SIGNS IN THE ANTERIOR EYE

Clinical spectrum of corneal abnormalities
1 Stigmata of systemic disease
 — Arcus senilis (hyperlipidemia*)
 — Band keratopathy (hypercalcemia‡)
 — Crystals (cystinosis, myeloma)
 — Clouding (lipid storage disorders)
 — Kayser–Fleischer rings (Wilson's)
2 Corneal dystrophies¶
 — Fuchs' dystrophy (in elderly)
 — Lattice-type dystrophy
 • Localized amyloid
 • Finnish amyloidosis (p. 185)
3 Post-keratitis scarring
 — Herpes simplex
 — Staphylococci, streptococci
 — *Pseudomonas* spp.
 — *Acanthamoeba* protozoal infections

* In young patients
‡ If long-standing
¶ Bilateral signs; usually autosomal dominant inheritance

Causes of a small pupil
1 Horner's syndrome
2 Neurosyphilis (Argyll Robertson pupils)
3 Myotonic dystrophy
4 Pontine lesions
5 Acute iritis
6 Opiates; organophosphate poisoning

Causes of a large pupil
1 Third nerve palsy (if due to compressive lesion)
2 Holmes–Adie syndrome
3 Midbrain lesions
4 Congenital syphilis
5 Trauma (local)
6 Anticholinergics, benzodiazepines, cocaine, mydriatics

Pupillary responses to mydriatics
1 Hyperactive (excessive mydriasis)
 — Holmes–Adie syndrome ('tonic' pupil; see below)
2 Hypoactive (sluggish response)
 — Myotonic dystrophy ('contratonic' pupil)
 — Argyll Robertson pupil

3 Autonomic neuropathy
— *Hyperactive* dilatation to topical adrenaline 1:1000, indicating denervation hypersensitivity*
— *Hypoactive* response to topical cocaine (2.5%) or hydroxyamphetamine, indicating depletion of endogenous noradrenaline

* Similarly, hyperactive constriction to 2.5% topical methacholine

Causes of Horner's syndrome
1 Pancoast tumor
2 Sympathectomy
3 Syringomyelia
4 Lateral medullary syndrome
5 Shy–Drager syndrome (may be alternating)

Double-barrelled eponymous pupillary anomalies
1 Holmes–Adie syndrome
— 'Tonic pupil'; usually unilateral; commoner in women
— Pupil reacts abnormally slowly to light (and accommodation), but exhibits denervation hypersensitivity to mydriatics
— Associated with hyporeflexia and peripheral anhidrosis
2 Argyll Robertson pupils
— Small irregular pupils, frequently unequal
— React to accommodation but not to light
— Hallmark of neurosyphilis; rarely seen in diabetes
3 Marcus–Gunn phenomenon
— Pupil constricts weakly to direct light, strongly to consensual illumination ('swinging light' test)
— Indicates relative afferent pupillary defect
— Hallmark of optic neuritis (hence, of multiple sclerosis)

Characteristic cataracts
1 'Snowflake'
— Insulin-dependent diabetes (rare)
2 'Sunflower'
— Wilson's disease (do not impair vision)
3 'Stellate' (punctate, radially distributed)
— Hypoparathyroidism
4 'Scintillatory' (polychromatophilic, dust-like)
— Myotonic dystrophy
5 Subcapsular posterior
— Steroid-induced (dose- and duration-dependent)
— Chronic uveitis (± steroid eyedrops)
— Irradiation

OCULAR PALSIES

Clinical characterization of ptosis
1 Bilateral
— Muscle disease (myasthenia; myotonic dystrophy)
2 Partial unilateral
— Horner's syndrome*
— Partial third nerve palsy
— Congenital ptosis (commonest cause in healthy people)

3 Complete unilateral
— Third nerve palsy

* 'Everything is smaller': ptosis, miosis, enophthalmos

Diplopia: signs favoring myopathic etiology
1 Bilateral ptosis or exophthalmos
2 Bifacial weakness (incl. orbicularis oculi)
3 Normal pupils; worsening of diplopia with fatigue
— Myasthenia gravis

Syndromes with impaired vertical gaze
1 Parinaud's
2 Richardson–Steele
3 Graves' disease
4 Thalamic hemorrhage

Painful ophthalmoplegic syndromes
1 Third nerve palsy
— Posterior communicating artery aneurysm
— Intracavernous internal carotid artery aneurysm
— Diabetes mellitus*, vasculitis*
— Migraine (esp. in children)
2 Sixth nerve palsy
— Tolosa–Hunt syndrome
— Gradenigo's syndrome
— Nasopharyngeal carcinoma
— Infraclinoid (extradural) carotid artery aneurysm
3 Total ophthalmoplegia (± proptosis)
— Superior orbital fissure syndrome

* Pupils may react normally due to separate blood supply

Varieties of nystagmus and their clinical significance
1 Physiologic (opticokinetic) nystagmus
— Reflex elicited by objects moving through fixed line of sight (e.g. looking out a train window)
— Mediated by angular/supramarginal gyri in posterior parietal lobe (independent of vestibular nuclei)
— Reduced (impaired) when looking at striped drum rotating *towards* side of destructive cerebral lesion
— Provides evidence of sightedness in infants, retarded or aphasic patients, hysterics and malingerers
2 Rotary nystagmus
— Usually due to *labyrinthine* lesions; hence, often accompanied by vertigo, deafness and/or tinnitus
— Horizontal direction defined by fast (saccadic) phase
— Maximal when eyes deviated in direction of fast phase
— Saccadic correction is made by the paramedian pontine reticular formation (PPRF) on the fast side e.g. benign positional nystagmus (due to utricle pathology)
— Fast phase towards dependent ear (e.g. clockwise rotation if left ear kept in dependent position)
— Nystagmus exhibits *latency* (10–20 sec prior to onset after repositioning) and *adaptation* (lessening of nystagmus following repeated repositioning)
3 Pendular nystagmus (i.e. no fast phase)
— Difficulty fixating and/or maintaining gaze

— Nystagmus evident even if gaze centered
— Usually congenital or familial; also seen in acquired amblyopia, myopathies (esp. myasthenia) and pontine/cerebellar lesions affecting PPRF
4 Vertical nystagmus
— Due to brainstem/cerebellar (not vestibular) pathology
— In diffuse cerebellar lesions, nystagmus may occur on fixation in *any* direction
— Upbeat nystagmus (fast phase up): lesions of pontine tegmentum or floor of fourth ventricle
— Downbeat nystagmus: cerebellar atrophy, or lesion at foramen magnum (may be surgically treatable)
5 Ataxic nystagmus
— i.e. Internuclear ophthalmoplegia (brainstem lesion)
— Bilateral horizontal nystagmus of abducting eye with paralysis of contralateral adductor
— (Almost) pathognomonic of multiple sclerosis
6 Ocular bobbing
— Indicates caudal pontine lesion
— Rapid downward movement of eyes, then slow return

Lateralization of pathologic eye signs
1 Nystagmus
— Maximal looking away from side of vestibular lesion
— Maximal looking towards side of cerebellar lesion
2 Homonymous hemianopia
— Hemianopic field defect on the side *opposite* the cortical lesion (i.e. on the *same* side as the hemiplegic arm or leg) in hemispheric disease
3 Diplopia
— When looking in direction of maximal diplopia, the more peripheral image disappears when the *abnormal* eye is covered

Lateralization of abnormal conjugate gaze
1 Hemispheric stroke
— Eyes turned *towards* side of CVA (i.e. away from hemiplegic arm or leg)
2 Lateral pontine lesion
— Eyes turned *away* from side of brainstem disease (i.e. towards hemiplegic limb)
3 Epileptic seizure
— Eyes turned *away* from side of irritative cortical (i.e. hemispheric) epileptogenic focus
4 Caloric testing
— Eyes turned towards ear irrigated with ice-cold water in patients with *intact* brainstem and labyrinth

THE FACE IN NEUROLOGIC DISEASE

Differential diagnosis of facial pain in trigeminal distribution
1 Trigeminal neuralgia
— Tends to occur in patients > 50 years
— Pain → maxillary and mandibular branches of CN V

2 Paratrigeminal neuralgia (Raeder's syndrome)
— May be caused by malignancy at skull base
— Pain in ophthalmic CN V; → orbit pain, Horner's
3 Post-herpetic neuralgia
— Tends to occur in elderly patients
— Pain → ophthalmic branch of CN V
4 Intracavernous internal carotid artery aneurysm
— May cause ophthalmoplegia, esp. CN III
— Pain/sensory loss → ophthalmic (± maxillary) CN V
5 Superior orbital fissure syndrome
— Often caused by tumor invasion; may cause proptosis
— Pain in ophthalmic CN V (± ophthalmoplegia)
6 Gradenigo's syndrome
— In petrous temporal lesions, e.g. chronic otitis media
— Pain → CN V; associated CN VI palsy; now rare

Non-trigeminal patterns of facial pain
1 Ramsay–Hunt syndrome (geniculate neuralgia)
— Varicella-zoster of the geniculate ganglion of CN VII
— 'Otic zoster': ear pain, facial paralysis, vesicles in ear and/or ipsilateral fauces, ± involvement of CN VIII
2 Costen's syndrome
— Affects patients with jaw malocclusion
— Pain → temporomandibular region
3 Tolosa–Hunt syndrome
— Usually due to granulomatous angiitis or tumors
— Painful ophthalmoplegia (palsies of CN III, IV or VI)
4 Glossopharyngeal neuralgia
— Similar pain to trigeminal neuralgia; affects elderly
— Pain → CN IX, provoked by speaking or swallowing
5 Jaw claudication
— Usually due to giant cell arteritis (elderly patients)
— Pain → jaw and/or tongue when eating or speaking

Clinical characterization of facial weakness
1 Unilateral upper motor neuron weakness (e.g. CVA)
— Upper face *spared* (bilateral innervation of frontalis and orbicularis oculi)
— No lower facial sagging (tone preserved)
— Facial paresis may disappear during emotion (mediated via extrapyramidal fibers)
— Often associated with ipsilateral hemiplegia
2 Unilateral lower motor neuron weakness (e.g. Bell's palsy)
— Upper face weak (loss of forehead wrinkling)
— Lower facial sagging (± mild dysarthria)
— Inability to voluntarily close eye (eye rolls up: Bell's sign) due to paralysis of orbicularis oculi → ectropion, conjunctivitis
— Progressively more proximal lesions
  • Loss of taste over ipsilateral anterior two-thirds of tongue ± sensory loss in external auditory meatus (chorda tympani involvement)
  • Hyperacusis (involvement of nerve to stapedius)

- Impaired or aberrant lacrimation during recovery (e.g. 'crocodile tears' while eating, due to greater petrosal nerve involvement)
  — Involvement of neighboring cranial nerves
  - CN VI (e.g. brainstem lesion)
  - CN VIII (e.g. in Ramsay–Hunt syndrome)
  - CN V, VIII (e.g. cerebellopontine angle tumor)*
3 Myopathy (e.g. myotonic dystrophy)
  — Symmetric facial wasting → long, haggard appearance
  - 'Transverse smile' (myotonic dystrophy)
  - 'Myasthenic snarl' (myasthenia gravis)
  — Periorbital edema/heliotrope rash (polymyositis)
  — Ptosis
  - May be asymmetric (i.e. albeit bilateral)
  - Absent in CN VII lesions
  — Fatiguability
  — Ophthalmoplegia‡
  - Usually asymmetric
  - Pupils normal (cf. CN III palsy)

* cf. CN VII palsy: more often due to surgery than tumor compression
‡ Complicates myasthenia gravis, *not* myasthenic syndrome or polymyositis

Facial presentations of systemic disease
1 Trigeminal neuralgia in a young patient
  — Multiple sclerosis
  — Cerebellopontine angle tumor
2 Bilateral lower motor neuron facial palsy
  — Guillain–Barré syndrome
  — Mikulicz syndrome (bilateral parotid infiltration, e.g. by sarcoidosis/tuberculosis/actinomycosis)
3 Facial neuromyopathy
  — Myotonic dystrophy
  — Facioscapulohumeral dystrophy
  — Myasthenia gravis

DISORDERS AFFECTING THE LOWER CRANIAL NERVES

Characterizing and lateralizing hearing loss
1 Weber's test
  — Lateralizes to deaf side
  - Conduction deafness, e.g. otosclerosis
  — Lateralizes to normal side
  - Nerve deafness, e.g. acoustic neuroma
2 Rinne's test
  — Bone > air conduction on affected side
  - Conduction deafness
  — Air > bone conduction on both sides
  - Nerve deafness

Clinical evaluation of vestibular function
1 Caloric testing
  — Tests integrity of one labyrinth at a time by slowly irrigating ear with hot (44°C) or cold (30°C) water
  — Patient lies flat with head elevated 30–45° to make horizontal semicircular canal vertical
  — Nystagmus induced exhibits one of two abnormalities

- Canal paresis (weaker nystagmus on affected side)
  - Directional preponderance, i.e. longer duration of nystagmus on stimulation of one labyrinth
  — Principal diagnostic uses
  - Menière's disease
  - Acoustic neuroma
  - Unconscious patients: tests brainstem integrity
2 Oculocephalic testing
  — Tests integrity of both labyrinths together by holding eyelids open and sharply rotating head to one side
  — *Doll's-eye movements* are those in which eyes lag behind head, but slowly regain original position
  — Doll's-eye movements indicate loss of hemispheric suppression but preservation of brainstem function

Distinction of acoustic neuroma from Menière's disease
1 Discrete symptomatic episodes unusual
2 Vertigo uncommon; rarely occurs in isolation
3 May be associated with post-auricular/suboccipital pain, facial spasms, paresthesiae or dysphonia/dysphagia
4 Physical signs may include limb ataxia, cranial nerve palsies (esp. V) or hemianesthesia/-paresis
5 Impaired oculovestibular (caloric) response
High frequency deafness with recruitment on audiometry
6 Radiology
  — MRI: best test for cerebellopontine angle tumors
  — SXR: widening of internal auditory meatus or erosion of petrous temporal (no longer routinely indicated)

Distinction of bulbar and pseudobulbar palsies
1 Bulbar palsy
  — Affect: normal
  — Swallowing: nasal regurgitation
  — Speech: nasal
  — Tongue: fasciculations
  — Jaw jerk: normal/absent
2 Pseudobulbar palsy
  — Affect: labile
  — Swallowing: dysphagia
  — Speech: 'Donald Duck'
  — Tongue: small (spastic)
  — Jaw jerk: increased

SPINAL CORD DISEASE: GENERAL

Clues to localizing a spinal cord lesion
1 Radicular pain (indicating myotome) and weakness
2 Pattern of reflex changes
3 Sensory level (indicating dermatome)
4 Spinal tenderness to percussion*
5 Vertebral bruit (indicating tumor/AVM)

* esp. acute epidural abscess, malignancy

Clinical sequelae of spinal cord lesions
1 Vital signs
  — Hypotension
  — Poikilothermia

2 Sphincter dysfunction
— Incontinence
— Chronic UTI → amyloidosis
3 Autonomic dysfunction
— Paralytic ileus
— Excessive sweating below lesion level
4 Musculoskeletal
— Pressure sores
— Contractures
5 Immobilization
— Hypercalcemia, renal calculi, osteoporosis
— Venous thrombosis

NEUROLOGY OF THE UPPER SPINE

Cranial nerve signs of high cervical cord disease
1 Ipsilateral hemifacial dissociated sensory loss*
2 Horner's syndrome
3 Rarely: nystagmus, optic neuritis/atrophy

* = isolated loss of pain and temperature sensation

Signs of craniocervical junction anomaly (e.g. Arnold–Chiari)
1 Occipital pain; facial sensory loss; ± Pagetoid appearance
2 Cerebellar signs (due to foraminal tonsillar herniation)
3 Downbeat nystagmus
4 Finger deafferentation (esp. proprioception) → pseudotremor
5 Bulbar palsy, spastic quadriparesis (may simulate MND)

Physical findings in cervical spondylosis
1 Limitation of neck movements
2 Absent tendon jerk(s) at level of lesion (root compression)
3 Increased tendon jerks below lesion (cord compression)
4 Inversion of reflexes
5 Dermatomal sensory loss in upper limbs
6 Dorsal column sensory loss in upper and lower limbs
7 Rombergism
8 Spastic paraparesis

Thoracic outlet syndrome: clinical features
1 Physical examination
— Supraclavicular 'fullness'/tenderness/bruit
— Dilated venous collaterals
— Arm pallor/cyanosis/edema
— Wasted interossei
— Sensory loss in C8–T1 distribution
2 Maneuvers
— Repetitive movements → arm claudication
— Arm abduction (to 90°) and external rotation lead to
  • Symptoms
  • Loss of radial pulse
  • Reduction of systolic BP in arm by > 15 mmHg
3 Investigation
— Plain X-ray of thoracic outlet and cervical spine
— Apical lordotic chest X-ray views
— Cervical MRI
— Consider angiography (bilateral) if cervical rib present

C4 root lesions: clinical findings
1 Ipsilateral hemidiaphragmatic paralysis
2 C4 sensory loss (abutting T2 dermatome) at shoulder

C5 root lesions
1 Total loss of shoulder abduction
2 Axillary nerve involvement
— Weak elbow flexion
— Reduced biceps jerk
— Larger sensory loss (lateral arm) than circumflex nerve palsy
3 Supraspinatus wasting ± scapula winging

THE MOTOR SYSTEM

Distinguishing upper and lower motor neuron lesions
1 Upper motor neuron lesions
— Increased tone ± clonus
— Increased tendon reflexes
— Absent abdominal reflexes
— Extensor plantar response(s)
— 'Pyramidal' pattern of weakness (see below)
2 Lower motor neuron lesions
— Prominent wasting
— Fasciculation (in anterior horn cell disorders)
— Reduced tone
— Reflexes may be reduced or absent

Patterns of weakness in upper motor neuron lesions
1 Upper limb extensors, esp.
— Elbow and wrist extension
— Finger extension and abduction
2 Lower limb flexors, esp.
— Hip and knee flexion
— Ankle dorsiflexion and eversion
3 Fine movements of fingers and feet (esp. in capsular lesions)

Absent abdominal reflexes: differential diagnosis
1 Upper motor neuron lesions, esp.
— Multiple sclerosis
— General paresis of the insane (neurosyphilis)
— Spinal cord lesions above T7
2 Non-specific ('false-positives')
— Old age
— Gross obesity
— Multiparity

NB: Superficial abdominal reflexes usually *preserved* in motor neuron disease

Signs suggesting upper motor neuron lesions
1 Babinski sign
— Dorsiflexion of great toe and fanning of other digits on stroking lateral sole of foot
2 Oppenheim's sign
— Dorsiflexion of great toe on applying pressure while sliding thumb and forefinger down anterior tibia

3 Hoffman's sign
— Adduction and flexion of all digits after passively flexing and releasing distal middle phalanx
4 Finger flexor
— Adduction and flexion of all digits on tapping palmar surface of relaxed fingers with tendon hammer

NB: Exaggerated finger flexion indicates hypertonia rather than an upper motor neuron lesion *per se*

Fasciculations: differential diagnosis
1 Neurologic
— Motor neuron disease (esp. in exams)
— Acute phase of poliomyelitis
— Localized fasciculations
  • Syringomyelia
  • Cervical spondylosis
  • Neuralgic amyotrophy
2 Metabolic
— Thyrotoxicosis
— Severe hyponatremia
3 Drugs
— Clofibrate
— Salbutamol (esp. IV)
— Lithium (if toxic)

THE SENSORY SYSTEM

Characteristic patterns of sensory loss
1 Symmetric 'glove-and-stocking' sensory loss to all modalities
— Peripheral neuropathy
2 Dermatomal sensory loss
— Nerve root lesion
3 Ipsilateral loss of pain and temperature, contralateral loss of proprioception/two-point discrimination
— Brown–Séquard syndrome
4 Bilateral loss of pain and temperature
Normal proprioception/two-point discrimination*
— Syringomyelia
— Anterior spinal artery thrombosis
5 Loss of proprioception/two-point discrimination/vibration
Loss of deep pain (e.g. in testes, Achilles' tendon)
Patchy loss of pinprick sensation (e.g. along side of nose)
— Tabes dorsalis

* cf. *unilateral* dissociated sensory loss: high cervical cord lesion (p. 264)

Symptoms suggesting dorsal column pathology
1 Difficulty with fine movements ('clumsy')
2 Limb 'tightness' (as though bandaged)
3 'Cotton-wool' sensation over skin

Causes of reduced dorsal column function
1 Subacute combined degeneration
2 Cervical spondylosis
3 Friedreich's ataxia
4 Tabes dorsalis*

* cf. syringomyelia, anterior spinal artery thrombosis: *normal* dorsal column function is usual

TESTING NERVE ROOT INTEGRITY

Clinical assessment of nerve root integrity: reflex levels
1 Biceps/supinator jerk present
— C6 intact
2 Triceps jerk present
— C7 intact
3 Finger flexor elicitable
— C8 intact
4 Abdominal reflexes present
— T7–12 intact
5 Cremasteric reflex present
— L1–2 intact
6 Knee jerk present
— L3–4 intact
7 Ankle jerk plantars present
— S1 intact
8 Anal reflex present
— S3–4 intact

Quick testing of nerve root integrity in the upper limb
1 C5: shoulder abduction (deltoid)
— 'Make wings, keep them up, don't let me push down'
2 C5–6: elbow flexion (biceps)
— 'Pull me towards you'
3 C7: elbow extension (triceps)
— 'Now push me away'
4 C8: finger flexion (long and short finger flexors)
— 'Squeeze my fingers; try to break them'
5 T1: finger abduction/adduction (intrinsics)
— 'Spread your fingers apart, don't let me push them in'

Quick testing of nerve root integrity in the lower limb
1 L1–2: hip flexion (iliopsoas)
— 'Push up against my hand, keep it up'
2 L2–3: hip adduction (adductors)
— 'Pull your knees together against my hands'
3 L3–4: knee extension (quadriceps)
— 'Try to straighten your knee; kick out against my hand'
4 L4: ankle dorsiflexion (tibialis anterior)
— 'Curl your ankle up, don't let me straighten it'
5 L5: great toe plantarflexion (extensor hallucis longus)
— 'Push your big toe down into my hand'
6 S1: ankle plantarflexion (gastrocnemius)
— 'Try to straighten your foot; don't let me bend it back'

NEUROLOGY OF THE UPPER LIMB

Clinical spectrum of radial nerve palsy
1 High axillary injury ('crutch palsy')
— All supplied muscles paralysed
— Paralysis includes triceps
  • Loss of elbow extension
  • Absent triceps jerk
— Sensory deficit may extend to posterolateral upper arm and dorsal forearm/hand

2 Humeral midshaft injury ('Saturday night palsy')
   — Wrist and finger drop
   — Triceps spared, normal elbow extension and triceps jerk
   — Paralyses brachioradialis/supinator/forearm extensors
   — Sensory deficit limited to dorsum of hand
3 Posterior interosseous nerve injury (distal to supinator)
   — Loss of thumb/index extension
   — Loss of thumb abduction
   — Brachioradialis/supinator/forearm extensors spared
   — No sensory deficit

Small hand muscles affected by median nerve lesion: 'LOAF'
1 **L**ateral two lumbricals
2 **O**pponens pollicis
3 **A**bductor pollicis brevis (best test of median nerve integrity)
4 **F**lexor pollicis brevis

Wasting of the small muscles of both hands
1 Disuse
   — Old age
   — Rheumatoid arthritis
2 Spinal cord disease
   — Syringomyelia
   — Motor neuron disease
3 Spinal cord compression
   — Cervical spondylosis
   — C8–T1 tumor
4 Bilateral nerve root compression
   — Cervical spondylosis
   — Thoracic outlet syndrome
5 Peripheral neuropathy
   — Charcot–Marie–Tooth disease
   — Lead poisoning, acute intermittent porphyria

NB: Myotonic dystrophy causes prominent forearm wasting but characteristically *spares* the small hand muscles

Wasting of the small muscles of one hand
1 Ulnar nerve lesion
2 T1 nerve root lesion (e.g. bronchogenic carcinoma)

Differentiation of T1 root lesion from ulnar nerve palsy
1 No sensory deficit in the hand*
2 Dermatomal sensory loss in medial arm
3 Weakness of opponens pollicis/abductor pollicis brevis (supplied by median nerve; i.e. T1 lesion → all intrinsics)

* NB: Ulnar nerve lesion at *wrist* (rare) also produces no sensory loss

NEUROLOGIC SIGNS IN THE LOWER LIMB

Absent ankle jerks with extensor plantar responses
1 Subacute combined degeneration
2 Friedreich's ataxia
3 Taboparesis

4 Rare causes
   — Meningeal carcinomatosis
   — Coexisting lumbar and cervical spondylosis
   — Motor neuron disease
   — Diabetic amyotrophy
   — Conus medullaris lesion
   — Spinal shock

Clinical assessment of paraparesis
1 Cauda equina compression
   — Early onset of lumbosacral pain, precipitated by walking
   — Flaccid paralysis → wasted calves/absent ankle jerks
   — Sphincter involvement/perianal anesthesia occur late
2 Conus medullaris lesion
   — Pain occurs late
   — Spastic paraparesis → wasted quadriceps/upgoing toes
   — Sphincter dysfunction occurs early
3 Parasagittal meningioma
   — Spastic paraparesis, extensor plantar response(s)
   — Distal weakness often prominent
   — Papilledema

Clinical assessment of footdrop
1 Lateral popliteal nerve palsy
   — Equinovarus deformity due to impaired eversion
   — Variable sensory loss (usually none)
   — Great toe: sensation/dorsiflexion usually normal
2 L5 root lesion
   — Eversion unimpaired (cf. S1 root lesion)
   — Dermatomal sensory loss (dorsum of foot)
   — Great toe: sensation/dorsiflexion usually impaired
3 Charcot–Marie–Tooth disease
   — Equinovarus deformity with pes cavus
   — 'Inverted champagne bottle' appearance of limbs
   — Mild glove-and-stocking sensory loss
   — Bilateral signs; possible hand involvement

GAIT ABNORMALITIES

Diagnostic significance of abnormal posture
1 Rombergism (loss of balance with eyes closed)
   — Proprioceptive deficit
2 Truncal ataxia (same with eyes open or closed)
   — Cerebellar (flocculonodular lobe) disease
3 Simian posture
   — Parkinsonism

Common pathologies underlying abnormal gait
1 Frontal gait apraxia
   — Cerebrovascular disease
   — Normal pressure hydrocephalus
2 Neurodegeneration
   — Parkinsonism
   — Encephalopathy (e.g. toxic)
3 Myelopathy
   — Cervical spondylosis
4 Cerebellar disease
5 Sensory neuropathy

Clinical characterization of abnormal gait

1 Wide-based ('drunken') gait
 — Cerebellar (vermis) disease
 — Same gait with eyes open or closed
2 Stamping ('footslapping') gait; may also be wide-based
 — Sensory (esp. dorsal column) ataxia
 — Worse with eyes closed
 — Associated with rombergism, e.g. in tabes dorsalis
3 High-stepping ('equine') gait
 — Footdrop, e.g. Charcot–Marie–Tooth disease
4 Circumducting ('sticky') gait
 — Hemiplegia
5 Scissors ('walking through mud') gait
 — Spastic paraparesis
6 Waddling ('duck-like') gait
 — Myopathy
7 Festinating gait (± pro-/retropulsion, turns-by-numbers)
 — Parkinsonism
8 Marche à petits pas ('sputtering'/apraxic gait), 'magnetic foot'
 — Pseudobulbar palsy
 — Alzheimer's disease
 — Normal pressure hydrocephalus

NB: In exams it is best to delay labelling the gait (if possible) until *after* the other signs have established the diagnosis!

PATTERNS OF PERIPHERAL NEUROPATHY

Important causes of hypertrophic (palpable) neuropathies
1 Charcot–Marie–Tooth disease
2 Acromegaly
3 Lepromatous leprosy
4 Amyloidosis

Predominantly motor neuropathies
1 Charcot–Marie–Tooth
2 Guillain–Barré syndrome
3 Acute intermittent (or variegate) porphyria
4 Diphtheria
5 Lead poisoning
6 Herpes zoster (common but usually subclinical)

Predominantly sensory neuropathies
1 Diabetes
2 Paraneoplastic
3 Nutritional (incl. B_{12}/folate deficiency, alcohol)
4 Uremia
5 Amyloid

Frequently painful neuropathies
1 Diabetic amyotrophy (p. 93)
2 Nutritional
 — Alcoholic neuropathy
 — Beri-beri, Strachan's syndrome
3 Toxic
 — Metronidazole
 — Thallium poisoning
4 AIDS-related neuropathy

Cranial nerve involvement in peripheral neuropathy
1 Diphtheria (CN IX)
2 Guillain–Barré (CN VI, VII)
 Miller–Fisher variant (III, IV)
3 Sarcoidosis (CN VII)
4 Diabetes (CN III)

Nerves frequently involved in leprosy
1 Upper limb
 — Radial (and radial cutaneous)
 — Ulnar, median
2 Lower limb
 — Common peroneal
 — Posterior tibial
3 Head and neck
 — Facial
 — Preauricular

Drugs commonly associated with peripheral neuropathy
1 Vincristine, vindesine, taxol
2 Nitrofurantoin
3 Metronidazole
4 Perhexiline maleate
5 Gold
6 Isoniazid (B_6 deficiency), ethambutol
 Phenytoin (folate deficiency)

Guillain–Barré syndrome: diagnostic criteria
1 Major criteria
 — Progressive lower motor neuron limb weakness*
 — Areflexia
 — Maximal deficit induced within 4 weeks of onset
 — No other cause of neuropathy demonstrable
2 Minor criteria
 — Lack of fever
 — Symmetrical weakness with only mild sensory signs
 — ↑ CSF protein with normal cell count
 — Segmental demyelination pattern of nerve conduction
 — Peripheral nerve myelin antibodies detectable acutely
 — Successful trial of plasmapheresis within first week
3 Factors tending to *exclude* the diagnosis
 — Sensory level
 — Marked asymmetry of signs
 — Bladder or bowel dysfunction
 — Elevated CSF cell count (> 50/mm³)

* Arms are also typically involved

AUTONOMIC NEUROPATHY

Principal causes of autonomic neuropathy
1 Diabetes mellitus
2 Uremia
3 Amyloidosis
4 Guillain–Barré syndrome
5 Liver disease ± alcoholism
6 Idiopathic (acquired): Shy–Drager syndrome
7 Idiopathic (congenital): Riley–Day syndrome

Presentations of autonomic neuropathy
1 Vital signs
   — Pulse
     • Fixed resting tachycardia (vagal paresis)
     • Postural tachycardia
   — Blood pressure*
     • Supine hypertension
     • Postural hypotension
2 Facial signs
   — 'Differential' gustatory sweating‡
   — Pupils: Horner's, anisocoria
3 Gastrointestinal
   — Epigastric pain (gastroparesis, esophageal reflux)
   — Nocturnal hyperdefecation; fecal incontinence
   — Chronic intestinal pseudoobstruction, causing either
     • Constipation, or
     • Diarrhea due to bacterial overgrowth
4 Pain unawareness
   — 'Silent' myocardial infarction
   — Loss of 'deep' pain (e.g. on compressing testis)
   — Loss of peripheral pain (small-fiber neuropathy)
5 Other functional losses
   — Hypoglycemic unawareness (e.g. in treated diabetics)
   — Urinary retention, overflow incontinence (urgency)
   — Impotence (NB: rarely presents in isolation)

* Differential diagnosis: antihypertensive therapy
‡ Associated with *anhidrosis* affecting non-facial skin

Assessment of autonomic neuropathy
1 Measurement of variation in heart rate/blood pressure, ECG R-R intervals and plasma noradrenaline/renin activity
   — Posturing using tilt-table
   — Valsalva maneuver (4-phase response)
   — Isometric handgrip
   — Mental arithmetic (serial 7, s)
   — Hands in iced water (for 90 sec)
   — Hyperventilation (for 30 sec)
   — Carotid sinus massage
   — Amyl nitrite/atropine/isoprenaline/noradrenaline
2 Pupillary responses
   — Intraocular adrenaline 1:1000 → *no* dilatation normally, but dilates in autonomic neuropathy (p. 261)
   — Intraocular cocaine 2.5%: dilatation normally, but *not* in autonomic neuropathy
   — Intraocular methacholine 2.5% → *no* constriction normally, but constricts in autonomic neuropathy (reflecting parasympathetic denervation)
3 Sweat tests
   — Heat patient to cause 1°C rise in oral temperature
   — Give IM pilocarpine or intradermal methacholine
4 Bladder urodynamics (cystometry)

EVALUATING THE CENTRAL NERVOUS SYSTEM

Markedly elevated CSF protein: differential diagnosis
1 Pyogenic meningitis
2 Meningeal carcinomatosis
3 Guillain–Barré syndrome
4 Froin's syndrome (spinal block)
5 Rare: alcoholism, amyloidosis, diabetes, acoustic neuroma

Meningitis with negative CSF Gram-stain?
1 Partly treated pyogenic meningitis
2 Unusual organism (not detected by routine measures)
   — Tuberculous meningitis
   — Cryptococcal meningitis
   — Neurosyphilis
   — Leptospirosis, brucellosis
3 Viral, e.g.
   — HSV#2; polio
   — HIV*
4 Non-infectious causes
   — Vasculitis (esp. SLE)
   — Meningeal carcinomatosis (p. 22)
   — Sarcoidosis
   — Behçet's/Whipple's disease; Vogt–Koyanagi syndrome

* Usually with a secondary meningitic organism; biopsy may be required

Differential diagnosis of cerebral mass lesions in AIDS
1 *Toxoplasma* encephalitis
2 Primary CNS lymphoma
3 Progressive multifocal leukoencephalopathy

CSF examination after suspected subarachnoid hemorrhage
1 Macroscopic blood staining
   — Reducing red cell count with serial aliquots suggests a 'traumatic tap'
2 Xanthochromia
   — Supports diagnosis of subarachnoid bleed
   — Insensitive test if macroscopic characterization relied upon (50% false-negative)
   — Spectrophotometric assay (peak at 450 nm) is very sensitive

Evoked responses: diagnostic utility
1 Visual evoked responses (VERs)
   — Multiple sclerosis: may be useful
     • Prior to firm diagnosis
     • Monitoring disease progress
   — Hemispheric disease, e.g.
     • 'Cortical' blindness vs hysteria (p. 258)
   — Retinal disease
   — Migraine (in children)
2 Brainstem auditory evoked responses (BAERs)
   — Suspected acoustic neuroma
   — Comatose patient

— Hysterical deafness
— Multiple sclerosis
3 Somatosensory evoked responses (SSERs)
— Peripheral nerve vs spinal cord/root lesion
— Multiple sclerosis

NB: *Any* of these electrophysiologic tests may be abnormal in HIV infection

Diagnosis of brain death
1 Sufficient cause
— Exclude hypothermia/sedative overdose
2 No response to noxious stimuli except spinal reflexes
3 Fixed pupils
4 Loss of oculovestibular and oculocephalic reflexes
5 Absent gag/corneal/cough reflexes
6 No spontaneous respiratory movements after ventilator disconnected and patient observed for 5 min with oxygen supplied via tracheal catheter

ELECTROENCEPHALOGRAPHY (EEG)

Normal EEG patterns
1 Awake (eyes closed)
— α waves (8–12 cps); over parietooccipital region
2 Non-REM sleep
— δ waves (0–3 cps)
3 REM sleep
— β waves (> 13 cps); over frontal region
4 Hyperventilation
— θ waves (4–7 cps)

Capabilities of the EEG
1 May diagnose epileptic activity
2 May confirm effect of metabolic disorder (e.g. liver failure)
3 May suggest focal pathology
4 May explain sleep disturbances and/or drop attacks
5 May help distinguish petit mal from temporal lobe epilepsy

Limitations of the EEG
1 Cannot exclude epilepsy
2 Cannot assess adequacy of antiepileptic treatment
3 Cannot exclude focal pathology
4 Cannot suggest structural nature of focal pathology

Principal indications for EEG
1 Diagnosis and management of epilepsy
2 Diagnosis of brain death
3 Unusual indications
— Unexplained organic brain syndrome
— Investigation of presenile dementia
— Evaluation of birth asphyxia

Suggestive diagnostic EEG patterns
1 Hepatic encephalopathy
— Triphasic waves (*not* in Wernicke's/DTs) ± δ waves
2 Barbiturate overdose
— Excess fast-wave (β) activity

3 'α coma'
— Follows infarction of midbrain tegmentum
4 Absence (petit mal) seizures
— Characteristic 3 cps spike-and-wave pattern
5 HSV encephalitis, SSPE, Creutzfeldt–Jakob
— Slow background repetitive sharp waves

The unconscious patient: utility of the EEG
1 Helps distinguish diffuse encephalopathy, e.g.
— Myxedema (→ diffuse slowing)
— Dialysis dementia (→ spike-and-wave pattern), *from*
2 Space-occupying lesions, e.g.
— Frontal lobe tumor (→ focal slowing), *or*
3 Other focal pathology, e.g.
— HSV encephalitis (→ temporal lobe slowing), *or*
4 Depressive pseudodementia (→ normal EEG)

INVESTIGATING CEREBROVASCULAR DISEASE

Techniques available for assessing carotid disease
1 Direct tests
— Angiography (incl. digital subtraction angiography)
— 'Duplex scan': B-mode (real-time) + pulsed Doppler
2 Indirect tests
— Ophthalmodynamometry
— Oculoplethysmography
— Periorbital directional Doppler ultrasonography
— Radionuclide angiography

Which investigation to choose in carotid disease?
1 Angiography
— Advantages
• Reveals location and severity of disease
• Still the 'gold standard' for preop diagnosis
— Disadvantages
• Invasive; may precipitate stroke
• May fail to reveal intramural pathology
2 'Duplex scan'
— Advantages
• Non-invasive; useful to monitor known disease
• May detect plaque hemorrhage or ulceration
• Normal study may obviate need for angiography
— Disadvantages
• Abnormal? may still require preop angiography
3 Indirect tests (ophthalmic artery flow/pressure studies)
— Advantages
• Non-invasive
— Disadvantages
• Only reliably detect unilateral disease
• Only reliably detect advanced (> 75% block) cases
• Only reliably detect occlusive (not ulcerated) cases

Indications for carotid duplex scanning
1 Carotid artery signs
— Hemiparesis, amaurosis, aphasia, *plus*

2   Good recovery, *plus*
3   Fit for carotid surgery

Imaging sequence in stroke patients
1   To distinguish hemorrhage from infarct, tumor, subdural
    — CT brainscan*
2   To assess carotid patency in patients who have recovered well from hemispheric TIA or minor stroke
    — Carotid ultrasound
3   To exclude cardiogenic source of emboli *if* carotid ultrasound normal *or* brainstem TIA/stroke + known cardiac disease
    — Cardiac echo
4   To evaluate extracranial and intracranial vessels if carotid ultrasound shows ≥ 50% stenosis and/or ulceration
    — Intraarterial digital subtraction angiography
5   To clarify infarct mechanism and prognosis in patients whose initial CT was normal
    — Follow-up non-enhanced CT at 10 days

* Non-enhanced unless tumor figures strongly in differential diagnosis

Indications for angiography in cerebrovascular disease
1   Operable patient, *plus*
2   Symptoms suggesting carotid pathology, *or*
3   Subclavian steal syndrome

INVESTIGATING THE PERIPHERAL NERVOUS SYSTEM

Investigation of peripheral neuropathy
1   Qualitative tests
    — Nerve conduction studies
    — Nerve biopsy
2   Etiologic tests
    — Blood film, MCV
    — B_{12}, folate
    — GGT/urate (ethanol)
    — Fasting blood sugar level, HbA_{1c}, GTT
    — Lead, mercury levels
    — Urinary porphobilinogen/δ-ALA
    — CSF protein and cell count
    — Carcinoma search (e.g. CXR) *only* if clinically indicated

Nerve conduction studies: diagnostic significance
1   General
    — Myopathy
      • Normal nerve conduction velocity
      • Reduced amplitude and duration of motor units
    — Neuropathy
      • Reduced nerve conduction velocity
      • Reduced number of motor units
2   Neuropathy: *segmental demyelination* (e.g. Guillain–Barré)
    — Marked slowing of conduction velocity
    — Amplitude may be normal
    — Early loss of reflexes and vibration sense
    — May → mononeuritis multiplex
    — Rapid recovery (often)

3   Neuropathy: *axonal degeneration* (e.g. nutritional deficiency)
    — Marked reduction of motor unit amplitude
    — Mild slowing of conduction velocity
    — Early onset of wasting
    — Incomplete recovery (usually)
4   Upper motor neuron lesion
    — Normal evoked muscle potentials
    — Low firing rate; slow to reach full interference pattern
    — Unexpected 'H' reflexes

Indications for nerve biopsy
1   Prognostic clarification (see above) of neuropathies due to
    — Axonal degeneration, *or*
    — Segmental demyelination
2   Definitive diagnosis of neuropathies due to
    — Polyarteritis/vasculitis
    — Amyloidosis, sarcoidosis
    — Leprosy
    — Déjerine–Sottas disease

DIAGNOSTIC ASPECTS OF MUSCLE DISEASE

Muscle biopsy: diagnostic value
1   Polymyositis
2   Polyarteritis
3   Myotonic dystrophy
4   Trichinosis, toxoplasmosis
5   Metabolic muscle disease (e.g. glycogen storage) Special myopathies (e.g. mitochondrial)

Pathologic patterns in electromyography (EMG)
1   Polymyositis
    — May cause *fibrillation* (brief low-amplitude action potentials due to denervation hypersensitivity), indicating pathology at the motor end-plate (i.e. in addition to the known muscle fiber pathology)
2   Myotonia
    — *'Dive-bomber'* EMG (high-frequency action potentials)
3   Myasthenia gravis
    — *Decremental* response to repetitive ('tetanic') stimuli
    — Increased 'jitter'
4   Myasthenic (Eaton–Lambert) syndrome
    — *Incremental* response to repetitive stimulation (= 'post-tetanic facilitation')

Myotonic dystrophy: recognition and diagnosis
1   General appearance
    — Frontal alopecia
    — Thick glasses (aphakia, cataracts)
    — Facial abnormalities, hyperostosis frontalis interna
2   Affect
    — Monotonous voice
    — Somnolent; subnormal intellect
3   Pattern of weakness/wasting
    — Myopathic facies
      • Ptosis, hanging jaw
      • Temporalis/sternomastoid wasting

— Weakness of neck flexion
— Distal limb weakness, wasted brachioradialis
4 Percussion myotonia
— Thenar eminence
— Forearm
— Quadriceps

Myotonic dystrophy: complications and management
1 Clinical complications
— Cardiac conduction defects; cardiomyopathy
— Hypoventilation; post-anesthetic respiratory failure
2 Biochemical complications
— Insulin resistance (impaired glucose tolerance)
— Gonadotrophin resistance ($\uparrow$ FSH/LH, hypogonadism)
— Hypogammaglobulinemia
3 Management includes
— Family screening using FSH levels and/or EMG
— Drugs: quinine, phenytoin, procainamide

NEURORADIOLOGY

Intracranial calcification on skull X-ray
1 Oligodendroglioma, meningioma
— 20% calcify ('ball of calcium')
— May be associated with overlying bony hyperostosis
2 Craniopharyngioma, esp. in children
— 75% calcify
— May be intra- or suprasellar
3 Pineal gland
— Calcified in 60% adults, 10% children
— Midline shift may indicate intracranial mass lesion
4 Tuberous sclerosis
— Multiple discrete lesions $\rightarrow$ temporal lobes
5 Sturge–Weber syndrome
— Subcortical 'tramline' calcification $\rightarrow$ parieto-occipital
— $\pm$ Ipsilateral facial hemangioma, contralateral paresis
6 Infection
— Toxoplasmosis
— CMV; TB
7 Vascular
— Aneurysm ('ring' calcification)
— Angioma (spotty flecks of calcification)
— Atheroma (curvilinear)
— Chronic subdurals (outlined by calcification; rare)
8 Basal ganglia calcification
— esp. Hypoparathyroidism
9 Cerebral calcifications and epilepsy
— Celiac disease

Characteristic CT scan appearances
1 Normal pressure hydrocephalus
— Large ventricles with minimal cortical atrophy
2 Benign intracranial hypertension
— Small ventricles
3 Intracerebral abscess
— Enhancing ring $\pm$ satellite edema

False-negative CT brainscans
1 Non-enhancing lesions < 1 cm diameter
2 Diffuse lesions (e.g. microgliomatosis)
3 Bilateral subdurals isodense with brain
4 Lesions near skull base or anterior optic pathways

Indications for CT brainscan in the stroke patient
1 Diagnostic uncertainty
— Young patient
— No history available
— Gradual/progressive onset of signs (?tumor/subdural)
— Atypical clinical course (esp. rapid deterioration)
2 Suspected intracranial hemorrhage
— Cerebellar hemorrhage (surgically evacuable)
  • Acute onset of ataxia
  • 'Stroke somewhere, stroke nowhere'*
— Subarachnoid hemorrhage‡
— Recent history of anticoagulant therapy¶
— Planned anticoagulant therapy¶

* i.e. no localizing signs
‡ CT = investigation of choice
¶ incl. antiplatelet and thrombolytic therapy

Other indications for CT brainscan
1 Head injury with disturbance of consciousness
2 Head injury with focal signs
3 Late-(adult) onset epilepsy, esp. with focal signs
4 Presenile dementia

MAGNETIC RESONANCE IMAGING (MRI)

Advantages of magnetic resonance imaging over CT
1 *No* ionizing radiation with MRI*
2 MRI can provide imaging sections in *any* anatomic plane
3 Compact bone does not produce any signal with MRI, hence no artefacts, e.g. in posterior cranial fossa (cf. CT)

* MRI consists of radiofrequency radiation emitted within magnetic field $\rightarrow$ resonance of magnetic elements (e.g. H_2) in body

Suspected diagnoses where MRI is superior to CT
1 Posterior fossa lesions, esp. tumors
2 Brainstem disease
3 Cerebellopontine angle disease, e.g. acoustic neuroma
4 Pituitary tumors; hydrocephalus
5 Craniocervical junction pathology, e.g. Arnold–Chiari
6 Demyelinating plaques*
7 Spinal cord/vertebral tumors, syrinxes
8 Disc disease, esp. herniation
9 Torn knee meniscus
10 Contrast allergy

* Gadolinium enhancement is used to demonstrate associated blood–brain barrier breakdown (due to perilesional inflammation)

Conditions in which CT may be superior to MRI
1 Acute skull trauma
2 Acute stroke, e.g. subarachnoid hemorrhage
3 Cerebral aneurysm or arteriovenous malformation

Contraindications to MRI
1 Cerebral aneurysm clips
2 Permanent pacemaker
3 Intraocular foreign bodies*
4 Shrapnel
5 Cochlear implants
6 Implanted infusion pumps
7 Pregnancy (esp. first trimester)

* esp. if visible on X-ray

Artificial implants usually not contraindicating MRI
1 Dental fillings (non-magnetic)
2 Intrauterine devices
3 Prosthetic heart valves (most)
4 Orthopedic prostheses

MANAGING NEUROLOGIC DISEASE

CEREBROVASCULAR DISEASE

Management considerations in cerebrovascular disease
1 In symptomatic patients, the more severe the stenosis, the higher the risk of stroke, *but*
2 Many severe (even occlusive) stenoses are asymptomatic; if so, the risk of stroke is < 2%
3 Atheromatous carotid lesions may regress
4 Absence of a bruit is not a contraindication to angiographic assessment (severe stenoses may be inaudible)
5 Hypertension is the biggest risk factor for a cerebrovascular event; in patients with TIAs, reducing diastolic BP by 5–10 mmHg may reduce stroke risk by up to 40–50%

Important therapeutic negatives in cerebrovascular disease
1 Endarterectomy is *not* indicated for asymptomatic bruits
   — esp. If < 30% stenosis
2 High-dose steroids are of *no* benefit in cerebral infarction
3 Extracranial-intracranial bypass grafting is *not* of proven benefit to symptomatic patients with internal/ carotid middle cerebral artery disease

Rationâle for aspirin prophylaxis in cardiovascular disease
1 Reduces morbidity and mortality of carotid TIAs in males
2 Reduces reinfarction (20%) and mortality (10%) following myocardial infarction
3 Reduces 'event rates' in unstable angina
4 Enhances coronary artery bypass graft patency
5 Helps prevent venous thrombosis after hip surgery in males
6 May retard progression of peripheral vascular disease

Indications for anticoagulation
1 TIAs associated with cardiac disease, e.g.
   — Mitral stenosis and/or atrial fibrillation
   — Post-infarct

2 Carotid-type TIAs
   — In a potentially operable patient prior to angiography
   — In a female unfit for surgery (or normal angiogram)
   — In a male unfit for surgery *and* unresponsive to aspirin
3 Vertebrobasilar insufficiency
   — In a female, *or*
   — In a male despite aspirin prophylaxis*
4 Relative need for anticoagulation is increased with
   — Recent onset (< 6/12) of TIAs
   — Increasing frequency or longer duration of attacks
   — Accumulating neurologic deficit with attacks

* Exception: subclavian steal syndrome may be surgically treated

SURGERY IN CEREBROVASCULAR DISEASE

Carotid endarterectomy: when should it be considered?
1 Logistic prerequisites
   — Fit patient with symptomatic carotid disease
   — Experienced vascular surgical team available*
2 Principal indication
   — > 70% stenosis (residual lumen < 2 mm) of cervical portion of internal carotid artery, *plus*
   — Symptoms
3 Other indications
   — Persistent symptoms of carotid stenosis (< 70%) despite appropriate medical therapy
   — Symptomatic carotid stenosis < 70%, *plus*
   — Contraindication to aspirin/warfarin
4 Less definite indications
   — Ulcerated (potentially embologenic) carotid lesion
   — Clots (luminal filling defects) ± tight stenosis
   — Acute phase occlusion with mild/fluctuating deficit
   — Severely reduced post-stenotic blood flow, thus making complete occlusion likely

* ≤ 5% operative stroke rate

Scenarios precluding carotid endarterectomy
1 Stenosis too mild
2 Symptoms related to contralateral cerebral hemisphere
3 Established total carotid occlusion
4 Patient unfit for general anesthesia

SPASTICITY

Antispasticity drugs: therapeutic considerations
1 General
   — Drug therapy tends to be more effective in spasticity of spinal rather than intracranial origin
2 Diazepam
   — CNS GABA agonist
   — Dosage limited by sedation
3 Baclofen
   — CNS GABA agonist
   — May cause depression

4 Dantrolene
— Peripheral effect on skeletal muscles; inhibits calcium release from sarcoplasmic reticulum
— May exacerbate weakness (therefore less popular)
— Occasionally associated with hepatotoxicity

Surgical measures in spasticity management
1 Neurolysis (or dorsal rhizotomy)
— Phenol/alcohol injection into nerve or nerve root
2 Tenotomy
— e.g. Hamstring, adductor, heel-cord
3 Myotomy
— e.g. Iliopsoas
4 Neurectomy
— e.g. Obturator; pudendal (for detrusor instability)
5 Myelotomy
6 Cordectomy
— A drastic measure for intractable symptoms, e.g. uncontrollable flexor/adductor spasms

Therapeutic indications for botulinum toxin (type A)
1 Adult focal dystonias*
— Blepharospasm
— Spasmodic torticollis
— Hemifacial spasm
— Spasmodic dysphonia
— Writer's cramp
2 Strabismus
3 Achalasia (inject into LES)
4 Investigational applications
— Tremor (some types)
— Spasticity (e.g. cerebral palsy)

* Toxin is injected into dystonic muscles

ANTICONVULSANT THERAPY

Choosing an anticonvulsant for epileptic disorders
1 Localization-related seizures*
— Drug of choice: carbamazepine
— Others: phenytoin‡, valproate, phenobarbitone
2 Idiopathic generalized seizures (usually genetic)
— Drug of choice: sodium valproate (see below)

* incl. complex partial seizures, tonic-clonic seizures, focal epilepsy
‡ NB: May worsen absence seizures

Epileptic disorders best treated by sodium valproate
1 Absence (petit mal) seizures
— Alternative: ethosuximide*
2 Tonic-clonic seizures associated with absence seizures
— Alternative: phenytoin
3 Myoclonic epilepsy
— Alternatives: clonazepam, nitrazepam
4 Febrile convulsions (prophylaxis)
— Alternative: phenobarbitone
5 Minor motor seizures (infantile spasms)
6 Lennox–Gastaut syndrome (epileptic encephalo-pathy)
— Alternatives: felbamate, lamotrigine

* NB: Worsens tonic-clonic seizures but fewer side-effects than valproate

Carbamazepine: indications and contraindications
1 Useful in
— Complex partial seizures (drug of choice)
— Tonic-clonic (grand mal) seizures
— Trigeminal neuralgia
2 *Not* indicated in
— Absence seizures
— Myoclonic epilepsy

Adjunctive ('add-on') antiepileptic drugs*
1 Vigabatrin (for partial epilepsy)
2 Lamotrigine
3 Gabapentin
4 Clobazam‡

* Especially useful in partial epilepsy. However, where possible, control with monotherapy is preferable
‡ A benzodiazepine used for *intermittent* back-up at times of high seizure incidence, e.g. menstruation, stress

Approach to management of status epilepticus
1 Initially: diazepam/lorazepam/clonazepam (slow IV)
2 At 10': paraldehyde (IM) → (15') phenobarbitone (IV)
3 At 20': phenytoin infusion (+ ECG/plasma monitoring)
4 At 30': chlormethiazole
5 At 40': thiopentone anesthesia (for 2 h)

Surgical treatment of epilepsy
1 Interventions
— Focal cortical resection
— Cerebral hemispherectomy
— Corpus callosotomy
2 Ideal patient profile
— Refractory to drug therapy*, *and*
— Typical complex partial seizures, *and*
— Unilateral temporal lobe ictal onset, *or*
— Focal cerebral lesion, esp.
• Hamartoma
• Cavernous vascular malformation

* A prerequisite

MECHANISMS OF ANTICONVULSANT ACTION

Drugs acting as GABA agonists*
1 Valproate
2 Benzodiazepines
3 Barbiturates
4 Vigabatrin
5 Lamotrigine
6 Gabapentin; baclofen‡

* i.e. act by enhancing GABA-mediated CNS inhibition
‡ NB: May reduce seizure threshold

Anticonvulsants acting as membrane stabilizers
1 Phenytoin
— Increases membrane binding of calcium
2 Carbamazepine
— Structurally related to tricyclics*
3 Lamotrigine
— Blocks voltage-sensitive sodium channels, thus reducing release of glutamate

* i.e. *not* to benzodiazepines

Pharmacokinetics of anticonvulsant therapy
1 Phenytoin
   — $t^{1/2} \approx 24$ h
   — Time to plateau ≈ 5 days
   — Once-daily dosage schedule is satisfactory
   — Children may require up to double the usual adult maintenance dose due to ↑ liver metabolism
   — Exhibits saturation kinetics (similar to aspirin, alcohol)
2 Phenobarbitone
   — $t^{1/2} \approx 100$ h
   — Time to plateau ≈ 2–3 weeks
   — Once-daily dosage schedule is satisfactory
3 Carbamazepine
   — $t^{1/2} \approx 12$ h
   — Time to plateau ≈ 3 days (may take longer since *initial* $t^{1/2} \approx 36$ h; shortens due to autoinduction)
   — Administered three times daily
4 Sodium valproate
   — Plasma $t^{1/2} \approx$ hours, but bears little relation to effect
   — Administered twice- or thrice-daily

PROBLEMS WITH ANTICONVULSANT THERAPY

Indications for monitoring anticonvulsant plasma levels
1 Phenytoin therapy, esp. if
   — Poor seizure control
   — Suspected toxicity
   — New drug added (e.g. valproate)
2 Carbamazepine therapy in initial stages
3 Renal or liver disease
4 Mentally retarded patients (if difficult to assess toxicity)
5 Suspected non-compliance

NB: For valproate, ethosuximide or phenobarbitone, 'therapeutic range' may need to be determined empirically on a patient-by-patient basis

Side-effects of phenytoin
1 Acute toxicity
   — Occurs with IV use (or overdose)
     • Hypotension
     • Arrhythmias
     • CNS depression
2 Acute toxicity with oral use
   — Dose-dependent; correlates with serum drug levels
     • Nystagmus → ataxia → drowsiness
3 Chronic toxicity with routine oral use
   — Dose-dependent, but may occur at therapeutic levels
     • Vitamin D deficiency: osteomalacia, hypocalcemia
4 Idiosyncratic
   — Not clearly dose-related
     • Nausea, vomiting, diarrhea
     • Skin rash
     • SLE; pseudolymphoma
5 Epilepsy-related
   — More common in high-dose therapy
     • Worsening of absence seizures
     • Increased frequency of tonic-clonic seizures

Side-effects of other anticonvulsants
1 Sodium valproate
   — Tremor (dose-dependent)
   — Polycystic ovaries*, hyperandrogenism, amenorrhea
   — Hair thinning (reversible), hair curling
   — Increased appetite, weight gain; ankle edema
   — Drowsiness (but less than most other anticonvulsants)
   — Stupor, encephalopathy ± hyperammonemia
   — Reye's-like hepatotoxicity (idiosyncratic)
     • Affects 1/10,000, esp. age < 3 years
     • Often preceded by increased seizure frequency
     • Potentially fatal
2 Carbamazepine
   — Drowsiness (esp. if coadministered with phenytoin)
   — SIADH with fluid retention (may → CCF in elderly)
   — Anticholinergic effects (structurally resembles tricyclics)
   — Leukopenia, agranulocytosis (rare)
3 Phenobarbitone and congeners (e.g. primidone)
   — Drowsiness/confusion, esp. in elderly
   — Hyperactivity in children
   — Megaloblastosis

* Affects 80% of women < 20 years taking valproate

Anticonvulsant interactions of clinical significance
1 Inducers of hepatic metabolism
   — Carbamazepine, phenytoin, phenobarbitone
     • Dosage may need to be increased due to autoinduction of drug metabolism
     • Starting any of these agents in a patient already stabilized on monotherapy (e.g. valproate) may lead to paradoxical initial deterioration
     • May antagonize oral contraceptives*, steroids, quinidine, warfarin and theophylline; toxicity of the latter may be precipitated by (say) carbamazepine withdrawal
2 Inhibitors of hepatic metabolism
   — Sodium valproate
     • Addition may precipitate *toxicity* of other anticonvulsants (e.g. phenobarbitone, CMZ) which may in turn antagonize valproate
     • Valproate may also precipitate phenytoin toxicity even in the absence of raised serum phenytoin levels, due to *plasma protein displacement* (i.e. ↑ free, not total, phenytoin)
   — Isoniazid, another P_{450} inhibitor, may also precipitate phenytoin toxicity (esp. in slow acetylators)

* Hence, patients using oral contraception should use *valproate* if possible

Considerations in managing the pregnant epileptic
1 Anticonvulsant usage is associated with 6% incidence of teratogenesis (about 3-fold increased), esp.
   — Phenytoin, phenobarbitone
     • Cleft palate, congenital heart disease
   — Valproate, carbamazepine
     • Spina bifida (1%), hypospadias

2 Always aim to use
— Monotherapy (where possible)
— Lowest possible dosage
3 Seizure control may deteriorate due to reduced drug concentration. If dosage is increased, toxicity may supervene in the puerperium unless levels are monitored
4 Antagonism of vitamin K-dependent coagulation factors by anticonvulsants, esp. barbiturates, may predispose to fetal or neonatal hemorrhage*
5 Phenytoin and phenobarbitone may reduce folate levels, which may in turn predispose to neural tube defects. Hence, women on anticonvulsants should take folic acid‡ prior to conception and for the first 12 weeks of pregnancy
6 A small but significant increased incidence of congenital malformations is seen in the offspring of epileptics, incl.
— Epileptic mothers *not* receiving anticonvulsants
— Epileptic fathers (i.e. married to non-epileptic mothers)

* cf. hemorrhagic disease of the newborn: no bleeding until ≥ 24 h post-partum
‡ Precise dose is controversial, varying from 0.4 to 5 mg/day

Contraindications to surgical management of epilepsy
1 Absolute
— Inadequate trial of medical therapies
2 Relative
— Bilateral interictal epileptiform discharges on EEG
— Non-temporal lobe epilepsy
— Dominant lobe epilepsy

PARKINSON'S DISEASE

Drug therapy in Parkinson's disease
1 Mild disease (symptoms without disability)
— Anticholinergics (e.g. benzhexol, orphenadrine)
• Avoid in elderly patients (→ confusion)
• Best for controlling salivation, tremor
• Confer additive benefit to levodopa
— Selegiline
• MAO inhibitor which may defer disability
• Prolongs dopamine action by blocking reuptake and breakdown
• Delays need for L-DOPA by ~ 9 months
— Amantadine
• Weak non-specific dopamine receptor agonist; modest efficacy
• Minimal toxicity: edema, livedo reticularis
• Amphetamine-like effect → insomnia, confusion
• Tolerance may be a problem
2 Moderately disabling disease
— L-DOPA
• Decarboxylated by neurons to dopamine
• Combined with peripheral decarboxylase inhibitor, e.g. carbidopa, benserazide
• Mainstay of therapy for bradykinesia, rigidity
• Antagonized by phenothiazines (e.g. prescribed for levodopa-induced nausea) or pyridoxine
3 Advanced or refractory disability
— Bromocriptine

• Dopamine agonist (like pergolide, lisuride)
• Prime indication: late failure of levodopa
• Longer duration of action than levodopa
• Expensive, toxic ('first-dose' reactions, psychosis)
— Catechol-*o*-methyltransferase inhibitors
• Entacapone, tolcapone
— Stereotactic surgery
• Rarely used; sole indication is incapacitating tremor (esp. unilateral) refractory to L-DOPA

Adjunctive measures in Parkinson's disease
1 Laxatives
— esp. if on anticholinergics
2 Tricyclic antidepressants
— Antidepressant + anticholinergic effects
3 β-blockers
— esp. for tremor
4 Benzodiazepines
— For myalgias
5 Counselling
— esp. for sexual problems
6 Handwriting assistance

PROBLEMS IN MANAGING PARKINSON'S DISEASE

Physical signs suggesting secondary parkinsonism
1 Blepharospasm or downward gaze palsy
2 Jerky tremor or myoclonus
3 Symptomatic orthostasis
4 Lower body parkinsonism
5 Cerebellar signs
6 Pyramidal signs

Primary L-DOPA resistance in parkinsonism: factors to exclude
1 Non-compliance (± dementia, depression)
2 Coadministration of phenothiazines or pyridoxine
3 Misdiagnosis
— Richardson–Steele (progressive supranuclear palsy)
• Associated downgaze palsy
— Multisystem atrophy
• Olivopontocerebellar atrophy
• Striatonigral degeneration
• Shy–Drager syndrome (autonomic failure)

Symptom-driven antiparkinsonian therapy
1 Treatment of mild bradykinesia only
— Amantadine (tremor may worsen)
2 Treatment of mild rigidity and bradykinesia
— Anticholinergics
— Selegiline
3 Treatment of moderate/severe rigidity, bradykinesia
— L-DOPA (+ carbidopa)
— L-DOPA + bromocriptine
4 Treatment of incapacitating tremor
— β-blockers
— Stereotactic surgery

Specific limitations of L-DOPA therapy
1 Episodic exacerbations of bradykinesia ('on-off' effect)

2 End-of-dose deterioration ('wearing-off' effect)
3 Dose-limiting effects
   — Confusion, nightmares
   — Depression, paranoid ideation
4 Dose-dependent toxicity
   — Vomiting (CNS effect and delayed gastric emptying)
   — Hypotension, orthostasis
   — Dyskinesias, blepharospasm, akathisia

The 'on-off' effect: therapeutic approaches
1 Add selegiline to L-DOPA
2 Substitute bromocriptine (or pergolide) for L-DOPA
3 L-DOPA 'drug holiday'
4 Transplantation of adrenal medulla or fetal substantia nigra

IATROGENIC NEUROLOGIC DISEASE

Neurologic sequelae of oral contraceptives
1 Migraine
2 Cerebral thrombosis/infarction
3 Hypertensive intracerebral hemorrhage
4 Subarachnoid hemorrhage
5 Dural sinus thrombosis
6 Chorea (Sydenham's); benign intracranial hypertension

Benign intracranial hypertension: iatrogenic causes
1 Tetracycline
2 Oral contraceptives, corticosteroids
3 Vitamin A
4 Nitrofurantoin; nalidixic acid; perhexiline

Varieties of drug-induced eye disease
1 Corneal microdeposits
   — Amiodarone (usually asymptomatic)
   — Chloroquine (reversible)
2 Cataracts
   — Steroids (incl. eyedrops)
   — Phenothiazines (usually asymptomatic)
3 Optic neuritis
   — Ethambutol
   — Chloramphenicol
4 Retinopathy
   — Chloroquine ('bull's-eye' macula)
   — Thioridazine (retinitis pigmentosa-like)
5 Stevens–Johnson syndrome
   — e.g. Sulfonamides

HEADACHE TREATMENTS

Serotonin receptors in migraine pathophysiology
1 5-HT$_1$ receptors
   — Inhibitory (cause vasoconstriction)
   — Agonists used for acute attacks
2 5-HT$_2$ receptors
   — Excitatory
   — Antagonists used for prophylaxis

Drugs useful in treating acute migraine
1 Serotonin-1 (5-HT$_1$) receptor agonists
   — Sumatriptan (most effective drug)
     • Oral (100 mg)
     • Subcutaneous (6 mg)
   — Ergotamine*
     • Oral, sublingual, suppository (2 mg)
     • Subcutaneous dihydroergotamine (1 mg)
2 Dopamine antagonists
   — IV metoclopramide 10 mg
   — IV prochlorperazine, chlorpromazine
3 NSAIDs
   — Aspirin (900 mg) + metoclopramide (10 mg)
   — Naproxen (750 mg)
   — Mefenamic acid, diclofenac, ibuprofen

* Contraindicated in patients with vascular disease

Drugs useful in migraine prophylaxis
1 Serotonin-2 (5-HT$_2$) receptor blockers
   — Methysergide*, pizotifen
   — Amitriptyline
2 β-blockers
   — Propranolol
   — Metoprolol, atenolol, nadolol
3 NSAIDs
   — Naproxen
   — Mefenamic acid, aspirin
4 Valproate

* May cause retroperitoneal, pleural or cardiac valvular fibrosis

Therapeutic modalities in cluster headache
1 Lithium
2 Sumatriptan, ergotamine
3 Steroids
4 Oxygen

Sumatriptan: properties and problems
1 Properties
   — Selective cerebral vasoconstrictor
   — 60% relief after oral dose, 80% after SC dose
2 Problems
   — 'Non-cardiac' chest pain
   — Facial flushing/tingling (esp. after SC dose)
   — Contraindicated in coronary atheroma/spasm
   — Expense

UNDERSTANDING NEUROLOGICAL DISEASE

Heritable neurologic diseases involving trinucleotide DNA repeats ('growing genes')
1 Fragile X syndrome
2 Myotonic dystrophy
3 Huntington's disease
4 Spinocerebellar ataxia #2
5 Adult-onset spinal and bulbar muscular atrophy

Amine neurotransmitters in CNS disease
1 Excitatory
   — Glutamate
   — Aspartate

2 Inhibitory
— Glycine
— GABA (decarboxylation product of glutamate)

Parkinson's disease vs Huntington's chorea: what's different?
1 Predominant site of neuronal loss in Parkinson's
— Pigmented nuclei: substantia nigra, locus ceruleus
Predominant site of neuronal loss in Huntington's
— Caudate nucleus (± frontal lobes, putamen)
2 Neurotransmitter loss in Parkinson's
— Dopamine
Neurotransmitter loss in Huntington's
— Acetylcholine (and GABA)
3 Pathophysiology of Parkinson's
— Relative excess of acetylcholine →
parkinsonism
Pathophysiology of Huntington's
— Relative excess of dopamine → chorea*
4 Dopamine receptor agonists (e.g. levodopa) in Parkinson's
→ Improvement of parkinsonism
Dopamine receptor agonists in Huntington's
→ Exacerbation of chorea
5 Dopamine receptor antagonists‡ in Parkinson's
→ Exacerbation of parkinsonism
Dopamine receptor antagonists in Huntington's
→ Improvement of chorea

* cf. *Tardive dyskinesia*: due to striatal supersensitivity to dopamine
‡ e.g. phenothiazines

Movement disorders: predominant sites of pathology
1 Kernicterus
— Caudate and lenticular nuclei
2 Hahervorden–Spatz disease
— Substantia nigra (zona reticulata)
3 Hemiballismus
— Subthalamus (contralateral)
4 Wilson's disease
— Putamen
Kayser–Fleischer rings*
— Descemet's membrane

* Absence of KFRs on slit-lamp examination reliably excludes Wilson's disease as a cause of neurologic, but not hepatic, dysfunction

Classical localization of selected intracranial pathologies
1 Herpes simplex encephalitis
— Temporal lobes
2 Wernicke's encephalopathy
— Mamillary bodies, mamillothalamic tracts
3 Pick's disease
— Anterior frontal and temporal lobes
4 Sturge–Weber syndrome
— Forehead hemangioma → occipital lobe involvement
— Facial hemangioma → frontoparietal involvement
5 Tuberous sclerosis
— Temporal lobe calcification

INTRACRANIAL BLEEDING DISORDERS

Predispositions to chronic subdural hematomata
1 Epilepsy
2 Alcoholism
3 Hemodialysis
4 Anticoagulant therapy
5 Poor socioeconomic status

Features of chronic subdurals
1 Headache occurs in 75%
2 History of head trauma in 50% (only)
3 Fluctuating level of consciousness in less than 25%

Predispositions to cerebral aneurysms
1 Aortic coarctation
2 Polycystic disease
3 Renal artery stenosis due to fibromuscular dysplasia
4 Essential hypertension
5 Ehlers–Danlos syndrome type IV
6 PAN/Wegener's/SBE

Sequelae of subarachnoid hemorrhage
1 Cerebral vasospasm
— Severity lessened by early (oral) use of nimodipine
— Nimodipine less useful for reversing delayed ischemia
2 Rebleeding
— 40% rebleed within 12 months
— 20% prove to have multiple aneurysms
3 Excessive catecholamine release (acute phase)
— Hypertension
— ECG abnormalities (e.g. T wave inversion)
— Glycosuria
4 Normal pressure hydrocephalus (long-term)

NEUROSYPHILIS

Clinical varieties of neurosyphilis
1 Meningovascular syphilis
— Non-specific mental changes
— Cranial nerve palsies
— Argyll-Robertson pupils, papilledema
— Cerebral infarction, limb paresis
2 Tabes dorsalis
— Symptoms: lightning pains, gastric crises, impotence
— Argyll-Robertson pupils, optic atrophy
— Pseudoptosis (overactive frontalis)
— Reduced vibration/proprioception/deep pain
— Patchy loss of temperature/pinprick → nose, tibia
— Charcot joints, trophic foot ulcers
— Rombergism, stamping gait (sensory ataxia)
— Hypotonia, hyporeflexia; flexor plantars
3 General paresis of the insane
— Dementia, incontinence, fits
— Argyll-Robertson pupils
— Dysarthria, tongue ('trombone') tremor
— Upper motor neuron signs, incl. extensor plantars

NEUROLOGY AND THE AIDS PATIENT

Neurologic indications for HIV serology
1 Unexplained mental deterioration
   — Encephalitis
   — Encephalopathy
   — Dementia
2 Myelopathy (aseptic meningitis, transverse myelitis)
3 Inflammatory neuropathy

Neurologic manifestations of AIDS
1 AIDS-dementia complex
   — Affects > 50% of AIDS patients with advanced disease
   — Causes ataxia, incontinence, mutism, paraplegia
   — Subacute encephalitis may be due to HIV (or CMV)
2 Opportunistic CNS infection
   — e.g. Toxoplasmosis, cryptococcosis, JC virus
3 Vacuolar myelopathy
   — Bilateral leg weakness, incontinence
4 Atypical aseptic meningitis
   — May be recurrent, involve cranial nerves or long tracts
5 Inflammatory demyelinating polyneuropathy
   — May mimic Guillain–Barré; mononeuritis multiplex
   — May precede AIDS diagnosis
6 CNS lymphoma (EBV-induced)
7 Zidovudine neurotoxicity (rare)
   — Idiosyncratic confusion, seizures
   — Dose-related ataxia/nystagmus
   — Symptom precipitation if drug abruptly withdrawn

MULTIPLE SCLEROSIS

Diagnosis of multiple sclerosis
1 Clinical
   — At least two remitting episodes of at least two focal lesions
2 Supporting investigations
   — Plaques on MRI (best test)
   — Delayed evoked responses, esp. VERs
   — Oligoclonal bands on CSF EPG in 90%*

* Also found in sarcoid, syphilis, SLE, etc; *not* routinely indicated

MRI correlations in multiple sclerosis
1 Positive detection of plaques in 98% of patients with *clinically convincing* MS; i.e. diagnostic role is purely supplementary to clinical evaluation
2 Gadolinium enhancement detects perivascular inflammation (*not* demyelination per se)
3 Enhancing and non-enhancing abnormalities change size rapidly; enhancing lesions last approximately 1 month
4 The incidence of new enhancing lesions far exceeds the number of clinical relapses
5 Standard MRI shows *poor* correlation with clinical deficit

6 Gadolinium-enhanced MRI is good for assessing treatment*

* e.g. showing that interferon-β reduces frequency of exacerbations (though not necessarily long-term disability)

Predictors of poor prognosis in multiple sclerosis
1 Advanced age at onset
2 Presents with acute brainstem syndrome (simulating stroke)
3 Incomplete recovery (esp. weakness) from initial attack
4 Early onset of cerebellar ataxia
5 Early loss of mental acuity (may be associated with euphoria)

Common presentations of multiple sclerosis
1 CN II involvement
   — Retrobulbar neuritis
2 Brainstem involvement
   — Diplopia (CN VI or internuclear palsy)
   — Nystagmus, vertigo
3 Spinal cord involvement
   — Asymmetrical leg weakness and/or numbness

Uncommon presentations of multiple sclerosis
1 Facial presentations
   — Trigeminal neuralgia
   — Facial palsy (*upper* motor neuron type)
   — Facial myokymia (continuous rippling of one side)
2 'Useless hand' with proprioceptive loss only
   — DD$_x$: hysteria
3 Lhermitte's sign
   — 'Electric' pains on flexing neck
4 Uhthoff's phenomenon
   — Worsening of weakness or vision with heat (e.g. hot bath or exercise)

Presentations suggesting alternative etiologic diagnoses
1 Peripheral neuropathy
2 Persistent loss of skin sensation
3 Epilepsy

Multiple sclerosis vs Friedreich's ataxia
1 Similarities
   — Optic atrophy
   — Nystagmus
   — Cerebellar signs
   — Extensor plantar responses
2 Factors favoring Friedreich's
   — Family history
   — Absent ankle jerks
   — Pes cavus/scoliosis
   — Cardiomegaly
3 Factors favoring multiple sclerosis
   — History of Lhermitte's or Uhthoff's phenomena
   — Trigeminal neuralgia (esp. bilateral)
   — Absent abdominal reflexes
   — Bladder enlargement
   — Brisk ankle jerks

SPINAL DISEASE

Transverse myelitis: features
1 Presentation
  — Pain (e.g. interscapular) localizing to final sensory level
  — Lower limb paresthesiae, ascending weakness
  — Sphincter dysfunction
2 Established clinical deficit
  — Flaccid paralysis
  — Complete sensory loss (typically to thorax)
3 Investigations
  — CT/MRI usually normal
  — CSF may reveal non-specific pleocytosis, ↑ protein
  — VERs usually normal
4 Features associated with poor prognosis
  — Fulminant onset
  — Pain
  — Spinal shock

Common vertebral levels of various pathologies
1 Cervical cord
  — Syphilitic myelitis
  — Syringomyelia
2 Thoracic cord
  — Subacute combined degeneration
  — Anterior spinal artery thrombosis (~ T4)
  — Pott's disease
3 Thoracolumbar
  — Ependymoma; metastatic tumors
  — Transverse myelitis
4 Lumbosacral
  — Tabes dorsalis

Neurologic deficits in cervical spondylosis
1 Lateral disc protrusion
  — Root compression
2 Foraminal osteophytes
  — Root compression
3 Osteophytes
  — Vertebral artery insufficiency
4 Posterior disc protrusion
  — Cord compression
5 Posterior disc protrusion
  — Vascular myelopathy

Predispositions to kyphoscoliosis and/or pes cavus
1 Friedreich's ataxia
  Hereditary spastic paraplegia
2 Charcot–Marie–Tooth disease
3 Polio
4 Neurofibromatosis
5 Syringomyelia

Pes cavus plus claw hands? Differential diagnosis
1 Reflexes depressed
  — Charcot–Marie–Tooth disease
2 Reflexes exaggerated
  — Syringomyelia

Associations of neurofibromatosis
1 Skin
  — Café-au-lait spots (> 5, > 1.5 cm diameter)
  — Axillary freckling
  — Melanoma
2 Neurogenic intracranial lesions
  — Optic glioma, cerebral glioma
  — Acoustic neuroma, meningioma
  — Ependymoma, malignant schwannoma
  — Syringomyelia
3 Vascular syndromes
  — Berry aneurysms
  — Aortic coarctation
  — Renal artery stenosis; pheochromocytoma
  — Mesenteric ischemia
4 Musculoskeletal
  — Limb deformities (tibial bowing, pes cavus)
  — Vertebral scalloping
5 Other associations
  — Pulmonary fibrosis
  — Diabetes insipidus
  — Hypospadias
  — Intellectual impairment

MOVEMENT DISORDERS

Patterns of cerebellar disease
1 Vermis involvement
  — Often due to alcoholism
  — Spinocerebellar tract connections involved
  — Signs
    • Wide-based gait (deviates to affected side)
    • Impaired tandem gait
    • Slurred speech
2 Flocculonodular lobe involvement
  — May be due to PICA syndrome/medulloblastoma
  — Vestibular connections involved
  — Signs
    • Truncal ataxia (unable to sit/stand unsupported)
    • Nystagmus (may be vertical)
    • Titubation
3 Posterior lobe involvement
  — Cortical connections involved (many causes)
  — Signs
    • Hypotonia
    • Limb ataxia ('drift')
    • Dysmetria ('past-pointing')
    • Dysdiadochokinesis
    • Intention tremor

Periodic paralysis: classification
1 Hypokalemic
  — Familial, or
  — Associated thyrotoxicosis (esp. in Oriental males), or
  — Associated with primary aldosteronism
  — Paralysis precipitated by
    • Carbohydrate meal (↑ insulin → ↓ K$^+$)
    • Rest after exertion (duration: hours – days)
  — Prophylaxis with
    • Potassium supplements
    • Acetazolamide
    • Spironolactone

2 Normokalemic
  — Paramyotonia (von Eulenberg's disease)
  — Weakness and/or myotonia inducible by cold
  — Treat with tocainide
3 Hyperkalemic (Gamstorp's disease)
  — Often familial
  — Typically affects eye muscles (duration ~ 30 min)
  — Precipitated by cold weather
  — Responds to intravenous calcium gluconate

MYASTHENIA GRAVIS

Myasthenia gravis: classification
1 Ocular
  — Lowest AChRAb levels (25% are normal)
  — Unresponsive to thymectomy; responds to steroids
2 Thymoma
  — Highest AChRAb levels
  — Non-pathogenic striated muscle antibodies
3 'Thymitis' (age < 40 years)
  — Female > male
  — HLA-B$_8$DRw$_3$ commonly
  — Associated with other autoimmune disease
  — Negative striated muscle antibodies
  — Best response to thymectomy (80%)
4 'Thymitis' (age > 40 years)
  — Male > female
  — HLA-A$_3$B$_7$DRw$_2$ commonly
  — Low levels of AChRAb
  — Best response to corticosteroids
5 Don't confuse with non-immune 'congenital myasthenia'
  — Associated with consanguinity
  — Absent AChRAb
  — No response to thymectomy/plasmapheresis

Clinical signs in myasthenia gravis: special maneuvers
1 Sustained lateral/upward gaze
  — Ptosis
  — Diplopia
  — Ophthalmoplegia
2 Count to 50
  — Slurring of speech
3 Drink water
  — Regurgitation, dysphagia
4 Abduct one shoulder repeatedly
  — Then compare other side
5 Elevate limb for long period, assess power
  — Then note improvement with rest*

* cf. psychogenic fatigue: rest doesn't help

Investigating the patient with suspected myasthenia gravis
1 Edrophonium ('Tensilon') test
  — Pretreat with atropine to prevent bradycardia, nausea
  — Give 1 mg test dose prior to 5 mg test proper
  — False-negatives in up to 10% (e.g. due to wasting)
2 EMG
  — Post-tetanic inhibition (p. 270)
3 AChRAb
  — 90% sensitivity (70% in ocular myasthenia)
  — False-positives
    • First-degree relatives
    • Myasthenics in remission
    • Rheumatoid patients on D-penicillamine

Approach to management of myasthenia gravis
1 Anticholinesterase therapy (losing popularity)
  — Commence with pyridostigmine 30 mg q.i.d.
  — Beware of cholinergic crisis when increasing dosage
  — May test integrity of bulbar/respiratory muscle power by injecting edrophonium 2 mg IV
2 Corticosteroid therapy (1 mg/kg alternate days) if
  — Seriously ill before thymectomy
  — Insufficiently improved after thymectomy
  — Ocular myasthenia
  — Now often used as initial therapy
  — Anticholinesterase potentiation may precipitate initial deterioration; hence, start treatment as inpatient
3 Azathioprine: best results if
  — Patient > 40 years
  — Male sex
  — Long-standing disease (> 10 years)
  — Absent HLA-B$_8$DRw$_3$
  — High AChRAb levels
4 Thymectomy
  — 80% of patients without thymoma improve
  — Improvement may be delayed up to 5 years
  — Less effective for thymoma (but all the more necessary)
  — Thymoma may be managed with transsternal thymectomy and/or thymic irradiation
5 Plasma exchange
  — Consider in myasthenic crisis or prethymectomy
6 Unexpected deterioration? Exclude
  — Thyrotoxicosis
  — Pregnancy
  — Sepsis
  — Drugs
    • Quin(id)ine, procainamide; phenytoin
    • Propranolol; lignocaine
    • Aminoglycosides
    • CNS depressants
    • D-penicillamine
    • Hypokalemia (e.g. due to diuretics)

9.1 Pomeroy SL et al (1990) Seizures and other neurologic sequelae of bacterial meningitis in children. N Engl J Med 323: 1651–1657

Follow-up study of 185 children with bacterial meningitis, showing that 37% had neurologic deficits during the acute illness but only 14% persisted at 12 months; of these, 10% had only sensorineural deafness. Epilepsy was uncommon, occurring in only 7%.

9.2 MRC Antiepileptic Drug Withdrawal Study Group (1991) Randomised study of antiepileptic drug withdrawal in patients in remission. Lancet 337: 1175–1180

Prospective randomized study of 1013 patients on anti-convulsants who had been seizure-free for at least 2 years; 60% of those who withdrew from therapy remained seizure-free, compared with 78% who continued. Patients on more than one drug were less likely to do well following withdrawal.

9.3 Friberg L et al (1991) Migraine pain associated with middle cerebral artery dilatation: reversal by sumatriptan. Lancet 338: 13–17

Study of 10 migraine patients by transcranial Doppler, showing that migraines were associated with reduced MCA flow rate (i.e. vasodilatation) on the affected side and that this was normalized with sumatriptan.

9.4 Beck RW et al (1992) A randomized, controlled trial of corticosteroids in the treatment of acute optic neuritis. N Engl J Med 326: 581–588

Beck RW et al (1993) The effect of corticosteroids for acute optic neuritis on the subsequent development of multiple sclerosis. N Engl J Med 329: 1764–1769

Both studies suggested that IV methylprednisolone, but not oral prednisolone, was useful – both in speeding the visual recovery from optic neuritis and in reducing the subsequent incidence of MS over a 2-year period.

9.5 Logigian EL et al (1990) Chronic neurologic manifestations of Lyme disease. N Engl J Med 323: 1438–1444

Even years post-infection, Lyme disease patients may develop chronic neurologic signs; these respond well to antibiotic therapy. Hence, Lyme disease provides a model of autoimmune disease pathogenesis.

9.6 Guillain–Barré Syndrome Steroid Trial Group (1993) Double-blind trial of intravenous methylprednisolone in Guillain–Barré syndrome. Lancet 341: 586–590

Nice study of 242 patients showing that a short course of high-dose methylprednisolone is of *no* benefit in GBS.

9.7 SALT Collaborative Group (1991) Swedish Aspirin Low-dose Trial (SALT) of 75 mg aspirin as secondary prophylaxis after cerebrovascular ischaemic events. Lancet 338: 1345–1349

Dutch TIA Trial Study Group (1991) A comparison of two doses of aspirin (30 mg vs 283 mg a day) in patients after a transient ischemic attack or minor ischemic stroke. N Engl J Med 325: 1261–1266

Both studies found that low-dose aspirin (75 or 30 mg) was effective in preventing vascular events post-TIA/stroke.

9.8 Veterans Affairs Stroke Prevention Investigators (1992) Warfarin in the prevention of stroke associated with nonrheumatic atrial fibrillation. N Engl J Med 327: 1406–1412

Randomized study of 571 male fibrillators treated with low-dose warfarin (to achieve INR 1.5–3) showing that cerebral infarction was preventable without a major increase in hemorrhage, even in patients older than 70.

9.9 European Carotid Surgery Triallists' Collaborative Group (1991) MRC European Carotid Surgery Trial: interim results for symptomatic patients with severe (70–99%) or with mild (0–29%) carotid stenosis. Lancet 337: 1235–1243

Prospective study of 2518 patients, showing that the benefits of surgery outweighed the risks in high-risk (but not low-risk) patients.

9.10 Spencer DD et al (1992) Unilateral transplantation of human fetal mesencephalic tissue into the caudate nucleus of patients with Parkinson's disease. N Engl J Med 327: 1541–1548

Report of four patients receiving brain grafts for parkinsonism. PET scanning with [18]Fluorodopa revealed caudate dopamine replenishment post-op, but persistent putaminal deficits. Symptoms were improved for 18 months follow-up, but disability persisted.

CHAPTER 10

Pharmacology and toxicology

Physical examination protocol 10.1   You are asked to examine a patient known to be a drug addict

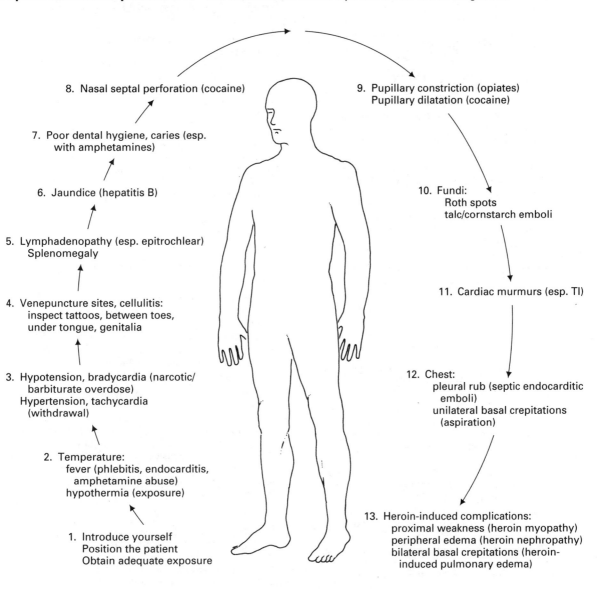

8. Nasal septal perforation (cocaine)

7. Poor dental hygiene, caries (esp. with amphetamines)

6. Jaundice (hepatitis B)

5. Lymphadenopathy (esp. epitrochlear) Splenomegaly

4. Venepuncture sites, cellulitis: inspect tattoos, between toes, under tongue, genitalia

3. Hypotension, bradycardia (narcotic/ barbiturate overdose) Hypertension, tachycardia (withdrawal)

2. Temperature: fever (phlebitis, endocarditis, amphetamine abuse) hypothermia (exposure)

1. Introduce yourself Position the patient Obtain adequate exposure

9. Pupillary constriction (opiates) Pupillary dilatation (cocaine)

10. Fundi: Roth spots talc/cornstarch emboli

11. Cardiac murmurs (esp. TI)

12. Chest: pleural rub (septic endocarditic emboli) unilateral basal crepitations (aspiration)

13. Heroin-induced complications: proximal weakness (heroin myopathy) peripheral edema (heroin nephropathy) bilateral basal crepitations (heroin-induced pulmonary edema)

CLINICAL ASPECTS OF PHARMACOLOGY AND TOXICOLOGY

Commonest toxicologic short cases
1 Heavy metal poisoning
2 Drug eruption

HEAVY METAL INTOXICATION

Clinical stigmata of mercury poisoning
1 Tremor ('hatter's shakes') → tongue, eyelids, legs
2 Erethism: irritability, easy embarrassment
3 Salivation, gingivitis, pharyngeal pain, bloody diarrhea
4 Nephrosis, renal tubular dysfunction (often reversible)
5 'Pink disease' (acrodynia) – skin hypersensitivity in infants exposed to topical mercury solutions (10% mortality)

Features of lead poisoning: acute vs chronic toxicity
1 Acute poisoning
   — Commoner in children
   Chronic poisoning
   — Commoner in adults
2 Musculoskeletal effects
   — Acute: arthralgias
   — Chronic: 'saturnine' gout
3 Renal effects
   — Acute: renal tubular dysfunction
   — Chronic: gouty nephropathy
4 Hematologic effects
   — Acute: hemolytic anemia ± basophilic stippling
   — Chronic: basophilic stippling ± hemolytic anemia
5 Gastrointestinal effects
   — Acute: colicky abdominal pain precipitated by alcohol and relieved by palpation or IV calcium
   — Chronic: constipation, gingival 'blue line' (adults), premature tooth loss (children)
6 Neurologic effects
   — Acute: headache, ataxia, fits, encephalopathy
   — Chronic: peripheral neuropathy (predominantly motor), psychiatric sequelae

Reversibility of complications in heavy metal poisoning
1 Lead poisoning
   — Chelation (p. 287) can reverse the GI and blood effects
   — R_x does *not* reverse the neurologic or renal sequelae
2 Wilson's disease (copper overload)
   — Penicillamine can reverse renal tubular dysfunction
   — R_x does *not* reverse end-stage liver/neurologic disease
3 Hemochromatosis (iron overload)
   — Phlebotomy may *prevent* all sequelae, incl. cardiac
   — Phlebotomy *prolongs life* in symptomatic patients
   — Phlebotomy is *not* effective in *reversing* established

• Hypogonadotrophic hypogonadism
• Diabetes mellitus
• Arthropathy
   — Phlebotomy does *not* reduce *hepatoma risk* in established *cirrhosis*

TOXIC OVERDOSE SYNDROMES

Clinical features of sympathomimetic overdose*
1 Paranoia, delusions
2 Tachycardia, hypertension, arrhythmias
3 Fever, sweating, piloerection
4 Mydriasis
5 Hyperreflexia
6 Stroke (esp. with cocaine), seizures

* e.g. due to cocaine, amphetamines (incl. 'ice'), theophylline, (pseudo)ephedrine, caffeine

Clinical features of anticholinergic overdose*
1 Tachycardia
2 Dry, flushed skin; mumbling speech
3 Mydriasis
4 Decreased bowel sounds
5 Urinary retention
6 Delirium, seizures

* e.g. due to tricyclics, antispasmodics, antihistamines, antiparkinsonian drugs, amantadine, mydriatics, certain plants

Clinical features of cholinergic overdose*
1 Salivation, lacrimation, fasciculation
2 Miosis
3 Weakness, sweating
4 Abdominal cramps, vomiting
5 Incontinence (urinary and fecal)
6 Pulmonary edema, confusion, fits

* e.g. organophosphate overdose, physostigmine, edrophonium

Clinical features of sedative/opiate/alcohol overdose
1 Hypotension, hypothermia, bradycardia
2 Respiratory depression, pulmonary edema
3 Miosis
4 Decreased bowel sounds
5 Needle marks
6 Coma

Clinical features of triazolam* overdosage
1 Hyperexcitability, behavioral disinhibition
2 Diurnal anxiety and confusion
3 Rebound insomnia, somnambulism
4 Excessive daytime sedation

* A benzodiazepine; common brand name is 'Halcion'

Odoriferous diagnosis of substance intoxication
1 Breath
   — Rotten apples (salicylism)
   — Bitter almonds (cyanide intoxication)
   — Mothballs (naphthalene)
   — Wintergreen (methylsalicylate)
   — Pears (paraldehyde, chloral hydrate)
   — Acetone (isopropyl alcohol)

2 Vomitus
— Garlic (arsenic poisoning, organophosphates)

MEDICAL COMPLICATIONS OF ILLICIT DRUG ABUSE

Complications of cocaine abuse
1 Agitation
2 Tachycardia, hypertension, fever
3 Priapism
4 Rhabdomyolysis ± acute renal failure
5 Inhalational sequelae
— (CSF) rhinorrhea
— Sinusitis, bronchitis, pneumonitis
— Pneumothorax (-mediastinum, -pericardium)
6 Obstetric sequelae
— Placental abruption
— Fetal abortion
— Prematurity
7 Infarctions
— Myocardial
— Bowel, skin
— Cerebral
8 Other cardiovascular sequelae
— Aortic dissection
— Subarachnoid hemorrhage
— Arrhythmias

Specific complications of parenteral drug abuse
1 Infective endocarditis
2 Chronic hepatitis; tetanus, botulism
3 AIDS
4 Osteomyelitis, septic arthritis, cellulitis
5 Thrombophlebitis; arteriovenous aneurysms
6 Pulmonary septic emboli/infarction
7 Renal failure

Symptoms and signs of narcotic withdrawal
1 Irritability, tremulousness, panic
2 Yawning
3 Runny nose, watery eyes
4 Chills, sweating, cramps, nausea ('cold turkey')

TOXIC OCCUPATIONAL EXPOSURES

Diseases due to occupational exposure to toxic agents
1 Asbestosis
2 Occupational asthma, industrial bronchitis
3 Hearing loss (noise-induced)
4 Contact dermatitis
5 Solvent poisoning
6 Lead poisoning (acute or chronic)
7 Toxic hepatitis
8 Silicosis
9 Miscellaneous poisoning
— Pesticides, carbon monoxide

Malignancies inducible by toxic workplace exposure
1 Mesothelioma, lung cancer
— Asbestos
2 Bladder cancer
— *p*-aminodiphenyl, benzidine, naphthalene dyes

3 Leukemia
— Ionizing radiation, benzene
4 Nasal sinus carcinoma
— Chromium, nickel, wood dust
5 Hepatoma
— Vinyl chloride monomer
6 Scrotal/skin cancer (e.g. in chimney sweeps)
— Aromatic hydrocarbons (e.g. in coal, creosote)

INVESTIGATING DRUG THERAPY

General reasons for checking plasma drug levels
1 Low toxic:therapeutic ratio
2 Substantial interpatient variability in drug metabolism
3 Efficacy difficult to monitor on clinical grounds

Specific indications for measuring drug levels
1 Life-threatening overdose
— Paracetamol (if urine screen +ve)
— Tricyclics, salicylate (peak levels occur late due to delayed gastric emptying)
— Methanol, salicylate (↑↑ levels → early hemodialysis)
2 Routine regular dose calibration
— Aminoglycosides
— Lithium
— Digoxin
— Anticonvulsants: phenytoin, carbamazepine
3 Initial calculation of maintenance dosage (esp. in cardiac, renal or liver failure)
— Quinidine, procainamide, disopyramide, lignocaine
— Theophylline
4 High probability of drug interaction, e.g.
— Adding quinidine to maintenance digoxin therapy
— Adding valproate to maintenance phenytoin
5 Treatment failure
— esp. Suspected non-compliance

Laboratory diagnosis of lead poisoning
1 ↑ Blood lead (esp. in children)
2 ↑ Urinary coproporphyrin III (good screening test)
3 ↑ Urine and serum ALA
4 ↑ Urine lead (EDTA-mobilization)
5 ↑ Serum iron and red cell protoporphyrin (→ ineffective erythropoiesis)

PHARMACOGENETICS

Genetic polymorphisms determining drug toxicity
1 Pseudocholinesterase deficiency (autosomal recessive)
— Causes suxamethonium (succinylcholine) sensitivity
— Leads to prolonged apnea post-anesthesia
2 Malignant hyperthermia (autosomal dominant)
— Hypercatabolic response to anesthetic agents, esp. halothane, suxamethonium; ± MAOIs, tricyclics

3 Favism (G6PD deficiency: X-linked dominant)
   — Manifests as hemolysis
   — Caused by primaquine, sulfonamides,
     nitrofurantoin
4 Acute intermittent porphyria (autosomal dominant)
   — Causes abdominal pain (acute), neuropathy
     (chronic)
   — Precipitated by many drugs, esp. barbiturates,
     alcohol
5 Steroid-induced glaucoma (autosomal recessive)
   — Precipitated by topical (or long-term systemic)
     steroids
   — Occurs in about 5% of the population
6 Slow acetylation (autosomal recessive)
   — Generally manifests as drug toxicity
     Rapid acetylation (autosomal recessive)
   — Generally manifests as drug insensitivity
7 Sulfonylurea flushing (autosomal dominant)
   — Precipitated by chlorpropamide or tolbutamide
   — Occurs in about 30% of Caucasians
8 Warfarin resistance (autosomal dominant)
   — Rare

METABOLIC POLYMORPHISMS

Rationâle for determining the acetylation phenotype*
1 Isoniazid
   — Slow acetylators
     • ↑ Peripheral neuropathy (B_6-responsive)
     • ↑ Iatrogenic SLE
     • ↑ Phenytoin/carbamazepine toxicity
     • ↑ Rifampicin-induced hepatotoxicity
   — Rapid acetylators
     • Failure of once-weekly TB therapy
     • ↑ Isoniazid-induced hepatitis
2 Sulfasalazine
   — Slow acetylators
     • ↑ Toxicity from sulfapyridine moiety, esp.
       headaches, leukopenia
     • ↑ Hemolysis in G6PD-deficient patients
3 Hydralazine
   — Slow acetylators
     • ↑ Iatrogenic SLE, esp. in females
   — Rapid acetylators
     • Failure of antihypertensive therapy
4 Procainamide
   — Slow acetylators
     • ↑ Iatrogenic SLE
5 Dapsone
   — Slow acetylators
     • ↑ Hemolysis in G6PD-deficient patients
   — Rapid acetylators
     • Failure of therapy for dermatitis
       herpetiformis

* 50% of the population are slow acetylators

Diseases associated with slow acetylation phenotype
1 Gilbert's syndrome
2 Sjögren''s syndrome
3 Arylamine-induced bladder cancer

Clinical sequelae of 'poor' debrisoquine oxidation phenotype*
1 Excessive hypotension with
   — Debrisoquine
   — Propranolol, metoprolol, timolol
2 Methemoglobinemia with phenacetin
3 Lactic acidosis with phenformin
4 Neuropathy/hepatotoxicity with perhexiline
5 Agranulocytosis with captopril
6 Confusion with nortriptyline (+ other anticholinergic
   effects)

* 50% of the population are poor metabolizers of debrisoquine –
i.e. they have homozygous monoxygenase deficiency

MANAGING DRUG THERAPY

APPROACH TO THE POISONED PATIENT

When to consider dialysis?
1 Methanol intoxication
2 Severe salicylate intoxication
3 Lithium poisoning (if plasma level > 5 mmol/L)
4 CCl_4 (within 48 h of ingestion)

Other treatment options in life-threatening overdosage
1 Forced alkaline diuresis (urine pH → 7.5–8.5)
   — (Pheno)barbitone
   — Salicylate
2 Forced acid diuresis (urine pH → 5.5–6.5)
   — Quin(id)ine
   — Amphetamine, phencyclidine
3 Charcoal hemoperfusion
   — Theophylline (if plasma level > 60 mg/L)
   — Barbiturates, methaqualone
   — Paraquat

Clinical use of oral activated charcoal ('gastrointestinal dialysis')
1 Technically simpler than hemoperfusion or dialysis
2 Suitable for use in district hospitals or remote
   locations
3 Most effective for weakly acidic drugs with small V_D

Drugs effectively eliminated by repeated oral charcoal
1 Phenobarbitone, carbamazepine, phenytoin
2 Salicylate, quinine, digoxin
3 Theophylline, aminophylline
4 Dapsone

Paracetamol (acetaminophen) overdose: principles of management
1 Gastric lavage ± charcoal adsorption, if
   — Ingestion of ≥ 10 g paracetamol within last 4 h, *or*
   — Time and/or quantity of ingested dose unknown
2 Specific therapy (if overdose taken within last 16 h)
   — Best guide: *paracetamol level* > 4 h post-ingestion
   — If above reference level for toxicity, infuse *N*-
     acetylcysteine according to nomogram‡
   — Therapy indicated if overdose taken within last
     24 h; may require continuation until
     72 h post-ingestion

3 If *N*-acetylcysteine unavailable, use oral methionine¶
4 *Prothrombin time* and *transaminases* should be monitored closely (may rise within 12 h of overdose)
5 In patients at risk of hepatic necrosis (esp. if massive overdose and/or late presentation), give 5% dextrose infusion to obviate risk of hypoglycemia
6 Liver transplant may be considered in otherwise fatal cases

‡ e.g. 150 mg/kg over 15 min, then 50 mg/kg over 4 h, then 100 mg/kg over 16 h
¶ Another glutathione precursor

Specific antidotes to inhaled or ingested poisons
1 Carbon monoxide (CO)
   — 100% oxygen (if carboxy-Hb > 30%)
   — *Hyperbaric* (2 atm./200 kPa) if unconscious
2 Cyanide (CN⁻)*
   — 100% oxygen ± sodium bicarbonate IV, *plus*
   — Dicobalt EDTA IV sodium thiosulphate IV, *or*
   — Amyl nitrite inhaled every 5 min, *or*
   — Hydroxocobalamin IV (in mild cases)‡
3 Organophosphate insecticides (cholinesterase inhibitors)
   — IV atropine every 10 min (to keep heart rate > 60)
   — Pralidoxime (PAM) slow IV hourly
4 Ethylene glycol or methanol
   — Gastric lavage, *plus*
   — 50 g ethanol IV loading dose, *plus*
   — IV 4-methylpyrazole, *or*
   — 5% ethanol IV + forced alkaline diuresis + hemodialysis

NB: Gastric lavage contraindicated following ingestion of paraffin, kerosene or petrol (due to risk of aspiration pneumonitis)
* Cyanide intoxication may occur secondary to smoke inhalation
‡ e.g. due to prolonged sodium nitroprusside therapy (p. 64)

Antidotes to metal or elemental poisoning
1 Lead (Pb; 'plumbism')
   — Calcium disodium EDTA slow IV b.d. + dimercaprol
   — Intramuscular administration is less hazardous in children at risk of encephalopathy
   — Oral or intragastric administration is *contraindicated*
2 Iron (Fe; presents with GI bleeding or hepatic necrosis)
   — Desferrioxamine (DFO) ± charcoal adsorption (by gastric lavage; then leave in stomach; then deep IM DFO loading dose; then *slow* infusion)*
3 Mercury (Hg), arsenic (As), gold (Au)
   — Dimercaptosuccinic acid, penicillamine
   — Dimercaprol (BAL) by deep IM injection (traditional)
4 Zinc (Zn; → 'metal-fume fever')
   — D-penicillamine p.o.
   — Also used in Pb, Hg, As, Au, Cu poisoning
   — Dimercaprol (BAL)
5 Thallium (used in rodenticides)
   — Prussian (Berlin) blue via nasogastric tube
   — Also used in Fe, CN⁻ poisoning

6 Bromism (Br)
   — Saline infusion
   — Also helpful in lithium poisoning

* NB: DFO should *not* be used in patients receiving vitamin C due to risk of cardiac damage. Also infusions longer than 24 h may cause excess free radicals leading to shock lung (ARDS); hence, keep them short

Antidotes to drug overdoses
1 Benzodiazepines
   — Flumazenil (0.2 mg over 30 sec)
2 Calcium channel blockers
   — Calcium (1 g over 5 min IV with ECG monitor)
3 Anticholinergics
   — IV neostigmine over 60 sec using ECG monitor
4 Tricyclics
   — Bicarbonate (1 mmol/kg IV for arrhythmias)
   — Physostigmine IV for anticholinergic effects
5 Isoniazid
   — Pyridoxine (5 g slow IV)
6 β-blockers
   — Glucagon (5 mg IVI)
7 Digoxin
   — Fab fragments (for arrhythmias)
8 Opiates
   — Naloxone (2 mg IVI to start with)
9 Nitrates
   — Methylene blue (if MetHb > 30%)
10 Warfarin
   — Vitamin K

SALICYLISM

Salicylate overdose: therapeutic options
1 Mild poisoning (salicylate level < 500 mg/L)
   — Fluid and electrolyte balance alone
2 Moderate (level < 500 mg/L + acidosis; or < 750 mg/L alone)
   — Forced alkaline diuresis, *or*
   — Oral activated charcoal
3 Severe (< 750 mg/L + renal impairment; < 900 mg/L alone)
   — Charcoal hemoperfusion, *or*
   — Hemodialysis

Metabolic complications of salicylate overdosage
1 Fever, sweating
   — Due to uncoupling of oxidative phosphorylation
2 Confusion
   — Due to neuroglycopenia, esp. in adults
3 Epigastric discomfort, vomiting
   — Due to delayed gastric emptying
4 Tachypnea (primary respiratory alkalosis)
   — Due to direct respiratory center stimulation (→ adults)
5 Primary metabolic acidosis (→ children)
   — Due to multifactorial pathogenesis, incl. lactic acidosis
6 Prerenal failure
   — Due to dehydration, renal vasoconstriction
7 Hypo- or hyperglycemia
   Hypo- or hypernatremia

8 Pulmonary edema and/or hypokalemia
   — esp. If forced alkaline diuresis
9 Gastrointestinal bleeding
   — *Unusual* despite gastric irritation, platelet dysfunction and/or hypoprothrombinemia

CLINICAL PHARMACOKINETICS

Drugs exhibiting saturation kinetics
1 Phenytoin
2 Salicylate
3 Alcohol

Important clinical contexts for drug interaction
1 Where dose and response are critically balanced
   — Anticoagulants
   — Oral hypoglycemics
2 Where major toxicity may supervene
   — Cytotoxics
   — Digoxin
   — Theophylline
   — Aminoglycosides
   — Lithium
3 Where loss of effect may be catastrophic
   — Antiarrhythmics (e.g. quinidine)
   — Anticonvulsants (e.g. valproate)
   — Corticosteroids (e.g. in temporal arteritis)
   — Oral contraceptives
4 Where indications for interacting drugs may be similar
   — Digoxin and loop diuretics ($\downarrow$ K$^+$→ $\uparrow$ digoxin toxicity)
   — Digoxin and quinidine, amiodarone ($\uparrow$ plasma digoxin)
   — Captopril and potassium-sparing diuretics ($\uparrow\uparrow$ K$^+$)
   — β-blockers and acetazolamide (acidosis may → CCF)
   — β-blockers and clonidine ($\uparrow$ risk of clonidine 'rebound')
   — Cimetidine and antacids ($\downarrow$ cimetidine absorption)
   — Azathioprine/6MP + allopurinol (4-fold potentiation)
   — Ketoconazole + cyclosporin A ($\uparrow$ CSA nephrotoxicity)
   — Tranylcypromine + clomipramine (hypertensive crisis)

Drugs often prescribed in slow-release formulations
1 Theophylline
2 Lithium
3 Morphine
4 Carbamazepine
5 L-DOPA

PHARMACOKINETIC FACTORS IN ELDERLY PATIENTS

Physiologic alterations affecting drug metabolism in elderly
1 Impaired renal excretion
2 Impaired hepatic metabolism

3 Impaired (oral) drug absorption
   — e.g. Due to achlorhydria
4 Altered drug distribution
   — Cardiac failure, dehydration
   — $\uparrow$ Fat, $\downarrow$ lean body mass
   — $\uparrow$ α_1-acid glycoprotein, $\downarrow$ albumin

Considerations in prescribing specific drugs for elderly patients
1 Reduced renal clearance
   — e.g. Digoxin, lithium, cimetidine, chlorpropamide
2 Reduced hepatic metabolism
   — e.g. Tricyclics, chlormethiazole, propranolol
3 Reduced volume of distribution (V_D; for water-soluble drugs)
   — e.g. Ethanol, digoxin, cimetidine
4 Reduced sensitivity
   — e.g. Some antihypertensives
5 Increased sensitivity
   — e.g. Benzodiazepines, warfarin, some diuretics

DRUG TOXICITY

Approximate incidences of some adverse drug reactions
1 Retroperitoneal fibrosis due to methysergide
   — 1 in 250
2 Pseudomembranous colitis due to clindamycin
   — 1 in 5000
3 Aplastic anemia due to chloramphenicol
   — 1 in 6000
   Aplastic anemia due to phenylbutazone
   — 1 in 10,000
4 Thrombotic complications of oral contraceptives
   Hepatitis due to halothane
   Vaginal carcinoma due to maternal stilbestrol
   — 1 in 10,000

Iatrogenic causes of gingival hypertrophy
1 Phenytoin
2 Cyclosporin
3 Nifedipine

Iatrogenic causes of priapism
1 Antihypertensives (esp. α-blockers)
   — Labetalol, hydralazine, prazosin, guanethidine
2 Phenothiazines
   — Chlorpromazine, fluphenazine
3 Cocaine

Associations of Reye's syndrome*
1 Aspirin ingestion
2 Influenza B

* Acute hypoglycemia, liver infiltration, coma in children

VENOMS AND TOXINS

Some venoms and toxins of clinical significance
1 Botulinum toxin (p. 273)
   — Used in some neurologic disorders

2 Hirudin (from leeches)
— Anticlotting agent
3 Venoms used in coagulation testing
— Batroxobin ('Reptilase')
— 'Stypven' (detects lupus anticoagulant)

UNDERSTANDING DRUG THERAPY

CLINICAL PHARMACOLOGY

Pharmacokinetics: principles underlying clinical practice
1 For a given dosage, the plasma level of any drug is inversely proportional to its volume of distribution (V_D)
2 The *loading dose* of any drug is directly proportional to its V_D
The *maintenance dose* of any drug is directly proportional to its clearance
3 Drugs with low V_D (i.e. high concentration in plasma relative to tissues) tend to be heavily protein-bound
The lower the V_D of a given drug, the more readily it is removed by dialysis
4 The steady-state plasma level of any drug is achieved following regular administration for a period approximating 3–5 half-lives of the drug
5 Biliary excretion tends to be of minor pharmacokinetic significance; enterohepatic recirculation will occur until hepatic metabolism produces polar drug metabolites able to be renally excreted

Clinical significance of plasma protein binding
1 Drug interactions due to displacement from plasma protein binding sites tend to be transient and of minor clinical significance
2 Changes in protein binding may greatly affect assayed *total* plasma concentrations of drug
3 If assay for *free* drug not available, *salivary* concentrations of phenytoin, isoniazid or theophylline may be used
4 Protein-bound drug molecules do not undergo glomerular filtration
Ionized drug molecules may undergo active tubular secretion irrespective of plasma protein binding status
Non-ionized (non-polar, liposoluble) drugs undergo passive renal tubular reabsorption and then hepatic metabolism
5 Acidic drugs tend to be highly protein-bound

Examples of significant alterations in plasma protein binding
1 Precipitation of kernicterus by sulfonamides displacing bilirubin
2 Precipitation of mucositis by aspirin displacing methotrexate (hence increasing free methotrexate levels)
3 Precipitation of hypoglycemia by phenylbutazone displacing tolbutamide
4 Precipitation of hemorrhage by clofibrate displacing warfarin
5 Precipitation of phenytoin toxicity by uremia, hepatic failure or concomitant valproate administration

6 Antagonism of lignocaine/propranolol/disopyramide effect due to major increases in α-1 acid glycoprotein (an acute phase reactant elevated in burns, trauma, surgery, etc.)

CHARACTERISTICS OF DRUG STRUCTURE AND FUNCTION

Polar vs non-polar drugs: the clinical distinction
1 Polar (ionized, water-soluble) drugs typically exhibit
— Heavy plasma protein binding
— Low V_D
— Long plasma $t^{1/2}$
— Low CNS penetration and toxicity
— Acidic pK_a
— Predominant renal excretion (via active tubular secretion without glomerular filtration)
— Examples: warfarin, frusemide
2 Non-polar (un-ionized, lipophilic) drugs typically exhibit
— Little plasma protein binding
— Large V_D
— Short plasma $t^{1/2}$
— High CNS penetration and toxicity
— Basic pK_a
— Predominant hepatic metabolism (via glomerular filtration and passive renal tubular reabsorption)
— Examples: propranolol, nortriptyline

Acidic vs basic drugs
1 Acidic
— 'ates': salicylate, clofibrate, valproate, barbiturate
— 'ins': warfarin, phenytoin, penicillins, cephalosporins*
— 'ides': frusemide, thiazides, sulfonamides, chlorpropamide, probenecid, most NSAIDs‡
2 Basic
— 'ines': chlorpromazine, imipramine, nortriptyline, morphine, propoxyphene, quinidine, cimetidine¶
— 'ols': propranolol, ethambutol, dipyridamole
— Other: verapamil, trimethoprim, diazepam

* NB: *Prazosin* is basic
‡ NB: *Procainamide, disopyramide, amiloride* are basic
¶ NB: *Theophylline* is acidic

Drugs yielding active hepatic metabolites responsible for efficacy
1 Aspirin; phenacetin ($\rightarrow$ paracetamol); phenylbutazone
2 Carbamazepine; diazepam
3 Verapamil; enalapril; lignocaine; procainamide
4 Carbimazole ($\rightarrow$ methimazole)
5 Amitriptyline; imipramine; chloral hydrate; L-DOPA
6 Cyclophosphamide; azathioprine ($\rightarrow$ 6MP)
Prednisone ($\rightarrow$ prednisolone)

Drugs yielding hepatic metabolites responsible for toxicity
1 Isoniazid ($\rightarrow$ acetylhydrazine, esp. in fast acetylators)
2 Methanol ($\rightarrow$ formaldehyde)
3 Phenacetin ($\rightarrow$ paracetamol); allopurinol ($\rightarrow$ oxypurinol)

4 Clofibrate, procainamide
5 Cyclophosphamide (acrolein metabolites → bladder toxicity)
6 Alcohol (→ acetaldehyde)

Drugs excreted by the kidney
1 β-blockers — atenolol
2 Antibiotics — penicillins, cephalosporins, aminoglycosides, tetracycline
3 Diuretics — frusemide, chlorothiazide
4 Cardiac drugs — digoxin, procainamide
5 CNS drugs — lithium
6 Hypoglycemics — chlorpropamide, metformin
7 Analgesics — aspirin (in overdosage only)
8 Other — cimetidine, ranitidine

MECHANISMS OF DRUG ACTION

Enzymes inhibited by drug therapy
1 Xanthine oxidase — allopurinol
2 Na^+/K^+-ATPase (cardiac) — digoxin
Na^+/K^+-ATPase (loop of Henle) — frusemide
3 H^+/K^+-ATPase (gastric) — omeprazole
4 Angiotensin-converting enzyme (ACE) — captopril, enalapril
5 Prostaglandin synthetase — aspirin
6 Monoamine oxidase — phenelzine, moclobemide
7 Carbonic anhydrase — acetazolamide
8 DOPA decarboxylase — carbidopa
9 DNA topoisomerase II (human) — VP-16 (etoposide)
DNA topo II (bacterial) — nalidixic acid, ciprofloxacin
10 Acetylcholinesterase — neostigmine

Receptors involved in drug action
1 Endorphin receptors
— Agonist: morphine
— Antagonist: naloxone
2 Aldosterone receptors
— Antagonist: spironolactone
3 Histamine receptors
— H_1 antagonists: chlorpheniramine, terfenadine
— H_2 antagonists: cimetidine, ranitidine, famotidine
4 Dopamine (CNS) receptors
— Agonist: bromocriptine
— Antagonist: chlorpromazine
5 α_1-adrenergic (post-synaptic) receptors
— Antagonist: prazosin
6 α_2-adrenergic (brainstem) receptors
— Agonist: clonidine
7 β_1-adrenergic receptors
— Agonist: dopamine
— Antagonist: metoprolol, atenolol
8 β_2-adrenergic receptors
— Agonist: salbutamol

DRUG METABOLISM BY HEPATIC MICROSOMAL ENZYMES

Drugs commonly inhibiting cytochrome P_{450}
1 Alcohol
— Acute binge

2 Antibiotics
— Isoniazid
— Erythromycin
— Sulfonamides
— Metronidazole
— Chloramphenicol
3 Anticonvulsants
— Valproate
4 Other drugs
— Cimetidine
— Allopurinol
— Chlorpromazine, imipramine
— Propranolol, metoprolol
— Dextropropoxyphene
— Disulfiram

Drugs commonly inducing cytochrome P_{450}
1 Alcohol
— Chronic ingestion
2 Antibiotics
— Rifampicin
3 Anticonvulsants
— Phenytoin
— Carbamazepine
— Phenobarbitone, primidone
4 Other
— Aminoglutethimide
— Spironolactone
— Griseofulvin
— Cigarette smoking

Drugs undergoing major hepatic metabolism
1 β-blockers
— Propranolol, labetalol, metoprolol, oxprenolol
β_2-agonists
— Salbutamol, terbutaline
2 Antibiotics
— Rifampicin, erythromycin
3 Diuretics
— Spironolactone
4 Cardiac drugs
— Nitrates, verapamil, nifedipine, lignocaine, prazosin
5 CNS drugs
— Chlormethiazole, tricyclics, phenothiazines, benzodiazepines, barbiturates, L-DOPA
6 Oral hypoglycemics
— Glibenclamide, tolbutamide
7 Analgesics
— Paracetamol, pethidine, pentazocine, propoxyphene
— Aspirin

PROSTAGLANDINS

Physiological actions of prostaglandins
1 PGI_2 (prostacyclin), PGE_1 (→ ↑ intracellular cAMP)
— Prevents calcium influx
— Relaxes vascular smooth muscle (i.e. vasodilates)
— ↓ Platelet aggregation
2 PGE_2
— Mediates edema in inflammation

— Mediates frusemide effect: inhibits renal tubule ADH
— Induces bronchodilatation
3 PGE_{2a}
— Abortifacient
— Induces bronchoconstriction
4 TXA_2 (thromboxane A_2)
— Induces vasoconstriction (incl. pulmonary arterial)
— ↑ Platelet aggregation
— Implicated in primary pulmonary hypertension, respiratory distress syndrome and renal vasoconstriction with proteinuria

Drugs interacting with prostaglandins
1 Cyclooxygenase inhibitors
— Include aspirin and other NSAIDs
— Do *not* inhibit lipooxygenase; hence arachidonate metabolism is redirected away from prostaglandin synthesis and towards leukotriene synthesis (incl. the bronchoconstrictor SRS-A)
— Latter mechanism may → aspirin-induced asthma
2 Phospholipase A_2 inhibitors
— Include high-dose steroids, hydroxychloroquine
— Block both prostaglandin and leukotriene synthesis
3 Selective TXA_2 synthetase inhibitors
— e.g. Dazoxiben (remain investigational)

DRUGS AND THE REPRODUCTIVE SYSTEM

Drugs contraindicated in pregnant women
1 Alcohol, nicotine, narcotics
2 Antithyroid drugs (esp. ^{131}I); sulfonylureas
3 Drugs predisposing to kernicterus
— Sulfonamides
— Aspirin
— Vitamin K
4 Vasoactive drugs
— Ergotamine, propranolol (placental insufficiency)
— ACE inhibitors (→ fetal death)
— Guanethidine (meconium ileus)
5 Antibiotics
— Tetracyclines (dental staining, enamel hypoplasia)
— Chloramphenicol ('grey syndrome': cardiovascular collapse in newborns)
— Aminoglycosides (esp. streptomycin): deafness
— Sulfonamides (fetal abnormalities in first trimester; kernicterus in late pregnancy)

Recognized teratogens
1 Warfarin ('koala bear' facies)
2 Phenytoin (digital hypoplasia)
Valproate (spina bifida)
Phenobarbitone (cleft palate)

3 Lithium (congenital heart disease; cretinism)
4 Thalidomide (phocomelia)
5 Ergometrine (Poland anomaly)
6 Cytotoxics (esp. methotrexate, alkylators)
7 Steroid hormones (DES → vaginal carcinoma in adolescent female progeny; androgens, cardiac/esophageal defects; low-dose prednisone probably safe)
8 Alcohol (acetaldehyde metabolite → 'fetal alcohol syndrome')
9 Isotretinoin (13-cis-retinoic acid), etretinate High-dose vitamin D or vitamin A
10 Radioisotopes, esp. ^{131}I
Live vaccines

Drugs contraindicated in breastfeeding mothers
1 Antibiotics
— Chloramphenicol, clindamycin, tetracycline
2 Vitamins
— Etretinate, high-dose vitamin A or D
3 Analgesics/antiinflammatories
— Aspirin, indomethacin, gold salts, penicillamine
4 Other
— Lithium, doxepin
— Amiodarone
— Atropine
— Ergotamine

Relatively safe drugs in pregnancy
1 Digoxin
2 Heparin (does not cross placenta)*
3 Insulin, thyroxine
4 Antibiotics
— Penicillins
— Cephalosporins
— Erythromycin
— Ethambutol; INH (plus pyridoxine)
— Nystatin
5 Salbutamol (by inhaler)
6 Antihypertensives
— Methyldopa
— Hydralazine

* Heparin does not appear teratogenic, but is associated with increased antepartum hemorrhage, prematurity and stillbirth and may contribute to maternal and fetal bone demineralization

Influences on drug metabolism in pregnancy
1 ↑ Glomerular filtration rate
→ ↑ clearance of digoxin, lithium
2 ↑ Hepatic microsomal (P_{450}) enzyme activity
→ ↑ anticonvulsant metabolism
3 ↑ Volume of distribution (e.g. for flucloxacillin)
4 ↓ Plasma protein binding (e.g. aspirin, phenytoin)
5 ↓ Gastric emptying

REVIEWING THE LITERATURE: PHARMACOLOGY AND TOXICOLOGY

10.1 Rolan PE (1994) Plasma protein binding displacement reactions – why are they still regarded as clinically important? Br J Clin Pharmacol 37: 125–128

Review making the point that plasma protein binding displacement is rarely if ever clinically considerate. Perhaps the only exception is in therapeutic drug monitoring, where transient alterations in free drug availability may occur due to binding interactions, but these alterations are quickly corrected by metabolism and excretion.

10.2 Vanherweghem J et al (1993) Rapidly progressive interstitial renal fibrosis in young women: association with slimming regimen including Chinese herbs. Lancet 341: 387–391

Description of nine women undergoing herbal slimming regimen which culminated in disastrous nephrotoxicity requiring dialysis in two cases.

10.3 De Silva HJ et al (1992) Does pralidoxime affect outcome of management in acute organophosphorus poisoning? Lancet 339: 1136–1138

Unique randomized study of 45 organophosphorus-poisoned patients from Sri Lanka, showing that atropine alone was as effective as atropine plus pralidoxime.

10.4 Frezza M et al (1990) High blood alcohol levels in women: the role of decreased gastric alcohol dehydrogenase activity and first-pass metabolism. N Engl J Med 322: 95–99

Comparative study of 43 alcoholic and non-alcoholic men and women, showing that alcoholic women had decreased gastric oxidation of ethanol associated with markedly impaired first-pass metabolism; thus perhaps explaining the apparent greater susceptibility of women to alcoholic liver disease and other complications of alcohol abuse.

10.5 Suter PM et al (1992) The effect of ethanol on fat storage in healthy subjects. N Engl J Med 326: 983–987

Ethanol reduced lipid oxidation and increased energy expenditure. Hence, regular ethanol intake exceeding energy requirements makes you fat.

10.6 O'Grady J et al (1991) Liver transplantation after paracetamol overdose. Br Med J 303: 221–223

Four out of six 'poor-prognosis' patients transplanted survived, whereas only one out of eight left untransplanted did.

10.7 Hertzman PA et al (1990) Association of the eosinophilia-myalgia syndrome with the ingestion of tryptophan. N Engl J Med 322: 869–873

Silver RM et al (1990) Scleroderma, fasciitis and eosinophilia associated with the ingestion of tryptophan. N Engl J Med 322: 874–881

Two back-to-back papers reporting an association between a suspected contaminant in proprietary tryptophan medications and development of the notoriously controversial syndrome.

10.8 Culpepper RC et al (1991) Natural history of the eosinophilia-myalgia syndrome. Ann Int Med 115: 437–442

No benefit from steroids in this study.

10.9 LaCroix AZ et al (1990) Thiazide diuretic agents and the incidence of hip fracture. N Engl J Med 322: 286–290

Prospective study of 9518 over-65s, suggesting that thiazide drugs reduced the probability of fracture by a third over 4 years follow-up.

CHAPTER 11

Psychiatry

Physical examination protocol 11.1   You are told to begin by asking the patient a few questions

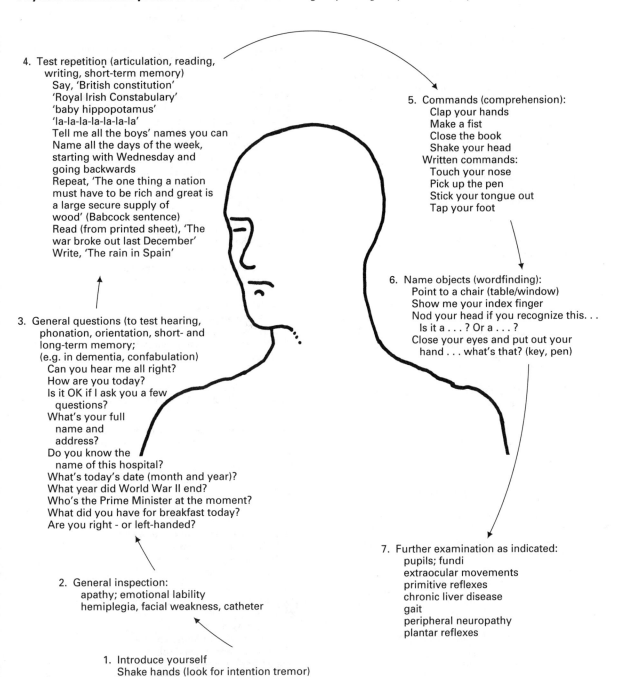

4. Test repetition (articulation, reading,
   writing, short-term memory)
   Say, 'British constitution'
   'Royal Irish Constabulary'
   'baby hippopotamus'
   'la-la-la-la-la-la-la'
   Tell me all the boys' names you can
   Name all the days of the week,
   starting with Wednesday and
   going backwards
   Repeat, 'The one thing a nation
   must have to be rich and great is
   a large secure supply of
   wood' (Babcock sentence)
   Read (from printed sheet), 'The
   war broke out last December'
   Write, 'The rain in Spain'

5. Commands (comprehension):
   Clap your hands
   Make a fist
   Close the book
   Shake your head
   Written commands:
   Touch your nose
   Pick up the pen
   Stick your tongue out
   Tap your foot

6. Name objects (wordfinding):
   Point to a chair (table/window)
   Show me your index finger
   Nod your head if you recognize this. . .
   Is it a . . . ? Or a . . . ?
   Close your eyes and put out your
   hand . . . what's that? (key, pen)

3. General questions (to test hearing,
   phonation, orientation, short- and
   long-term memory;
   (e.g. in dementia, confabulation)
   Can you hear me all right?
   How are you today?
   Is it OK if I ask you a few
   questions?
   What's your full
   name and
   address?
   Do you know the
   name of this hospital?
   What's today's date (month and year)?
   What year did World War II end?
   Who's the Prime Minister at the moment?
   What did you have for breakfast today?
   Are you right - or left-handed?

7. Further examination as indicated:
   pupils; fundi
   extraocular movements
   primitive reflexes
   chronic liver disease
   gait
   peripheral neuropathy
   plantar reflexes

2. General inspection:
   apathy; emotional lability
   hemiplegia, facial weakness, catheter

1. Introduce yourself
   Shake hands (look for intention tremor)

CLINICAL ASPECTS OF PSYCHIATRIC DISORDERS

Commonest psychiatric short cases
1 Wernicke–Korsakoff (alcohol amnesia) syndrome
2 Tardive dyskinesia

HIGHER CEREBRAL DYSFUNCTION

Common presentations of organic brain syndromes
1 Impaired consciousness (esp. acute pathologies)
2 Impaired short-term memory (esp. chronic pathologies)
3 Disorientation
4 Disinhibition
5 Visual hallucinations

Signs favoring organic (rather than affective) psychosis
1 Positive suck/pout reflex
2 Positive palmar-mental reflex
3 Positive (tonic) grasp reflex

Psychiatric disease with thyroid dysfunction?
1 Hypothyroidism*
   — Depression
   — (Pseudo)dementia
   — Coma
2 Thyrotoxicosis
   — Delirium

* May arise *secondary* to lithium therapy of MDP; alternatively, 'rapid-cycling' MDP patients often develop hypothyroidism which deteriorates symptomatically with antidepressants; carbamazepine or T_4 may be useful

Psychiatric presentations of Parkinson's disease
1 Frontal-subcortical cognitive dysfunction (affects 70%)
   — May improve with levodopa
2 Frank dementia (affects 10%)*
   — Secondary (reversible) causes require exclusion
3 Depression
   — May be prevented by good control of motor symptoms
   — Alternatively, may *mask* motor benefit of levodopa
   — Tricyclics, ECT may improve mood *and* motor function
4 Psychosis (usually drug-induced)
   — Withdraw anticholinergics
   — Reduce dose of levodopa, bromocriptine

* NB: Alzheimer's patients develop parkinsonism in about 60%

Common causes of confusion in elderly patients
1 Hypoxemia (any cause)
2 Sepsis (e.g. UTI, pneumonia)
3 Depression
4 Drugs (e.g. digoxin, indomethacin, cimetidine, L-DOPA)
5 Dementia (diagnosis of exclusion)

DEMENTIA

Prerequisites for the diagnosis of dementia
1 Acquired memory defect
2 Associated non-memory cognitive defect* interfering with normal social or work abilities, e.g.
   — Dysphasia
   — Visuospatial impairment
3 Arousal state normal

* Severity of cognitive impairment tends to be *underestimated* (or not recognized at all: anosognosia) by demented patients, unlike in depression

Differential diagnosis of dementia in the AIDS patient*
1 Primary cerebral HIV infection
   → Basal ganglia; tends to spare cortex
2 Secondary cerebral infection
   — Cerebral toxoplasmosis or cryptococcosis
   — Herpes simplex encephalitis
   — JC virus (progressive multifocal leukoencephalopathy)
3 Cerebral neoplasm
   — Cerebral lymphoma
   — Cerebral Kaposi's

* Affects 50% of patients dying with AIDS

Disorders causing dementia and gait disturbance
1 Normal pressure hydrocephalus
2 Vascular
   — Multiinfarct dementia/pseudobulbar palsy
   — Binswanger's encephalopathy
3 Parkinson's disease
4 Progressive supranuclear palsy (Richardson–Steele syndrome)

NORMAL PRESSURE HYDROCEPHALUS

Clinical features of normal pressure hydrocephalus
1 Gait apraxia (most consistent feature; absent in Alzheimer's)
2 Dementia
3 Incontinence (usually a late feature)
4 Signs: extensor plantar responses, suck/grasp reflexes

Predispositions to normal pressure hydrocephalus
1 Subarachnoid hemorrhage
2 Meningitis, esp. if chronic
3 Paget's disease

Diagnostic confirmation of normal pressure hydrocephalus
1 CT brainscan
   — Marked ventricular enlargement
   — Minimal cortical atrophy
2 Lumbar puncture
   — Symptomatic improvement after CSF sampling
   — Pressure monitoring: intermittent high-pressure waves
3 Clinical response to ventricular shunting

ALZHEIMER'S DISEASE

Clinical significance of Alzheimer's disease
1 Accounts for up to 75% of dementias
2 Responsible for up to 50% of nursing home admissions

Clinical features of Alzheimer's disease
1 Early stage
   — Mild memory impairment
   — Anomia
   — Impaired calculation
   — Reduced insight and judgement
   — EEG and PET scan often abnormal
2 Intermediate stage
   — Severe amnesia
   — Agitation
   — Impaired language function
   — Delusions
3 Advanced stage
   — Mute
   — Bedfast
   — Extrapyramidal deficit
   — CT: cerebral atrophy
   — EEG: frank slowing

Features suggesting dementias other than Alzheimer's
1 *Sudden* onset
2 *Early* onset of
   — Gait disturbance
   — Seizures
3 *Focal* neurologic signs

Key disorders to exclude prior to diagnosing Alzheimer's*
1 Depression
2 Drug toxicity
   — Alcohol, sedatives
   — L-DOPA
   — Antihypertensives

* NB: Definitive diagnosis is only possible by brain biopsy (which is rarely indicated; hence, this is a clinical diagnosis)

AFFECTIVE DISORDERS

Potentially misleading presentations of depression
1 Anorexia, weight loss
2 Fatigue
3 Constipation
4 Loss of libido
5 Amenorrhea
6 Sleep disturbance

Features of seasonal affective disorder (SAD)
1 Winter
   — Hypersomnia, fatigue*
   — Increased appetite (esp. carbohydrate craving)
2 Summer
   — Well (unipolar SAD)
   — Mania or hypomania (bipolar SAD)

* May improve with bright morning light (phototherapy) during winter

Differential diagnosis of hypersexuality
1 Manic phase of manic-depressive psychosis (MDP)
2 Huntington's chorea
3 Kleine–Levin syndrome

ALCOHOLISM

Confusion in the alcoholic patient: differential diagnosis
1 Acute intoxication
2 Delirium tremens (48–72 h post-withdrawal)
3 Hypoglycemia (6–36 h post-binge)
4 Head injury → subdural hematoma
5 Post-ictal
6 Wernicke–Korsakoff syndrome
7 Ketoacidosis or lactic acidosis
8 Hepatic encephalopathy
9 Sepsis (e.g. *Klebsiella* pneumonia, aspiration pneumonia)
10 Unusual neurological syndromes
   — Central pontine myelinolysis
   — Marchiafava–Bignami disease*

* Callosal demyelination; rarely diagnosed premortem

Neuropsychiatric manifestations of alcoholism
1 Epilepsy; may complicate
   — Acute alcohol intoxication
   — Chronic heavy alcohol ingestion
   — Alcohol withdrawal
   — Subdural hematoma
2 Withdrawal-related
   — Tremulousness
   — Agitation
   — Delirium tremens
3 Toxic neuronal degeneration
   — Cerebral atrophy ± dementia
   — Cerebral atrophy
   — Central pontine myelinolysis (typically precipitated by use of hypertonic saline or lactulose)
   — Callosal demyelination (Marchiafava–Bignami)
4 Nutrition-related (hypovitaminemic)
   — Wernicke's encephalopathy
   — Korsakoff's psychosis
   — Pellagra
   — Neuropathy (typically painful)
   — 'Tobacco-alcohol' amblyopia

The confused alcoholic: DTs rather than encephalopathy?
1 Severe agitation
2 Gross tremulousness without asterixis
3 Autonomic overactivity (sweats, fever, miosis, ↑ HR/BP)
4 Visual hallucinations
5 EEG: *no* triphasic waves
6 Improvement with sedation*

* NB: This is *not* a diagnostic test

Features of Korsakoff's (alcohol amnesia) syndrome
1 Loss of past memories
2 Inability to form new memories

3 Loss of insight
4 Confabulation*
5 Apathy
6 Limited response to thiamine‡

* *Not* invariable; may disappear with disease progression. 'Provoked' confabulation may also occur in Alzheimer's and other dementias
‡ cf. Wernicke's; Korsakoffian neuropathology tends to be far more severe, hence only 25% respond completely (50% partial)

ANXIETY STATES

Differential diagnosis of recurrent acute anxiety attacks
1 Anxiety neurosis
2 Agoraphobia
3 Hyperventilation syndrome
4 Thyrotoxicosis
5 Pheochromocytoma
6 Drug withdrawal (incl. alcohol)

Presentations of functional anxiety states
1 Panic attacks: sweating, palpitations
  Headaches
  — May simulate
    • Pheochromocytoma
    • Insulinoma
2 Presyncopal episodes, visual disturbance
  Paresthesiae, tetany
  — May simulate
    • Epilepsy
    • TIAs
3 Fatigue, breathlessness, tremulousness
  Atypical chest pain
  — May mimic
    • Thyrotoxicosis
    • Pulmonary emboli
    • Mitral valve prolapse
4 Poor concentration
  Sleep disturbance
  — May simulate
    • Intracranial tumor
    • Sleep apnea
    • Hepatic failure
5 Feelings of unreality; fear of madness
  Difficulty swallowing
  — May simulate
    • Schizophrenia
    • Hysteria
    • Aerophagy
    • Agoraphobia

Diagnosis of hyperventilation syndrome
1 High index of suspicion
2 Relief of symptoms following use of rebreathing bag
3 Reproduction of symptoms by forced voluntary overbreathing (best test)

NB: Measuring the $PaCO_2$ during an attack is *not* a reliable test

'Funny turns': features favoring epilepsy
1 Clouding of consciousness
2 Prodromal irritability; premonitory stereotyped 'aura'

3 *Witnessed* absence or transiently impaired consciousness
  Regular, stereotyped tonic-clonic activity
  Tongue-bite, cyanosis or incontinence
4 Post-ictal paresis or confusion but *no* retrograde amnesia*
5 Abnormal EEG during attack

* cf. hysterical fugue

HYSTERIA

Clinical spectrum of somatoform disorders
1 Hysteria
2 Psychogenic pain
3 Hypochondriasis
4 Münchausen's syndrome
5 Dermatitis artefacta
6 Compensation neurosis

Manifestations of hysteria
1 Conversion or dissociative symptoms, e.g.
  — Paralysis
  — Pseudoseizures
  — Sensory disturbance
  — Abnormal gait
2 Symptoms associated with
  — *Belle indifference*
  — Secondary gain
3 Briquet's (familial) syndrome
  — Multiple recurrent somatic complaints
4 Ganser syndrome
  — Amnesia, pseudodementia
  — Fugue state, hallucinations
  — Absurd answers, abrupt termination
5 Multiple personality
6 Mass hysteria

ANOREXIA NERVOSA

Physical findings in the patient with anorexia nervosa
1 Vital signs
  — Bradycardia
  — Hypotension
  — Hypothermia
2 Musculoskeletal
  — Marked weight loss
  — Myopathy (nutritional)
  — Weakness (hypokalemic)
3 Cardiovascular
  — Pallor (normochromic anemia)
  — Peripheral cyanosis
  — Arrhythmias
4 Skin
  — Carotenemia
  — Excessive lanugo hair
  — Edema (secondary hyperaldosteronism)
5 Gastrointestinal
  — Parotidomegaly
  — Rectal prolapse
6 Hypothermia

NB: Secondary sexual development is *normal* in anorexia nervosa

Investigating anorexia nervosa: potential abnormalities
1 Elevated plasma urea
2 Abnormal LFTs
3 'Sick euthyroid' (p. 98)
4 Elevated growth hormone, reduced somatomedin C
5 Multifollicular cystic ovaries on pelvic ultrasound

Complications of anorexia nervosa other than amenorrhea
1 Dental caries
2 Gastric dilatation or atrophy
3 Constipation, cathartic colon
4 Renal calculi
5 Osteoporosis

INVESTIGATING PSYCHIATRIC DISORDERS

INVESTIGATION OF DEMENTIA

Investigation of the patient with presenile dementia
1 Looking to exclude reversible etiologies
   — CT brainscan (see below)
   — Thyroid function tests/TSH
   — Vitamin B_{12} assay
   — VDRL
2 HIV serology (in 'at-risk' patients)

Prerequisites for CT scanning in dementia
1 Presenile onset
2 Less than 2 years' duration
3 Mild to moderate in severity
4 Patient fit for neurosurgery if indicated

Reversible pathologies excluded by CT scanning
1 Space-occupying intracerebral lesion (tumor, abscess)
2 Subdural hematoma
3 Normal pressure hydrocephalus

NB: *Unilateral* cerebral abnormalities usually do not affect conscious state

THE ABNORMAL BRAIN BIOPSY

Definitive histological confirmation of Alzheimer's disease
1 Cerebral amyloid (A4) angiopathy, *plus*
2 Neuritic β-amyloid plaques*, *and/or*
3 Neurofibrillary tangles*

* Correlate quantitatively with dementia severity

Dementia: neurofibrillary tangles in autopsied brain?
1 Alzheimer's disease
2 Post-encephalitic parkinsonism*
3 Dementia pugilistica ('punch-drunk' syndrome)
4 Creutzfeldt–Jakob disease
5 SSPE

* cf. sporadic Parkinson's disease → Lewy bodies

MANAGING PSYCHIATRIC DISEASE

IATROGENIC ORGANIC BRAIN SYNDROMES

Drugs commonly causing confusion in the elderly
1 Digoxin (may also → fatigue, euphoria)
2 Propranolol (also → nightmares, insomnia); methyldopa
3 Indomethacin (also → vertigo, headache)
4 Cimetidine (esp. in renal or hepatic insufficiency)
5 Amantadine, L-DOPA (esp. if used with anticholinergics)
6 Sedative-hypnotics, tricyclics, phenothiazines; alcohol

Psychiatric side-effects of steroid therapy
1 Commoner in
   — High-dose treatment
   — Prolonged duration of treatment
   — Patient with psychiatric history
2 Commonest symptom
   — Euphoria*
3 Frank psychosis
   — Affects about 5%

* cf. primary Cushing's disease → depression

TACRINE

Rationâle for tacrine* in Alzheimer's disease
1 Tacrine is a non-competitive acetylcholinesterase inhibitor active in the CNS
2 Prolongs CNS cholinergic activity, thus reversing one of the key neurotransmitter defects in Alzheimer's (p. 300)
3 High-dose effects on Na^+/K^+ channel blockade, muscarinic agonism and alteration of MAO metabolism are probably not clinically relevant

* Tetrahydro-9-acridinamine-monohydrochloride

Limitations of tacrine therapy for Alzheimer's disease
1 Side-effects
   — Hepatotoxicity*
   — Nausea, diarrhea
2 Efficacy
   — Cognitive benefits are mild
   — Course of disease is unchanged

* Must monitor ALT; withdraw drug if ALT > 3 x normal

ANTIPSYCHOTIC DRUG THERAPY

Clinical spectrum of lithium toxicity (level > 1.5 mmol/L)*
1 CNS toxicity
   — Lethargy → drowsiness → seizures → coma
2 Gastrointestinal toxicity
   — Nausea, vomiting, diarrhea
3 Cerebellar toxicity
   — Tremulousness; dysarthria; ataxia

4 Renal toxicity
— Polyuria, polydipsia (nephrogenic diabetes insipidus)
— Affects 30% but usually subclinical; may → renal failure
5 Thyroid toxicity
— Goiter, hypothyroidism
6 Cardiovascular
— ECG → T wave flattening/inversion
— Cardiovascular collapse in massive overdose

* Lower plasma levels may cause toxicity, esp. in *sodium-depleted* patients (e.g. on diuretics) or in *dehydration* due to vomiting, diarrhea or polyuria

Drug classes used to treat endogenous depression
1 Tricyclic antidepressants
— e.g. Protriptyline, lofepramine
2 Tetracyclic antidepressants
— e.g. Mianserin
3 Selective serotonin reuptake inhibitors (SSRIs)
— e.g. Fluoxetine (Prozac™), paroxetine
4 Monoamine uptake inhibitors (MAOIs)
— e.g. Phenelzine, moclobemide

Clinical pharmacology of mianserin
1 Tetracyclic structure bears no similarity to tricyclics
2 Fewer arrhythmogenic and anticholinergic side-effects
3 Safer in overdose: an advantage in treating suicidal patients
4 Agranulocytosis (1:5000) and aplasia limit enthusiasm

MONOAMINE OXIDASE INHIBITORS

Pharmacologic classification of MAOIs
1 Irreversible MAOIs
— Phenelzine, tranylcypromine (antidepressants)
— Isoniazid
2 Selective MAO-B inhibitors
— Selegiline
3 Reversible (and selective) MAO-A inhibitors
— Moclobemide, toloxatone, clorgyline

Important interactions with MAOIs
1 (Tyr)amine-rich foods (flavor often enhanced by age)
— Mature cheese
— Yeast extracts (e.g. Marmite, packet soups)
— Soya bean, broad bean pods
— Pickled herring
— Alcoholic (or dealcoholized) drinks, esp. red wine
2 Drugs
— Pethidine (may be lethal)
— Tricyclics, levodopa, terbutaline
— Amine-containing drugs, esp. cold remedies*
— SSRIs (e.g. fluoxetine‡; see below)

* Contain (pseudo)ephedrine, phenylpropanolamine
‡ cf. Paroxetine: short half-life, hence can start MAOI after 2 weeks

Life-threatening MAOI interactions
1 Pseudopheochromocytoma
— Seen with SSRIs *or* drugs listed above

— Noradrenaline-mediated paroxysmal hypertension
— Other symptoms: confusion, sweating, abdominal pain
2 Serotonin syndrome (see below)
— Seen with SSRIs *or* serotoninergic tricyclics*
— Consists of CNS irritability, seizures, myoclonus
3 Management implications of these interactions
— Lethal combination; SSRIs must *never* be co-prescribed, even when 'selective' MAOIs used
— Cease MAOI ≥ 2 weeks before starting SSRI
— Cease fluoxetine ≥ 5 weeks before starting MAOI

* e.g. clomipramine, amitriptyline

Management of MAOI-induced hypertensive crisis
1 IV phentolamine 5–10 mg
2 IV chlorpromazine 25 mg

SELECTIVE SEROTONIN REUPTAKE INHIBITORS (SSRIs)

Advantages of SSRIs (e.g. fluoxetine) over tricyclic antidepressants
1 Less muscarinic receptor blockade
— Fewer anticholinergic side-effects
2 No membrane-stabilizing effects on the heart
— Fewer arrhythmias, lower suicide risk (i.e. safer)
3 Less sedation
4 Less weight gain
5 Effective for obsessive-compulsive symptoms

Side-effects of SSRIs
1 CNS hyperstimulation
— Insomnia, 'nervy' sensation, tremor, headache
— ?Aggressive behavior, ?precipitation of mania
2 Gastrointestinal toxicity (more so than tricyclics)
— Weight loss*
— Nausea, diarrhea, abdominal discomfort
3 Sexual problems
— Reduced libido
— Delayed ejaculation
4 General malaise ± cognitive impairment
5 Sweating
6 Hyponatremia

* Or, less often, weight gain

Major drug interactions with SSRIs
1 SSRI potentiation (esp. CNS excitation)
— MAOIs
— Lithium
— Selegiline*
— Sumatriptan
2 Potentiation of interacting drug
— Tricyclics (cardiotoxicity)
— Warfarin (hemorrhage)

* esp. if using fluoxetine

ANTISCHIZOPHRENIC DRUG THERAPY

Drugs used in schizophrenia
1 Conventional strategies
   — Dopamine-blocking neuroleptics
     • Phenothiazines (e.g. chlorpromazine)
     • Butyrophenones (e.g. haloperidol)
2 Refractory cases ('atypical' neuroleptics)
   — Clozapine‡
     • 5-HT$_2$ receptor blocker
     • Minimal if any extrapyramidal toxicity
     • Lowest risk for tardive dyskinesias
     • Agranulocytosis occurs in 0.5% (i.e. *a lot*), hence must monitor blood count weekly
     • Dose-dependent seizure induction
   — Risperidone
     • Catecholamine*/5-HT$_2$ receptor blocker
     • Low incidence of extrapyramidal toxicity
     • Minimal sedation (cf. clozapine)
   — Sulpiride
     • Less sedation and extrapyramidal toxicity
     • Good for apathetic patients
     • May cause major increase in prolactin levels

* incl. dopamine D$_2$ receptors
‡ Effective in 30–60% of cases refractory to conventional neuroleptics

NEUROLEPTIC SIDE-EFFECTS

Distinguishing features of drug-induced movement disorders
1 Neuroleptic-induced pseudoparkinsonism
   — Usually appears after several months therapy
   — Commoner in high dosage and in *elderly* patients, esp. if demented
   — May remit with continued treatment, respond to conventional antiparkinsonian therapy or persist despite total drug withdrawal
   — May be indistinguishable from Parkinson's disease
   — Occurs in 20–30% of treated patients
   — Treat with anticholinergics
2 Neuroleptic-induced acute dystonic reactions
   — Usually occur within 24 h of (usually initial) dosage; occasionally precipitated by drug withdrawal
   — May be due to metoclopramide*
   — Commoner in *men* than women, *young* > old
   — Occur within 48 h of administration; duration variable
   — May be preceded by akathisia, grimacing, hyperreflexia
   — May → oculogyric crisis, opisthotonus, trismus/torticollis
   — Responsive to IV benztropine, diphenhydramine
   — Affect approximately 2% of treated patients
3 Neuroleptic-induced tardive dyskinesia
   — Insidious onset; may be unmasked after dose reduction
   — Affects 30% after 4 years' therapy‡
   — Commoner in *women* than men, *elderly* > young

   — Probably reflects dopamine receptor hyper-sensitivity
   — *No* subjective patient distress; disappears during sleep
   — 40% remit after drug ceased; 60% persist or worsen
   — Treat with tetrabenazine (also used in Huntington's)
   — Continued treatment with offending drug does *not* increase severity of dyskinesia, but *does* reduce likelihood of remission (disorder not progressive)

* cf. *rarely* causes parkinsonism or tardive dyskinesia; avoid in children
‡ But *may* occur as early as 3 months

Neuroleptic drug toxicity: major associations
1 Sedation
   — Chlorpromazine, clozapine, thioridazine
2 Hypotension
   — Chlorpromazine, clozapine
3 Extrapyramidal effects
   — Haloperidol, fluphenazine, trifluoperazine
4 Anticholinergic effects
   — Clozapine, thioridazine

Clinical features of tardive dyskinesia
1 Orofacial dyskinesia: hyperkinesis of cheeks/tongue/mouth
   — 'Fly-catcher's tongue'
   — 'Bon-bon' sign
   — Rumination, pouting
2 Glottal dyskinesia
   — Grunting
3 Blepharospasm, increased blink frequency
4 Torticollis
5 Upper limbs
   — 'Piano-playing' fingers
   — Choreiform or ballistic movements
   — Shoulder shrugging
6 Lower limbs
   — Foot-tapping
   — Great toe dorsiflexion

Differential diagnosis of tardive dyskinesia
1 Huntington's disease
  Wilson's disease
   — Patients may be receiving phenothiazines for psychiatric disorder, but develop extrapyramidal symptoms de novo
2 Tourette's syndrome
   — Grimacing and profanities in children
   — Important to diagnose, since treatable with haloperidol

Features of neuroleptic malignant syndrome*
1 Clinical signs
   — Fever
   — Rigidity
   — Autonomic dysfunction
     • Fluctuations of heart rate, blood pressure
     • Sphincter disturbance
     • Sweating, salivation
   — Clouding of consciousness

2 Diagnosis
— Elevated plasma CPK ± renal failure (p. 305)
— Leukocytosis
3 Therapy
— Dantrolene
— Bromocriptine
4 Outcome
— Up to 50% die

* = malignant hyperthermia (p. 234)

DRUGS USED IN ALCOHOLISM

Drugs used to control alcohol withdrawal symptoms
1 Benzodiazepines
2 β-blockers
3 Chlormethiazole

Drugs used to promote alcohol abstinence
1 Disulfiram (an aldehyde dehydrogenase inhibitor)
2 Acamprosate* (a GABA agonist)
3 Citalopram (an SSRI)

* calcium acetyl homotaurinate

CANNABINOIDS

Side-effects of cannabis use
1 Anxiety, panic
Paranoia, visual hallucinations
Predisposition to schizophrenia in chronic users
2 Tachycardia
Supine hypertension with postural hypotension
3 Bronchitis, emphysema
4 'Amotivational syndrome'

Potential therapeutic scenarios for cannabinoid use
1 Nausea (e.g. prior to cancer chemotherapy)
2 Glaucoma
3 Spasticity

ELECTROCONVULSIVE THERAPY (ECT)

Indications for ECT
1 Severe depression in patients resistant to tri-/
tetracyclics
2 Severe depression complicated by dehydration or
weight loss
3 Depression associated with suicidal ideation or
delusions
4 Drug-resistant mania
5 Puerperal psychosis (treatment of choice)

Contraindications to ECT
1 Increased intracranial pressure
2 Known cerebral aneurysm
3 Past history of
— Cerebrovascular disease
— Myocardial infarction
— Aortic aneurysm
4 Unfit for general anesthesia

PSYCHOSURGERY

Potential indications for psychosurgery
1 Cingulotomy
— Refractory incapacitating obsessional neurosis
2 Ventromedial frontal lobe surgery
— No longer used for schizophrenia
— Occasionally still used for severe refractory
depression
3 Temporal lobectomy, callosal sectioning,
commissurotomy
— Drug-resistant epilepsy

UNDERSTANDING PSYCHIATRIC DISEASE

Spectrum of self-inflicted diseases
1 Münchausen syndrome
2 Diuretic and/or laxative abuse*
3 Factitious fever
4 Factitious hypoglycemia
5 Thyrotoxicosis factitia
6 Dermatitis artefacta

* Results in symptomatic hypokalemia, nephropathy

NEUROTRANSMITTER ABNORMALITIES

Neurotransmitter abnormalities in schizophrenia
1 ↓ Somatostatin ⎫
2 ↓ CCK   ⎬ — In the hippocampus

Neurotransmitter abnormalities in Huntington's chorea
1 Preservation of *aspiny* neurons in caudate
— ↑ Somatostatin
— ↑ Dopamine
2 Depletion of striatal *spiny* neurons
— ↓ GABA
— ↓ Substance P
— ↓ Metenkephalin
— ↓ Acetylcholine

Neurotransmitter abnormalities in Alzheimer's disease
1 ↓ Acetylcholine (neuronal degeneration in nucleus
basalis)
2 ↓ Somatostatin (cortical degeneration of *aspiny*
neurons)
3 ↓ Noradrenaline (neuronal degeneration in locus
ceruleus)
4 ↓ Dopamine (neuronal degeneration in ventral
tegmentum)
5 ↓ Serotonin (degeneration of raphe nucleus)

SPONGIFORM ENCEPHALOPATHIES

Classification of spongiform encephalopathies
1 In animals
— Scrapie
— Bovine spongiform encephalopathy

2 In humans
— Kuru
— Creutzfeldt–Jakob disease (CJD)

Pathogenesis of human spongiform encephalo-pathies
1 Kuru
— Only ever described in one New Guinea tribe
— Speculatively linked to cannibalism (i.e. said to be orally transmissible), but this could also be explained by sporadic introduction of CJD
2 Creutzfeldt–Jakob disease
— Not orally transmitted
— Vectors include pituitary extracts, corneal grafts, contaminated brain electrodes
— Corresponding familial (Gerstmann–Sträussler–Schenker) syndrome is due to mutation affecting a protease-resistant glycoprotein (*prion protein*)

REVIEWING THE LITERATURE: PSYCHIATRY

11.1 Suddath RL et al (1990) Anatomical abnormalities in the brains of monozygotic twins discordant for schizophrenia. N Engl J Med 322: 789–794

MRI study of 15 pairs of identical twins discordant for schizophrenia, in which small anterior hippocampi and enlarged lateral/third ventricles were found associated with schizophrenia.

11.2 Jobst KA et al (1992) Detection in life of confirmed Alzheimer's disease using a simple measurement of medial temporal lobe atrophy by computed tomography. Lancet 340: 1179–1183

Controversial study of 44 patients with biopsy-proven Alzheimer's, suggesting a narrowing of the medial temporal lobe in affected patients – thus raising the possibility that neuroradiology may provide non-invasive diagnostic info.

11.3 Eagger SA et al (1991) Tacrine in Alzheimer's disease. Lancet 337: 989–992

Randomized placebo-controlled study of 89 Alzheimer patients, 19 of whom were withdrawn due to toxicity. A mild relative cognitive benefit – equivalent to the deterioration normally expected over 6–12 months – was apparent in the tacrine-treated cohort.

11.4 Davis KL et al (1992) A double-blind, placebo-controlled multicenter study of tacrine for Alzheimer's disease. N Engl J Med 327: 1253–1259

Six-week study of 215 patients, showing a reduction in the rate of cognitive decline, albeit not reaching conventional levels of statistical significance.

11.5 Tonnesen H et al (1992) Postoperative morbidity among symptom-free alcohol misusers. Lancet 340: 334–337

Comparative study of 15 heavy drinkers (> 60 g alcohol/day) undergoing colorectal surgery; compared with a control group, the rate of post-operative complications was increased more than 3-fold, while length of hospital stay was almost doubled.

11.6 Walsh DC et al (1991) A randomized trial of treatment options for alcohol-abusing workers. N Engl J Med 325: 775–782

Inpatient treatment was significantly more effective than AA attendance in this randomized study of 227 working alcoholics.

11.7 Godfrey P et al (1990) Enhancement of recovery from psychiatric illness by methylfolate. Lancet 336: 392–395

Interesting study suggesting that CNS methylation abnormalities may be linked to mental illness.

11.8 Landay AL et al (1991) Chronic fatigue syndrome: clinical condition associated with immune activation. Lancet 338: 707–712

One of many conflicting and inconclusive studies searching for an organic basis for chronic fatigue syndrome.

CHAPTER 12

Renal medicine

Physical examination protocol 12.1   You are asked to examine a patient for signs of renal disease

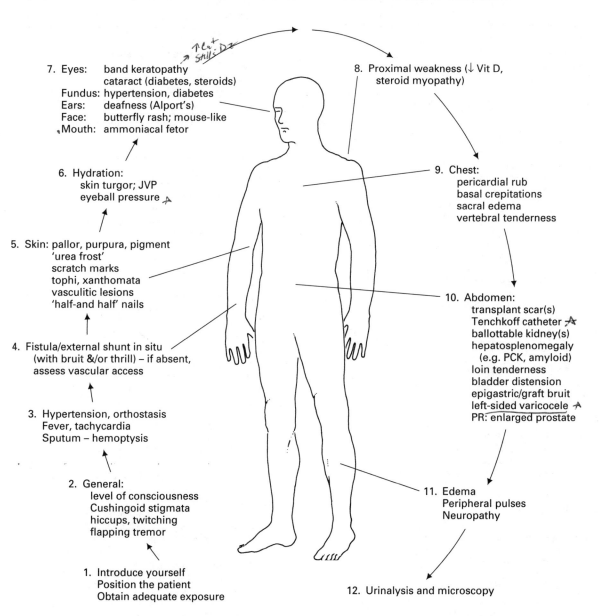

7. Eyes: band keratopathy
          cataract (diabetes, steroids)
   Fundus: hypertension, diabetes
   Ears: deafness (Alport's)
   Face: butterfly rash; mouse-like
   Mouth: ammoniacal fetor

6. Hydration:
      skin turgor; JVP
      eyeball pressure

5. Skin: pallor, purpura, pigment
         'urea frost'
         scratch marks
         tophi, xanthomata
         vasculitic lesions
         'half-and half' nails

4. Fistula/external shunt in situ
   (with bruit &/or thrill) – if absent,
   assess vascular access

3. Hypertension, orthostasis
   Fever, tachycardia
   Sputum – hemoptysis

2. General:
      level of consciousness
      Cushingoid stigmata
      hiccups, twitching
      flapping tremor

1. Introduce yourself
   Position the patient
   Obtain adequate exposure

8. Proximal weakness (↓ Vit D,
   steroid myopathy)

9. Chest:
      pericardial rub
      basal crepitations
      sacral edema
      vertebral tenderness

10. Abdomen:
       transplant scar(s)
       Tenchkoff catheter
       ballottable kidney(s)
       hepatosplenomegaly
          (e.g. PCK, amyloid)
       loin tenderness
       bladder distension
       epigastric/graft bruit
       left-sided varicocele
       PR: enlarged prostate

11. Edema
    Peripheral pulses
    Neuropathy

12. Urinalysis and microscopy

CLINICAL ASPECTS OF RENAL DISEASE

Commonest renal short cases
1 Polycystic kidneys
2 Renal transplant (± cushingoid)

The abdominal mass: why do you think it's a kidney?
1 Able to get above it
2 Moves little with respiration
3 Bimanually ballottable
4 Resonant on percussing above

Clinical assessment of hydration status
1 Vital signs
— Heart rate, blood pressure
— Marked orthostatic response if dehydrated
2 Weight loss
— Mildly dehydrated: < 3%
— Profoundly dehydrated: > 10%
3 Skin turgor/elasticity
— Test over tibiae, scapulae, sternum
— Reduction implies at least moderate dehydration
Eyeball pressure
4 CNS signs
— Confusion (may reflect severe dehydration)
5 Urine output
— Less than 30 mL/h suggests hypovolemia
6 Signs of fluid overload
— Tachycardia, tachypnea
— Elevated JVP
— S_3, gallop
— Aortic incompetent murmur (e.g. if dialysis overdue)
— Pulmonary and/or peripheral edema

RENAL FAILURE

Features indicating chronicity of renal failure
1 Band keratopathy
2 Peripheral neuropathy
3 Bilaterally shrunken kidneys on plain abdominal film or IVP
4 CXR: annular calcification of mitral/aortic valve(s)
5 Renal osteodystrophy on X-ray and biopsy

Potentially reversible precipitants of renal failure
1 Vascular
— Prolonged hypotension (e.g. dehydration, shock, CCF)
— Malignant hypertension
— Vasculitis (esp. Goodpasture's syndrome)
— Renal vein thrombosis
2 Obstruction (exclude with ultrasound)
— Prostatomegaly
— Bladder atony (e.g. in diabetic autonomic neuropathy)
— Calculi
— Idiopathic retroperitoneal fibrosis
— Tumor infiltration (e.g. Ca bladder → ureteric orifices)

3 Infection*
— Pyelonephritis (? secondary to subacute obstruction)
— Septicemia → acute tubular necrosis
— Glomerulonephritis (see below)
— Genitourinary TB → upper tract obstruction
— Amyloidosis (e.g. due to chronic UTI in paraplegic)
4 Metabolic derangement
— Acute hyperuricemia (e.g. tumor lysis syndrome)
— Hypercalcemia
— Chronic hypokalemia (laxative abuse, Conn's)
— Heavy metal poisoning
5 Iatrogenic
— Radiographic contrast examination, esp. IVP
— Drug toxicity (e.g. NSAIDs, aminoglycosides)

* esp. in patients with single kidneys or preexisting renal impairment

Renal failure due to glomerulonephritis?
1 Intrinsic renal disease
— Normal serum complement
• IgA nephropathy (commonest nephritis)
— Low serum complement
• Acute (post-infectious) GN
• Membranoproliferative GN
2 Systemic disease
— Normal serum complement
• PAN, Wegener's (ANCA-positive)
• Anti-GBM disease (Goodpasture's)
• Henoch–Schönlein purpura
— Low serum complement
• SLE
• SBE
• *Staph albus*: 'shunt nephritis'

Clinical evolution of renal dysfunction
1 Reduced renal reserve (creatinine clearance 60–100 mL/min)
— Asymptomatic
2 Renal insufficiency (creatinine clearance 30–60 mL/min)
— Nocturia; leg cramps
— Hypertension
— Hyperuricemia: elevated blood urea nitrogen
3 Renal failure (creatinine clearance 15–30 mL/min)
— Nausea, anorexia, diarrhea
— Edema; infections; occult bleeding, mouth ulcers
— Phosphate retention; metabolic acidosis
— Anemia (exception: polycystic disease)
4 Uremia (creatinine clearance < 15 mL/min)
— Lethargy, irritability (→ fits, coma)
— Pruritus, hiccups, flapping tremor
— Pericarditis; pulmonary edema
— Bone pain
— Hyperkalemia
— Hypocalcemia, ↑ alkaline phosphatase

RENAL DISORDERS IN MULTISYSTEM DISEASE

Renal failure with hemoptysis: differential diagnosis
1 Goodpasture's syndrome

Wegener's granulomatosis
Henoch–Schönlein purpura
PAN, SLE, cryoglobulinemia
2 Renal vein thrombosis with pulmonary embolism
3 Acute renal failure with pulmonary edema
4 Right-sided infective endocarditis with septic pulmonary emboli and immune-complex nephritis
5 Infection: tuberculosis, Legionnaire's disease

Renal disease with jaundice: differential diagnosis
1 Hemolytic-uremic syndrome
2 Hepatorenal failure (hepatic nephropathy)
3 Leptospirosis (Weil's disease)
4 Hepatitis B with nephrotic syndrome
5 Alcoholic cirrhosis with IgA nephropathy
6 Polycystic disease with congenital hepatic fibrosis
7 Stauffer's syndrome: renal cell carcinoma with non-metastatic hepatic dysfunction (e.g. cholestasis)
8 Toxic: CCl_4, methoxyflurane

Hepatorenal failure: clinical features
1 Occurs in advanced liver failure
2 Precipitated by
   — Diuretics, paracentesis
   — Portocaval shunt
   — Biliary contrast radiography
3 Characterized by
   — Oliguria
   — Normal urinary sediment
   — Urinary sodium < 5 mmol/L
4 No improvement following IV volume repletion*
5 Transplanted kidneys work well in host with normal liver

* cf. prerenal failure

Diagnostic significance of skin lesions in renal failure
1 Impetigo, erythema nodosum
   — Suggest post-streptococcal glomerulonephritis
2 Purpura
   — Amyloid ('pinch'; post-proctoscopic periorbital type)
   — Vasculitis (palpable)
   — Henoch–Schönlein ($\rightarrow$ thigh, buttock)
   — Cryoglobulinemia ($\pm$ ulceration, gangrene)
3 Inherited nephropathies
   — Scrotal angiokeratomata (Fabry's disease)
   — Carotenemic pigmentation (Balkan nephropathy)
   — Hypoplastic nails (nail-patella syndrome)
   — Adenoma sebaceum, ash-leaf macules (tuberous sclerosis; angiomyolipomata $\rightarrow$ massive hematuria)

SYMPTOMS AND SIGNS OF RENAL DISEASE

Renal disease with small kidney(s) size
1 Chronic glomerulonephritis
   — Symmetrically smooth
2 Chronic pyelonephritis
   — Asymmetrically scarred
   — Cortical scars opposite dilated calices, esp. upper poles
3 Medullary cystic disease

4 Post-obstructive atrophy
5 Renovascular insufficiency
6 Late stage of many diseases causing large kidneys initially

Renal disease with bilateral renal enlargement
1 Polycystic disease
2 Medullary sponge kidneys
3 Obstructive uropathy (bilateral hydronephrosis)
4 Acute nephropathies
   — Acute glomerulonephritis
   — Acute interstitial nephritis
   — Acute tubular necrosis
   — Acute urate nephropathy
5 Other
   — Amyloidosis
   — Renal vein thrombosis ($\pm$ nephrosis, amyloid)
   — Insulin-dependent diabetes
   — Acromegaly (renal function typically normal)
   — Radiation nephritis

Common features of interstitial nephritis
1 Fever, arthralgias, rash
2 Renal failure with microhematuria $\pm$ polyuria/pyuria
3 Eosinophilia (esp. if drug-induced), eosinophiluria > 5%
4 Abnormal liver function tests
5 Radiographically enlarged kidneys

Differential diagnosis of loin pain
1 Calculus; sloughed papilla
2 Pyelonephritis; perinephric abscess
3 Acute glomerulonephritis (esp. proliferative)
4 Vesicoureteric reflux
5 Hemorrhage into cyst; infected cyst
6 Segmental infarction (sickle-cell disease, embolism)

Nocturia: diagnostic significance
1 Prostatism
2 Edematous states
3 Salt-losing nephropathies, e.g.
   — Analgesic nephropathy
   — Medullary sponge kidneys
   — Sickle-cell disease
4 Polyuric states, e.g.
   — Diabetes mellitus/insipidus
   — Primary polydipsia
   — Post-ATN
5 Bladder pathology
   — Tumor, fibrosis, infection
   — Loss of reflex inhibition (e.g. multiple sclerosis)
   — Vesicoureteric reflux ('double micturition' in children)

INVESTIGATING RENAL DISEASE

URINARY ABNORMALITIES

Highly diagnostic features on urine microscopy
1 Red cell casts (acute glomerulonephritis)
2 Doubly refractile oval fat bodies (nephrotic syndrome)

Urinary stigmata of glomerular disease
1 Red cell casts
2 Heavy proteinuria (> 2 g/day)
3 Pleomorphic red cells on phase-contrast microscopy

Clinically important causes of 'sterile pyuria'
1 Inadequately treated urinary tract infection
2 Genitourinary TP or other fastidious organism, e.g.
   — *Strep. morbillorum/agalactiae/milleri*
   — *Corynebacteria,* lactobacilli
3 Inflammatory non-infective disease
   — Papillary necrosis (esp. analgesic nephropathy)
   — Calculi (renal or bladder)
   — Interstitial nephritis/polycystic disease (light pyuria)
4 Lower tract inflammation
   — Prostatitis
   — Chemical cystitis (e.g. due to cyclophosphamide)
5 Dysuria-pyuria ('urethral') syndrome
   — Pathogenic bacteriuria $< 10^5$ organisms/mL
   — Bacterial urethritis, e.g. chlamydial
   — Periurethral herpes simplex
6 'False pyuria' (i.e. nil on suprapubic tap)
   — Primary vaginal infection, poor specimen collection
   — e.g. *Gardnerella vaginalis, C. albicans, Trichomonas* spp.

Urinary tract infection: factors favoring pyelonephritis
1 Clinical
   — Loin pain/tenderness, fever, tachycardia, rigors
2 Urine microscopy
   — White blood cell casts
3 Blood
   — Leukocytosis ± positive blood cultures
4 IVP
   — Poor excretion of contrast on affected side
5 Therapy
   — Failure of appropriate single-dose antibiotics

Iatrogenic causes of reddish urine
1 Drug excretion products
   — Rifampicin
   — Metronidazole
   — Sulfasalazine
   — Doxorubicin
   — Desferrioxamine
2 Drug toxicity
   — Drugs inducing acute intermittent porphyria (p. 286)
   — Drugs inducing rhabdomyolysis (e.g. clofibrate, heroin)
   — Drugs inducing hematuria (e.g. warfarin, urokinase)

Myoglobinuria: precipitants and laboratory features
1 Causes
   — Muscle crush injury
   — Hyperthermia (e.g. malignant) ± convulsions
   — Polymyositis
   — McArdle's syndrome
   — Meyer–Betz (familial) disease
   — Haff disease
   — Drugs: acute alcoholic binge; heroin; 'angel dust' (phencyclidine, PCP); clofibrate

2 Features
   — Acute oliguric renal failure with red urine
   — Urinalysis 'heme +', but no red cells on microscopy
   — Serum clear*
   — Initial hypocalcemia → 'rebound' hypercalcemia
   — ↑ Serum potassium, phosphate, urate

* Myoglobin does not bind haptoglobin and is thus renally cleared immediately; cf. intravascular hemolysis (p. 173)

Crystalluria: differential diagnosis
1 Cystinuria (autosomal recessive)
2 Xanthinuria (hereditary *or* allopurinol-induced)
3 Orotic aciduria (hereditary)
4 Uricosuria (acquired, hereditary or drug-induced)
5 APRT* deficiency (→ 2,8-dihydroxyadenine urolithiasis)
6 Hyperoxaluria
   — Autosomal recessive (pyridoxine-responsive)
   — Ileal disease‡ (e.g. Crohn's, resection)
   — Toxic: ethylene glycol ingestion, methoxyflurane
7 Drugs
   — Sulfadiazine, nitrofurantoin
   — Acetazolamide, triamterene
   — Acyclovir; 5-FC

* adenine phosphoribosyltransferase
‡ Calculous tendency partly due to *hypocitruria* → alkaline urine

PROTEINURIA

Clinical sequelae of heavy proteinuria
1 Edema
2 Weakness (muscle catabolism ± diuretic-induced ↑ K^+)
3 Frothy urine
4 Postural hypotension
5 Thromboembolism (incl. renal vein thrombosis)
6 Hypercholesterolemia (xanthomata, vascular disease)

Laboratory characterization of proteinuria
1 *Selective* (glomerular) proteinuria is characterized by urinary losses of albumin and/or transferrin primarily
2 *Non-selective* proteinuria leads to loss of IgG; *selectivity* may therefore be quantified by urinary albumin:IgG ratio
3 Similarly, *tubular* proteinuria may be confirmed by the urinary β_2 microglobulin:albumin ratio
4 Low IgG:transferrin (albumin) ratios predict steroid responsiveness in nephrotic syndrome (e.g. 'minimal lesion' with selective proteinuria)
5 *Microalbuminuria* is excessive urinary protein excretion which is persistently less than that detectable by conventional dipstick testing

Clinical significance of microalbuminuria
1 Defined as overnight urinary albumin excretion in the range 20–200 µg/min
2 Predicts impending nephropathy in diabetes mellitus
3 Correlates with hypertension in diabetics and in the general population
4 Predicts morbidity and death from cardiovascular causes in both diabetics and the general population

Characteristics of benign orthostatic proteinuria
1 Non-selective
2 Benign sediment
3 < 1 g/day
4 Typical diurnal fluctuation
5 No increase with time

NEPHROTIC SYNDROME

Laboratory manifestations of the nephrotic syndrome
1 ↓ Albumin
2 ↓ Transferrin
   → Iron-resistant hypochromic anemia
3 ↓ IgG, ↑ α_2 globulins
   → Hypogammaglobulinemia
4 ↓ Plasma volume, ↑ fibrinogen, V, VII, VIII, X
   → Hypercoagulable state (e.g. → renal vein thrombosis)
5 ↓ 25-hydroxyvitamin D (due to urinary losses)
   → Secondary reduction in 1,25 dihydroxyvitamin D
6 ↑ Cholesterol*
   → Accelerated atherosclerosis

NB: GFR may be overestimated by creatinine clearance. Reduced GFR (reflecting hypovolemia rather than renal damage) is more accurately measured using ^{51}Cr-EDTA clearance
* Occurs due to ↑ synthesis of LDL apoprotein B

Prognostic variables in the nephrotic syndrome
1 Clinical features portending poor prognosis
   — Oliguria; hematuria
   — Hypertension
   — Purpura
2 Results portending poor prognosis
   — Non-selective proteinuria
   — Hypocomplementemia
3 Etiologic significance of steroid-resistance in minimal change disease
   — Hodgkin's disease
   — Amyloid
   — Focal sclerosis (i.e. biopsy sampling error)
4 Indications for alkylator therapy in minimal change disease
   — At least two relapses after initial response to steroids

GLOMERULAR DISEASE

Investigation of unexplained glomerular disease
1 Urinalysis: blood, protein, glucose, nitrites
2 Careful microscopic examination of freshly voided urine
3 Urine screen for opiate derivatives
4 Serum albumin and 24-h urine protein
5 Infection screen
   — ASO titer, HBsAg, VDRL
   — Thick/thin film (if history of travel/malarial exposure)
   — Blood cultures
     • Infective endocarditis
     • 'Shunt' (*Staph. albus*) nephritis

     • Pneumococcal peritonitis
     • Brucellosis, leptospirosis
6 CXR
   — Sarcoid
   — Malignancy
7 Immunologic screen
   — ANA, rheumatoid factor; C_3, C_4
   — Cryoglobulins
   — Anti-GBM
   — EPG/IEPG/urinary BJP (± marrow pending result)
8 Rectal biopsy
   — Congo red
9 Renal biopsy
   — Light microscopy
   — Immunofluorescence, Congo red
   — Electron microscopy

NB: A low *carbamylated hemoglobin* measurement may indicate acute rather than chronic renal failure, thus clarifying desirability of urgent intervention

Spectrum of renal pathology in diabetes
1 Renal enlargement (in early insulin-dependent diabetes)
   Osmotic polyuria
2 Diffuse glomerulosclerosis
   Nodular glomerulosclerosis (Kimmelstiel–Wilson lesion)*
3 Glycogen deposition in tubules (Armanni–Ebstein lesion)
4 Interstitial nephritis
   Pyelonephritis, papillary necrosis
   Recurrent urinary tract infections
5 Hyporeninemic hypoaldosteronism (↑ K^+, ↑ Cl^-)

* Suggests insulin-dependent diabetes

WHO grading of renal pathology in SLE
1 Normal light microscopic appearances
   Positive mesangial immunofluorescence
2 Mesangial changes only
3 Focal proliferative glomerulonephritis
4 Diffuse proliferative glomerulonephritis
5 Membranous glomerulonephritis
6 Advanced sclerosis*

* Important diagnosis, since absent inflammation contraindicates treatment

Electron microscopy of renal disease
1 Minimal lesion nephrosis
   — Epithelial podocyte fusion
2 Fanconi syndrome, congenital nephrosis
   — 'Swan-neck' deformity, dilatation of proximal tubule
3 Alport's syndrome
   — Splitting of lamina densa and lamina propria of glomerular basement membrane*
4 Medullary cystic disease
   — Cystic dilatation at corticomedullary junction
5 Medullary sponge kidneys, infantile polycystic kidneys
   — Dilatation of collecting ducts‡

* Similar to chronic rejection
‡ cf. adult polycystic kidneys – abnormality involves entire nephron

IMMUNOPATHOLOGY OF THE NEPHRON

Some causes of membranous nephropathy
1 Paraneoplastic
2 Autoimmune disease, esp. SLE
3 Sarcoidosis
4 Infections
 — Hepatitis B, syphilis
 — *P. malariae**
5 Drugs
 — Gold, penicillamine
 — Captopril (high-dose only)

* Cure of malaria will *not* necessarily lead to resolution of the nephropathy

Immunofluorescence of glomerular disease
1 Helpful in diagnosing early membranous nephropathy
 — Diffuse IgG $\pm$ C_3
2 Distinguishes
 — Minimal change disease (IF-)
 — Mesangial nephropathy (+IgM, weak +C_3)
3 Focal sclerosis
 — +IgM, +C_3
4 Mesangiocapillary GN
 — Bright C_3 staining
 — Modest Ig/C_{1q} staining
5 SLE
 — Heavy IgG, A, M deposits
 — +C_{1q}, C_3
 — +ANA $\rightarrow$ 5–10% (pathognomonic)
6 IgA nephropathy/HSP
 — Mesangial IgA + C_3 $\pm$ IgM/G, but *without* C_{1q} (cf. SLE)
7 Goodpasture's (associated with circulating anti-GBM)
 — *Linear* IgG in kidney, lung (rarely $\rightarrow$ SLE, rejection)
8 Post-infectious (e.g. post-strep)
 — 'Lumpy-bumpy' electron-dense deposits with +C_3

Complement levels in glomerulonephritis
1 Reduced ($\downarrow$ C_3)
 — Post-infectious (SBE, 'shunt', post-strep)
 — SLE; cryoglobulinemia
 — Mesangiocapillary type I and (esp.) II
 • May be low even with quiescent nephritis
 • C_3-nephritic factor may be detectable in type II
2 Normal
 — Minimal lesion
 — IgA nephropathy
 — Goodpasture's syndrome; rapidly progressive GN
 — PAN, HSP, Wegener's
 — Membranous

Associations of IgA nephropathy
1 Cirrhosis
2 Celiac disease
3 Tuberculosis
4 Seronegative arthritis

INVESTIGATING RENAL FAILURE

Diagnostic approach to unexplained acute renal failure
1 Clinical
 — Hypovolemia (favors prerenal cause)
 — Fluid overload (favors renal/post-renal cause)
2 Urine microscopy/urinalysis/MSU
 — Helps exclude glomerulonephritis, UTI
3 Renal ultrasound
 — Excludes post-renal obstruction
4 Blood cultures, coagulation screen
 — Helps exclude septicemia, DIC
5 Renal biopsy $\pm$ high-dose IVP
 — Confirms or refutes diagnosis of glomerulonephritis

Disproportionate elevation of blood urea vs creatinine
1 Increased catabolism: trauma, infection, fever
2 Dehydration (loss of water and sodium): nephrosis, CCF
3 Gastrointestinal hemorrhage (with volume loss)
4 High protein intake
5 Drugs: tetracycline, corticosteroids, cyclosporin

Disproportionate reduction of blood urea vs creatinine
1 Liver disease
2 Pregnancy (expanded plasma volume)
3 Starvation
4 Selective increase of creatinine (muscle trauma, cimetidine)

Acute renal failure: 'prerenal' or acute tubular necrosis?
1 Prerenal
 — Urinary sodium < 10 mEq/L
 — Urinary osmolality > 500 mosm/L
 — Urine: plasma osmolality > 1.1
 — Urine: plasma creatinine concentration > 20
2 ATN
 — Urinary sodium > 20 mEq/L
 — Urinary osmolality < 400 mosm/L
 — Urine: plasma osmolality = 0.9–1.05
 — Urine: plasma creatinine concentration < 15

RENAL BIOPSY

Indications for renal biopsy
1 Hematuria with proteinuria
2 Hematuria with negative cystoscopy and IVP
3 Proteinuria > 1 g/day, esp. with renal impairment
4 Nephrotic syndrome in adults
5 Acute renal failure (esp. oliguric/nephritic type) following exclusion of pre- and post-renal causes
6 Chronic renal failure* with radiographically normal kidneys
7 Renal vasculitis (before and during therapy)
8 Malfunctioning transplant kidney

* But *not* end-stage, irreversible renal failure

Renal biopsy: complications and contra-indications
1 Complications
 — Persistent gross hematuria

— Pain ('clot colic,' perinephric hematoma)
— Hypotension (transient), brady-/tachycardia
— Intrarenal AV fistula
— Urinoma, urinary fistula
— Hypertension (chronic)
2 Contraindications
— Inadequate immunofluorescence/electron microscopy
— Coagulopathy; ↓ platelet number and/or function
— Bilaterally small kidneys on IVP
— Diastolic BP > 120 mmHg
— Solitary (functioning) kidney
— Diabetic glomerulosclerosis clinically suspected
— Established uremia

TUBULAR DISORDERS

Indicators of proximal tubular dysfunction
1 Glycosuria (i.e. without hyperglycemia)
2 Phosphaturia
3 Uricosuria
4 Aminoaciduria

Indicators of distal tubular dysfunction
1 Urinary concentration defect
— Screen: overnight urine < 700 mosm/L is abnormal
— Water deprivation test: < 900 mosm/L is abnormal
— DDAVP stimulation: < 800 mosm/L is abnormal
2 Urinary acidification defect: ammonium chloride test
— pH > 5.0 is abnormal

Pathological spectrum of renal tubular dysfunction*
1 Defective tubular responsiveness to hormones
— Nephrogenic diabetes insipidus (XR; distal tubular dysfunction)
— Bartter's syndrome (AR, distal)
— Liddle's syndrome (AD, distal)
— Pseudohypoparathyroidism (XD, proximal)
— Hypophosphatemic rickets (XD, proximal)
2 Primary tubular defects (± intestinal transport defects)
— 'Renal' glycosuria (AD, proximal)
— Hartnup disease (AR, proximal; p. 233)
— Cystinuria (AR, proximal)‡
— Cystinosis (AR, proximal; → uremia, childhood death)
— Fanconi's (AR, proximal)¶
— Renal tubular acidosis type I (AD, distal)
3 Secondary tubular transport defects
— Distal tubule defects
• Liver disease
• Medullary sponge kidneys
• Infantile polycystic disease
• Amphotericin B
• Cyclosporin A toxicity
• Lithium
— Proximal tubule defects
• Wilson's disease; heavy metal poisoning
• Medullary cystic disease
• Fanconi's syndrome; cystinosis
• Acetazolamide use

— Distal and/or proximal defects
• Myeloma
• Sjögren's syndrome, other autoimmune disorders
• Renal transplant rejection
• Long-standing hypercalciuria/-emia or hypokalemia
• Obstructive uropathy
• Analgesic nephropathy, chronic pyelonephritis

* X = X-linked, A = autosomal, R = recessive, D = dominant
‡ Recurrent calculi due to **c**ystine loss, though **o**rnithine, **a**rginine and **l**ysine – 'COAL' – are also lost
¶ Aminoaciduria, glycosuria, phosphaturia, natriuria, hypercalciuria, uricosuria, 'tubular' proteinuria

Renal tubular acidosis: clinical presentations in adults
1 Weakness (hypokalemia)
2 Bone pain (osteomalacia)
3 Constipation
4 Renal calculi
— Calcium phosphate (± nephrocalcinosis)
— Struvite (due to associated hypocitruria)
5 Renal failure

When to suspect renal tubular acidosis (RTA)
1 General
— High urine pH relative to plasma pH, *and*
— Negative urine culture
2 Distal and proximal RTA
— Hyperchloremic hypokalemic acidosis ($\uparrow$ Cl⁻, $\downarrow$ HCO₃⁻)
— Normal anion gap (i.e. $Na^+ - Cl^- - HCO_3^- = 8–12$; p. 236)
— Symptomatic hypokalemia
3 Distal RTA (acidification defect)
— Urine pH > 5.4 following oral acid load*
— Nephrocalcinosis, calculi
4 Proximal RTA (bicarbonate-wasting)
— Urine pH < 5.4 after oral acid load
— Hypouricemia and hypophosphatemia
— ± Fanconi's syndrome
5 RTA type 4
— Hyporeninemic hypoaldosteronism
— Urine pH < 5.4 after oral acid load
— Occurs in elderly diabetics or obstructive uropathy
— Causes *hyperkalemia* and acid urine

* Ammonium chloride 100 mg/kg

Possible constituents of 'tubular proteinuria'
1 'Physiological'
— Tamm–Horsfall protein
— β₂ microglobulin
— IgA
2 Pathological
— Myoglobin
— Lysozyme
— Bence-Jones protein

How to distinguish urinary concentrating defects
1 Water deprivation*/DDAVP → > 1000 mosm/L
— Normal
2 Water deprivation/DDAVP → *no* increase
— Nephrogenic diabetes insipidus

3 Water deprivation → no increase
   DDAVP → *major* increase
   — Pituitary diabetes insipidus
4 Water deprivation/DDAVP → *submaximal* increase
   — Long-standing primary polydipsia

* i.e. for 12 h; plasma osmolality should be ~ 295 mosm/kg

DISORDERS OF WATER METABOLISM

Primary polydipsia: its clinical significance
1 80% of primary polydipsia patients are schizophrenic
2 Commonest presentation of primary polydipsia is fitting
3 10% of primary polydipsics die within 2 years of diagnosis

Features of nephrogenic diabetes insipidus
1 The diagnosis may be effectively *excluded* if any voided urine specimen has an osmolality exceeding 600 mosm/L or specific gravity exceeding 1.015. Conversely, if an overnight voided specimen has an osmolality less than 350 mosm/L, a water-deprivation test may be indicated
2 Distinction from 'central' diabetes insipidus may be made if concentration defect persists after bilateral intranasal instillation of 20 μg DDAVP
3 Primary polydipsia tends to be associated with a low plasma osmolality (~275 mosm/L) whereas diabetes insipidus is associated with higher readings (~295 mosm/L). In long-standing primary polydipsia, however, definitive distinction from nephrogenic diabetes insipidus may not be possible on the basis of osmolalities alone
4 Nephrogenic diabetes insipidus may occur as an X-linked recessive (XR) disorder or, more commonly, as a manifestation of other disorders including sickle-cell disease/trait, obstructive uropathy, chronic hypercalcemia/hypokalemia or drugs (e.g. lithium)
5 Potentially useful management options include
   — Treatment of underlying cause
   — Thiazides (or ethacrynic acid) ± dietary salt restriction

NB: Chlorpropamide, which is of potential benefit in incomplete central diabetes insipidus, is *ineffective* in nephrogenic diabetes insipidus

Drug-induced disturbances of water metabolism
1 SIADH
   — Chlorpropamide
   — Carbamazepine
   — Amitriptyline
2 Nephrogenic diabetes insipidus
   — Lithium
   — Demeclocycline
   — Amphotericin B

Diagnosis of inappropriate ADH secretion
1 Plasma osmolality* < 275 mosm/L
2 Urinary osmolality inappropriately high‡ (see below)

3 Urinary sodium > 20 mmol/L

* plasma osmolality = BUN + glucose + 2 x Na^+
‡ *Normal* waterloading causing urine flow of 10 mL/min should cause urine osmolality ~ 100 mosm/kg and serum osmolality ~ 280 mosm/kg

Inappropriate ADH secretion: features
1 Remains a diagnosis of exclusion
   — Measurement of plasma ADH is *not* useful
2 Not characterized by significant edema, weight gain or hypertension despite hypervolemia*
3 Development of symptoms may be more dependent on *rate* of decline of serum sodium than on absolute level‡
4 Unlike other hyponatremias (see below), may also cause
   — Hypouricemia
   — ↓ Albumin
   — ↓ Creatinine/BUN
   — ↓ Hematocrit
5 Important differential diagnoses of ↓ Na^+
   — Myxedema (ADH-independent ↓ free water clearance)
   — Addison's disease (but associated with ↑ K^+)
   — Chlorpropamide (→ ↑ ADH secretion *and* sensitivity)
6 Therapeutic options include
   — Treatment of underlying cause
   — Water restriction ± frusemide ± ↑ dietary NaCl
   — Demeclocycline (or lithium)
   — V_2-receptor (renal tubular ADH receptor) antagonists
   — Hypertonic saline (a desperation measure; p. 242)

* NB: Elderly patients may develop cardiac failure
‡ Urinary osmolalities need only be *inappropriately* elevated for the diagnosis to be entertained; e.g. a urinary osmolality of 250 mosm/L would be consistent with SIADH in association with an identical plasma value (provided that urinary Na^+ was also elevated)

RENAL RADIOLOGY

Intravenous pyelography: predispositions to renal failure*
1 Myeloma
2 Diabetes (controversial)
3 Old age (esp. if hypovolemic, e.g. nephrotic) Infants (esp. if dehydrated, since unable to concentrate urine)

* NB: May be prevented by avoiding routine preparatory dehydration

Retrograde pyelography: causes of 'spidery infundibula'
1 Polycystic kidneys
2 Intrarenal space-occupying lesion (e.g. tumor)
3 Renal vein thrombosis

Pelviureteric junction translucency: differential diagnosis
1 **C**arcinoma (TCC)
2 **C**lot
3 **C**alculus (radiolucent; p. 316)
4 **C**rystals (p. 316)

Differential diagnosis of papillary necrosis
1   Analgesic abuse
2   Diabetes mellitus
3   Sickle-cell disease
4   Tuberculosis

Common congenital renal abnormalities on IVP*
1   Duplex collecting systems
    — Commoner in females
    — Upper pole ureter → lower bladder (and vice versa)
    — Lower pole ureter is prone to vesicoureteric reflux
2   Horseshoe kidney
    — Fused lower poles
3   Pelvic (ectopic) kidney
    — May interfere with parturition
    — May simulate a pathological pelvic mass
4   Crossed renal ectopia
    — Ectopic kidney lies directly below orthotopic partner
    — Fusion may occur
    — Collecting system of ectopic kidney crosses midline to enter bladder on correct side

* All may predispose to infection, obstruction and calculi

Rationâle of isotope renal scans
1   ^{131}Iodo-hippuran scan
    — 80% excreted by renal tubular secretion
    — Helps assess effective renal plasma flow (RPF) and, thereby, functional status of renal homograft
    — Renography may be useful in follow-up of (diagnosed) obstructive uropathy and/or assessment of pelviureteric junction obstruction
2   ^{99m}Tc-DTPA or ^{51}Cr-EDTA (inulin analog) scans
    — Help assess renal perfusion (varies with GFR)
    — *Dynamic* (vascular phase) studies
      • Useful for checking post-transplant anastomosis
      • Gross hypoperfusion in a non-functioning graft favors rejection over tubular necrosis
      • Also useful in assessment of suspected renovascular trauma
    — *Static* (parenchymal phase) studies may be useful in
      • Assessing renal cortical function in severe renal failure (more sensitive than IVP)
      • Evaluating suspected intrarenal trauma
3   ^{66}Gallium scan
    — Helpful in excluding graft infection, usually in conjunction with ultrasound or transplant biopsy

MANAGING RENAL DISEASE

THERAPY OF RENAL FAILURE

Immediate management priorities in acute renal failure
1   To treat life-threatening hyperkalemia and/or pulmonary edema (e.g. by continuous arteriovenous hemofiltration)
2   To establish the nature, hence reversibility, of renal disorder

Therapeutic considerations in end-stage chronic renal failure
1   Exclude reversible factors contributing to azotemia
2   Treat hypertension
3   Reduce protein intake if symptomatically uremic*
4   Administer bicarbonate (unless sodium restricted), phosphate binders and/or vitamin D analogs as needed
5   Modify drug intake for degree of azotemia
6   Realistically assess age, general condition, mental capacity and overall prognosis prior to definitive intervention
7   Assess patient suitability for chronic ambulatory peritoneal dialysis (CAPD) or hemodialysis
    — Will the patient cope?
    — How adequate is vascular access?
    — When would a fistula be created?
    — How is the patient's cardiovascular stability?
8   Document HBsAg status
9   Determine age and number of siblings and document degree of 'matching' between patient and siblings with respect to
    — ABO compatibility (essential)
    — HLA (B and DR: 'cytotoxic' crossmatch) compatibility
    — MLC compatibility‡
10 Ensure regular blood transfusion if transplantation feasible

* Also assists in controlling acidosis and hyperkalemia
‡ Helps distinguish relative suitability of similar HLA matches

Treating the complications of chronic renal failure
1   Anemia
    — Folate, multivitamins
    — Ferrous sulfate
    — Erythropoietin
    — Dialysis
2   Acidosis
    — Sodium bicarbonate
    — Dialysis
3   Hyperuricemia
    — Allopurinol
4   Renal bone disease
    — Phosphate binders (aluminium hydroxide)
    — Vitamin D analogs (dihydrotachysterol)
    — Calcium supplements, high-calcium dialysate
    — Parathyroidectomy

ERYTHROPOIETIN

Specific indications for erythropoietin in renal failure
1   Transfusion often required
    — e.g. > six times per year
    — Risk of iron overload, hepatitis C
2   Symptoms due to recurrent anemia
    — Angina, CCF
    — Reduced quality of life (any cause)
3   Absolute level of hemoglobin
    — Consistently < 8 g/dL

Differential diagnosis of erythropoietin-resistant anemia
1   Iron deficiency

— Occult blood loss, menorrhagia
— Responds to iron dextran infusion (diagnostic test)
2 Aluminium toxicity
— Diagnose by bone biopsy
— R_x: desferrioxamine; minimize aluminium exposure
3 Occult infection
— May reduce response to erythropoietin
4 Occult hemopoietic insufficiency or hemolysis
— e.g. Coexisting myeloma, thalassemia
5 Non-compliance
— If self-administered by subcutaneous injection

Side-effects of erythropoietin treatment
1 Injection site pain, 'flu-like syndrome
2 Rapid changes in hematocrit
— Exacerbation of hypertension
— Headaches, seizures
— Thrombosis of shunts or fistulae
3 Hyperkalemia

PRESCRIBING IN RENAL DISEASE

Drugs competing for renal excretion: clinical significance
1 Probenecid
— Reduces tubular secretion of penicillin (aspirin, indomethacin, AZT) → potentiation
2 Quinidine, verapamil, spironolactone
— Decrease tubular secretion of digoxin → toxicity
3 Thiazides, frusemide
— Increase lithium reabsorption → toxicity
4 Aspirin
— Reduces tubular secretion of methotrexate → toxicity

'Safe' drugs in chronic renal failure
1 Antihypertensives — β-blockers
2 Antiarrhythmics   — Disopyramide
3 Antibiotics   — Amoxicillin, co-trimoxazole, cephalexin, doxycycline
4 Analgesics   — Paracetamol (low-dose)
5 Gastrointestinal   — Cimetidine, metoclopramide
6 Hypnotic   — Temazepam

Popular antihypertensives in chronic renal disease
1 Frusemide
— Used in preference to thiazides* once renal function falls to < 50% normal
2 β-blockers
— esp. Metoprolol
3 Calcium antagonists
— Efficacy maintained as GFR falls
— Nifedipine may increase microalbuminuria
4 ACE inhibitors
— Oppose high-renin hypertension‡, hence very effective
— Toxicity (e.g. captopril neutropenia) worse in uremia

— Appear to reduce proteinuria and slow renal disease

* Exception is the thiazide-like drug *metolazone*, which can be combined with frusemide in refractory hypervolemia
‡ NB: May catastrophically reduce GFR and thus precipitate acute renal failure if inadvertently used in patients with bilateral renal artery stenosis

Principles of corticosteroid use in renal disease
1 Renal biopsy precedes steroid use in adult renal disease
2 Steroids may lead to rapid resolution of
— Minimal lesion nephrosis (esp. in children)
— Acute interstitial nephritis
— Mesangial proliferative glomerulonephritis
— Idiopathic retroperitoneal fibrosis (exclude TB first)
3 Steroids usually need to be combined with other drugs in
— RPGN (including Goodpasture's)
— PAN
— Multiple relapses of minimal-lesion nephrosis
4 Steroids may help membranous nephropathy if used early
5 Steroids are rarely useful in sclerodermatous nephropathy

DIURETICS

Mechanisms of diuretic action
1 Acetazolamide
— Carbonic anhydrase inhibitor
— ↓ Proximal tubular transport of NaCl/bicarbonate
— *Ineffective* if serum bicarbonate < 20 mEq/L
— Toxicity: hyperchloremic acidosis due to 'bicarbonate wasting' (p. 309); nephrocalcinosis if long-standing
— Useful short-term treatment of edema, esp. if pregnant, premenstrual or with metabolic alkalosis
— Also useful in urate nephropathy and in salicylism (i.e. as part of forced alkaline diuresis)
2 Mannitol
— Acts by delivering osmotic load to proximal tubule
— Used in head trauma, etc.
3 Frusemide
— Blocks Cl⁻ pump (thick ascending limb, loop of Henle)
  → Blocks countercurrent multiplier system
  → Blocks water reabsorption from collecting system
— Also increases renal cortical perfusion
— Systemic venodilator (acts acutely in heart failure)
— Effective at low clearances
4 Thiazides
— Act on thin ascending limb (cortical diluting segment) of distal tubule → block active sodium reabsorption
— *Reduce* renal perfusion
— Also useful in proximal renal tubular acidosis
— *Not* effective at clearance < 20 mL/min

5 Potassium-sparing diuretics
— Triamterene → ↓ permeability of distal tubule/collecting ducts
— Amiloride → ↓ sodium/H_2O reabsorption, ↓ K^+ loss (mainly used as diuretic for patients on digoxin)
— Spironolactone: inhibits aldosterone action on distal tubule and collecting ducts; antiandrogenic side-effects (mainly used for cirrhotics with ascites)

Opposing indications for frusemide and thiazides
1 SIADH
— Frusemide (+ sodium supplements)
Nephrogenic diabetes insipidus
— Thiazides (+ sodium restriction)
2 Hypercalcemia
— Frusemide
Idiopathic hypercalciuria
— Thiazides

Clinically significant diuretic side-effects in elderly patients
1 Commoner with potassium-sparing diuretics
— Hyperkalemia (esp. in renal impairment)
— Hyponatremia (symptomatic in up to 20%)
— Precipitation of prerenal failure
2 Commoner with thiazides/frusemide
— Hypokalemia (esp. significant in patients on digoxin)
— Precipitation of gout (esp. in females)
— Precipitation of clinical diabetes
— Precipitation of incontinence

DRUG TOXICITY IN RENAL DISEASE

Nephrotoxicity of non-steroidal antiinflammatory drugs
1 Electrolyte disturbances
— Sodium retention (edema)
— Hyponatremia ± SIADH
— Hyperkalemia, esp. in diabetics (↓ renin release)
2 Acute renal failure in volume-contracted patients due to antagonism of prostaglandin-mediated renal arteriolar vasodilatation (reversible)
3 Acute tubular necrosis
4 Interstitial nephritis (drug hypersensitivity)
5 Papillary necrosis (due to medullary ischemia)
6 Minimal change nephrosis (indomethacin, naproxen)
7 Antagonism of antihypertensive therapy (e.g. frusemide, ACE inhibitors) by indomethacin

Patient subsets at increased risk of NSAID nephrotoxicity
1 Elderly
2 Preexisting renal impairment
3 Volume contraction
— Diuretics
— Cardiac failure
— Cirrhosis, nephrosis
— Hypertension
— Perioperative

Spectrum of antibiotic-induced nephrotoxicity
1 Antianabolic effect (→ ↑ BUN)
— Tetracyclines (exception: doxycycline)

2 Interstitial nephritis
— Penicillins (esp. methicillin)
— Cephalosporins, sulfonamides
— Rifampicin (esp. intermittent)
3 Hypokalemic alkalosis
— Penicillins (esp. ticarcillin)
4 Proximal tubular necrosis
— Aminoglycosides (potentiated by frusemide)
Distal tubular necrosis
— Amphotericin B
5 Nephrogenic diabetes insipidus
— Demethylchlortetracycline (demeclocycline)
6 Crystalluria (→ collecting duct obstruction)
— Sulfadiazine (for nocardiosis)
— Nitrofurantoin
— 5-FC, acyclovir

Accumulation of toxic drug metabolites in chronic renal failure?
1 Allopurinol
2 Digoxin
3 Methyldopa, metoprolol
4 Clofibrate
5 Opiates; propoxyphene

ALTERING DRUG REGIMENS IN RENAL DISEASE

Modification of drug therapy in renal failure
1 Avoid due to toxicity
— K^+-sparing diuretics (esp. in elderly or diabetics)
— ACE inhibitors
→ Life-threatening hyperkalemia
— Tetracyclines (except doxycycline)
→ Worsen azotemia
— Nitrofurantoin
→ Neuropathy; also ineffective
— Chloramphenicol
→ Accumulate myelotoxic inactive metabolites
— Lithium carbonate
→ Toxicity potentiated by diuretic therapy
— Metformin
→ Lactic acidosis
— Clofibrate
→ Toxic myopathy
— Methotrexate
2 Avoid due to ineffectiveness
— Thiazides
— Nalidixic acid, mandelamine
3 Major dose reduction required*
— Digoxin, procainamide
— Cimetidine, amantadine
— Vancomycin, aminoglycosides, amphotericin B
— Penicillin G, ampicillin, ticarcillin
— Sulfonamides, cephalosporins
— 5-FC (→ crystalluria)
— Ethambutol (→ optic neuritis)
4 *No* dose reduction usually required
— Digitoxin, frusemide (but beware of ototoxicity)
— Prazosin, minoxidil, hydralazine
— Tolbutamide, glibenclamide
— Prednisone, azathioprine, heparin
— Doxycycline

— Flucloxacillin, erythromycin, fusidic acid
— Isoniazid, rifampicin
— Griseofulvin, miconazole, ketoconazole, clotrimazole

NB: A rare example in which dosage may require *increase* in renal failure is that of phenytoin: ↓ plasma protein binding of phenytoin in renal failure → ↑ free drug → ↑ liver metabolism; renal excretion of phenytoin is insignificant
* i.e. according to nomogram or serum level

Drugs requiring repeat dosage following dialysis*
1 After *either* peritoneal dialysis or hemodialysis
    — Aminoglycosides
    — Ticarcillin
    — Cefuroxime, cephalothin
    — Isoniazid, ethambutol
    — 5-FC
    — Methyldopa
    — Aspirin
2 After hemodialysis only
    — Penicillins (except cloxacillin)
    — Cephalosporins
    — Metronidazole, trimethoprim
    — Acyclovir
    — Allopurinol
    — Paracetamol
    — Azathioprine, cyclophosphamide, prednisolone
    — Captopril, metoprolol, minoxidil, nadolol

* cf. heavily *protein-bound* drugs – *not* dialysable

HEMODIALYSIS

Indications for dialysis in renal failure
1 Symptomatic uremia (despite conservative management)
2 Fluid overload (diuretic-resistant)
3 Refractory hyperkalemia (after diet, resins, bicarbonate)
4 Unacceptable decline in quality of life (esp. if due to long-term complication, e.g. neuropathy, pericarditis)

Biochemical consequences of a hemodialysis treatment
1 Reduction in
    — Plasma creatinine/BUN
    — Plasma potassium
    — Plasma phosphate
    — Plasma osmolality
2 Increase in
    — Plasma bicarbonate/pH
    — Plasma sodium
    — Plasma calcium

Conditions with poor prognosis when treated by hemodialysis
1 Diabetes mellitus
2 Amyloidosis
3 Scleroderma
4 SLE
5 Hypertensive nephrosclerosis

Acute complications of hemodialysis
1 Hypotension

2 Arrhythmias (± digoxin toxicity)
3 Cramps; nausea; headaches
   Fever (e.g. due to Staph bacteremias)
4 Air embolism (due to IV bags with airways)
5 Exsanguination (due to external shunts)
6 Disequilibrium syndrome
    — Headaches, hypertension, confusion, fitting
    — Occurs during first few dialyses due to rapid reduction of extracellular osmolarity → cerebral edema

Chronic complications of hemodialysis
1 Accelerated atherosclerosis*
2 Hepatitis B
3 Sexual dysfunction, infertility, depression
4 Wernicke's syndrome; central pontine myelinolysis
5 Vascular
    — Fistula thrombosis or endarteritis
    — Hemorrhage (subdural, pericarditis, stroke, GI bleeding)
6 Dialysis dementia (due to cerebral aluminium overload)
7 Arthropathy (amyloidosis)
8 Nephrogenic ascites (indicates *dire* prognosis unless transplanted or switched to CAPD)

* 60% die from myocardial/cerebral infarction

ALTERNATIVES TO HEMODIALYSIS

Relative indications for chronic ambulatory peritoneal dialysis (CAPD) in renal failure
1 Unsuitability for hemodialysis
    — Extremes of age
    — Cardiovascular instability
    — Inadequate vascular access
    — Heparin contraindicated (e.g. in pericarditis)
    — Geographical remoteness
    — Religious conviction (Jehovah's Witness)
2 Symptomatic progression while on hemodialysis
3 Diabetic retinopathy
4 Scleroderma

NB: CAPD precluded by previous laparotomy (→ adhesions)

Problems encountered in CAPD patients
1 Peritonitis (esp. due to *Staph albus*; Gram-negatives may indicate visceral perforation by catheter); loculated ascites
2 Catheter blockage
3 Hyperglycemia, hypertriglyceridemia
   → Obesity, accelerated atheroma, worsening of diabetic control (necessitating intraperitoneal insulin)
4 Protein and amino acid depletion
5 Basal atelectasis, pleural effusions
6 Hernias; ileus (constipation)

Advantages of CAPD over hemodialysis
1 Early benefits
    — Better blood pressure control
    — Higher Hb
    — Less muscle wasting and weight loss

— Less acidosis
— No dialysis disequilibrium
2 Long-term benefits
— Loss of pigmentation
— Return of menstruation
— Improved calcium/phosphate balance

RENAL TRANSPLANTATION

Specific indications for transplantation
1 Severe renal osteodystrophy
2 Inability to cope with dialysis, esp. in young patient

Contraindications to transplantation
1 Lack of compatible kidney donor
2 Advanced age or debility
3 Chronic infection (TB, HBV, bronchiectasis, osteomyelitis)
4 Malignancy
5 Peptic ulceration
6 Primary disease known to recur in grafts

Significance of hypertension in the renal transplant patient
1 Fluid overload
2 Chronic rejection
3 Steroid-induced
4 Stenosis of donor renal artery
5 Renin production from remnant kidneys (rare)
6 Cyclosporin A toxicity (i.e. *independent* of nephrotoxicity)

Features of cyclosporin nephrotoxicity
1 Acute toxicity
— ↓ GFR/renal blood flow
2 Chronic toxicity
— Interstitial fibrosis, tubular atrophy
3 Toxicity may be potentiated by other drugs
— esp. Ketoconazole

Graft complications related to surgery in renal transplantation
1 Ureteric obstruction
2 Lymphocele
3 Renal vein thrombosis
4 Renal artery stenosis

Prolonged post-transplant oliguria; differential diagnosis
1 Acute rejection
2 Acute tubular necrosis
3 Arterial (anastomotic) stenosis* or thrombosis
4 Ureteric obstruction (lymphocele, hematoma ischemia)
5 Cyclosporin A nephrotoxicity
6 Sepsis (e.g. CMV, UTI)

* May be non-invasively detected by magnetic resonance angiography

Management of prolonged post-transplant oliguria if rejection suspected
1 Exclude vascular and ureteric obstruction
2 Transplant biopsy: is rejection confirmed?

3 If not, measure intrarenal pressure manometrically using 25 G needle (abnormally elevated in rejection)
4 If diagnosis still in doubt, decrease cyclosporin A dose
5 If no improvement in serum creatinine within 48 h of CSA reduction, proceed with therapeutic trial of steroids or azathioprine (i.e. as for confirmed graft rejection)

Features of cytomegalovirus graft infection
1 Manifests with post-transplant azotemia and/or oliguria
2 Most severe infections occur in seronegative patients receiving grafts from seropositive donors (a relative contraindication to matching)
3 Other mechanisms of infection include reactivation in seropositive hosts (occurs in 90%, mild) and transmission by granulocyte transfusions
4 Biopsy reveals diffuse glomerular lesions with minimal interstitial inflammatory response (cf. rejection)
5 The helper:suppressor (CD4:CD8) T cell ratio in peripheral blood is generally lower in CMV graft infection than in rejection, but this is inconsistently affected by the immunosuppressive regimen

Clinical stigmata of graft rejection
1 Hyperacute
— May occur within minutes
— Irreversible; graft nephrectomy mandatory
2 Acute
— May occur at *any* time
— Graft swelling, tenderness, fever
— Oliguria, azotemia
— ↓ Urinary sodium
— Active urine sediment
— May respond to immunosuppression
3 Chronic
— Occurs after months to years
— Inexorable, irreversible decline in GFR
— May manifest as interstitial nephritis or proliferative glomerulonephritis

Late problems following renal transplantation
1 Recurrent glomerulonephritis (contraindicates further attempts at transplantation; see below)
2 Reflux nephropathy
3 Avascular necrosis of bone (usually head of femur) Other steroid-related morbidity, e.g. cataracts
4 Infections
5 Malignancy
— Non-Hodgkin's lymphoma (incl. cerebral)
— Skin BCC or SCC (incl. vulva, perineum)
— SCC cervix (in situ)
— Hepatobiliary carcinoma
— Kaposi's sarcoma

Renal biopsy patterns classically recurring in transplants
1 Dense deposit disease*
2 Focal sclerosis and hyalinosis
— e.g. Due to reflux heroin or analgesic abuse
3 Oxalosis, cystinosis, amyloidosis
4 Severe diabetic glomerulosclerosis

5 Vasculitis
— Anti-GBM disease (Goodpasture's syndrome)
— Cryoglobulinemia
6 IgA nephropathy

* Mesangiocapillary glomerulonephritis type II

Graft biopsy in transplant rejection: implications for therapy
1 Acute rejection refractory to steroids
— Biopsy → cellular infiltrate
• Increase the steroids
— Biopsy → intimal proliferation
• Organize graft nephrectomy
2 Chronic rejection provisionally diagnosed
— Biopsy → recurrence of original disease process
• Abandon graft (further transplant contraindicated)
— Biopsy → confirmation of chronic rejection
• Prepare for dialysis (± retransplantation)

RENAL CALCULI

Radiological appearances predicting stone composition
1 Opaque stones
— Calcium oxalate
— Calcium phosphate
— Struvite ('infection' stones, 'triple phosphate': magnesium ammonium phosphate, MAP), esp. if large staghorn
2 Semiopaque
— Cystine
3 Lucent
— Urate
— Xanthine
— Orotic acid
— 2,8 dihydroxyadenine*

* Responsive to allopurinol prophylaxis

Determining the etiology of renal calculi
1 Family history
— Cystinuria, xanthinuria, hyperoxaluria
— Gout
— Multiple endocrine neoplasia (→ 1° HPT)
2 Medication history
— Megadose vitamin therapy
— Milk-alkali syndrome
— Acetazolamide (→ alkaline urine → urea-splitting bugs)
— Probenecid
3 Strain urine for passed stone fragments
— Quantitative chemical analysis: calcium, magnesium, ammonium, phosphate, oxalate, carbonate, urate
— Qualitative chemical analysis (cystine)
— Bacteriological analysis, esp. for *Proteus* spp.
4 Urine specimen analysis
— pH
— Microscopy
— Culture (esp. for urea-splitting organisms*)
— Sodium nitroprusside test (for cystine)
— Crystal counts (cystine, struvite) in fresh sample

5 Quantitative 24-h urine analysis
— Volume
— Oxalate
— Calcium, phosphate, urate
— Cystine (if qualitative tests positive)
— cAMP (if hyperparathyroidism suspected)
6 Plasma biochemistry
— Calcium, bicarbonate
— Urate (abnormally low? Exclude xanthinuria)
— Creatinine
— iPTH (if calcium elevated)
7 IVP
— Polycystic kidneys
— Medullary sponge kidneys
— Duplex collecting system

* *Proteus mirabilis, Pseudomonas aeruginosa, Klebsiella* spp.

Stone composition as a pointer to pathogenesis
1 Uric acid
— Hyperuricosuria (± hyperuricemia)
2 Struvite
— Infection with urease-splitting organisms
3 Cystine
— Cystinuria
4 Calcium phosphate
— Renal tubular acidosis
5 Calcium oxalate
— Idiopathic hypercalciuria
— Primary hyperparathyroidism
— Hypocitruria, hyperoxaluria, hyperuricosuria

Children with renal stones: diagnoses to exclude
1 Cystinuria
2 Distal RTA (calcium phosphate stones)
3 Hereditary hyperoxaluria
4 Medullary sponge kidneys (calcium oxalate stones in adolescents)

Long-term management of recurrent renal calculi
1 High fluid intake (indicated for all stone types)
2 Calcium oxalate stones (50%)
— Thiazides
— Allopurinol
— Low-oxalate diet
— Pyridoxine (*if* hereditary hyperoxaluria)
— Cholestyramine (*if* ileal disease present)
3 Calcium phosphate stones (25%)
— Thiazides (→ ↓ urinary calcium)
— Urinary acidification (oral citrate)
— Cellulose phosphate (binds calcium in gut)
— Low-calcium diet
4 Struvite stones (15%)
— Surgery
— Percutaneous shock wave lithotripsy
— Percutaneous nephrostomy with lavage chemolysis
— Antibiotics
— Urinary acidification (pH < 5.5)
— Acetohydroxamic acid (a urease inhibitor)
5 Urate stones (5–10%)
— Allopurinol
— Urinary alkalinization (pH > 6.5): bicarbonate + acetazolamide
— Low purine diet

6 Cystine stones (0.5–3%)
  — Aggressive hydration (3–5 L/day)
  — D-penicillamine (beware of drug-induced nephrosis)
  — Urinary alkalinization (pH > 7.5); less effective than for urate stones

IMMEDIATE THERAPY OF RENAL CALCULI

Prerequisites for ureteroscopic* removal of ureteric stones
1 Stone diameter < 5 mm, *and*
2 Stone situated < 5 cm from ureteric orifice, *and*
3 Stone impacted < 5 weeks duration

* i.e. using Dormia basket

Potential indications for surgical management of renal stones
1 Symptoms
2 Obstruction
3 Infection

EXTRACORPOREAL SHOCK WAVE LITHOTRIPSY (ESWL)

Factors favoring use of ESWL
1 Stones < 2 cm diameter
2 Renal pelvis or upper ureteric stones
3 Opaque stones* (most types), incl.
  — Calcium oxalate dihydrate
  — Calcium phosphate
  — Struvite

* Tend to fragment well

Relative contraindications to ESWL
1 Large (> 3 cm diameter) staghorn stones*
2 Stone(s) in lower third of ureter‡
3 Risk of precipitating renal failure
  — Obstruction preventing passage of fragments
  — Simultaneous treatment of bilateral stones
4 Stone composition (if known)
  — Radiolucent stones, esp. urate
    • May be dissolved by alkalinization
    • Catheterization or contrast required for fluoroscopic localization
  — Some opaque stones
    • Cystine¶ (may dissolve with penicillamine/H_2O)
    • Calcium oxalate monohydrate¶
5 Pregnancy, bleeding diathesis

* Best treated by percutaneous nephrolithotomy; for stag-horns, ESWL can be combined with surgery. *All* residual struvite must be removed to eliminate infective nidus
‡ Best treated by ureteroscopy
¶ Tend *not* to break up into fine fragments

Complications of ESWL
1 Renal colic
2 Perirenal hematoma*
3 Newly acquired hypertension
4 Pancreatitis (rare)

* Bowel hematomas have also been reported

MASSIVE BLADDER HEMORRHAGE

Precipitants of massive bladder hemorrhage
1 Trauma
2 Bladder tumors (esp. post-radiotherapy)
3 Long-term cyclophosphamide therapy (hemorrhagic cystitis)
4 Amyloidosis

Management modalities in massive bladder hemorrhage
1 Intravesical vasopressin
  — Works only for as long as infusion continued
2 Intravesical alum irrigation
  — Precipitates mucosal protein; no toxicity (cf. formalin)
3 Helmstein balloon compression
  — May cause fibrosis (similar to formalin instillation)
4 Arterial embolization
  — Effective measure in trauma cases
5 Supravesical urinary diversion
  — For intractable bleeding
6 Emergency cystectomy
  — For life-threatening hemorrhage resistant to above measures

UNDERSTANDING RENAL DISEASE

COMPLICATIONS OF RENAL DISEASE

Major pathogenetic mechanisms of anemia in renal failure
1 ↓ Erythropoietin secretion
2 ↓ Utilization of iron (anemia of chronic disease) due to ?'uremic toxins'
3 ↓ Production of glutathione by pentose phosphate pathway leading to shortened erythrocyte survival (hemolysis)
4 Marrow fibrosis due to secondary hyperparathyroidism
5 Occult blood loss due to
  — Impaired platelet function
  — Heparinization during hemodialysis
  — Loss of blood and folate during hemodialysis
  — Surreptitious ongoing aspirin ingestion
6 Diagnostic phlebotomies

Mechanisms of impotence in chronic renal failure
1 Depression
2 Reduced serum testosterone
3 Hyperprolactinemia
4 Autonomic neuropathy
5 Antihypertensive medications

Psychiatric etiologies in chronic renal failure
1 Uremia
2 Water intoxication
3 Rapid electrolyte shifts
4 Dialysis disequilibrium syndrome (?cerebral edema)
5 Dialysis dementia (?aluminium-induced)

Manifestations of disturbed calcium homeostasis in renal disease
1. Proximal myopathy (vitamin D deficiency)
2. Hyperparathyroidism: bone pain and deformity
3. Osteopenia
4. Osteomalacia: bone pain, deformity, pathological fracture
5. Avascular necrosis of the femoral head (in transplants)
6. Extraskeletal calcification
   — Band keratopathy
   — Pruritus
   — Vascular calcification
   — Periarticular soft tissues

RENAL OSTEODYSTROPHY

Pathogenesis of renal bone disease
1. Nephron loss $\rightarrow \downarrow$ GFR
    $\rightarrow$ Phosphate retention
2. Nephron loss $\rightarrow \downarrow$ dihydroxylated vitamin D (25-HCC)
   — $\downarrow$ 1,25-DHCC $\rightarrow$ osteomalacia
3. Skeletal PTH resistance + phosphate retention + $\downarrow$ 1,25-DHCC
    $\rightarrow \downarrow$ Ionized serum calcium (Ca^{2+})
4. $\downarrow Ca^{2+}$ $\rightarrow \uparrow$ PTH
   — Secondary hyperparathyroidism
   — Osteosclerosis and/or osteitis fibrosa cystica
5. Dialysate
   — Aluminium* $\rightarrow$ osteomalacia
   — Heparin $\rightarrow$ osteoporosis
6. Anorexia
    $\rightarrow$ Dietary deficiencies

* NB: Aluminium also present in oral phosphate binders

Radiographic features of renal osteodystrophy
1. 90% of biopsy-proven cases exhibit radiological abnormalities
2. 50% have vascular calcification
3. 50% have 'rugger-jersey' spine
4. 25% have subperiosteal lesions

Factors predicting incidence and severity of osteomalacia
1. Duration of dialysis (cf. transplant: osteomalacia *rare*)
2. Bone aluminium content

Approach to management of renal osteodystrophy
1. GFR < 30 mL/min
   — Prophylactic calcium (5 g/day $CaCO_3$ = 2 g/day Ca^{2+})
2. Development of significant hyperphosphatemia
   — Add oral phosphate binders
3. Indications for oral 1,25-DHCC/dihydrotachysterol
   — Development of hypocalcemia
   — Development of myopathy and/or bone pain
   — Radiographic erosions or fractures
   — Elevation of serum alkaline phosphatase
4. Tertiary (or severe secondary) hyperparathyroidism
   — Regular calcitriol (1,25-DHCC) *infusions*
   — Subtotal parathyroidectomy
5. Use aluminium-free dialysate when dialysing

INCONTINENCE

Urinary incontinence: important physical signs
1. Fever, cachexia; foul urine
   — Urinary tract infection
2. Suprapubic tenderness
   Bladder enlargement to percussion
   — Retention with overflow
3. Pelvic and rectal examination
   — Tumors, fistulae, uterine prolapse
4. $\downarrow$ Anal sphincter tone
    $\downarrow$ Bulbocavernosus reflex
   Perianal anesthesia ± fecal incontinence
   — Cauda equina syndrome
5. Pyramidal signs + sensory level
   — Cord compression
6. Peripheral neuropathy; optic atrophy
   Postural hypotension
   — Autonomic neuropathy
7. Gait apraxia, dementia; primitive reflexes
   — Normal pressure hydrocephalus
8. Urinalysis (glycosuria, hematuria, nitrites)

Adjunctive drugs for urinary incontinence
1. Stress incontinence
   — Phenylpropanolamine, imipramine
   — Systemic or topical estrogens if post-menopausal
2. Urge incontinence (detrusor instability)*
   — Oxybutinin, propantheline
   — Emepronium bromide
   — Imipramine
   — Intranasal desmopressin
3. Overflow incontinence
   — Bethanechol (may exacerbate symptoms in elderly)
4. Functional (e.g. dementia)
   — No specific drug therapy

* Best response to treatment

Other measures in treating urinary incontinence
1. Pelvic floor exercises
   Bladder retraining
   Biofeedback
2. Pessary
   Penile clamp
   Intermittent catheterization
3. Surgical repair (for stress incontinence)
   Electrical sphincter stimulation
   Artificial sphincters

THERAPY OF BENIGN PROSTATIC HYPERPLASIA

Medical therapies in prostatism*
1. α_1-blockers ($\rightarrow \uparrow$ flow by relaxing prostatic smooth muscle)
   — Alfuzosin, terazosin
   — Indoramin
2. Drugs which may shrink benign prostatic hypertrophy (BPH)
   — Finasteride (5-α-reductase inhibitor‡)
   — Flutamide (antiandrogen)

3 Antispasmodics (for detrusor instability)
   — Oxybutinin
4 β-sito sterol (plant steroids)

* Note that *surgery* remains the mainstay of treatment for severe symptoms
‡ 5-α-reductase converts testosterone to the active dihydrotestosterone (DHT); hence, finasteride reduces libido and causes impotence and gynecomastia

Morbidity of transurethral resection of the prostate (TURP)
1 Retrograde ejaculation (50%)
2 Impotence (5%)
3 Incontinence (5%)
4 Intraoperative reactions
   — Hypertension, tachypnea, bradycardia

RENAL CYSTIC DISEASE

Clinical spectrum of renal cystic disease
1 Medullary sponge kidneys (sporadic inheritance)
   — Manifests with stones or UTI in adults
   — Normal life expectancy
2 Medullary cystic disease (adult type = autosomal dominant)
   — Causes renal failure and osteodystrophy in childhood
   — Associated with liver fibrosis and retinitis pigmentosa
3 Infantile polycystic disease (autosomal recessive)
   — Causes renal failure in childhood
   — Associated with liver fibrosis and portal hypertension
4 Adult polycystic disease (autosomal dominant)
   — Causes renal failure in middle life
   — Associated with cysts in liver, pancreas, spleen, lungs

Features of medullary sponge kidneys
1 Asymmetrically enlarged kidneys
2 Probably underdiagnosed (as idiopathic hypercalciuria) in calcium stone-formers; IVP → 'grapelike clusters'
3 Presents between 10 and 40 years of age (bimodal) 60% get calculi; usually oxalate*
4 30% get
   — Hematuria
   — Urinary tract infections
   — Papillary necrosis/nephrocalcinosis
5 Does not usually lead to uremia; may be totally asymptomatic
6 Instrumentation should be avoided if possible

* *Staph albus* infections may cause struvite stones

Features of medullary cystic disease
1 Asymmetrically shrunken kidneys
2 Histology similar to chronic interstitial nephritis
3 Hypertension rare
4 Urinalysis typically normal
5 No calcification on IVP
6 Progresses inexorably to uremia via proximal RTA (p. 309) and/or salt-losing nephropathy

ADULT POLYCYSTIC KIDNEY DISEASE

Polycystic kidney disease: features
1 Episodic loin pain
   — Cyst hemorrhage
   — Cyst torsion
   — Clot colic
   — Calculi
2 Hematuria ± nocturia, mild proteinuria
3 Hypertension
4 Urinary tract infections
5 Anemia (normochromic *or* hypochromic) *or* polycythemia

Associations of polycystic kidney disease
1 Extrarenal cysts
   — Liver (30%)
   — Spleen, pancreas
2 Saccular aneurysms, esp. cerebral (10%)
   — Present with subarachnoid hemorrhage
3 Gastrointestinal manifestations
   — Colonic diverticulosis
   — Herniae
4 Cardiac valve disease
   — Aortic root dilatation, aortic incompetence
   — Mitral valve prolapse, mitral incompetence
5 Rare associations
   — Myotonic dystrophy
   — Hereditary spherocytosis
   — Peutz–Jeghers syndrome

Principles of managing adult polycystic disease
1 Prompt treatment of hypertension or urinary tract infection
2 Non-nephrotoxic analgesics for recurrent flank pain
3 Transplant work-up (if azotemia supervenes)
4 Genetic counselling‡
5 Rarely, cyst puncture or nephrectomy may be indicated

‡ Normal IVP ± ultrasound at age 20 makes future polycystic disease unlikely

MISCELLANEOUS RENAL DISORDERS

Pathogenetic mechanisms implicated in 'heroin nephropathy'
1 Nephritis due to contaminants (e.g. lead)
   — Typically focal sclerosing glomerulonephritis
2 Immune-complex mediated nephritis
   — Heroin acting as a hapten
3 Post-infective
   — Staphylococcal bacteremias
   — Hepatitis B
4 Myoglobinuric nephropathy
   — Due to associated rhabdomyolysis

Clinical spectrum of analgesic-related disease
1 General
   — Psychiatric disorder; passive aggression; headaches
   — Premature aging; pigmentation
   — Dementia

2 Anemia
 — Normochromic (often disproportionate to azotemia)
 — Hypochromic (occult gastric bleeding)
 — Megaloblastic (post-gastrectomy)
3 Gastrointestinal symptoms
 — Dyspepsia, esophagitis
 — Gastric ulcer
4 Cardiovascular associations
 — Hypertension (± renovascular component)
 — Ischemic heart disease
5 Renal complications
 — Sterile pyuria, hemoproteinuria
 — Salt-losing nephropathy, nocturia
 — Nephrogenic diabetes insipidus
 — Renal tubular acidosis
 — Renal colic
 — Osteomalacia
 — Ureteric strictures
 — Frequent UTI (esp. *Proteus*)
 — Chronic renal failure
6 Malignancy
 — Transitional cell carcinoma of renal pelvis

Spectrum of heredofamilial renal disease
1 Alport's syndrome (AD)
 — Females are mildly affected; no nerve deafness
 — Associated with
  • Lens abnormalities
  • Platelet dysfunction
  • Hyperprolinemia, cerebral malfunction
 — Does *not* recur after transplantation
2 Fabry's disease (AR; galactosidase A deficiency)
 — Affected females have isolated renal impairment
 — Associated (in affected males) with
  • 'Bathing trunk' punctate spots (angiokeratomas)
  • Corneal dystrophy
  • Ischemic heart disease
  • Acroparesthesiae
3 Nail-patella syndrome (AD)
 — Often presents with nephrotic syndrome

 — 'Moth-eaten' glomerular basement membrane
 — Associated stigmata
  • Dystrophic nails, esp. thumb and index
  • Absent patellae
  • Absent iliac horns on plain pelvic X-ray
4 Cystinosis (AR)
 — Lysosomal storage disease → intracellular cystine excess
  • Fanconi's syndrome, renal failure ~ age 10
  • Dysphagia in adulthood (esophageal dysfunction)
 — Oral cystamine depletes cystine and arrests disease

Retroperitoneal fibrosis: associations and features
1 Etiologic associations (usually idiopathic)
 — Methysergide, dexamphetamine, ergotamine
 — Carcinoma; Crohn's disease
 — Connective tissue disorders, Raynaud's
 — Middle-aged males; HLA-B27
2 Clinical associations
 — Mediastinal fibrosis (→ aortic/caval involvement)
 — Sclerosing cholangitis
 — Fibrosing alveolitis
 — Riedel's thyroiditis
 — Peyronie's disease
 — Pseudotumor oculi
 — Coronary arterial fibrosis
 — Constrictive pericarditis
3 Pathologic features
 — Periaortic inflammation: mononuclear infiltration commencing in lower abdomen/mediastinum
 — Ureters fibrosed, but lumen *not* occluded
4 Radiographic features (IVP)
 — Medial deviation of lower two-thirds of both ureters
5 Therapeutic features
 — May respond dramatically to corticosteroids, *but*
 — Genitourinary TB must first be *actively* excluded

NB: *Sclerosing peritonitis* due to practolol or carcinoid syndrome is a distinct entity

REVIEWING THE LITERATURE: RENAL MEDICINE

12.1 Locatelli F et al (1991) Prospective randomised multicentre trial of effect of protein restriction on progression of chronic renal insufficiency. Lancet 337: 1299–1304

Zeller K et al (1991) Effect of restricting dietary protein on the progression of renal failure in patients with insulin-dependent diabetes mellitus. N Engl J Med 324: 78–84

Two studies with different conclusions: the former offered little support for the hypothesis that protein restriction substantially retards progression of chronic renal failure, whereas the latter study showed that diabetic patients restricted in protein and phosphorus intake experienced significantly slower deterioration of renal function.

12.2 Mathiesen ER et al (1991) Efficacy of captopril in postponing nephropathy in normotensive insulin dependent

diabetic patients with microalbuminuria. Br Med J 303: 81–87

Falk RJ et al (1992) Prevalence and pathologic features of sickle cell nephropathy and response to inhibition of angiotensin-converting enzyme. N Engl J Med 326: 910–915

These two studies are typical of many over the last decade which have demonstrated the benefits of ACE inhibitors in retarding progression of renal disease in diabetes and other nephropathic disorders.

Madhavan S et al (1995) Renal function during antihypertensive treatment. Lancet 345: 749–751

Negative study which failed to confirm a relationship between blood pressure control and renal function, thus keeping alive the controversy.

12.3   Mutti A et al (1992) Nephropathies and exposure to perchloroethylene in dry-cleaners. Lancet 340: 189–193

Staessen JA et al (1992) Impairment of renal function with increasing blood lead concentrations in the general population. N Engl J Med 327: 151–156

Two studies confirming an association between environmental exposure to nephrotoxins and development of renal impairment in individuals without other predisposition to renal disease.

12.4   Hossack KF et al (1988) Echocardiographic findings in autosomal dominant polycystic kidney disease. N Engl J Med 319: 907–912

Patients with adult polycystic kidney disease (and their relatives) had an unexpectedly high incidence of mitral valve prolapse, mitral incompetence, aortic incompetence, tricuspid incompetence and tricuspid valve prolapse, suggesting that the pathophysiology of adult PCK is related to a defect of extracellular matrix production.

12.5   Perneger TV et al (1994) Risk of kidney failure associated with the use of acetaminophen, aspirin, and nonsteroidal antiinflammatory drugs. N Engl J Med 331: 1675–1679

Uremia was significantly associated with chronic ingestion of paracetamol and NSAIDs, but not with aspirin, in this case-control study of 716 patients.

12.6   British Association for Paediatric Nephrology (1991) Levamisole for corticosteroid-dependent nephrotic syndrome in childhood. Lancet 337: 1555–1557

Encouraging study of 61 steroid-dependent children, showing more than 3-fold increase in the number of prolonged remissions following addition of alternate-day levamisole to a tapering steroid regimen.

12.7   Goldstein AR et al (1992) Long-term follow-up of childhood Henoch–Schönlein nephritis. Lancet 339: 280–282

Study of 78 HSP patients showing that hypertension and/or renal impairment affected 44% of those presenting 23 years earlier with proteinuria or nephritis, while pregnancy-associated hypertension/proteinuria was common even in those presenting with hematuria alone.

12.8   van der Heide J et al (1993) Effect of dietary fish oil on renal function and rejection in cyclosporine-treated recipients of renal transplants. N Engl J Med 329: 769–773

Donadio JV et al (1994) A controlled trial of fish oil in IgA nephropathy. N Engl J Med 331: 1194–1199

Two more testaments to the benefits of fish oil, one for preventing transplant rejection and the other for slowing IgA nephropathy.

12.9   Rosenlof K et al (1990) Erythropoietin, aluminium, and anaemia in patients on haemodialysis. Lancet 335: 247–249

Salusky IB et al (1991) Aluminum accumulation during treatment with aluminum hydroxide and dialysis in children and young adults with chronic renal disease. N Engl J Med 324: 527–531

The first study suggested that aluminium antagonizes erythropoietin action by interfering with haem synthesis; while the second indicated that calcium carbonate is superior to aluminium hydroxide in preventing phosphate retention and osteodystrophy.

12.10   Jardin A et al (1991) Alfuzosin for treatment of benign prostatic hypertrophy. Lancet 337: 1457–1461

While this and other studies have suggested a symptomatic benefit from α-blockers in BPH, the most significant finding of this report may have been the very significant symptomatic improvement seen with prescription of placebo.

CHAPTER 13

Respiratory medicine

Physical examination protocol 13.1 You are asked to examine the respiratory system

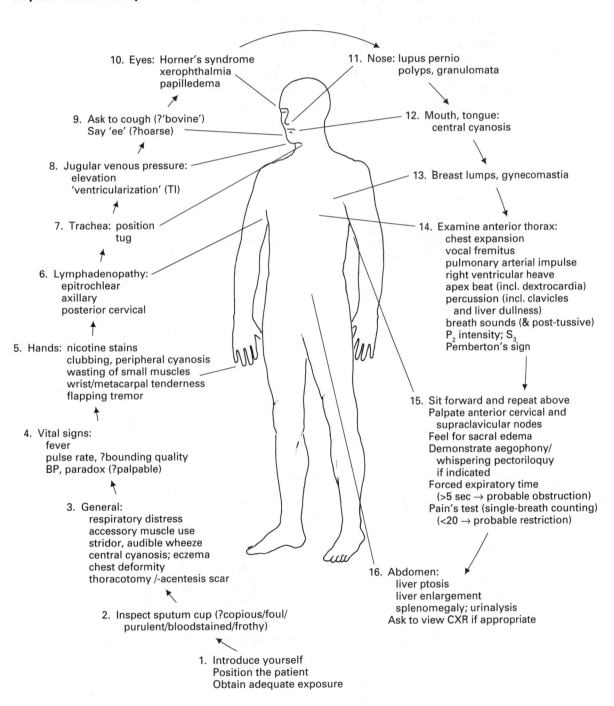

10. Eyes: Horner's syndrome
    xerophthalmia
    papilledema

11. Nose: lupus pernio
    polyps, granulomata

9. Ask to cough (?'bovine')
   Say 'ee' (?hoarse)

12. Mouth, tongue:
    central cyanosis

8. Jugular venous pressure:
   elevation
   'ventricularization' (TI)

13. Breast lumps, gynecomastia

7. Trachea: position
   tug

14. Examine anterior thorax:
    chest expansion
    vocal fremitus
    pulmonary arterial impulse
    right ventricular heave
    apex beat (incl. dextrocardia)
    percussion (incl. clavicles
        and liver dullness)
    breath sounds (& post-tussive)
    P_2 intensity; S_3
    Pemberton's sign

6. Lymphadenopathy:
   epitrochlear
   axillary
   posterior cervical

5. Hands: nicotine stains
   clubbing, peripheral cyanosis
   wasting of small muscles
   wrist/metacarpal tenderness
   flapping tremor

15. Sit forward and repeat above
    Palpate anterior cervical and
        supraclavicular nodes
    Feel for sacral edema
    Demonstrate aegophony/
        whispering pectoriloquy
        if indicated
    Forced expiratory time
        (>5 sec → probable obstruction)
    Pain's test (single-breath counting)
        (<20 → probable restriction)

4. Vital signs:
   fever
   pulse rate, ?bounding quality
   BP, paradox (?palpable)

3. General:
   respiratory distress
   accessory muscle use
   stridor, audible wheeze
   central cyanosis; eczema
   chest deformity
   thoracotomy /-acentesis scar

16. Abdomen:
    liver ptosis
    liver enlargement
    splenomegaly; urinalysis
    Ask to view CXR if appropriate

2. Inspect sputum cup (?copious/foul/
   purulent/bloodstained/frothy)

1. Introduce yourself
   Position the patient
   Obtain adequate exposure

Diagnostic pathway 13.1 This patient is breathless. Why do you think that might be?

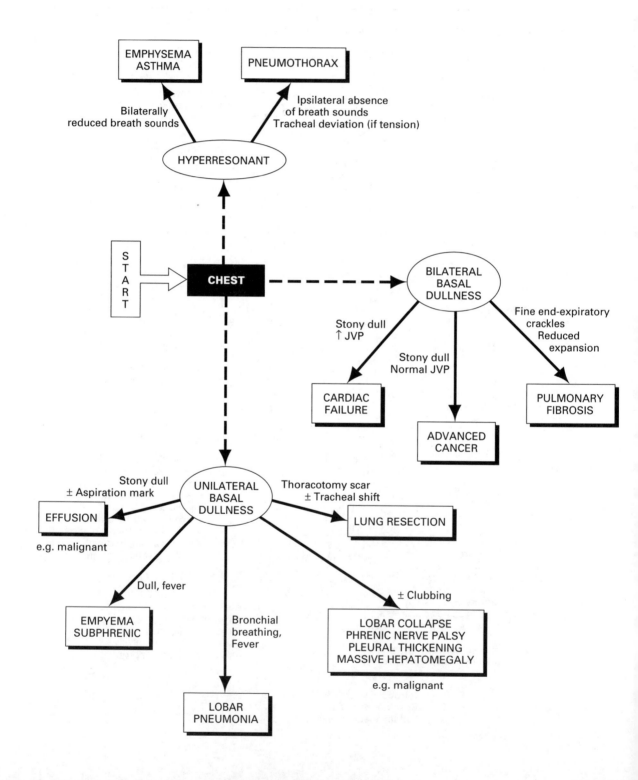

CLINICAL ASPECTS OF RESPIRATORY DISEASE

Commonest respiratory short cases
1 Pleural effusion
2 Chronic obstructive airways disease (± cor pulmonale)
3 Lobar consolidation

DYSPNEA

Grading of exertional dyspnea by clinical history: MRC criteria
1 Grade I
   — Breathless hurrying on level ground or walking uphill
2 Grade II
   — Breathless walking flat with people of one's own age
3 Grade III
   — Breathless enough to stop walking at one's own pace

Dyspnea: typical rates of onset
1 Maximal within seconds
   — Pneumothorax
   — Pulmonary embolism*
2 Maximal within hours
   — Asthma
   — Hypersensitivity pneumonitis
   — Pneumonia
   — Cardiac failure
   — Hemorrhage
3 Maximal within days to months
   — Progressive anemia (any cause)
   — Progression of restrictive lung disease
   — Exacerbation of obstructive airways disease
   — Enlarging pleural effusion(s)
   — Primary or secondary malignancy

* Symptoms will worsen, perhaps gradually, with subsequent emboli; hence, small emboli may *not* be associated with rapid symptom onset

'Blue bloater' or 'pink puffer'? Features favoring the latter*
1 Severe subjective dyspnea
2 Scanty sputum, few infections
3 CXR: hyperlucent lungs, 'thin' heart
4 $PaCO_2 < 40$ mmHg
   $PaO_2 > 60$ mmHg
5 Hematocrit not elevated
6 No signs of pulmonary hypertension or cor pulmonale

* i.e. features suggesting dominant emphysema rather than chronic bronchitis

PRESENTATIONS OF RESPIRATORY DISEASE

Differential diagnosis of recurrent hemoptysis
1 Bronchiectasis; chronic bronchitis

2 Bronchial adenoma
3 Mitral stenosis; recurrent left ventricular failure
4 Recurrent pulmonary embolism with infarction
5 Telangiectasia (arteriovenous malformation)

Predispositions to recurrent lower respiratory tract infections
1 Hypogammaglobulinemia
2 Ciliary dysfunction
   — Cystic fibrosis
   — Immotile cilia syndrome
   — Pulmonary alveolar proteinosis
   — Bronchiectasis
3 Autoimmune disease
   — Sjögren's syndrome
   — Relapsing polychondritis
4 Esophageal disease
   — Achalasia
   — Scleroderma
   — Riley–Day syndrome
   — Pharyngeal pouch
5 Cardiovascular disease
   — Atrial septal defect
   — Mitral stenosis
   — Pulmonary emboli

Lifestyle clues to unusual lung infections
1 Bird fanciers
   — Psittacosis
2 Abattoir or farm workers
   — Brucellosis
   — Q fever (*Coxiella burneti*)
3 Florists, gardeners
   — Sporotrichosis (from rose thorns)
4 Camping enthusiasts
   — Tularemia
5 Wool classers, leather workers
   — Anthrax

Diagnostic considerations in refractory pneumonia
1 Wrong antibiotics
2 Multiple or unusual organisms
3 Immunosuppressed patient (e.g. myeloma, AIDS, transplant)
4 Empyema/abscess formation
5 Recurrent aspiration (e.g. pharyngeal pouch)
6 Proximal endobronchial neoplasm
7 Misdiagnosis
   — Lymphoma, alveolar cell carcinoma
   — Pulmonary infarction/hemorrhage
   — Adult respiratory distress syndrome
   — Hypersensitivity pneumonitis
   — Pulmonary eosinophilia
   — Pulmonary edema
   — Iatrogenic (incl. antibiotic) reaction

Differential diagnosis of unexplained pleuritic pain
1 **P**leurodynia (Bornholm's disease, epidemic myalgia)
2 **P**neumonia
3 **P**neumothorax
4 **P**ulmonary infarction
5 **P**ericarditis
6 (Sub)**p**hrenic abscess
7 **P**ancreatitis
8 **P**athologic rib fracture

CLINICAL SIGNS OF RESPIRATORY DISEASE

Diagnostic clues from sputum examination
1 Copious, purulent, pungent
   — Bronchiectasis, lung abscess
2 Copious, pink, frothy
   — Acute left ventricular failure
3 Copious, clear, watery
   — Alveolar cell carcinoma
4 Rubbery brown plugs
   — Allergic bronchopulmonary aspergillosis
5 'Anchovy sauce'
   — Amebic abscess
6 Melanoptysis (jet-black fibrotic particles)
   — Pneumoconiosis with progressive massive fibrosis
7 'Blood oyster' (blood within mucopurulent sputum)
   — TB
8 Rusty staining of mucoid sputum
   — Early pneumococcal pneumonia

Clinical components of clubbing
1 Soft tissue swelling
2 Loss of nailfold angle (> 150°)
3 Exaggerated curvature of long axis of nail
4 Increased nailbed fluctuation ('boggy') on pressure
5 May be associated with wrist metacarpal tenderness (HPO)

Differential diagnosis of basal crackles with clubbing
1 Bronchiectasis
   — Coarse crackles (may be unilateral)
2 Asbestosis; idiopathic fibrosing alveolitis
   — Bibasilar fine end-inspiratory crackles

Clinical significance of basal dullness
1 'Stony' dullness
   — Pleural effusion
2 'Non-stony' dullness
   — Loss of aeration (consolidation, abscess)
   — Loss of lung volume (collapse, severe fibrosis)

Examination of the patient with bronchiectasis
1 Copious purulent sputum (foul-smelling? Anaerobic)
2 Clubbing, coarse crackles
3 Nasal discharge and/or polyps
4 Dextrocardia
5 Hepatosplenomegaly; enlarged kidneys
   — Indicative of secondary (reactive) amyloidosis

Causes of hepatomegaly in respiratory disease
1 Chronic venous congestion
   — In cor pulmonale
2 Metastatic liver disease
   — In lung cancer
3 Spurious (ptosed liver)
   — In emphysema

Peripheral edema: pathogenesis in respiratory disease
1 Right ventricular failure
2 Sequelae of chronic systemic venous congestion
   — 'Cardiac cirrhosis'
   — Protein-losing enteropathy
   — Nephrosis

3 Membranous nephropathy (paraneoplastic)
4 Yellow nail syndrome (lymphedema)
5 Fluid retention due to corticosteroid administration

OBSTRUCTIVE SLEEP APNEA

Sleep apnea: presenting complaints
1 Snoring (in obstructive variety); insomnia
   Nocturnal choking and/or panic attacks
   Hypnagogic hallucinations; nightmares
2 Disorientation after waking
   Excessive daytime somnolence (→ car accidents)
3 Morning headaches (CO_2 retention)
4 Depression, personality change
5 Impotence; nocturnal enuresis; reduced libido
6 Related to etiology, e.g. myxedema, acromegaly

Complications of sleep apnea
1 Systemic hypertension*
   — Present in 70%
2 Left ventricular disease
   — Left ventricular hypertrophy
   — Dilated cardiomyopathy
3 Ischemic heart disease
   — Myocardial infarction
   — Nocturnal cardiac arrhythmias (incl. bradycardia)
   — Unexpected death during sleep
4 Secondary cardiovascular sequelae
   — Pulmonary hypertension
   — Cor pulmonale (40%)
   — Polycythemia
5 Respiratory sequelae
   — Impaired (diurnal) pulmonary function (70%)
   — Respiratory failure

* Due to increased sympathetic activity

INVESTIGATING RESPIRATORY DISEASE

Electrophoretographic clues in respiratory diagnosis
1 α_1 pallor
   — Emphysema due to α_1AT deficiency
2 Hypogammaglobulinemia
   — May underlie chronic bronchitis
3 Polyclonal gammopathy
   — Sarcoidosis (inter alia)

Diagnosis of α_1-antitrypsin deficiency
1 Family history of emphysema or childhood liver disease*
2 Emphysema in a young patient (< 40 years) or non-smoker‡
3 *Basal* hyperlucency on CXR
4 Panacinar (panlobular) emphysema on lung biopsy
5 α_1 pallor on electrophoresis
   ↓ α_1AT levels on quantitative assay

* Neonatal hepatitis ± infantile cirrhosis
‡ Rarely may present with mesangiocapillary glomerulonephritis

Sputum microscopy in atopic asthma: features
1 Eosinophils

2   Charcot–Leyden crystals (eosinophil derivatives)
3   Creola bodies (clumps of bronchiolar epithelial cells)
4   Curschmann's spirals (bronchiolar casts)

Differential diagnosis of pulmonary eosinophilia*
1   Allergic bronchopulmonary aspergillosis (ABPA; p. 334)
2   Vasculitis
    — PAN
    — Churg–Strauss syndrome
3   Hypereosinophilic syndrome
4   Tropical eosinophilia
    — Filariasis
5   Löffler's syndrome (in temperate zones)
    — Helminth infestation
6   Drug reactions

* Lung infiltrates on CXR and eosinophil count $> 0.5 \times 10^9$/L

TESTING LUNG FUNCTION

Lung function tests: typical disease patterns
1   Obstructive airways disease
    — ↑ Residual volume (RV)
    — ↓ FEV_1/VC (< 70%)
    — ↑↑ RV/TLC (total lung capacity)
2   Restrictive lung disease
    — ↓ RV, VC, TLC
    — N, ↑ FEV_1/VC
    — N, ↑ RV/TLC

NB: VC and TLC may be normal in 'pure' emphysema

Lung function monitors in large airway disease
1   FEV_1 /VC
2   PEFR (peak expiratory flow rate)
3   V_{max} (density-dependence of maximal expiratory flow)
4   Airways resistance

Lung function monitors in small airway disease*
1   Maximal mid-expiratory flow rate (MMFR)
    — At 50% and 25% VC
2   Single-breath nitrogen washout studies
    — Slope of phase III
3   Closing volume
4   Flow-volume curves
    — Also useful in extrathoracic obstruction
5   Frequency-dependence of dynamic compliance
    — Most sensitive test, but esophageal balloon required
6   Other tests
    — $V_{max\,50}$
    — ↑ RV
    — ↓ $FEV_{3.0}$
    — ↓ DL_{CO}
    — Postural changes in PaO_2

* e.g. subclinical lung dysfunction in smokers with normal FEV_1

Abnormalities of the peak expiratory flow rate (PEFR)
1   Reduced
    — Obstructive airways disease (e.g. asthma)
    — Respiratory muscle weakness
    — Poor technique

2   Normal or increased
    — Restrictive lung disease (e.g. fibrosis)

Indicators of reversible obstruction on lung function testing
1   Post-bronchodilator increase in FEV_1 > 200 mL
2   Post-bronchodilator increase in PEFR > 60 L/min*

* NB: Lesser improvements do *not* preclude a therapeutic trial of bronchodilators or steroids if clinical suspicion of 'asthma' remains

ARTERIAL BLOOD GAS ANALYSIS

Diagnostic scenarios for arterial blood gas measurement
1   Suspected sedative overdose
2   Suspected CO_2 narcosis in 'blue bloater'
3   Suspected pulmonary embolism
4   Assessment of severe asthma
5   Suspected surreptitious vomiting*

* Associated with metabolic alkalosis

Clues to the interpretation of arterial blood gases
1   ↓ PaO_2 normalizing on 100% oxygen; > PaO_2
    — Alveolar hypoventilation (overdose, Guillain–Barré)
2   ↓ PaO_2 normalizing on 100% oxygen; normal or low $PaCO_2$
    — V/Q mismatch*
3   ↓ PaO_2 *not* correcting with 100% oxygen; normal $PaCO_2$
    — Shunting (intrapulmonary *or* intracardiac)
4   Normal or slightly reduced PaO_2; ↓↓ PaO_2 on exercise, normalizing with 100% oxygen; normal or low $PaCO_2$
    — Diffusion defect (rare)
    — Altitude
5   PaO_2 < 60 mmHg, $PaCO_2$ > 45 mmHg
    — Inadvertent venous (non-arterial) blood sample

* NB: *Severe* mismatching may cause ↑ $PaCO_2$

Significance of increased alveolar-arterial (A-a) oxygen gradient*
1   Ventilation/perfusion mismatching, e.g.
    — Airways obstruction
    — Pulmonary embolism
2   Shunt
    — Intrapulmonary (e.g. ARDS, pulmonary edema)
    — Intracardiac (e.g. Eisenmenger's syndrome)
3   Diffusion defect‡

* PaO_2/R, where R = 0.8 normally; normal A-a gradient < 15 mmHg
‡ Only *minor* contribution to pathophysiology of fibrotic and emphysematous lung disease; V/Q mismatch is more important

Tissue hypoxia with normal cardiorespiratory capacity
1   Hypoxemia despite normal A-a gradient
    — Alveolar hypoventilation
    — ↓ FiO_2 (e.g. altitude)
2   Normal PaO_2 with increased oxyhemoglobin affinity
    — Massive stored blood transfusion (↑ citrate → ↓ 2,3DPG)

— Bicarbonate administration in ketoacidosis
— Profound hypothermia/acidemia/hypophosphatemia
— Myxedema
— High-affinity Hb (e.g. Köln, Chesapeake)
— Carbon monoxide poisoning
3 Cyanide intoxication
4 Hyperviscosity
5 Anemia

Acid-base disturbances in respiratory disease

1 Acute respiratory acidosis (ventilatory failure)
— 10 mmHg $\uparrow$ $PaCO_2 \rightarrow$ 1 mEq/L $\uparrow$ HCO_3^- (tissue buffer)
2 Chronic respiratory acidosis (incl. 'acute-on-chronic' exacerbations, e.g. of chronic bronchitis)
— 10 mmHg $\uparrow$ $PaCO_2 \rightarrow$ 3 mEq/L $\uparrow$ HCO_3^- ($\uparrow$ renal reabsorption of HCO_3^- and $\uparrow$ acid excretion)
— High base excess
3 Acute respiratory alkalosis (e.g. secondary to ketoacidosis)
— 10 mmHg $\downarrow$ $PaCO_2 \rightarrow$ 2 mEq/L $\uparrow$ HCO_3^-
4 Chronic respiratory alkalosis (e.g. 'pink puffer')
— 10 mmHg $\downarrow$ $PaCO_2 \rightarrow$ 5 mEq/L $\downarrow$ HCO_3^-
— *Rarely* does bicarbonate level drop to < 15 mmol/L

Clinical manifestations of carbon dioxide retention

1 $PaCO_2$ > 80 mmHg
— Progressive impairment of consciousness
— Central cyanosis seen at rest *if* Hb O_2 saturation < 85%
2 Neurological
— Flapping tremor
— Hyporeflexia; muscle twitching
— Headache
3 Vascular
— Hypertension
— Bounding pulse
— Warm extremities (cf. peripheral cyanosis), sweating
— Edema, tender pulsatile liver if cor pulmonale present
4 Ocular
— Miosis
— Retinal vein distension
— Papilledema
5 $PaCO_2$ > 120 mmHg
— Extensor plantar responses
— Coma

Clinical significance of central cyanosis

1 Alveolar hypoventilation (type II respiratory failure)
— e.g. Sedative overdose
2 Right-to-left shunting
— i.e. $\uparrow$ FiO_2 fails to cause $\uparrow$ PaO_2
3 Mechanical
— Superior vena caval obstruction
4 Normal PaO_2
— Polycythemia vera
— Low-affinity Hb (e.g. Kansas, Hammersmith)
5 *Severe* V/Q mismatching (type I respiratory failure)
— e.g. Massive pulmonary embolism

SLEEP STUDIES

Indications for sleep studies

1 Suspected sleep apnea (p. 326)
— Loud snoring plus daytime somnolence
— Cor pulmonale, central cyanosis
— Observed apneas
2 Unexplained progressive clinical deterioration in a patient with chronic obstructive airways disease

Measurements made during sleep studies

1 Measurement of sleep stages ($\geq$ 3 h sleep required)
— EEG (p. 269)
— Submental EMG
— Bilateral electrooculograms*
2 Airflow measurement
— Nasal/oral thermistors
— CO_2 sensor or pneumotachography
— Airway pressure (CPAP‡ study)
3 Respiratory effort measurement
— Chest/abdominal strain gauges
— Surface EMG of respiratory muscles
— Esophageal balloon (pleural pressure changes)
4 Arterial blood gases
— Skin oximetry
— Transcutaneous CO_2 electrodes
5 ECG (single lead)
— Detects rate/rhythm disturbances linked to apnea

* To detect bilateral conjugate eye movements during REM sleep
‡ Continuous positive airways pressure

RESTRICTIVE LUNG DISEASE

Lung function monitors in restrictive lung disease

1 Post-exercise A-a (alveolar-arterial oxygen) gradient, *or* Hb O_2 desaturation
2 DL_{CO}
3 Static compliance
4 VC, TLC (e.g. in myasthenia gravis)

Additional disease monitors in fibrosing alveolitis

1 Cellularity of bronchoalveolar lavage (see below)
2 [67]Gallium scanning (macrophage uptake; semi-quantitative)
3 Transbronchial biopsy (restricted to initial diagnosis)

Conditions affecting measurement of diffusing capacity

1 $\uparrow$ DL_{CO}
— Alveolar hemorrhage (Hb sequestered in alveolae)
• Goodpasture's syndrome (if *recent* bleed)
• Idiopathic pulmonary hemosiderosis
• Mitral stenosis
— Acute asthma (hyperinflation)
— Physiological
• High-output states: exercise, altitude
• Supine position
— Polycythemia
2 $\downarrow$ DL_{CO}
— Pulmonary fibrosis (restrictive lung disease), e.g.
• Asbestosis

- Sarcoidosis
- Fibrosing alveolitis
- Connective tissue diseases, PAN
— Severe V/Q mismatching
- Emphysema
- Pulmonary embolism
- Pneumonectomy
— Smoking (↑ carboxyhemoglobin)
— Anemia*

* NB: May complicate alveolar hemorrhagic states

BRONCHOALVEOLAR LAVAGE (BAL)

Indications for bronchoalveolar lavage
1 Diagnostic (saline) lavage
   — Opportunistic infections
   — Alveolar hemorrhagic syndromes
   — Alveolar proteinosis
   — Dust diseases, e.g. asbestosis
   — Histiocytosis X
2 Prognostic lavage
   — Fibrosing alveolitis
   — Sarcoidosis
   — Hypersensitivity pneumonitis
   — ARDS
   — Drug-induced lung disease
3 Therapeutic (heparin/acetylcysteine) lavage
   — Pulmonary alveolar proteinosis
   — Cystic fibrosis/bronchiectasis
   — Asthma with mucus plugging

Normal composition of BAL fluid
1 Total leukocyte count
   — Non-smokers: 5–10 x 10^6/µL
   — Smokers: 20–50 x 10^6/µL
2 Leukocyte differential
   — Macrophages
     - 80–90% (non-smokers)
     - 95% (smokers)
   — Lymphocytes
     - 5–15% (non-smokers)
     - 1–10% (smokers)
   — Neutrophils
     - 0–2% (non-smokers)
     - 2–5% (smokers)
   — Eosinophils: < 1%
3 T cell subsets
   — Helpers* (T_H, CD4+) ~ 50%
   — Suppressors (T_S, CD8+) ~ 30%
   — Killers ~ 5–10%
   — B cells, plasma cells ~ 5–10%
   — Null cells ~ 5%

* cf. bronchoalveolar T_{H2} lymphocytes: normal number, but functionally activated in atopic asthma

Lymphocytosis vs granulocytosis on BAL?
1 Predominant lymphocytosis
   — Sarcoidosis (unless chronic)
   — Hypersensitivity pneumonitis
   — Berylliosis, silicosis
   — Tuberculosis

   — Sjögren's syndrome
   — Drug-induced lung disease
2 Predominant granulocytosis
   — Cryptogenic fibrosing alveolitis*
   — ARDS
   — Bacterial infection
   — Asbestosis
   — Scleroderma, rheumatoid arthritis

* More responsive subtypes may be associated with lymphocytosis (see below)

BAL cell counts in disease
1 Smokers
   — Overall increase in cellularity (up to 5-fold)
   — Reduced number of activated T cells
   — Reduced function of macrophages and lymphocytes
2 Fibrosing alveolitis
   — Increased neutrophils (5–50%) in active disease
   — Worse if > 10% neutrophils (esp. if + ^{67}Ga scan)
   — Prognosis better *if* lymphocytosis (> 25%) present
3 Sarcoidosis
   — Lymphocytosis (up to 40%)
   — May be predictive of steroid responsiveness
   — Marked excess of T_H cells* indicates poor prognosis
   — Neutrophil excess associated with advanced disease
4 Hypersensitivity pneumonitis
   — Lymphocytosis (cf. fibrosing alveolitis)
5 Histiocytosis X
   — Histiocytosis X cells (containing 'X bodies')
   — Cholesterol-laden macrophages ('foam cells')
6 Eosinophilic pneumonia
   — Eosinophils
7 Drug-induced lung disease
   — Lymphocytosis, macrophages
8 Chronic lipoid pneumonia
   — Fat globules in macrophages
9 Asbestosis
   — Ferruginous bodies
10 Alveolar proteinosis
   — PAS-positive alveolar cell lipoprotein

* cf. peripheral blood: lymphopenia, relative excess of suppressor T cells

Therapeutic significance of BAL counts in fibrosing alveolitis
1 Lymphocytosis
   — Better response to steroids
2 Neutrophil/eosinophil granulocytosis
   — Worse response to steroids
   — Better response to cyclophosphamide

BRONCHOSCOPY

Indications for bronchoscopy
1 Rigid (under general anesthesia)
   — Removal of foreign body
   — Therapeutic lavage
   — Large biopsy required

2 Fiberoptic
   — CXR suggesting primary endobronchial neoplasm
   — Hemoptysis and/or positive sputum cytology
   — Assessment of stridor or localized wheeze
   — Unexplained diffuse lung disease or CXR opacities
   — Diagnosis of suspected opportunistic (e.g. invasive fungal) infection, esp. if immuno-suppressed

Contraindications to bronchoscopy
1 Severe hypoxemia (any cause, esp. respiratory)
2 Severe asthma
3 Severe pulmonary hypertension
4 Severe hemoptysis
5 Cardiovascular instability (e.g. recent infarct)
6 Hepatitis B, HIV infection or untreated TB
7 Unavailability of experienced bronchoscopist

Contraindications to transbronchial biopsy
1 Coagulopathy
2 Uremia
3 PEEP

NB: SVC obstruction is *not* generally regarded as a contraindication to bronchoscopic biopsy

Diagnostic significance of lung granulomata
1 Infection
   — Caseating
     • Tuberculosis
     • Some atypical mycobacteria
   — Non-caseating
     • Histoplasmosis, other fungi
2 Hypersensitivity
   — Sarcoidosis
   — Hypersensitivity pneumonitis
   — Berylliosis
3 Vasculitis
   — Wegener's granulomatosis
   — Churg–Strauss syndrome*
4 Neoplasm
   — Histiocytosis X (p. 235)
   — Lethal midline granuloma
   — Lymphomatoid granulomatosis

* Associated with peri- or extravascular granulomata

Indications for bronchography in suspected bronchiectasis*
1 Prerequisite
   — Potentially operable (i.e. fit) patient
2 Severe symptoms
   — Recurrent localized pneumonia
   — Severe hemoptysis
3 Unavailability of high-resolution CT (p. 332)

* i.e. as work-up for possible surgery

PLEURAL DISEASE

Diagnostic aspects of pleural effusions
1 Transudate (< 30 g/L protein; often bilateral)
   — Cardiac failure, constrictive pericarditis
   — Cirrhosis, nephrosis
   — Myxedema
   — Meigs' syndrome (i.e. transudate and/or peripheral edema suggest that local pathology is unlikely)
2 Uniformly bloodstained effusion
   — Metastatic carcinoma (i.e. to pleura)
   — Pulmonary infarction
   — Primary TB (parapneumonic effusion)
3 Chylous effusion (positive Sudan III stain)
   — Trauma (esp. endoscopy or surgery)
   — Lymphomas
   — Other masses compressing the thoracic duct
   — Nephrosis, cirrhosis (uncommon)
   — Spurious ('pseudochylous' effusions due to cholesterol in TB/rheumatoid effusions; Sudan III negative)
4 Elevated amylase
   — Esophageal perforation (salivary isoenzyme)
   — Pancreatitis
5 Low glucose
   — Rheumatoid arthritis
   — Empyema formation in parapneumonic effusion
6 pH
   — < 6.0: esophageal rupture
   — < 7.2: implies empyema, hence need for thoracostomy

Possible indications for pleural biopsy
1 Suspected tuberculosis (biopsy should be cultured)
2 Suspected malignant pleural effusion; cytology negative
3 Suspected granulomatous disorder

RADIOGRAPHIC DIAGNOSIS OF LUNG DISEASE

Upper zone CXR infiltrates: differential diagnosis
1 Infection
   — Tuberculosis
   — Aspergillosis
   — *Klebsiella* pneumonia
2 Fibrosis
   — Silicosis
   — Radiation fibrosis
   — Ankylosing spondylitis
   — Hypersensitivity pneumonitis (long-standing)
3 Histiocytosis X

Lower zone CXR infiltrates: differential diagnosis
1 Idiopathic pulmonary fibrosis
2 Pulmonary fibrosis due to connective tissue disease
3 Asbestosis
4 Bronchiectasis
5 Cytotoxic-induced lung disease
6 Pulmonary hemosiderosis
7 Aspiration
8 Hypersensitivity pneumonitis (acute)

Radiographic localization of mediastinal masses
1 Superior mediastinum
   — Thymoma
   — Retrosternal thyroid
   — Zenker's diverticulum

2 Anterior/middle
— Dermoid cyst/teratoma
— Bronchogenic/pericardial cyst
— Morgagni diaphragmatic hernia
— Sarcoidosis
3 Posterior
— Neurogenic tumors (and other paravertebral masses)
— Bochdalek diaphragmatic hernia (cf. Morgagni)
— Achalasia, hiatus hernia (may also be in middle)
4 Any mediastinal compartment
— Aortic aneurysm (usually middle)
— Lymphoma, teratoma (usually anterior)
— Metastatic carcinoma (usually middle)

Indications for special CXR projections
1 (Lateral) decubitus
— Suspected small pleural effusion, esp. if subpulmonic
2 Expiratory
— Suspected pneumothorax
— Suspected bronchial occlusion (? inhaled foreign body)
3 Erect
— Suspected perforation of abdominal hollow viscus
4 Penetrated PA
— Suspected left atrial enlargement
— Suspected left lower lobe collapse
5 Oblique
— Visualization of pleural plaques
— Suspected rib fracture(s)
6 Apical lordotic
— Visualization of lesions in lung apex

Differential diagnosis of unilateral hemithorax transradiancy
1 Pneumothorax
2 Mastectomy
3 Pulmonary embolism
4 Emphysematous bullae
5 Macleod's syndrome, Swyer–James

Significance of the apparently elevated hemidiaphragm
1 Phrenic nerve palsy
2 Segmental/lobar collapse (→ tracheal deviation) or resection
3 Subpulmonic effusion (decubitus film → diagnosis)
4 Subphrenic collection
5 Massive hepatomegaly
6 Diaphragmatic rupture (e.g. post-traumatic) or dysfunction (e.g. herpes zoster affecting C4 nerve root)

Interstitial vs alveolar infiltrates
1 Interstitial ('honeycombing,' e.g. sarcoidosis)
— 'Ground glass' appearance (e.g. asbestosis, berylliosis)
— Reticular appearance (e.g. pulmonary fibrosis)
— Nodular (e.g. histoplasmosis, pneumoconiosis)
2 Alveolar (e.g. pulmonary edema, pneumonia)
— Fluffy opacities
— Air bronchograms
— Lobar or segmental distribution
— Rapid evolution

Clinically important causes of 'honeycomb lung'
1 Cryptogenic fibrosing alveolitis
2 Granulomatous lung diseases
— Sarcoidosis
— Histiocytosis X
— Hypersensitivity pneumonitis (long-standing)
3 Vasculitis
— Scleroderma
— Rheumatoid arthritis (± effusion)
4 Dust diseases
— Organic dusts
• Hypersensitivity pneumonitis
— Inorganic dusts
• Pneumoconiosis; silicosis; berylliosis
• Asbestosis (± 'holly-leaf' pleural plaques)
5 Neoplasia
— Lymphangitis carcinomatosa
— Alveolar cell carcinoma

Clinically important causes of bilateral hilar adenopathy
1 Sarcoidosis
— Typically symmetrical lymphadenopathy
— Patient usually looks well
2 Lymphoma
— Typically asymmetrical lymphadenopathy
— Patient often looks ill
3 Unusual causes
— TB, fungal infections
— Carcinomatosis

Differential diagnosis of hilar calcification
1 TB
2 Silicosis ('egg-shell' appearance)
3 Histoplasmosis

Disseminated interstitial nodules: differential diagnosis
1 Previous varicella pneumonia, esp. if adult-onset
2 Histoplasmosis; hydatid disease
3 Miliary TB
4 Mitral stenosis
— Microlithiasis due to 2° pulmonary hemosiderosis
5 Malignancy
— Metastases, e.g. from germ-cell primary
— Lymphangitis carcinomatosa
— Bronchoalveolar cell carcinoma
6 Sarcoidosis, pneumoconiosis, Caplan's syndrome

Common causes of pulmonary cavitation
1 Infection
— TB
— Anaerobes (± aspiration)
— *Klebsiella pneumoniae, Staph. aureus*
— Pneumococcal (serotype 3)
— Invasive aspergillosis, nocardiosis, actinomycosis, histoplasmosis, coccidioidomycosis, blastomycosis
— Amebiasis
2 Pulmonary infarction
— Septic emboli
— Bland emboli (with secondary infection)
— Vasculitis (e.g. PAN, Wegener's)
3 Malignancy

Radiographic pointers to bacterial diagnosis of pneumonia
1 Lobar consolidation with pleural effusion
— Pneumococcus
2 'Bulging' fissure
— *Klebsiella* (classical)
— Pneumococcus (common)
3 Periosteal reaction
— *Actinomyces* spp.
4 Superior segment of right lower lobe involved
— Aspiration
5 Right middle lobe collapse/consolidation
— Malignancy

Investigation of bronchiectasis
1 CXR
— 'Tramline' bronchial thickening
— Dextrocardia (Kartagener's)
2 High-resolution lung CT
— If available
3 Bronchography, *if*
— Severe hemoptysis
— Recurrent localized pneumonia
— Optimization of postural drainage required
— Lobectomy being considered in fit young patient
4 Etiology
— Sweat test, immunoglobulins (in children)
— Nasal biopsy for electron microscopy (immotile cilia)
— AFBs; *Aspergillus* precipitins/skin test
5 Complications
— Sputum culture (for *Staph aureus*, *Ps. aeruginosa*)
— Protein electrophoresis; biopsy (for amyloid)

Radiographic features of miscellaneous disorders
1 Asbestosis
— Calcified pleural plaques (esp. diaphragmatic)
— Bibasilar interstitial fibrosis
— 'Shaggy' pericardial silhouette
2 Pulmonary infarction
— Usually normal
— Area(s) of linear atelectasis
— (Small) pleural effusion(s)
— Wedgeshaped peripheral lesion(s), apex towards hilum
— Elevated hemidiaphragm (if collapse)
— Enlarged pulmonary artery, reduced peripheral vascular caliber
3 Emphysema
— Hyperinflation (DD_x = asthma)
• Hyperlucent lungfields ('black lungs')
• 'Flat' low hemidiaphragms
• Visible 11th rib
• Small, narrow heart shadow
— Bullae
— Pulmonary artery > 2 cm (pulmonary hypertension)

Potential indications for high-resolution chest CT
1 Diagnosis of diffuse infiltrative lung disease
— Diagnostic sensitivity of 95%*
— Distinguishes
• Sarcoidosis
• Pulmonary fibrosis (fibrosing alveolitis)
• Lymphangitis carcinomatosa

• Lymphangioleiomyomatosis
• Hypersensitivity pneumonitis
• Histiocytosis X (p. 235)
2 Prognosis and follow-up of diffuse infiltrative lung disease
— Quantifies severity
— Distinguishes active from irreversible fibrosis
— Useful for monitoring therapy‡
3 Early diagnosis of CXR-negative disorders, e.g. in AIDS
— *P. carinii* pneumonia
— Invasive aspergillosis
— Pulmonary Kaposi's
4 Non-invasive diagnosis
— Bronchiectasis (supplants bronchography)
— Suspected radiation pneumonitis
— Suspected drug-induced lung diseases
— Emphysema (if firm diagnosis needed)

* i.e. with 100% sensitivity for biopsy; CXR is only 80%
‡ e.g. steroids for fibrosing alveolitis

Indications for invasive diagnosis of pulmonary infiltrates
1 Percutaneous needle aspiration
— Cavitating infiltrates
— Peripheral infiltrates
2 Bronchoscopy
— Infiltrate of presumed infective etiology
— Infiltrate of presumed neoplastic etiology
3 Bronchoalveolar lavage
— Presumed opportunistic infection*
— Cytology of peripheral infiltrates
4 Open lung biopsy: histopathology required, e.g.
— Drug-induced lung fibrosis
— Radiation pneumonitis

* May also require open lung biopsy

MANAGING RESPIRATORY DISEASE

ASTHMA

Unexpected death in acute asthma: risk factors
1 Recent discharge from hospital
2 Overdependence on inhaled sympathomimetics
   Underutilization of systemic steroids
3 Inadequate monitoring of lung function at night
4 Intravenous administration of aminophylline in patients already receiving maintenance oral theophylline

Considerations in assessing asthma severity
1 Patient's assessment of severity
   Request for admission by patient or family
2 Previous admission(s) for stabilization
3 History of steroid requirement, esp. if recent reduction
4 Rapid symptomatic development (labile disease)
5 Insufficient lung function to use usual inhalers
6 Iatrogenic factors
— Inappropriate sedation
— Precipitation by aspirin or β-blockers

Clinical criteria favoring hospitalization in acute asthma

1 General demeanor
   — Difficulty speaking
   — Sweaty, anxious, irritable
   — Exhausted; confused; sitting forward
2 Vital signs
   — Tachycardia > 150/min
   — Tachypnea > 28/min
   — Forced expiratory time > 4 sec
   — Blood pressure
     • Paradox* > 20 mmHg
     • Pulsus paradoxus (i.e. palpable paradox)
     • Hypotension (ominous)
3 Signs of respiratory distress
   — Stridor, audible wheezing
   — Accessory muscle use (e.g. sternomastoids)
   — Intercostal recession (chest wall indrawing)
   — Tracheal tug (descends on inspiration)
4 Signs of ventilatory failure
   — Central cyanosis
   — Sleepiness
   — 'Quiet' (grossly hyperexpanded) chest
5 Pulmonary function tests
   — PEFR < 200 L/min
   — FEV_1 < 1 L *or* too incapacitated to perform adequately
   — $PaCO_2$ > 40 mmHg
6 CXR
   — Pneumothorax
7 ECG
   — P pulmonale ± right ventricular strain

NB: Presence of one or more of these signs on presentation may justify admission; persistence of any sign following bronchodilators makes admission mandatory
* defined as systolic drop of > 12 mmHg on inspiration

Therapeutic approach to the young patient with asthma

1 Occasional mild symptoms, no severe acute attacks
   — β_2-agonist (e.g. salbutamol inhaler), *or*
   — Antimuscarinics (e.g. ipratropium bromide)
2 Occasional symptoms with some severe acute attacks
   — Intermittent inhaled β_2-agonist supplemented with short-course oral steroids as needed
3 Frequent (> twice-weekly) attacks
   — Prophylaxis: inhaled sodium cromoglycate
   — No benefit? Inhaled beclomethasone
   — Inhaled long-acting β_2-agonist (e.g. salmeterol) p.r.n.
   — Supplement with steroids during acute exacerbations
4 Refractory nocturnal symptoms
   — Oral long-acting β_2-agonist
   — Oral cromakalim (K^+ channel activator)
   — Bedtime dose of slow-release theophylline may help (also useful in patients unable to use inhalers)
   — Oral steroids

Novel arachidonate-pathway drug classes for extrinsic asthma

1 Leukotriene receptor antagonists
2 5-lipoxygenase inhibitors
3 Kinin (bradykinin/tachykinin) receptor blockers

Pharmacokinetic considerations in theophylline therapy

1 *Higher* dose may be required in
   — Cigarette smokers
   — Chronic alcohol ingestion without liver damage
   — Children < 12 years
   — Treatment with phenytoin, carbamazepine, barbiturates; rifampicin, isoniazid; sulfinpyrazone
2 *Reduce* dose in
   — Hepatic insufficiency
   — Cardiac failure; fever; pregnancy
   — Elderly patients
   — Treatment with erythromycin; cimetidine; propranolol; oral contraceptives; allopurinol
3 *Overdosage* may precipitate hypokalemia*; hyperglycemia; acidosis; convulsions
   — If supportive measures fail, hemoperfusion may be used if plasma theophylline levels exceed 50 mg/L

* Parenteral β_2-agonists may also cause hypokalemia

Indications for inhaler therapy in pulmonary disease

1 Sodium cromoglycate (at least 4–8 weeks)
   — Prophylaxis for children with extrinsic (i.e. allergic or exercise-induced) asthma
2 Anticholinergics (e.g. ipratropium bromide)
   — COAD > asthma (prophylaxis)
3 β_2-agonists (e.g. salbutamol, salmeterol)
   — Asthma (acute)
4 Corticosteroids (e.g. beclomethasone, budesonide)
   — Asthma > COAD (prophylaxis)
5 Amiloride/N-acetylcysteine
   — Cystic fibrosis

Side-effects of inhaled steroids

1 Hoarseness, irritative cough
   — Due to laryngeal myopathy*
2 Oropharyngeal thrush
   — esp. Elderly patients
   — Commoner if given more than twice daily

* Hence, may contraindicate use in singers
NB: Metabolic (systemic) effects of inhaled steroids remain largely theoretical

PRINCIPLES OF VENTILATORY SUPPORT

Potential hazards of oxygen therapy

1 Carbon dioxide retention
2 Reduced bronchial ciliary activity; drying of secretions
3 Adult respiratory distress syndrome
4 Potentiation of radiation or cytotoxic-induced pneumonitis
5 Retrolental fibroplasia in neonates

Indications for assisted ventilation

1 Apnea
2 Ineffective cough
3 Inadequate ventilation ($PaCO_2$ > 45 mmHg) due to
   — Unconsciousness (any cause, incl. post-anesthesia)
   — Flail segment, asynchronous respiration
   — Guillain–Barré, myasthenia gravis

— Severe asthma
— ARDS (p. 335)

Therapeutic benefits of mechanical ventilation
1 Subjective benefits
— Relieves respiratory distress
— Permits sedation
2 Objective benefits
— Improves gas exchange/oxygenation
— Reverses respiratory acidosis
— Eliminates respiratory muscle oxygen debt
— Reverses atelectasis

Neurological precipitants of respiratory failure
1 Neuromuscular
— Myasthenia gravis
— Polymyositis, myotonic dystrophy
2 Neuropathy
— Guillain–Barré syndrome
— Diphtheria, acute intermittent porphyria
3 Anterior horn cell disease
— Polio
— Motor neuron disease
4 Spinal cord lesion
— Trauma
— Tumor; demyelination
5 Brainstem
— Cerebrovascular accident
— Encephalitis; polio; tumor; demyelination

DOMICILIARY OXYGEN

Indications for long-term low-flow oxygen therapy
1 Prerequisites
— Age < 70 years
— No other major illness
— Cessation of smoking (carboxyhemoglobin < 3%)
2 Stable chronic airflow obstruction with
— PaO_2 < 55 mmHg on room air
— $PaCO_2$ > 45 mmHg (esp. if associated with edema)
— FEV_1 < 1.5 L and FVC < 2 L
3 Controversial
— Palliation of severe hypoxemic lung disease
— Stable airflow obstruction without elevated $PaCO_2$
— Advanced restrictive lung disease

Benefits of long-term oxygen therapy in chronic lung disease
1 Subjective relief from dyspnea
2 Improved exercise tolerance
3 Reduced pulmonary artery pressure
4 Fewer hospital admissions
5 Prolonged survival

Contraindications to long-term low-flow oxygen therapy
1 Obstructive sleep apnea (see below)
2 Respiratory muscle weakness
3 Ventilatory impairment due to kyphoscoliosis

Treatment modalities in obstructive sleep apnea
1 Weight loss
2 Nocturnal nasal CPAP*

3 Medroxyprogesterone acetate
4 Mandibular advancement dental prostheses
5 Uvulopharyngoplasty
6 Tracheostomy

* continuous positive airways pressure; incl. BiPAP, 'smart' CPAP

DRUG THERAPY OF RESPIRATORY DISEASE

General principles of steroid therapy in respiratory disease
1 Allergic bronchopulmonary aspergillosis
— Maintenance prednisolone up to 10 mg/day may be indicated if frequent exacerbations
2 Hypersensitivity pneumonitis
— Maintenance therapy may be justified *only* if avoidance of antigen proves impossible
3 Fibrosing alveolitis
— Some benefit from 40 mg/day prednisolone, esp. if
• Cellular biopsy with desquamation
• > 10% lymphocytosis on lavage (unusual)
4 Adult respiratory distress syndrome
— Probably no value in established disease
5 Wegener's granulomatosis
— Prednisolone useful if used with cyclophosphamide
— This combination also of value in Churg–Strauss syndrome and lymphomatoid granulomatosis

Presumptive management of pneumonia in adults
1 Mild community-acquired pneumonia, treatable at home
— Amoxycillin 500 mg t.d.s. orally
2 Severe community-acquired pneumonia, in hospital
— Erythromycin 1 g IV q 6 h
— Covers *Mycoplasma*, pneumococci, *Legionella*, most staphylococci and *C. psittaci*)
— ± Ampicillin 1 g IV q 6 h
— Provides additional cover for pneumococci and for *H. influenzae*)
3 *Legionella* strongly suspected
— Erythromycin 1 g q 6 h *plus* rifampicin 600 mg b.d.
4 Staphylococcal pneumonia suspected (e.g. post-influenza)
— Flucloxacillin 2 g IV q 4–6 h (± aminoglycoside)
5 Hospital-acquired pneumonia
— IV β-lactamase (e.g. ampicillin) + amino-glycoside
Aspiration pneumonia suspected
— Add metronidazole to cover anaerobes (or penicillin)
6 Pneumonia in the neutropenic patient
— Antipseudomonal β-lactamase + amino-glycoside
7 Pneumonia in patients with weight loss, lymph-adenopathy and/or oral candidiasis (i.e. ?AIDS)
— Consider co-trimoxazole/pentamidine for *P. carinii*

NB: Chest physio is of *no* proven value in lobar pneumonia

ALTITUDE-INDUCED DISORDERS

Pathogenesis of acute mountain sickness (AMS)
1 Altitude-induced *hypoxemia*
2 *Respiratory alkalosis* limits ventilatory response to hypoxia*
3 *Pulmonary edema* due to high pulmonary artery pressures
4 *Cerebral edema* causes the typical AMS symptoms

* Limits ventilatory response to hypoxemia, i.e. until acclimatization occurs with reduction of extracellular fluid bicarbonate levels

Prevention of acute mountain sickness
1 Physical factors in prevention of AMS
— Slow ascent
— Temporary (immediate) descent if symptoms develop
2 Medical prophylaxis (NB: adjunctive only to above measures)
— Acetazolamide 250 mg b.d. from 48 h preascent
— Slow-release nifedipine 20 mg q 8 h during ascent

Treatment of acute mountain sickness
1 Treatment of incipient AMS
— Add 3% CO_2 to inhaled air, thus increasing $PaCO_2$ levels and abolishing respiratory alkalosis → Secondary improvement in ventilation, oxygenation and cerebral perfusion
2 Treatment of established AMS
— Dexamethasone (for cerebral edema)

LUNG TRANSPLANTATION

Potential indications for single-lung transplantation
1 End-stage pulmonary fibrosis
— Prior to irreversible pulmonary hypertension
2 End-stage pulmonary emphysema
— esp. α_1-antitrypsin deficiency

Potential indications for heart–lung transplantation*
1 Combined cardiopulmonary disease
— Pulmonary hypertension (primary or Eisenmenger's)
2 Diffuse lung disease with chronic bronchial infection‡
— esp. Cystic fibrosis¶, bronchiectasis

* Heart–lung transplants en bloc are technically easier than double-lung procedures, since the latter require tracheal anastomosis
‡ Single-lung transplant *contraindicated* here due to inevitable contamination of allograft with flora from remaining (septic) lung
¶ Consider when FEV_1 falls below 30% of expected

Problems with lung transplantation
1 Infection
— CMV, *P. carinii*
— *Aspergillus, Candida* spp.
2 Rejection
— Acute (< 6 months post-transplant)

— Obliterative bronchiolitis (= chronic rejection)
• esp. Heart–lung transplants (→ 40–50%)
3 Technical concerns
— Bronchial dehiscence/stenosis
• esp. Single-lung transplants
— Prior chest surgery or pleurodesis (= contraindications)
4 Expense
— Initial procedure *plus* follow-up care
5 Shortage of donor organs

UNDERSTANDING RESPIRATORY DISEASE

ADULT RESPIRATORY DISTRESS SYNDROME (ARDS)

Diagnostic criteria for adult respiratory distress syndrome
1 History
— Previously normal lung function
— Acute respiratory distress after a precipitating event
2 CXR
— Diffuse infiltrates (sparing apices, costophrenic angles)
3 Blood gases
— PaO_2 < 60 mmHg despite FiO_2=60% (due to shunting)
— $PaCO_2$ normal or low
— Arterial-alveolar (A-a) oxygen tension ratio < 0.25
4 Pulmonary investigations
— Reduced pulmonary compliance ('stiff lungs')
— Pulmonary hypertension (> 30/15 mmHg) usual
— Pulmonary wedge pressure normal (< 18 mmHg)
— Thoracic compliance < 30 mL/cmH$_2$O
5 Therapeutic rationâle
— Assisted ventilation (volume-cycled, patient-initiated) using positive end-expiratory pressure (PEEP) of 8–15 cmH$_2$O to increase the functional residual capacity (and hence increase compliance and thus reduce intrapulmonary shunting)

Common antecedents of adult respiratory distress syndrome
1 Sepsis (incl. pneumonia, Gram-negative septicemia)
2 Aspiration (incl. drowning)
3 Inhalation (smoke, oxygen, chlorine)
4 Multiple trauma
5 Massive transfusion

NB: ARDS *may* also occur in neutropenic patients even though neutrophils are implicated in the pathogenesis

Treatment modalities in ARDS
1 High-frequency PEEP (see above)
2 Early commencement of steroids
3 Exogenous surfactant
4 *N*-acetylcysteine
5 Prostaglandin E$_1$
6 Inhaled nitric oxide

GRANULOMATOUS LUNG DISEASE

Main features distinguishing chronic from acute sarcoidosis
1 Age of presentation
   — Older (> 30 years) patients
2 CXR
   — Pulmonary infiltrates
   — No hilar adenopathy
3 Skin
   — Lupus pernio common
   — Erythema nodosum unusual
4 Mikulicz syndrome (parotidomegaly and facial palsy)
   — Common
5 Therapeutic response
   — Steroid-resistant
6 Prognosis
   — Poor

Cardiac manifestations of sarcoidosis
1 Heart block: first-degree/RBBB/complete heart block
2 Arrhythmias: SVT/VT/ventricular ectopic beats
3 Mitral valve disease
4 Pericarditis
5 Congestive cardiac failure
6 Sudden death

Indicators of disease activity in sarcoidosis
1 Symptoms
2 Investigations of organ involvement, e.g. lung
   — CXR
   — DL_{CO}
3 Bronchoalveolar lavage
   — Increased overall cellularity
   — Up to 40% lymphocytes (predominantly T_H)
   — ↓ IgG:albumin ratio (cf. allergic alveolitis)
4 ^{67}Gallium scan
   — A sensitive index of disease activity
   — Extrapulmonary uptake (parotid, nodes) supports diagnosis but does *not* exclude lymphoma
5 Serum angiotensin-converting enzyme (ACE)
   — Elevated in 70% of patients with active (acute) disease
   — Useful in monitoring response to steroids
   — *Not* specific for initial diagnosis (↑ in granulomatous diseases, e.g. Gaucher's, silicosis, miliary TB)
   — Serum lysozyme and transcobalamin II are similar indices of disease activity, but less sensitive
6 Other laboratory associations
   — Serum and/or urinary calcium (if elevated)
   — Hypergammaglobulinemia (polyclonal)
   — Lymphopenia (relative excess of T_S cells; cf. BAL)

Differential diagnosis of elevated ACE with lung infiltrates
1 Dust diseases (antigenic reactions)
   — Asbestosis
   — Silicosis
   — Berylliosis
2 Infections
   — Miliary TB
   — Coccidioidomycosis

3 Hypersensitivity pneumonitis
4 ARDS (see above)
5 Lymphoma

Indications for corticosteroids in sarcoidosis
1 Intractable constitutional symptoms
2 Progressive lung disease
3 Hypercalcemia* and/or persisting hypercalciuria
4 Hypersplenism
5 Vital organ involvement
   — Heart
   — CNS
   — Eye

* May also respond to chloroquine

Hypersensitivity pneumonitis*: making the diagnosis
1 Clinical
   — Recurrent dyspnea 4–6 h after antigen exposure
   — Dry cough; typically *no* wheezing
   — Fevers, progressive weight loss
   — Occurs *less* commonly in smokers
2 CXR
   — Mid- and lower zone mottling (in acute phase)
   — Upper zone mottling (in chronic fibrosis)
3 Lung function tests
   — Restrictive (transient in acute phase)
4 Blood gases
   — Low PaO_2 and $PaCO_2$
   Diffusion capacity
   — Low DL_{CO}
5 Precipitins
   — Do *not* indicate pathogenicity‡
   — Do *not* correlate with disease activity
   — Tend to *exclude* diagnosis if negative
6 Immune profile
   — Total serum IgE levels typically *normal*
   — Eosinophilia *absent*
7 Bronchoalveolar lavage
   — Lymphocytosis
   — ↑ IgG:albumin ratio
8 Transbronchial biopsy
   — Granulomata
   — Bronchiolitis, mononuclear infiltrate
9 Inhalation provocation (the definitive diagnostic test)
   — Improvement on cessation of exposure
   — Relapse on rechallenge

* Extrinsic allergic alveolitis
‡ Exception: budgerigar exposure

ASPERGILLUS-RELATED LUNG DISEASE

Diagnosis of allergic bronchopulmonary aspergillosis (ABPA)
1 Clinical
   — Exacerbation of asthma in an atopic patient
   — Expectoration of rubbery brown sputum plugs which repeatedly yield aspergilli on culture
2 CXR
   — Upper lobe pulmonary infiltrates
   — Peripheral linear shadowing
3 Immune profile
   — Peripheral eosinophilia > 1000/mL

— Elevated total serum IgE (> 2000 ng/mL)
— Elevated specific IgE to *A. fumigatus*
  • Typically negative in aspergilloma
— Elevated specific IgG to *A. fumigatus* (IgE:IgG > 2)
  • Often negative in invasive aspergillosis
— Immediate skin reactivity to *A. fumigatus* (prick test +)
— Precipitating antibodies to *A. fumigatus* (weak +)
4 Confirmatory investigation*
— High-resolution CT (p. 332)
— Bronchoscopy/bronchography to demonstrate proximal saccular upper lobe bronchiectasis
5 Therapy and course
— Resolution of symptoms, eosinophilia, sputum positivity and CXR appearances with long-term systemic steroids (prednisone 0.5 mg/kg daily x 2 weeks, then alternate days x 2 months, then taper)
— Undiagnosed (untreated) ABPA may progress to refractory asthma, lung fibrosis and respiratory failure

* cf. *invasive* aspergillosis: diagnose by lung biopsy or by serum/ urine *Aspergillus* antigen detection

Therapeutic spectrum of *Aspergillus*-related pulmonary disease
1 Allergic bronchopulmonary aspergillosis
— Treat with bronchodilators and/or steroids
2 Aspergilloma ('fungus ball')
— Treat conservatively or surgically
3 Invasive aspergillosis
— Treat urgently with IV amphotericin B + 5-FC
— Mortality approaches 95% in transplant patients

LUNG INFECTIONS

Predispositions to specific pulmonary infections
1 Tuberculosis (incl. reactivation)
— Silicosis
— Alcoholism
— Gastrectomy or jejunoileal bypass
— Active measles; uncontrolled diabetes mellitus
— Iatrogenic immunosuppression
2 *M. kansasii/avium-intracellulare*
— Preexisting lung disease
3 Anaerobic infections (abscess, aspiration pneumonia)
— Obtunded consciousness; anesthesia, alcoholism
— Poor dental hygiene
— Achalasia, scleroderma, Riley–Day syndrome
4 *Klebsiella* spp.
— Alcoholism, derelict lifestyle
5 *Ps. aeruginosa*
  Staph aureus
— Cystic fibrosis (bronchial colonization)
6 *Ps. pyocyanea*
— Humidifier/ventilator therapy
7 *Nocardia asteroides*
— Pulmonary alveolar proteinosis
— Chronic granulomatous disease of childhood
8 *Staph aureus*
  Serratia marcescens
  Candida spp.
— Heroin addiction

9 *P. carinii*
  Cytomegalovirus
— Immunosuppression: transplant or AIDS
10 Aspergilloma
— Old tuberculous cavities
— Emphysematous bullae, lung cysts
— Apical cavities in ankylosing spondylitis
— Cystic fibrosis, atopic asthma
11 *Moraxella catarrhalis*
— Chronic obstructive airways disease

Differential diagnoses in pneumonic presentations
1 Failure of ampicillin/penicillin in community pneumonia
— 'Atypical' pneumonias (q.v.)
— Viral (e.g. adenovirus, varicella, measles)
— *Staph aureus*, *Klebsiella*
— Tuberculosis
2 Pneumonia in recent Asian migrant
— Tuberculosis
— *Ps. pseudomallei* (melioidosis)*
3 Pneumonia in bird-fanciers
— Psittacosis (exclude allergic alveolitis)
4 Pneumonia in meatworkers
— Q fever
5 Post-influenza pneumonia
— *Staph aureus*, pneumococci
6 Eosinophilic pneumonia
— Tropical diffuse: filariasis (*Wuchereria bancrofti*)
— Tropical localized: ascariasis (Löffler's syndrome)
— Non-tropical localized: aspergillosis
— Toxic (e.g. nitrofurantoin, toluene)

* Also seen in travellers to South-East Asia or South America

ATYPICAL PNEUMONIA

The atypical pneumonias: which ones are they?
1 Common
— Mycoplasma (*M. pneumoniae*)
— Viral pneumonias
2 Unusual
— Legionnaire's disease (*L. pneumophila*)
— Q fever (*Coxiella burneti*)
— Psittacosis (*Chlamydia psittaci*)
— TWAR (*Chlamydia pneumoniae*: p. 228)
— Histoplasmosis, coccidioidomycosis
— Tuberculosis

Clinical aspects of *Mycoplasma* pneumonia
1 Occurrence
— Slowly spreading epidemics
— Long incubation period, insidious onset
2 Course
— Initial URTI transforms to LRTI
— Family members often also affected
— Clinical relapse following treatment often occurs
3 Extrapulmonary manifestations
— Arthralgias/-itis
— Headaches, meningism ± aseptic meningitis
— Substernal discomfort (tracheobronchitis)
— 'Cold' autoimmune hemolysis ± anemia
— Ear pain due to bullous or hemorrhagic myringitis*

— Erythema multiforme
— Myopericarditis
4 Diagnosis
— Routine sputum non-diagnostic
— Throat swab may (eventually) yield positive cultures
— Diagnosis established by serology (CFT)
— Resistant to β-lactams

* Classic but rare

Distinguishing features of psittacosis
1 History
— Avian exposure
2 Symptoms
— Epistaxis
— Photophobia
— Thrombophlebitis
— Myalgias, confusion, stupor
3 Signs
— Splenomegaly (± anicteric hepatomegaly)
— Horder's spots (may simulate rose spots of typhoid)
— Proteinuria
4 Investigations
— Positive serology (CFT)*
— Transbronchial biopsy → cytoplasmic inclusions (LCL bodies) within macrophages

* Even low-titer generally suffices for diagnosis in acute phase

Distinguishing features of Q ('query') fever
1 Distinction from other rickettsioses
— Not transmitted from arthropods
— No rash
— Negative Weil–Felix reaction
2 Pleuritic chest pain
3 Weight loss (may be dramatic)
4 Granulomatous hepatitis (→ about 20%)
5 Culture-negative endocarditis (usually de novo) requiring valve replacement (typically aortic)

Clinical spectrum of Legionnaire's disease
1 Commoner in
— Smokers
— Debilitated patients
— Males aged about 50–60 years
— Moderate (about 30 g/day) alcohol intake
2 Transmission
— No documented person-to-person spread
— Nosocomial transmission not infrequent
— Water-containing receptacles may be disease reservoir
3 Distinguishing clinical features
— High fever, rigors
— Encephalopathy ± headache
— Gastrointestinal upset
— Transient azotemia; hemoproteinuria
4 Investigations
— Hyponatremia (SIADH); also → other pneumonias
— Hypophosphatemia
— Transient liver function test abnormalities
— Negative routine cultures
5 Diagnosis
— Most rapid: direct fluorescence on lung biopsy*

— Dieterle silver impregnation stain on sputum
— *Culture* of lung biopsy or pleural fluid in medium containing charcoal yeast-enriched (CYE) agar with alphaketoglutarate or cysteine/iron in 5% CO_2
— Serology (indirect fluorescent antibody)
  • 4-fold rise to > 1:128 (usually takes 2 weeks)
  • Single titer of > 1:256? Infection at some stage
6 Management
— IV fluids if hypovolemic (diarrhea, sweats)
— Electrolyte homeostasis
— Erythromycin 2–4 g/day IV ± rifampicin 600 mg/day (continue for 2 weeks, even though defervescence occurs within 48 h)
— PEEP if in respiratory failure (→ 10–20%)

* Or pleural fluid

PATHOGENESIS AND FEATURES OF RESPIRATORY DISEASE

Pathogenesis of pulmonary emphysema
1 Protease-antiprotease imbalance in alveolar epithelial lining fluid causes proteolytic destruction of alveolae, thus reducing pulmonary gas-exchanging interface
2 Cigarette smoke efficiently inactivates the key antiprotease α_1-antitrypsin (α_1AT), thus predisposing to emphysema
3 Free radical production from activated neutrophils (e.g. in chronic inflammation) may also contribute to damage
4 2% of emphysema patients have a detectable reduction in circulating α_1AT, reflecting a genetic mutation (ZZ) which causes impaired α_1AT release after hepatic synthesis
5 The extent to which heterozygotes (MZ) are predisposed to cigarette-induced emphysema is unclear
6 Recombinant aerosolized α_1AT is being used on an investigational basis

Pathogenesis of cystic fibrosis (CF)
1 Mutation of transmembrane conductance regulator (CFTR)
2 CFTR mutation causes defective chloride (Cl^-) transport, which in turn causes increased sodium (Na^+) and water resorption from duct and bronchial lumen
3 Thick, tenacious secretions and sputum result, leading to high frequencies of *Pseudomonas* spp. superinfection*
4 Point mutation of phenylalanine at position 508 (ΔF_{508}), the ATP-binding site, is the underlying defect in 70%; the other 30% of cases are due to hundreds of mutations
5 The heterozygote frequency of this mutation (about one in 40) has been suggested to reflect evolutionary selection due to increased resistance to *V. cholerae*
6 Severe phenotypes (meconium ileus, pancreatic insufficiency) usually imply two defective alleles (e.g. ΔF_{508} homozygotes)

Therapeutic approaches to cystic fibrosis
1 Amiloride
— ↓ Na^+ reabsorption → ↓ sputum viscosity

2 High-dose ibuprofen
— Reduces lung destruction by reducing inflammation
3 Mucolytics
— incl. Inhaled DNases or α_1-antitrypsin
4 CFTR gene therapy
— esp. Using adenovirus-like vectors
— Remains investigational

* Either *Ps. aeruginosa* or *Ps. cepacia*

Clinical features of immotile cilia syndrome
1 Genetic etiology; includes Kartagener's (in 50%)
2 Other manifestations include otitis media, nasal polyposis and infertility (esp. in males: 95%)
3 Affected females may develop salpingitis, but usually remain fertile (as in cystic fibrosis)
4 Electron microscopy confirms ultrastructural defect of dynein arms in bronchial/nasal cilia and in sperm

Clinical features of yellow-nail syndrome
1 Usually presents in old age
2 Greenish-yellow nail discoloration and dystrophy
3 Associated with recurrent pleural effusions, peripheral lymphedema, chronic chest infections, myxedema

Clinical features of pulmonary alveolar proteinosis
1 Protean clinical manifestations, variable prognosis
2 Sputum $\rightarrow$ PAS-positive lipoprotein in epithelial cells
3 CXR $\rightarrow$ diffuse infiltrates, perihilar 'rosette'
4 Often complicated by opportunistic infection, esp. *Nocardia* (which may in turn metastasize to brain)
5 Therapeutic lavage may help avoid need for steroids

Clinical features of idiopathic pulmonary hemosiderosis
1 Age of onset < 20 years
2 Sputum $\rightarrow$ hemosiderin-laden macrophages
3 Presents with hemoptysis $\pm$ iron-deficiency anemia
4 Diffuse (predominantly basal) infiltrates on CXR
5 No renal disease; negative immunofluorescence and anti-GBM Ab (cf. Goodpasture's)
6 Subclinical disease activity is proportionate to the DL_{CO}

REVIEWING THE LITERATURE: RESPIRATORY MEDICINE

13.1 Sporik R et al (1990) Exposure to house-dust mite allergen (Der p I) and the development of asthma in childhood. N Engl J Med 323: 502–507

Young S et al (1991) The influence of a family history of asthma and parental smoking on airway responsiveness in early infancy. N Engl J Med 324: 1168–1173

Two studies examining causative factors in asthma pathogenesis. The former study of 67 children showed that 16 of 17 atopic children were sensitized to house-dust mite, with most having been exposed from age 1; the latter showed that bronchial hyperresponsiveness (BHR) is commoner in infants whose parents smoke.

13.2 Sears MR et al (1990) Regular inhaled beta-agonist treatment in bronchial asthma. Lancet 336: 1391–1396

O'Connor BJ et al (1992) Tolerance to the nonbronchodilator effects of inhaled β_2-agonists in asthma. N Engl J Med 327: 1204–1208

Progressive loss of effect of β-agonist medication (as measured by methacholine provocation) was documented in these two studies, thus cautioning against relying on this class of drugs for regular treatment maintenance (and see below).

13.3 Molfino NA et al (1991) Respiratory arrest in near-fatal asthma. N Engl J Med 324: 285–288

Spitzer WO et al (1992) The use of β-agonists and the risk of death and near death from asthma. N Engl J Med 326: 501–506

The first of these studies showed that asphyxia (rather than arrhythmias) was the cause of respiratory arrest, suggesting that undertreatment may be at least as hazardous as overtreatment. The second study indicated that patients receiving nebulized β-agonists (esp. fenoterol) were at increased risk of arrest – though whether this association reflects drug toxicity or disease severity remains unclear.

13.4 Chapman KR et al (1991) Effect of a short course of prednisone in the prevention of early relapse after the emergency room treatment of acute asthma. N Engl J Med 324: 788–794

Huib AM et al (1992) A comparison of bronchodilator therapy with or without inhaled corticosteroid therapy for obstructive airways disease. N Engl J Med 327: 1413–1419

These studies were among the first to validate the early use of corticosteroids in patients with severe asthma. However, the first showed that relapse prevention was improved only for as long as the period of (oral) steroid administration. The second confirmed the additive efficacy of inhaled steroids (but not inhaled ipratropium bromide) over terbutaline alone, especially in young (< 40 yrs) patients, allergic patients and non-smokers.

13.5 Bersten AD et al (1991) Treatment of severe cardiogenic pulmonary edema with continuous positive airway pressure delivered by face mask. N Engl J Med 325: 1825–1830

Prospective study of 39 patients showing a reduction in the need for intubation and ventilation in patients randomized to receive CPAP. Mortality was reduced, but not significantly (perhaps due to small numbers).

13.6 Malone S et al (1991) Obstructive sleep apnoea in patients with dilated cardiomyopathy: effects of continuous positive airway pressure. Lancet 338: 1480–1484

Small study of eight obese snorers, showing that nasal CPAP at night significantly improved LV function.

Hung J et al (1990) Association of sleep apnoea with myocardial infarction in men. Lancet 336: 261–264

Case-control study of 101 infarct patients, showing a relative 20-fold increased risk for individuals with sleep apnea.

13.7 Stradling JR et al (1990) Effect of adenotonsillectomy on nocturnal hypoxemia, sleep disturbance, and symptoms in snoring children. Lancet 335: 249–253

Study of 61 children with recurrent tonsillitis requiring adenotonsillectomy, 60–65% of whom had abnormal sleep studies. Surgery resulted in resolution of nocturnal hypoxemia, hyperactivity, aggression and learning difficulties.

13.8 Grossman RF et al (1990) Results of single-lung transplantation for bilateral pulmonary fibrosis. N Engl J Med 322: 727–733

Twenty patients with severe restrictive lung diseases were treated with lung transplants and nine survived more than 1 year. These survivors did well functionally, with none requiring supplemental oxygen.

13.9 Hedlund JU et al (1992) Risk of pneumonia in patients previously treated in hospital for pneumonia. Lancet 340: 396–397

Of 573 consecutive pneumonia patients, the risk of a further episode was 5–6 times higher than for controls. It is suggested that pneumococcal vaccination is probably cost-effective in such individuals.

13.10 Sutherland G et al (1992) Randomised controlled trial of nasal nicotine spray in smoking cessation. Lancet 340: 324–329

Placebo-controlled study of 227 smokers trying to quit, showing that 26% of the nicotine-spray cohort became abstinent within a year, compared with only 10% of placebo patients; benefit was greatest in the heaviest smokers.

ICRF General Practice Research Group (1993) Effectiveness of a nicotine patch in helping people stop smoking. Br Med J 306: 1304–1308

The use of nicotine patches (as opposed to gum) resulted in a doubling of cigarette abstinence after 6–12 months, confirming the (relative) efficacy of nicotine supplements in this setting.

CHAPTER 14

Rheumatology

Physical examination protocol 14.1   You are asked to examine a patient with rheumatoid arthritis

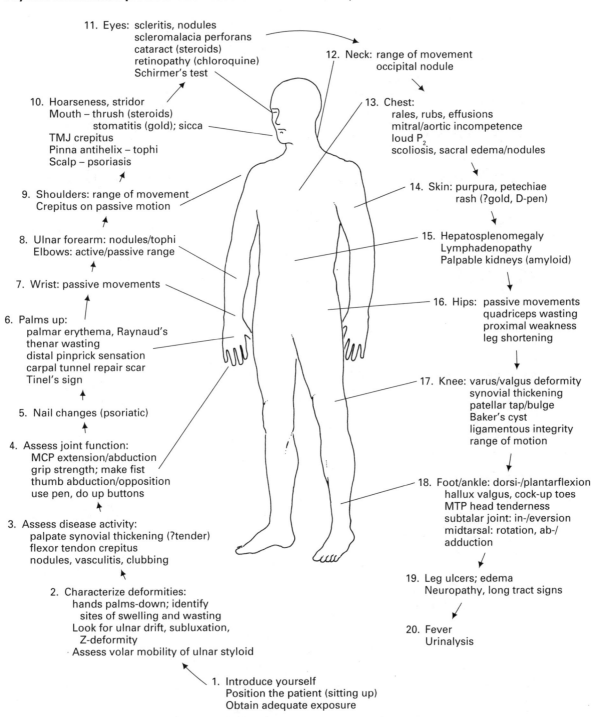

11. Eyes: scleritis, nodules
    scleromalacia perforans
    cataract (steroids)
    retinopathy (chloroquine)
    Schirmer's test

12. Neck: range of movement
    occipital nodule

13. Chest:
    rales, rubs, effusions
    mitral/aortic incompetence
    loud P_2
    scoliosis, sacral edema/nodules

10. Hoarseness, stridor
    Mouth – thrush (steroids)
      stomatitis (gold); sicca
    TMJ crepitus
    Pinna antihelix – tophi
    Scalp – psoriasis

9. Shoulders: range of movement
   Crepitus on passive motion

14. Skin: purpura, petechiae
    rash (?gold, D-pen)

8. Ulnar forearm: nodules/tophi
   Elbows: active/passive range

15. Hepatosplenomegaly
    Lymphadenopathy
    Palpable kidneys (amyloid)

7. Wrist: passive movements

6. Palms up:
   palmar erythema, Raynaud's
   thenar wasting
   distal pinprick sensation
   carpal tunnel repair scar
   Tinel's sign

16. Hips: passive movements
    quadriceps wasting
    proximal weakness
    leg shortening

5. Nail changes (psoriatic)

17. Knee: varus/valgus deformity
    synovial thickening
    patellar tap/bulge
    Baker's cyst
    ligamentous integrity
    range of motion

4. Assess joint function:
   MCP extension/abduction
   grip strength; make fist
   thumb abduction/opposition
   use pen, do up buttons

18. Foot/ankle: dorsi-/plantarflexion
    hallux valgus, cock-up toes
    MTP head tenderness
    subtalar joint: in-/eversion
    midtarsal: rotation, ab-/
      adduction

3. Assess disease activity:
   palpate synovial thickening (?tender)
   flexor tendon crepitus
   nodules, vasculitis, clubbing

19. Leg ulcers; edema
    Neuropathy, long tract signs

2. Characterize deformities:
   hands palms-down; identify
     sites of swelling and wasting
   Look for ulnar drift, subluxation,
     Z-deformity
   Assess volar mobility of ulnar styloid

20. Fever
    Urinalysis

1. Introduce yourself
   Position the patient (sitting up)
   Obtain adequate exposure

Physical examination protocol 14.2   You are asked to examine a young man with chronic low back pain

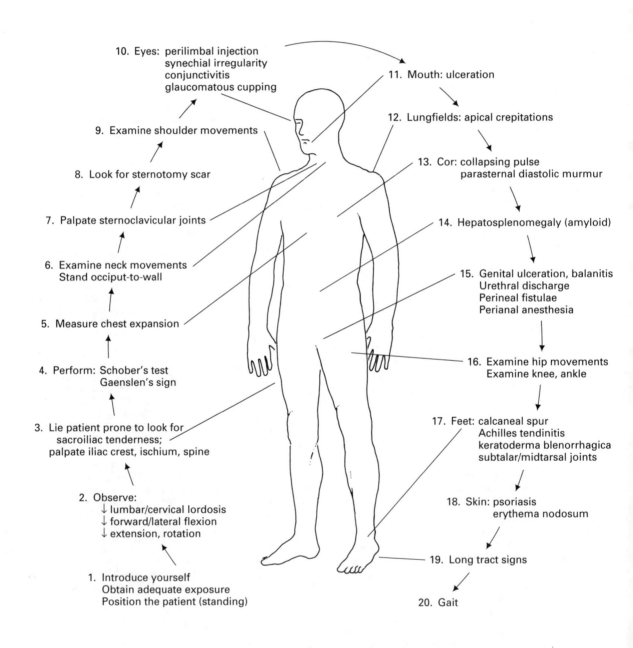

10. Eyes: perilimbal injection
    synechial irregularity
    conjunctivitis
    glaucomatous cupping

11. Mouth: ulceration

12. Lungfields: apical crepitations

9. Examine shoulder movements

13. Cor: collapsing pulse
    parasternal diastolic murmur

8. Look for sternotomy scar

14. Hepatosplenomegaly (amyloid)

7. Palpate sternoclavicular joints

6. Examine neck movements
   Stand occiput-to-wall

15. Genital ulceration, balanitis
    Urethral discharge
    Perineal fistulae
    Perianal anesthesia

5. Measure chest expansion

4. Perform: Schober's test
   Gaenslen's sign

16. Examine hip movements
    Examine knee, ankle

3. Lie patient prone to look for
   sacroiliac tenderness;
   palpate iliac crest, ischium, spine

17. Feet: calcaneal spur
    Achilles tendinitis
    keratoderma blenorrhagica
    subtalar/midtarsal joints

2. Observe:
   ↓ lumbar/cervical lordosis
   ↓ forward/lateral flexion
   ↓ extension, rotation

18. Skin: psoriasis
    erythema nodosum

1. Introduce yourself
   Obtain adequate exposure
   Position the patient (standing)

19. Long tract signs

20. Gait

Diagnostic pathway 14.1 This patient has unusual hands. What sort of process do you think is responsible?

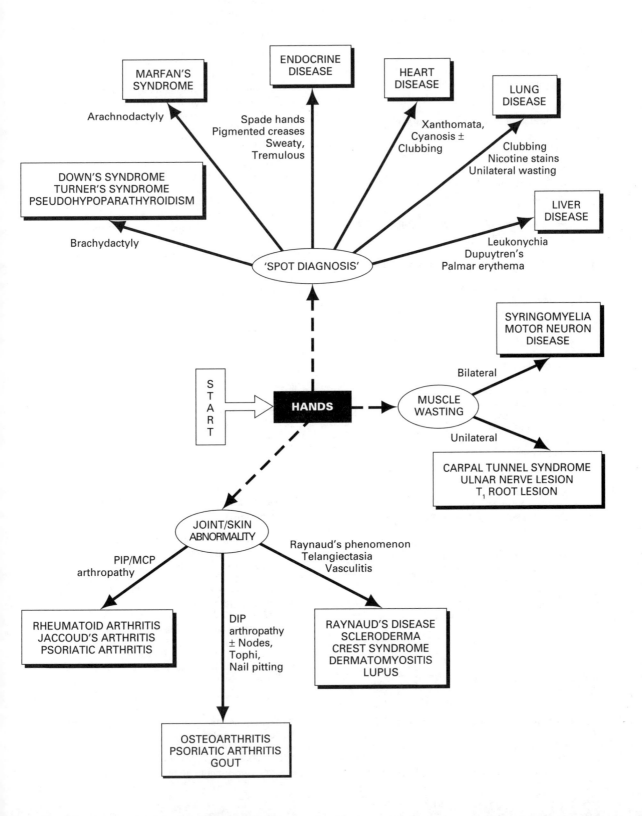

Commonest rheumatological short cases
1 Rheumatoid hands
2 Seronegative spondyloarthropathy

Clinical assessment of joint function: modified ARA criteria*
1 ARA I
— Normal joint function (= no disease)
2 ARA II
— Adequate function despite symptoms (= early disease)
3 ARA III
— Reduced function, but self-care possible (= disease)
4 ARA IV
— Self-care precluded by dysfunction (= severe disease)

Systematic characterization of joint dysfunction
1 Dysfunction
— Loss of normal joint function
2 Disability
— Impairment of an activity by joint dysfunction
3 Handicap
— Effect of joint dysfunction on fulfilment of a role

Chronic arthritis: assessment of daily functional capacity
1 Mobility
— Getting out of bed
— Floor to chair; chair to bed
— Negotiating stairs
— Using public transport; shopping
2 Ability to wash
— Using toilet
— Shaving; brushing teeth; cutting nails
— Bathing
3 Dressing
— Using buttons and zips
— Doing up laces; putting on shoes, socks
— Combing hair
4 Feeding
— Preparing food; making tea
— Using cutlery; administering medications
— Chewing; eating apples; swallowing
5 Housework
— Turning taps, keys, dials
— Making beds; using telephone
— Hanging washing

Patterns of joint involvement in rheumatic disease
1 Rheumatoid arthritis (F:M = 3:1)
— MCPs, PIPs, wrists
— Knees, ankles
— Lateral MTPs, subtalar/midtarsal joints
— Cervical spine, incl. atlantoaxial joint
— TMJs (pain on chewing); cricoarytenoids (hoarseness)
2 Osteoarthritis (F:M = 3:1)
— DIPs and PIPs
— Base of thumb (first carpometacarpal joint)
— Knees, hips
— First MTP joint (involvement may be asymptomatic)
— Lumbosacral spine (i.e. apophyseal joints)
3 Seronegative spondyloarthropathies (M > F)
— Hips, knees, ankles (asymmetric, oligoarticular)
— Sacroiliac joints
— Spondylitis: often begins at thoracolumbar junction
4 Gout (M:F = 8:1)
— First MTP joint (at onset in 75%; eventually → 90%)
— Ankles and tarsal bones
— Knees, elbows (incl. olecranon bursa)
— DIPs and PIPs (much less commonly)

Key factors predisposing to osteoarthritis of specific joints
1 Hand
— Bad genes (e.g. collagen gene 2A mutation)
2 Knee
— Trauma
— Obesity*
3 Hip
— Abnormal joint shape

* Note that obesity has also been linked to osteoarthritis of the hands

Nodes and nodules in rheumatic disease
1 Heberden's nodes (DIP osteophytes in primary OA)
  Bouchard's nodes (PIP osteophytes in primary OA)
2 Rheumatoid nodules
3 Gouty tophi (DIPs, PIPs, elbows, ears, heels)
4 Xanthomata

Differential diagnosis of morning stiffness
1 Rheumatoid arthritis
— Difficulty doing up buttons, etc.
— May improve with nocturnal NSAID suppositories
2 Ankylosing spondylitis
— Low back pain/stiffness radiating to buttocks and thighs
— Improved with exercise, NSAIDs
3 Polymyalgia rheumatica
— Difficulty getting out of bed
— *Marked* diurnal variation*
4 Osteoarthritis
— Short duration of stiffness (< 15 min)
— Pain may be worsened by prolonged use
5 Myxedema

* May be asymptomatic by evening (cf. rotator cuff syndrome)

Differential diagnoses of miscellaneous presentations
1 Young patient with joint deformity
— Hemophilia (if male)
— Juvenile chronic arthritis
— Syringomyelia, Riley–Day (i.e. Charcot joint)

2 Charcot's joints
— Tabes dorsalis (→ knee)
— Syringomyelia (→ shoulder, elbow)
— Diabetes mellitus (→ foot)
— Leprosy (lepromatous)
— Overzealous administration of intraarticular steroids
3 Acute monarthritis
— Septic
— Seronegative (incl. 'reactive')
— Hemarthrosis (± trauma)
— Crystal-induced
  • (Pseudo) gout
  • Triamcinolone*
4 Transient polyarthritis
— SLE
— Rheumatic fever, SBE, serum sickness
— Parainfectious: e.g. hepatitis B, gonorrhea
— Reiter's syndrome, 'reactive' arthritides
— Henoch–Schönlein purpura
5 Arthropathy affecting DIPs
— Primary (familial) osteoarthritis
— Psoriatic arthritis
— Other arthropathies (if extensive)
  • Juvenile chronic arthritis; RA
  • Gout
  • Sarcoidosis
  • Hemochromatosis
  • Multicentric reticulohistiocytosis
6 Sternoclavicular arthritis
— Ankylosing spondylitis
— Narcotic addiction
— Tietze's syndrome
7 Chondrocalcinosis
— Old age
— Joint trauma (e.g. menisceal injury of knee)
— Familial
— Gout, OA, RA, Paget's
— Metabolic predisposition
  • Hyperparathyroidism; hypophosphatasia
  • Hemochromatosis; ochronosis
  • Acromegaly; myxedema
  • Wilson's disease

* Typically causes arthritis a few hours after joint injection

Clinical patterns suggesting misdiagnosis
1 'Osteoarthritis' with MCP (esp. 2nd and 3rd) involvement ± chondrocalcinosis on X-ray
— Hemochromatosis
— Wilson's disease
2 'Psoriatic arthritis' with pustular skin lesions and/or prominent eye involvement
— Reiter's syndrome
'Psoriatic arthritis' with positive rheumatoid factor
— Rheumatoid arthritis (i.e. with psoriasis)
3 'Ankylosing spondylitis' with negative HLA-B27 in a female
— Psoriatic arthritis
— Inflammatory bowel disease
4 Post-diarrheal 'reactive arthritis' followed by development of mucocutaneous lesion
— Reiter's syndrome
— Inflammatory bowel disease

Characteristics of benign (mechanical) back pain
1 Symptoms
— Previous similar episode(s)
— Sudden onset
2 Examination
— Asymmetrical or uniradicular findings
— Abnormal femoral stretch/straight leg raise

EXAMINATION OF SPECIFIC JOINTS

Examination of the hip
1 Check for leg *shortening*
— e.g. Collapsed femoral head in OA
2 Test *movements*
— Flexion, abduction, rotation
3 Test for fixed flexion deformity of the hip (*Thomas's test*)
— With the patient supine, flex the contralateral hip to straighten lumbar spine (tilting pelvis to neutral)
— Flexion of ipsilateral hip? = fixed flexion deformity
4 Look for *Trendelenburg sign* (downward tilt of contralateral pelvis when weight-bearing on affected hip)
→ Severe joint or (esp. if bilateral) neuromuscular disease

Differential diagnosis of elbow lesions
1 Rheumatoid nodule
2 Gouty tophus
3 Olecranon bursa (e.g. due to gout, trauma)
4 Synovial cyst (different location to above)
5 Skin lesions
— Tendon xanthoma
— Pseudoxanthoma elasticum
— Psoriasis
— Subcutaneous calcification in CREST syndrome

Clinical diagnosis of shoulder pain
1 All movements restricted (incl. passive abduction, rotation)
— *Articular/capsular disease*
  • 'Frozen shoulder' (adhesive capsulitis)
  • Rheumatoid arthritis
  • Other synovitis, e.g. septic arthritis
2 Active abduction/rotation only restricted (passive normal)
— *Rotator cuff injury* (→ 'painful arc')
  • Supraspinatus tendinitis
  • Infraspinatus tendinitis: pain on active external rotation
  • Subscapularis tendinitis: pain on active internal rotation
  • Bicipital tendinitis: local tenderness, pain on supination

SOFT-TISSUE SYNDROMES

Adhesive capsulitis ('frozen shoulder'): course and therapy
1 *Pain* usually worsens within the first year of onset

2 *Function* usually improves over the first 2 years
3 > 50% of patients are left with some residual dysfunction
4 Best managed with gentle active movements

Repetitive strain injury*: clinical features
1 Usually unilateral
2 Pain most often affects hand, shoulder girdle and neck
3 Common symptoms
   — Proximal muscular 'tightness'
   — Weakness of handgrip
   — Hand numbness and/or paresthesiae
4 *Not* associated with muscle wasting
   No objective reproducible neurological deficit
5 Best treated by continuing normal limb activity

* Also called 'chronic regional pain syndrome' or 'localized fibromyalgia syndrome', i.e. *not* true tenosynovitis/tendinitis

Carpal tunnel syndrome: physical findings
1 Numbness (± pain) of the first three digits
   — Sensory loss involves half* of middle/ring finger
   — 'Flick test': subjective relief on shaking hand
2 Weakness
   — Thumb opposition and abduction
   — Wasting of thenar eminence
3 Provocative bedside tests
   — Positive Tinel's sign
   — Positive Phalen's test‡
   — Direct pressure over median nerve
   — Median nerve sensory loss after tourniquet applied
4 Predisposing stigmata, e.g.
   — Rheumatoid arthritis, pregnancy (common)
   — Acromegaly, myxedema (in exams)

* cf. proximal nerve root lesion (e.g. due to coexisting cervical spondylosis): sensory loss involves entire finger
‡ Numbness/pain reproduced by flexing wrists for 1 min

RHEUMATOID ARTHRITIS (RA)

Clinical assessment of disease activity
1 History
   — Presence of constitutional symptoms
   — Duration of morning stiffness
   — Recent involvement of new joints
   — Recent reduction in range of joint movement
2 Physical examination
   — Number of *tender* swollen joints
   — Degree of soft-tissue swelling/tenderness
   — Ring size at proximal interphalangeal joints
   — Grip strength
   — Walking time for given distance

Differential diagnosis of impaired hand function in RA
1 Active disease
   — Synovitis
   — Tendinitis
2 Joint deformity
3 Tendon rupture
4 Carpal tunnel syndrome
5 Mononeuritis

6 Cervical vertebral compression
   — T1 nerve root
   — Spinal cord

Differential diagnosis of impaired walking in RA
1 Active disease
   — Metatarsal head involvement esp.
2 Inactive disease
   — Joint deformity, muscle contractures
3 Muscle wasting
   — Secondary to synovitis/deformity/steroids
4 Spastic paraparesis
   — Cervical myelopathy
5 Peripheral nerve lesions
   — Neuropathy, mononeuritis multiplex

Diseases which may mimic rheumatoid arthritis
1 Psoriatic arthritis
   — Must be rheumatoid factor negative
2 Juvenile chronic arthritis
   — Polyarticular RF+ subtype
3 Rheumatic fever
   — Arthritis typically spares neck and PIP joints
   Post-rheumatic fever (Jaccoud's) arthritis
4 Collagen diseases
   — SLE, MCTD, scleroderma
5 Other
   — Relapsing polychondritis
   — Multicentric reticulohistiocytosis
   — Erosive osteoarthritis
   — Calcium pyrophosphate deposition disease

Rheumatoid arthritis or osteoarthritis? Some comparisons
1 RA — Predominant DIP involvement rare
   OA — Predominant MCP involvement rare
2 RA — Disease → ulnar deviation at MCPs
   OA — Disease → first carpometacarpal joint involvement
3 RA — Tender dorsally subluxed ulnar styloid ('piano key')
   OA — Tenderness of first carpometacarpal joint
4 RA — Elbow → ↓ extension (ulnar-humeral joint disease)
   OA — Elbow → ↓ supination (radiohumeral involvement)
5 RA — First sign of neck involvement is ↓ rotation
   OA — First sign of neck involvement is ↓ lateral flexion

DISEASE MECHANISMS IN RHEUMATOID ARTHRITIS

Mechanisms of splenomegaly in rheumatoid arthritis
1 Primary disease manifestation (normal neutrophil count)
2 Felty's syndrome (↓ neutrophil count)
3 Sjögren's syndrome
4 Amyloidosis

Mechanisms of muscle wasting in rheumatoid arthritis
1 Systemic hypercatabolism
   — Wasting parallels weight loss

2 Disuse atrophy
3 Inflammatory (vasculitic) myositis
4 Neuropathic
— Vasculitis
— Entrapment
— Splint-induced nerve compression (shouldn't happen)
5 Iatrogenic
— Corticosteroid myopathy
— Polymyositis/myasthenia gravis due to penicillamine

Mechanical basis of rheumatoid deformities
1 *Rupture* of flexor/extensor tendons
— Indicated by loss of active (but not passive) movements beginning in one finger and progressing (without treatment) to involve all
— Therapy = repair ruptured tendon, wrist synovectomy + excision of ulnar head to prevent further rupture
2 Ulnar deviation
— Subluxation of extensor tendons at MCP joints due to synovitic capsular ligamentous stretching
3 Swan-neck deformity
— PIP joint hyperextension and compensatory DIP joint flexion due to interossei contractures and/or shortening of extensor tendon(s)
4 Bouttonière deformity
— PIP fixed flexion contracture (with DIP hyperextension) due to division of extensor hood with volar slipping (± detachment and rupture) of extensor tendon from middle phalanx
5 Mallet finger deformity
— Stretching or rupture of the extensor insertion into the dorsum of the terminal phalanx
6 Z-deformity of the thumb
— MCP flexion and IP hyperextension due to prolapse of metacarpal head between the long and short extensor tendons or to rupture of the thumb flexor
7 'Piano-key' sign
— Hypermobility of a dorsally subluxated ulnar styloid due to laxity of the radioulnar joint (often painful)

Pathogenesis of anemia in rheumatoid arthritis
1 Active inflammatory ('chronic') disease‡
2 Felty's syndrome
3 Iatrogenic
— Aspirin/NSAID-induced GI bleeding*
— Gold/penicillamine-induced hypoplastic anemia
— Sulfasalazine-induced hemolysis or folate deficiency

‡ NB: Anemia reflects disease *activity,* not *chronicity*
* Parenteral iron may cause arthritic 'flare'

COMPLICATIONS OF RHEUMATOID ARTHRITIS

Classic stigmata of rheumatoid vasculitis
1 Skin infarcts
2 Episcleritis
3 Neuropathy

Renal disorders in rheumatoid arthritis‡
1 Amyloidosis (nephrosis)
2 Renal tubular acidosis (in Sjögren's syndrome)
3 Analgesic nephropathy
4 NSAID-induced (usually benign) renal disease*, e.g.
— Interstitial nephritis ($\rightarrow$ hematuria ± proteinuria)
— Nephrosis (rare)
5 Other iatrogenic renal syndromes
— Transient reversible proteinuria (gold, penicillamine)
— Nephrosis due to gold, penicillamine
— Goodpasture's syndrome due to penicillamine

‡ NB: *Glomerular* disease as a primary disease manifestation of RA is quite rare
* See also p. 313

Pulmonary manifestations of rheumatoid arthritis
1 Pleural disease (pleurisy, effusions)
2 Fibrosing alveolitis, interstitial fibrosis
3 Bronchiolitis obliterans ($\rightarrow$ acute, often fatal, lung syndrome)
4 Pulmonary arteritis/hypertension
5 Nodules: may lead to
— Cavitation
— Bronchopleural fistulae
— Caplan's syndrome
6 Stridor due to
— Cricoarytenoid arthritis
— Nodule on vocal cords
7 Recurrent lower respiratory tract infections (Sjögren's)
8 Iatrogenic
— Asthma (salicylates)
— Allergic/fibrosing alveolitis (gold)
— Goodpasture's (D-penicillamine)
— Interstitial fibrosis (methotrexate, chlorambucil)

Rheumatoid complications with male predilection
1 'Rheumatoid lung' (fibrosis, effusions, nodules, pleurisy)
2 Accelerated vasculitis (e.g. $\rightarrow$ mononeuritis multiplex)
3 Mitral valvular regurgitation*

* Commoner post-mortem than aortic regurgitation, but *rarely* of clinical significance (unlike aortic regurgitation)

Diagnosis of Felty's syndrome
1 Defining criteria
— Seropositive rheumatoid arthritis, *plus*
— Splenomegaly, *plus*
— Neutropenia
2 Frequent concomitants
— Serious infections
— Leg ulcers (vasculitic)
— Mononeuritis multiplex
— Anemia, thrombocytopenia
— Lymphadenopathy, hepatomegaly
— Sjögren's syndrome
— Pigmentation, weight loss
3 Laboratory clues
— Thrombocytopenia despite active disease
— Hypocomplementemia
— Positive ANA, high-titer RF (IgM)

4   Response to medical therapy
   — Leukocyte count may (paradoxically) improve after gold
5   Response to splenectomy
   — Arthritis not affected
   — Leukopenia usually improves at least temporarily
   — Infections may increase in frequency or severity

Bad prognostic indicators in rheumatoid arthritis
1   History
   — Male sex
   — Insidious onset
   — Polyarticular presentation
   — Marked (> 10%) weight loss
   — Disability within 1 year of onset
2   Signs
   — Fever; nodules; necrotizing scleritis
   — Lung fibrosis; neuropathy
   — Lymphadenopathy, splenomegaly (± Felty's/ Sjögren's)
   — Purpura (any cause)
3   Complications
   — Early onset (< 3 yrs) of erosions
   — Development of amyloidosis
4   Routine laboratory testing
   — Marked normochromic anemia
   — Thrombocytosis; eosinophilia (unless gold-induced)
   — Hypoalbuminemia, polyclonal gammopathy
   — Markedly elevated ESR/acute phase reactants
5   Specific tests
   — Markedly elevated rheumatoid factor (IgM)
   — Positive neutrophil-specific ANA
   — Cryoglobulinemia
   — HLA-DR3 or -DR4 (research use only)

Prevalence of Raynaud's in autoimmune diseases
1   Scleroderma   —   95%
2   Sjögren's
    Systemic lupus   }   —   25%
    Dermatomyositis
3   Rheumatoid arthritis   —   5%

CRYSTAL ARTHROPATHIES

Presentations of calcium pyrophosphate deposition disease
1   Asymptomatic X-ray chondrocalcinosis   —   30%
2   Pseudogout (→ knee, wrist)   —   30%
3   Accelerated symmetric osteoarthritis   —   30%
4   Pseudorheumatoid arthritis   —   5%
5   Pseudoneuropathic (Charcot) arthritis —   rare

Clinical spectrum of abnormal hydroxyapatite deposition
1   Supraspinatus tendinitis
2   Periarthritis in chronic hemodialysis
3   Milwaukee shoulder (destructive crystal arthritis)
4   Calcinosis associated with scleroderma, dermatomyositis
5   Myositis ossificans
6   Repeated articular steroid injections into small finger joints

SERONEGATIVE SPONDYLOARTHROPATHIES

Ankylosing spondylitis: maneuvers on clinical examination
1   Chest expansion
   — If < 5 cm, indicates costovertebral involvement)
2   Schober's test
   — Positive if full lumbar flexion fails to increase by > 5 cm the distance between L_5 and a point 15 cm above
   — Indicates lumbar disease
3   Occiput to wall
   — Positive if failure of approximation
   — Indicates loss of cervicothoracic lordosis
4   Straight leg raising
   — Indicates malingering if normal in patient complaining of impaired forward flexion
5   Examination of peripheral joints, esp. hips and sternoclavicular joints

Potential complications of ankylosing spondylitis
1   HLA-B27 covariables
   — Enthesopathy
     • Plantar fasciitis
     • Achilles tendinitis
   — Anterior uveitis
   — Chronic prostatitis
2   Chest
   — Chest pain due to costovertebral joint disease
   — Aortic incompetence (due to aortitis*)
   — Pericarditis; cardiac conduction defects
   — Restrictive lung function
     • Impaired chest wall excursion
     • Apical pulmonary fibrosis
3   Cauda equina syndrome
4   Amyloidosis
5   Leukemia (esp. CGL), bone sarcomas
   — If previously treated with spinal irradiation

* cf. RA, where valve dysfunction arises due to valvulitis or nodules

Ankylosing spondylitis in females
1   Neck involvement and peripheral arthritis more common
2   Extraarticular manifestations more common
3   Radiological changes milder
4   True incidence may be underestimated

Clinical patterns of psoriatic arthritis
1   Oligoarticular asymmetric type (70%)
   — 'Sausage' digits = flexor tendon sheath effusions*
   — Indicate underlying dactylitis
2   Distal interphalangeal joint type (15%)
   — Accompanies psoriatic nails
     • Pitting, hyperkeratosis, onycholysis
3   Pseudorheumatoid type
   — Seronegative; affects males and females equally
   — Arthritis severity varies with skin disease
4   Ankylosing spondylitis-type
   — HLA-B27 + in 75% (less common than AS/Reiter's)
5   Arthritis mutilans
   — Often associated with sacroiliitis
   — 'Telescoping' digits

— 'Opera-glass' deformity (may be painless)
— X-ray: 'pencil-in-cup' appearance

* Also found in Reiter's syndrome

Rheumatic aspects of inflammatory bowel disease (IBD)

1 A *non-deforming asymmetric arthritis*, principally affecting knees, ankles and PIPs, occurs in 15%
2 This peripheral arthritis occurs at least 6 months following onset of bowel disease. Its severity reflects that of IBD; colectomy abolishes it
3 *Erythema nodosum, uveitis, mouth ulcers* and *pyoderma* occur in association with peripheral arthritis in IBD
4 *Spondylitis/sacroiliitis* occurs in 5%, may predate onset of bowel symptoms and is associated with HLA-B27. It is independent of IBD activity and unaffected by colectomy; no sex predilection
5 Arthritis and spondylitis in *Whipple's disease* remit with appropriate antibiotics and have *no* HLA association

Differential diagnosis of genital and oral ulceration

1 Reiter's syndrome; Behçet's syndrome
2 Crohn's disease
3 Pemphigus
4 Erythema multiforme
5 Syphilis, herpes simplex
6 Strachan's (orogenital) syndrome

Reiter's vs Behçet's syndrome: the clinical distinction

1 Reiter's
— Male:female = 10:1
— Painless ulcers
— Predominant ocular manifestation: conjunctivitis
— Long-term ocular disability rare
— Long-term joint disability frequent (→ 50%; often mild)
— Spondylitis/sacroiliitis frequent
— HLA association: B27
— Infection seems important in pathogenesis
— R$_x$: NSAIDs
2 Behçet's
— Male:female = 2:1
— Painful ulcers
— Predominant ocular manifestation: uveitis
— Long-term ocular disability almost invariable
— Long-term joint disability rare
— Spondylitis/sacroiliitis uncommon
— HLA associations
• B12
• B5 (eye disease, esp. in Japanese; colitis)
— Racial/genetic factors seem important in pathogenesis
— R$_x$ immunosuppressives (e.g. CSA, azathioprine)

Clinical spectrum of Behçet's syndrome

1 Mouth ulceration (98%)
2 Genital ulceration*
3 Skin lesions
— Erythema nodosum*
— Thrombophlebitis (in 30%; → sterile pustules at venepuncture sites)
4 Eye disease (esp. in males, Japanese; HLA-B5 in 80%)

— Uveitis → pain, photophobia, blurred vision
— Hypopyon; conjunctivitis, scleritis, phthisis bulbi
— Retinal venulitis → 'battlefield' fundus
— Optic neuritis, CRV occlusion
5 CNS disease (30%)
— Aseptic meningitis
— TIA-like episodes
— Cranial nerve palsies
6 Colitis (in 30%; associated with HLA-B5)
— May lead to perforation
— Clinically overlaps with inflammatory bowel disease

NB: Spondylitis/sacroiliitis, when present, are linked to HLA-B27
* Associated with non-deforming arthritis

OCULAR SEQUELAE OF RHEUMATIC DISEASES

Uveitis: etiological categorization

1 Seronegative arthritides (incl. inflammatory bowel disease)
— *Severe* in
• Behçet's
• Juvenile chronic arthritis (ANA+, pauciarticular)
— *Common* in
• Ankylosing spondylitis
• Reiter's syndrome (conjunctivitis commoner)
— *Rare* in psoriatic arthropathy
2 Infection
— Toxoplasmosis, toxocara
— Leptospirosis, syphilis, TB, brucellosis, gonorrhea
3 Sarcoidosis
4 Vogt–Koyanagi syndrome
→ Chronic uveitis, recurrent aseptic meningitis, vitiligo
5 Idiopathic (60%) ± HLA-B27

Anterior vs posterior uveitis

1 Anterior uveitis (iritis)
— Uniocular (acute) presentation usual
— Painful red eye
• Circumcorneal ('ciliary') hyperemia
• Photophobia
• Discharge
— Visual acuity unaffected *unless* complicated by
• Vitreous inflammation (iridocyclitis, hypopyon)
• Corneal opacification (band keratopathy)
• Cataracts, glaucoma (esp. if topical steroids used)
— Slit-lamp examination: posterior synechiae
— Signs of chronicity
• Miosis
• Keratopathy
• Cataracts
• Glaucoma
— R$_x$: *topical* steroids; mydriatics*
2 Posterior uveitis (choroidoretinitis)
— Binocular (chronic) presentation usual
— Painless white eye
— Reduced visual acuity
• Vitreous debris ('floaters')
• Macular edema
• Retinopathy

— Fluorescein angiography: retinal venous leakage
— R$_x$: *systemic* steroids, cyclosporin; azathioprine

* Prevent formation of posterior synechiae

Ocular manifestations of rheumatoid arthritis
1 Keratoconjunctivitis sicca (in 20–30%)
2 Scleral disease
— Episcleritis (hyperemia): good prognosis, sclera heals
— Scleritis: intermediate prognosis, sclera scars
— Scleromalacia perforans: poor prognosis, sclera sloughs
3 Scleral nodules and/or vasculitis
4 Iatrogenic
— Corneal opacity, pigmentary retinopathy (chloroquine)
— Cataracts (steroids)

Differential diagnosis of band keratopathy
1 Juvenile chronic arthritis (ANA+, RF-, pauciarticular type)
2 Long-standing hyperparathyroidism
3 Long-standing renal failure
4 Long-standing sarcoidosis
5 Long-term chloroquine treatment*

* NB: Corneal microdeposits also occur with amiodarone or chlorpromazine

Ocular complications of corticosteroid therapy
1 Herpes simplex keratitis ($\rightarrow$ *topical* steroids)
2 Papilledema (benign intracranial hypertension)
3 Cataract (p. 261)
4 Glaucoma

INVESTIGATING RHEUMATIC DISEASES

SEROLOGIC ASSESSMENT OF RHEUMATIC DISEASE

The acute phase reactants
1 Grossly elevated in inflammatory conditions*
— C-reactive protein
— Serum amyloid-A (SAA) component
2 Moderately elevated in inflammatory conditions
— α_1AT, orosomucoid, α_1 acid glycoprotein
— Haptoglobin, ceruloplasmin, AT III
— C_3 (C_4, C_9); $C_{1\text{-INH}}$
— Fibrinogen, plasminogen; factors V, VIII
— Ferritin
3 Decreased in inflammatory conditions
— Albumin, prealbumin
— Transferrin, iron, TIBC
— Fibronectin

* Increased in RA/JCA, normal in SLE; rise quickly (within 6–10 h of inflammatory insult) unlike, say, fibrinogen (24–48 h)

Clinical utility of C-reactive protein estimations
1 Correlates more closely than ESR with
— Radiographic progression of joint damage
— Disease response to gold/penicillamine (in RA)

2 Useful in monitoring activity of
— Ankylosing spondylitis
— Juvenile chronic arthritis
3 Helpful in distinguishing infective episodes* in
— SLE
— Sicca syndrome
4 Grossly elevated values may aid in distinguishing
— Rheumatoid arthritis (from SLE)
— Crohn's disease (from ulcerative colitis)
— Bacterial meningitis (from viral)
— Pyelonephritis (from cystitis)

* $\uparrow\uparrow$ CRP in infection; normal in active disease

Rheumatoid factors: clinical correlations
1 RA latex (human IgG)
— Most sensitive test
2 Rose–Waaler (rabbit IgG)
— Most specific test
3 Marked elevation in RA
— Rheumatoid lung disease
— Felty's, Sjögren's
4 Marked elevation in non-rheumatic conditions
— SBE
— Myeloma
— Cryoglobulinemia

Grossly elevated ESR in rheumatoid arthritis
1 Highly active synovitis
2 Extraarticular vasculitis
3 Development of amyloidosis
4 Sjögren's syndrome
5 Septic arthritis

RADIOLOGICAL ASSESSMENT OF RHEUMATIC DISEASE

Classical X-ray signs of common rheumatic disorders
1 Rheumatoid arthritis
— Cortical erosions in MCPs, ulnar styloid, carpals*
— Early: soft-tissue swelling, juxtaarticular osteoporosis
— Late: joint (incl. atlantoaxial) subluxation, deformity
2 Primary (familial) osteoarthritis
— Osteophyte formation
— Subchondral sclerosis (no periarticular osteoporosis)
— Joint space narrowing; loose bodies
— Sparing of metacarpophalangeal joints
3 Chondrocalcinosis: calcification of cartilage in
— Knee, wrist
— Symphysis pubis
— Intervertebral discs
4 Reiter's syndrome
— Periostitis contiguous with affected joints
— Calcaneal spurs
— Asymmetric erosions (sparing hands) and sacroiliitis
5 Charcot (neuropathic) joint
— Both sides exhibit destructive changes and sclerosis
— Loose bodies; soft tissue swelling; no osteoporosis

* Most diagnostic sign

Differential diagnosis of radiographic erosions in hands
1 Rheumatoid arthritis
2 Gout
3 Psoriatic arthritis
4 Sarcoidosis
5 Miscellaneous
   — Gaucher's
   — Albright's (polyostotic fibrous dysplasia)
   — Osteitis fibrosa cystica ('brown tumors')
   — Aneurysmal bone cyst, non-ossifying fibroma

The abnormal spinal radiograph: features and diagnosis
1 Ankylosing spondylitis
   — Vertebral 'squaring'
   — Syndesmophyte formation ($\rightarrow$ 'bamboo spine')
   — Romanus lesion (erosion of anterosuperior vertebra)
   — Apophyseal joint fusion
   — Sacroiliac joint erosion, sclerosis or fusion
   — Hip joint erosions
2 DISH (diffuse idiopathic skeletal hyperostosis = Forestier's)
   — Heavy ossification of paraspinal ligaments
   — Olecranon and/or calcaneal spurs
   — Preservation of disc height
   — Normal sacroiliac joints
3 Pott's disease (spinal TB)
   — Gibbus (acute anterior angulation)
   — Paraspinal mass
   — Narrowing of disc space
   — Vertebral collapse (often affects contiguous vertebrae)
4 Metastatic carcinoma
   — Obliteration of pedicle in PA view
   — Discrete lytic (and/or sclerotic) spinal lesions
   — Multiple levels of vertebral collapse
5 (Old) Scheuermann's disease (adolescent osteochondritis)
   — Residual signs of vertebral epiphyseal osteochondritis
6 Straight back syndrome (± marfanoid habitus)
   — Marked reduction of AP chest diameter on lateral CXR

Differential diagnosis of sacroiliitis
1 Ankylosing spondylitis
2 Other seronegative arthritides
   — Psoriatic
   — Reiter's
   — Juvenile chronic arthritis
3 Inflammatory bowel disease, 'reactive' spondyloarthritis
4 Infection
   — Septic arthritis
   — TB
   — Brucellosis
5 Recurrent polyserositis (familial Mediterranean fever)
6 Ochronosis

Atlantoaxial subluxation: diagnosis and management
1 Pathogenesis
   — Odontoid erosion
   — Ligamentous destruction
2 Occurrence
   — Rheumatoid arthritis
   — Juvenile chronic arthritis
   — Ankylosing spondylitis
3 Diagnosis: lateral flexion (+ extension) cervical spine X-ray
   — Odontoid peg > 2.5 mm displaced on atlas
   — MRI: may show inflammatory mass
4 Management if symptomatic
   — If positive MRI scan, proceed to surgery
     • Transoral anterior approach, *plus*
     • Posterior cervical fusion
5 Management if asymptomatic
   — Cervical collar when driving
   — Check for A-a subluxation prior to anesthesia
   — Choose spinal rather than general anesthesia

INVASIVE ASSESSMENT OF JOINT DISEASE

Indications for joint aspiration
1 Diagnosis
   — Septic arthritis
   — Crystal synovitis
2 Therapy
   — Massive effusion interfering with joint function
3 Diagnosis and therapy
   — Hemarthrosis (± coagulation cover)

Indications for joint injection
1 Diagnosis
   — Arthrogram for suspected menisceal (knee) tears
   — Arthrogram for suspected (ruptured) Baker's cyst
2 Therapeutic
   — Intraarticular corticosteroids
   — 'Medical synovectomy' (yttrium^{90})

Indications for diagnostic arthroscopy
1 Unexplained monarthritis
2 Suspected injury (e.g. $\rightarrow$ meniscus, cruciates)
3 Histologic diagnosis sought (e.g. villonodular synovitis)

Important diagnoses on synovial biopsy
1 Tuberculous arthritis
2 (Pigmented) villonodular synovitis
3 Amyloidosis
4 Ochronosis (alkaptonuria)
5 Synovial tumors (e.g. hemangioma)

ANALYSIS OF SYNOVIAL FLUID

Non-inflammatory effusions: characteristics and causes
1 Characteristics
   — Synovial fluid white cell count < 2 x 10^9/L
   — High viscosity
   — Negative fibrin clot
2 Causes
   — Osteoarthritis
   — Post-traumatic
   — Sympathetic (e.g. adjacent to osteomyelitis)
   — Myxedema

— Amyloidosis
— Sickle-cell disease
— Hypertrophic pulmonary osteoarthropathy

Synovial fluid leukocyte counts in health and disease
1 Normal
— < 0.2 x 10^9/L
2 'Non-inflammatory' synovitis (e.g. osteoarthritis)
— < 2.0 x 10^9/L; 10–30% polymorphs
3 Inflammatory synovitis
— Septic arthritis
• 5–500 x 10^9/L (av. 50 x 10^9/L)
• 80–100% polymorphs
— Gout
• 2–200 x 10^9/L (av. 15 x 10^9/L)
• 60–95% polymorphs
— Reiter's syndrome
• 2–50 x 10^9/L (av. 20 x 10^9/L)
• 50–90% polymorphs
— Rheumatoid arthritis
• 2–100 x 10^9/L (av. 10 x 10^9/L)
• 50–75% polymorphs

Other joint fluid abnormalities
1 ↓ Glucose level
— Septic arthritis
— Reiter's syndrome
— Rheumatoid arthritis (*also* low in RA effusions)
2 Complement levels
— ↑ In Reiter's syndrome
— ↓ In RA, SLE, gout, sepsis*
3 Cytology
— Phagocytosed leukocytes
• Reiter's syndrome
— 'Ragocytes'
• Rheumatoid arthritis
— Hemosiderin-laden *macrophages*
• Recurrent hemarthroses
— Hemosiderin-laden *synovial* cells
• Hemochromatosis

* NB: *Plasma* complement levels may be similarly low in active SLE, but elevated in active rheumatoid arthritis. Hence, synovial:serum complement ratio is typically < 10% in RA without systemic vasculitis. When RA is complicated by systemic vasculitis, however, plasma complement levels are usually also low

Differential diagnosis of hemarthrosis
1 Hemophilia
2 Major trauma (e.g. fracture communicating with joint)
Minor trauma in anticoagulated patient
3 Joint tumors, incl. pigmented villonodular synovitis
4 Charcot joint; arthritis mutilans
5 Calcium pyrophosphate deposition disease
6 'Traumatic tap'*

* Distinguish from true hemarthrosis by centrifuging aspirate and demonstrating absent xanthochromia

Crystal arthropathies: findings on joint aspiration
1 Gout
— Needleshaped urate crystals
— Strongly negative birefringence (polarized microscopy)

— Angle of extinction: parallel
— Crystals may → non-inflamed joints in gouty patients
2 Pseudogout
— Rhomboid-shaped pyrophosphate crystals
— Weakly positive birefringence
— Angle of extinction: oblique
3 Rheumatoid arthritis may mimic crystal synovitis due to cholesterol crystals in chronic effusions
4 Hydroxyapatite crystals may be seen on electron microscopy in OA or other arthritides, especially if bone destruction
5 Post-steroid injection flare (4–12 h later) due to steroid crystals

HLA IN RHEUMATIC DISEASE

Relative indications for tissue typing in rheumatic disease
1 Older male child (11–16 years) with oligoarthritis, if diagnosis of ankylosing spondylitis is neither certain nor unlikely
— B27-positive
• 90% risk of ankylosing spondylitis
• ↓ Risk of chronic anterior uveitis
— B27-negative
• 15% probability of ankylosing spondylitis
• ↑ Risk of chronic anterior uveitis
2 Controversial
— DR3 screening to predict patients at increased risk of renal toxicity from gold/penicillamine

NB: *No* absolute – or routine – indications currently exist

HLA associations in rheumatoid arthritis
1 DR4
— 6-fold ↑ (seropositive) disease
— ↑ Felty's syndrome
2 DR3
— ↑ Incidence of major side-effects (esp. proteinuria, cytopenia) from gold, penicillamine
— ↑ Sjögren's syndrome
3 DR2
— ↓ Incidence of disease (? protective)

MANAGING RHEUMATIC DISEASE

Therapeutic emergencies in rheumatic disease
1 Atlantoaxial subluxation
— Tends to affect RA patients on long-term steroids
— R_x: surgical decompression and fusion (if symptomatic)
2 Temporal arteritis
— Draw blood for ESR as soon as diagnosis suspected
— R_x: prednisone 20–60 mg/day (high dose if eye disease)
— Commence treatment as soon as ESR drawn*
3 Septic arthritis
— Drain joint, Gram-stain, culture, sensitivity
— R_x: intravenous antibiotics

4 Vasculitic complications
— Mononeuritis multiplex
— Digital gangrene, bowel infarction
— R$_x$: high-dose steroids, cytotoxic drugs
5 Iridocyclitis
— Complicates seronegative arthropathies (*not* RA)
— R$_x$: mydriatics, topical/systemic steroids
Episcleritis
— Complicates RA (*not* seronegative arthropathies)
— R$_x$: topical steroids, NSAIDs or systemic steroids
6 Iatrogenic: GI bleed, blood dyscrasia, adrenal dysfunction
— Identify and cease offending medication
— R$_x$: supportive

* Biopsy results unaffected by up to 48 h of steroids

GENERAL MEASURES IN RHEUMATIC DISORDERS

Rationâle of exercise in joint disease
1 To maintain or restore muscle strength around joint
2 To maintain or restore range of joint movement
3 To prevent or minimize periarticular osteoporosis

Principles of occupational therapy in rheumatic disease
1 Provision of appliances to reduce joint strain
— Work splints (for wrists)
— Removable splints (for unstable knees)
— Cervical collars (hard or soft)
2 Provision of appliances to improve function
— Special shoes and insoles, non-slip mats
— Walking sticks, wheelchairs, walking frames
— Shopping cart
3 Home visits to adapt house for activities of daily living
— Toilet aids, handrails, electric toothbrush
— Tap turners, electric can opener, large-handled cutlery
— Book rest, page turner, push-button phone

Principles of physiotherapy in rheumatoid arthritis
1 *Night splinting* to rest knees, wrists in position of function
Serial splinting to reverse early deformities*
2 *Passive exercises* to maintain range of joint movement
Isometric exercises to maintain muscle power
Active exercises to maintain power and range of movement
3 Facilitation of exercise using
— Ultrasound
— Heat
— Hydrotherapy

* e.g. knee flexion; bedrest may exacerbate deformity in active disease

How to treat nerve/tendon compression in rheumatoid arthritis
1 **S**plinting (esp. wrist or knee)
2 **S**ystemic treatment (e.g. gold)
3 **S**teroid injection (soluble preparation → ↓ risk of neurolysis)

4 **S**ynovectomy (esp. wrist or knee)
5 **S**urgical decompression

Effects of posture or physiotherapy on ankylosing spondylitis
1 *No* effect on rate of ankylosis
2 *Mild* reduction in pain
3 *Major* reduction in disability*

* e.g. eventual ankylosis → erect, not kyphotic, posture

NON-STEROIDAL ANTIINFLAMMATORY DRUGS (NSAIDs)

Points to consider in NSAID prescribing
1 NSAIDs may improve joint *function* by reducing pain and inflammation; they do not reverse the arthropathy
2 The maximum tolerated dose of any given NSAID should be prescribed before being discarded as ineffective
3 Several NSAIDs may need to be tried to find the best
4 In general, different NSAIDs should *not* be combined

Non-steroidal antiinflammatory drugs: toxicity
1 Gastrointestinal (esp. with high-dose aspirin, indomethacin)
— Dyspepsia, gastritis, ulceration*
2 CNS (esp. with indomethacin)
— Headache, confusion, dizziness
3 Blood dyscrasias (esp. with phenylbutazone†)
— Aplastic anemia, agranulocytosis, thrombocytopenia
4 Nephrotoxicity
— Precipitation of acute renal failure
— Edema (sodium retention); nephrosis
— Papillary necrosis
— Interstitial nephritis
5 Other: bullous dermatoses, hepatitis, aseptic meningitis

* Sulindac and ibuprofen are probably the least ulcerogenic of these drugs (p. 134). In general, however, patient tolerance of any one drug is unpredictable
† Phenylbutazone now *only* indicated for refractory ankylosing spondylitis

ASPIRIN

Aspirin as first-line therapy
1 Juvenile chronic arthritis
2 Rheumatic fever
3 Rheumatoid arthritis
Seronegative spondyloarthropathies (not AS)
Soft tissue rheumatism
— In USA
4 Osteoid osteoma

NB: The association of aspirin with Reye's syndrome makes monitoring mandatory in children younger than 12 requiring aspirin therapy

Predispositions to aspirin hepatotoxicity
1 Juvenile chronic arthritis

2 Reiter's syndrome
3 Chronic active hepatitis
4 Rheumatic fever
5 SLE

Presentations of aspirin sensitivity
1 Urticaria, bronchospasm, anaphylaxis
2 Pyrexia of unknown origin
3 Pneumonitis
4 Pancreatitis
5 Proctocolitis
6 Ulceration of the esophagus

Aspirin toxicity: the clinical spectrum
1 Antiinflammatory action requires daily dosage of 2–4 g/day
2 Gastrointestinal intolerance is main cause of non-compliance
3 Tinnitus and vertigo are dose-related toxicities which may be clinically useful in regulating drug dosage. Hearing loss may necessitate treatment cessation; salicylate levels and/or audiograms may be useful in monitoring
4 Iron-deficiency anemia may occur in the absence of gastrointestinal symptoms; hypoprothrombinemia rare
5 High-dose regimens are uricosuric, whereas low-dose administration may lead to hyperuricemia and gout
6 Hepatotoxicity manifests as asymptomatic transaminase elevation which often normalizes if drug continued; it occurs more commonly in young patients

REMITTIVE DRUG THERAPY

Diseases treatable with remittive drug therapy
1 Gold
— Rheumatoid arthritis
— Sjögren's syndrome
• Higher incidence of drug reactions
• Sicca syndrome alone may not respond
— Psoriatic arthritis
— Juvenile chronic arthritis
— Pemphigus (steroid-sparing)
2 D-penicillamine
— Rheumatoid arthritis
— Cystinuria → proteinuria in 25%
— Wilson's disease → proteinuria in 5%
— Psoriatic arthritis
— Heavy metal poisoning
3 Chloroquine
— SLE (esp. joint and skin involvement)
— Juvenile chronic arthritis
— Rheumatoid arthritis
— *Contraindicated* in psoriatic arthritis
4 Sulfasalazine
— Rheumatoid arthritis
— Seronegative spondyloarthropathies

Gold: toxicity
1 Pruritic rash
— Occurs in 30% of treated patients

— May mimic lichen planus, pityriasis rosea
— Frequently preceded by peripheral eosinophilia
— Aurothiomalate (IMI) > triethylphosphine gold (oral)
2 Gastrointestinal
— Stomatitis, mouth ulcers
— Diarrhea (triethylphosphine gold)
3 Leukopenia, thrombocytopenia
— An absolute indication for treatment cessation
— Heavy metal chelators may be indicated if acute
4 Proteinuria
— Occurs in 5% of treated patients
— If < 1 g/day, drug may be cautiously reintroduced *after* normalization of protein excretion
— If > 1 g/day, cease gold therapy indefinitely
5 Nephrosis
— Occurs in 1% of treated patients
— Recovery may take 18 months
6 Rare
— Fibrosing alveolitis
— Enterocolitis, cholestasis
— Neuropathy

D-penicillamine: toxicity
1 Loss of taste, anorexia, nausea
— Occurs in 25%
— Improves with continued treatment
2 Proteinuria (25%), nephrosis (5%)
3 Thrombocytopenia (10%)
4 Early rash (10%) in first month: may reintroduce R_x
Wrinkly skin (elastosis serpiginosa perforans)
Late (pemphigus-like) rash in 5%; if severe, cease R_x
5 Rare
— SLE, myasthenia gravis, polymyositis
— Goodpasture-like syndrome
6 Lack of efficacy (25%)
— Similar incidence to gold
— More likely if previously unresponsive to gold

Indications for methotrexate in non-malignant disease
1 Rheumatoid arthritis*
2 Juvenile chronic arthritis
3 Psoriasis‡
4 Crohn's disease

* Second- or third-line treatment
‡ Hepatotoxicity may be dose-limiting

TREATING RHEUMATOID ARTHRITIS

Rheumatoid arthritis: indications for remittive therapy
1 Symptomatic young patients (esp. females) with polyarticular disease and high levels of rheumatoid factor
2 Radiological erosions developing in the first year of disease
3 Troublesome symptoms despite NSAIDs for 6 months
4 Extraarticular disease affecting vital organ function

Prescribing strategy in rheumatoid arthritis
1 First-line therapy: symptomatic treatment only
— NSAIDs
— Aspirin 3–4 g/day (popular in USA only)

2   Remittive drugs ($\rightarrow$ $\downarrow$ erosions)
— Methotrexate (oral weekly dose: 7.5–10 mg)
— Gold (intramuscular or oral)
— D-penicillamine (oral)
— Sulfasalazine (oral)
— (Hydroxy)chloroquine (oral)
3   Failure of conventional remittive drugs?
— Cytotoxics (azathioprine, cyclophosphamide)
— Systemic corticosteroids

NB: Nocturnal slow-release NSAIDs (oral or suppositories) may help minimize morning stiffness in RA

Relative efficacy of remittive drugs
1   High efficacy
— Methotrexate
— Sodium aurothiomalate
2   Intermediate efficacy
— Penicillamine
— Sulfasalazine*
3   Mild efficacy
— Antimalarials
— Triethylphosphine gold

* But often used before other drugs due to good tolerance

Relative toxicity of remittive drugs
1   High toxicity
— Sodium aurothiomalate
2   Intermediate toxicity
— Penicillamine
— Methotrexate*
3   Mild toxicity
— Sulfasalazine
— Triethylphosphine gold
— Antimalarials

* Patients should avoid alcohol (due to risk of liver toxicity) and take supplementary folate

Indications for systemic steroids in rheumatoid arthritis
1   Development of stridor
2   Necrotizing scleritis
3   Pleuropericarditis
4   Other signs of extraarticular vasculitis threatening vital organ function, e.g. mononeuritis multiplex
5   Persistent arthritis despite adequate trial of remittive drugs

SYSTEMIC STEROIDS IN RHEUMATIC DISEASE

Prescribing steroids in rheumatoid arthritis
1   Uncommonly indicated; if necessary, treatment should be aimed at a specific goal (i.e. a temporizing measure only)
2   Treatment should be low-dose: 5–7.5 mg prednisone/day max.
3   To minimize adrenal suppression, use a single a.m. dose only
4   Alternate-day steroids don't work in RA; if symptoms appear well-controlled on alternate-day steroids, then the patient probably doesn't need steroids at all

Potency and toxicity of various corticosteroids
1   30 mg cortisone acetate
= 25 mg hydrocortisone
= 5 mg (methyl)prednis(ol)one, triamcinolone
= 1 mg dexamethasone, betamethasone
2   Hydrocortisone causes sodium retention; hence, useful in adrenal replacement therapy, but not otherwise
3   Triamcinolone, given systemically, is the most myopathic of the corticosteroids; therefore only used topically
4   Prednisone is a prodrug; hence, in severe liver disease, better to use prednisolone (the active metabolite)

ACTH or prednisone? Pros and cons of ACTH therapy
1   Disadvantages of ACTH
— Expensive
— Painful (daily intramuscular injections)
— Difficult to adjust or taper dosage
— Greater salt/fluid retention than prednisone (reflecting greater mineralocorticoid effect)
— Pigmentation; bruising; severe allergic reactions
2   Advantages of ACTH
— For juvenile chronic arthritis patients
$\rightarrow$ $\downarrow$ Growth stunting
— For hospitalized patients with inflammatory arthritis
$\rightarrow$ No adrenal suppression (hence, easy to stop)
— For polymyositis/dermatomyositis/multiple sclerosis
$\rightarrow$ $\downarrow$ Muscle wasting (androgen effect)
— For post-menopausal female patients
$\rightarrow$ $\downarrow$ Osteoporosis ($\uparrow$ androstenedione $\rightarrow$ $\uparrow$ estrone)

INTRAARTICULAR STEROIDS

Potential indications for intraarticular steroids
1   Systemic treatment contraindicated (e.g. blood dyscrasia)
2   Systemic treatment inadequate to control inflammation at one or more joints (incl. Baker's cyst)
3   Troublesome oligoarticular inflammation not warranting systemic therapy (e.g. in seronegative arthropathy)
4   To mobilize (and reduce deformity) in rehabilitation
5   Rapid analgesia required

Intraarticular steroids: which joints?
1   Common
— Knee, shoulder
2   Less often
— Ankle, elbow, fingers
3   Rare
— Hip

Intraarticular steroid therapy: potential morbidity
1   Crystal-induced synovitis (a 'flare' of pain and swelling a few hours after injection; esp. with triamcinolone)

2 Charcot-like arthropathy (i.e. severe joint destruction, though probably **not** due to loss of pain sensation)
3 Cushing's syndrome
4 Septic arthritis, *or*
 Suppression of inflammatory signs (e.g. in septic arthritis complicating RA)

ANTIMALARIALS IN RHEUMATIC DISEASE

Potential hazards of antimalarial chemotherapy
1 Chloroquine is avoided in psoriatic arthritis due to the risk of a pustular exacerbation (which may be indistinguishable from keratoderma blenorrhagica of Reiter's syndrome)
2 Chloroquine should not be administered in full dosage to SLE patients with porphyria cutanea tarda. If the drug is prescribed in this context, the patient should be phlebotomized on at least two prior occasions and the drug given in low-dose twice-weekly schedule
3 Oculotoxicity includes cycloplegia ($\rightarrow$ transient blurring) and corneal microdeposits (rarely culminating in band keratopathy) in addition to the well-known retinopathy

Features of chloroquine retinopathy
1 Occurrence is commoner with
 — Renal impairment
 — SLE
 — Concomitant probenecid therapy
 — Daily dosage > 150 mg *base* per day*
2 Occurrence *cannot* be predicted by onset of visual symptoms (more commonly due to presbyopia or cycloplegia)
3 Slit-lamp examination every 4–6 months is mandatory, but benefit remains unproven. Best screening tests are
 — Observation of the foveal reflex
 — Charting the pericentral visual fields to a red object
4 The classic 'bull's eye' macula may supervene despite early cessation of therapy

* i.e. > 250 mg chloroquine phosphate/sulfate or 400 mg hydroxychloroquine

THE HYPERURICEMIC PATIENT

Etiology of hyperuricemia in childhood
1 Associated with gout in childhood
 — HGPRTase deficiency (Lesch–Nyhan syndrome)
 — PRPP synthetase overactivity
2 Not associated with gout in childhood
 — Acute leukemia ($\rightarrow$ lymphoblastic, post-chemo)
 — Chronic hemolysis (e.g. sickle-cell disease)
 — Lead poisoning
 — Von Gierke's; Gaucher's
 — Severe diabetes mellitus, hypertriglyceridemia

Management aspects of gout and hyper-uricemia
1 Modalities available for treating acute gouty arthritis

 — Colchicine (traditional remedy; major GI toxicity)
 — NSAIDs (now more popular than colchicine)
 — Joint aspiration
 — Intraarticular corticosteroids
2 Modalities available for long-term gout prophylaxis
 — Allopurinol
 — Uricosurics: probenecid, sulfinpyrazone
3 Drugs inhibiting uricosurics (avoid in gouty patients)
 — Thiazides
 — Ethambutol
 — Low-dose salicylate
 — Cyclosporin

Exclusive indications for allopurinol administration
1 Tophaceous gout, *or*
 Gouty bony erosions
2 Recurrent troublesome acute gouty attacks
3 Recurrent urate calculi, *or*
 Recurrent oxalate calculi with hyperuricosuria
4 Prevention of uric acid nephropathy in patients at risk for tumor lysis syndrome (p. 169) prechemo-therapy
5 *Massive* urate overproduction (> 7.2 mmol/24 h urine) despite low-purine alcohol-free diet, esp. if family history of renal disease

NB: Asymptomatic hyperuricemia or uncomplicated gout are *not* indications for maintenance allopurinol

Allopurinol: toxicity
1 Major hypersensitivity reactions (toxic epidermal necrolysis, vasculitis, eosinophilia) may be heralded by rash or fever
2 Major reactions are commoner in renal impairment and/or diuretic therapy and may lead to renal failure
3 Hepatotoxicity is an uncommon but serious sequela
4 Ampicillin rashes are more frequent
5 Allopurinol potentiates
 — 6MP, azathioprine (4-fold)
 — Warfarin (weak effect)

OPERATIVE OPTIONS IN JOINT DISEASE

Rheumatoid arthritis: the place of surgery
1 Resection of metatarsal heads
 — For forefoot pain due to MTP subluxation
2 Total articular arthroplasty
 — Ideal for hip
3 Excision arthroplasty
 — Excision of radial head in severe erosive elbow arthritis
 — Resection of distal ulna as part of wrist synovectomy
4 Synovectomy (improves symptoms for about 2 years)
 — Knee: for refractory Baker's cyst
 — Wrist: for refractory nodular tenosynovitis
5 Miscellaneous
 — Silastic MCP joint replacement (deformity recurs)
 — Immediate tendon reanastomosis for rupture
 — Posterior cervical fusion for atlantoaxial subluxation
 — Decompression of entrapment neuropathies
 — Splenectomy in Felty's syndrome

Total hip replacement: indications and complications
1 Indications
   — Patient > 50 with unrelieved severe hip arthritis
   — *Any* patient with permanent loss of hip mobility
   (< 45° flexion, < 10° abduction) leading to reduced
   activity
2 Complications
   — Implant loosening
   — Infection of bone-cement interface
   — Metal sensitivity ($\rightarrow$ loosening)
   — Mechanical failure
   — Post-operative thromboembolism despite
   prophylaxis

Arthrodesis or osteotomy? Clinical considerations
1 Arthrodesis
   — Favored joints: wrist, ankle (subtalar joint only)
   — Less popular: knee, hip, tarsal, first MCP
   — Best for young (20–30) patients
   — Best for monarthritis ($\downarrow$ mobility less significant)
   — Preferred to osteotomy if joint architecture
   destroyed
2 Osteotomy
   — Favored joints: hip, knee
   — Best for patients younger than 50
   — Best for painful stable joints ($\uparrow$ mobility not a
   priority)
   — Preferred to arthrodesis if X-ray confirms
   asymmetrical disruption of joint architecture

Anesthetic considerations in patients with rheumatic disease
1 Rheumatoid arthritis
   — If cervical spine X-ray shows atlantoaxial subluxation and/or odontoid erosion in an asymptomatic patient, use soft collar and spinal anesthesia
   — If atlantoaxial subluxation or odontoid erosion
   occurs in a patient with symptoms of cord compression, assess with MRI and consider cervical
   spine surgery (pp. 351, 353) *prior* to elective
   operation
   — If temporomandibular joint disease evident,
   anticipate difficult endotracheal intubation
   (though rarely a major problem in RA; cf. in JCA)
2 Ankylosing spondylitis
   — Lower cervical spondylosis and/or TMJ disease
   may make intubation difficult
   — Costovertebral involvement may restrict
   ventilation
3 Juvenile chronic arthritis
   — Intubation may be difficult due to micrognathia

Patient selection for 'medical synovectomy'*
1 Most effective for recurrent inflammatory knee
   effusions
2 Any risk of pregnancy is an absolute contraindication
3 Youth is a relative contraindication (risk of
   leukemogenesis)
4 Ideally, the joint to be injected should be devoid of
   gross synovial thickening or severe destructive
   changes
5 Adequate rest, physiotherapy, drugs and intraarticular
   steroids should precede use of medical synovectomy

* i.e. intraarticular instillation of, say [90]yttrium

PAGET'S DISEASE

Treatable causes of pain in Paget's disease
1 Osteoarthritis (hip, knee) due to limb deformity
2 Pseudogout
3 Nerve entrapment
4 Microfractures due to cortical expansion
5 Pathological fracture
   — Disease-related
   — Supervening osteosarcoma
   — Diphosphonate use

Indications for commencement of specific chemotherapy
1 Serum alkaline phosphatase > 1000 U/L
2 Severe bone pain unresponsive to conservative
   measures
3 Intractable angina or heart failure (if due to Paget's)
4 Progressive deformity of weight-bearing long bones
   or skull base, esp. in relatively young patients
   Osteolytic lesions affecting long bones, esp. if
   painful
5 Hypercalcemia (precipitated by immobilization or
   trauma) and/or radioopaque renal calculi
6 Neurological sequelae
   — Spinal cord compression
   — Peripheral nerve entrapment
   — Visual failure due to macular degeneration
   — Progressive deafness accompanied by tinnitus

Drug treatment: relative indications and contraindications
1 Calcitonin
   — Indications
     • Severe bone pain requiring rapid relief
     • Painful osteolytic lesions
     • Hypercalcemia/symptomatic hypercalciuria
     • Failure or toxicity of alternative therapy
   — Contraindications
     • Resistance due to neutralizing antibodies
     • Unsuitability of parenteral administration;
       expense
2 Biphosphonates (clodronate, pamidronate,
   etidronate)
   — Indications
     • Predominant skull involvement
     • Mild to moderate bone pain
     • Incomplete clinical/biochemical response to
       calcitonin
   — Contraindications
     • Severe bone pain (may be worsened)
     • Development of fractures*
     • Known (preexisting) osteolytic lesions
     • Development of diarrhea while on treatment
3 Mithramycin
   — Indications
     • Failure or toxicity of first-line agents
     • Severe or life-threatening hypercalcemia
   — Contraindications
     • Thrombocytopenia
     • Severe renal or hepatic dysfunction

* With etidronate only

POLYMYALGIA RHEUMATICA

Diagnostic criteria for polymyalgia rheumatica (PMR)
1 Age > 50
2 ESR > 50 mm/h
3 Bilateral shoulder/pelvic girdle morning stiffness
   — Symptomatic episodes > I h duration, *and*
   — Clinical history > 1 month duration
4 Response to low-dose (~ 15 mg/day prednisone) steroids
5 Minor criteria
   — Weight loss, night sweats, fever
   — Symmetrical proximal muscle tenderness
   — ↑ Alkaline phosphatase/GGT, ↓ Hb
   — Positive joint scintigraphy*
   — Normal CPK, EMG, muscle biopsy

* i.e. synovitis, but *no* myositis or vasculitis/arteritis, in 'pure' PMR

Exclusion of coexisting temporal arteritis
1 50% of temporal arteritis patients have symptoms of PMR
2 50% of *all* PMR patients (± symptoms of temporal arteritis) will have giant cell arteritis on temporal artery biopsy
3 10–20% of patients with *clinically pure* PMR will be found to have temporal arteritis on biopsy
4 False-negative biopsies may occur due to 'skip lesions' (i.e. the *abnormal* arterial segments) causing sampling error; for a 2 cm biopsy, however, false-negative rate is < 5%
5 Height of initial ESR *does not* predict disease severity or likelihood of complications
6 With proper management, the diagnosis of giant cell arteritis is *not* associated with reduced life expectancy

INFECTION AND JOINT DISEASE

Infections commonly associated with arthritis
1 *Staph aureus*, esp. in intravenous drug abusers
2 *Staph albus*, esp. in prosthetic joints
3 *Salmonella* spp., esp. in hyposplenic patients*
4 *H. influenzae*, esp. in children
5 *N. gonorrheae*, esp. in young women
6 Lyme disease (spirochetal etiology)

* Causes osteomyelitis or spondylitis

Infections commonly associated with arthralgias
1 Associated with arthralgias alone
   — Influenza A
   — Coxsackie B, EBV, mumps
   — Mycoplasmas
   — Brucellosis
2 Associated with arthralgias ± arthritis
   — Hepatitis B
   — Rubella (incl. rubella vaccine)

— Parvovirus
— Alphaviruses (arboviruses)
  • Ross River, Sindbis, Chikungunya, Barmah Forest
— Disseminated gonococcal infection

Reactive arthritis: occurrence and manifestations
1 Etiology
   — Post-dysenteric
     • *Shigella flexneri*
     • *Salmonella* spp.
     • *Yersinia enterocolitica*
     • *Campylobacter jejuni*
   — Venereal: *Chlamydia trachomatis*
2 Symptoms
   — Knee and ankle pain 1–3 weeks following infection
   — Enthesopathy (tenosynovitis, plantar fasciitis)
   — Low back pain
3 Urethritis may occur with post-dysenteric syndrome
   — e.g. In prepubertal children
4 Joint fluid is sterile
5 The initial episode generally settles over about 3 months
6 Long-term prognosis is good, but 50% will have recurrence

Rheumatologic manifestations of HIV infection
1 Seronegative spondyloarthropathy
   — Heel pain, enthesopathy
   — Remains associated with HLA-B27
   — Tends to be more severe than in HIV-negative disease
2 Septic arthritis
   — Typically affects axial joints
   — Pathogen may be transferred by sex or needles
3 AIDS-associated arthritis
   — Often very painful
   — Lower limb oligoarthritis or symmetric polyarthritis
   — Synovial fluid: 'non-inflammatory' profile (p. 351)

OTHER ARTHROPATHIES

Juvenile chronic arthritis: a working classification
1 Systemic onset ('Still's disease')
   — RF–, ANA–
   — Age of onset < 16 years
   — Quotidian fever usual ± ↑ WCC
   — Non-pruritic rash, Koebner phenomenon (p. 363)
   — ± Polyserositis, hepatosplenomegaly, adenopathy
   — 50% → polyarticular disease, 50% remit
   — Acute phase associated with significant mortality
   — Commonest cause of death is amyloidosis
2 Polyarticular non-systemic ('juvenile rheumatoid arthritis')
   — RF+ (100%) ANA+ (75%)
   — 90% female
   — Late childhood onset → severe adult disease
3 Pauciarticular disease (→ knee) and/or chronic uveitis (50%)
   — RF–, ANA+ (50%)

— 90% female, early childhood onset
— Major joint disability unusual
— Severe eye disease common
4 Pauciarticular disease (→ hip), sacroiliitis, acute uveitis (10%)
— RF–, ANA–, HLA-B27+ (75%)
— 90% male
— May progress to typical ankylosing spondylitis

Clinical aspects of miscellaneous arthropathies
1 Jaccoud's (post-rheumatic fever) arthropathy
— Moderately severe rheumatic heart disease
— History of severe or prolonged rheumatic fever
— Mildly symptomatic but deforming arthropathy
— Reducible ulnar deviation and PIP hyperextension
— Good hand function despite extent of deformity
— No erosive or destructive changes on X-ray
— Rheumatoid factor negative
2 Palindromic rheumatism
— Equal incidence in males and females
— Asymptomatic between exacerbations
— Typically affects hand, wrists, carpal tunnel
— 90% rheumatoid factor negative at diagnosis
— May evolve to typical RA (and become seropositive)
3 Relapsing polychondritis
— Associated with autoimmune disease in 30%
— Fever, arthralgias, episcleritis, swollen floppy ears
— Nasal septum involvement/collapse ('saddle nose')
— Laryngeal disease → hoarseness, respiratory obstruction
— Tracheobronchial degeneration, sudden death
— Approx. 10% →
  • Aortic valvular incompetence/aneurysm
  • Mitral valve prolapse
— Responds to corticosteroid administration

Rheumatologic manifestations of sickle-cell disease
1 Gout
2 Sickle crisis →
— Lower limb arthralgias, myalgias
— Acute synovitis with non-inflammatory effusion
3 'Hand-foot' syndrome*

4 Secondary hemochromatotic arthropathy (transfusional)
5 Septic arthritis/osteomyelitis from *Salmonella* (hyposplenic)
6 Aseptic (avascular) necrosis

* Dactylitis due to periostitis, marrow expansion and/or infarction

AVASCULAR NECROSIS OF BONE

Avascular necrosis of the femoral head: predispositions
1 Primary (Perthes' disease: epiphyseal osteochondritis)
2 Local trauma
— Slipped epiphysis (often bilateral in fat children)
— Femoral neck fractures
— Traumatic dislocation
3 Sickle-cell disease (including sickle trait)
4 Hypercoagulable states, e.g.
— Hb C disease
— Paroxysmal nocturnal hemoglobinuria
— Nephrotic syndrome; pregnancy
5 SLE, rheumatoid arthritis
  Corticosteroid administration
  Renal transplantation
6 Alcoholism, cirrhosis, pancreatitis
7 Myxedema
8 Gaucher's disease
9 Caisson (decompression) disease; hyperbaric oxygen
10 Therapeutic irradiation

Diagnosing avascular necrosis of the femoral head
1 X-ray of abducted hip
— Irregular femoral head, translucent band, sclerosis
2 ^{99m}Tc diphosphonate scan
— Low isotope uptake (only useful post-trauma)
3 CT scan
— Subchondral rarefaction
4 MRI
— Clear definition of area of ischemic necrosis

REVIEWING THE LITERATURE: RHEUMATOLOGY

14.1 Byrn C et al (1993) Subcutaneous sterile water injections for chronic neck and shoulder pain following whiplash injuries. Lancet 341: 449–452

Sterile water injected over tenderpoints (T-points) was significantly better than saline in this randomized study of 40 long-standing whiplash injury victims.

14.2 Carette S et al (1991) A controlled trial of corticosteroid injections into facet joints for chronic low back pain. N Engl J Med 325: 1002–1007

Randomized comparison of injecting either steroids (methylprednisolone) or saline into the facet joints of patients reporting relief from the same procedure using local anesthetic. No significant benefit was recorded in the steroid group, thus invalidating the use of this approach.

14.3 Malmivaara A et al (1995) The treatment of low back pain – bed rest, exercises, or ordinary activity? N Engl J Med 332: 351–355

Randomized study of 185 Finnish patients, showing that continuing normal (albeit limited) activities was more fruitful than either bedrest or back exercises.

14.4 Bradley JD et al (1991) Comparison of an antiinflammatory dose of ibuprofen, an analgesic dose of ibuprofen, and acetaminophen in the treatment of patients with osteoarthritis of the knee. N Engl J Med 325: 87–91

Interesting study showing that paracetamol was as effective as high- or low-dose ibuprofen for symptomatic knee osteoarthritis.

March L et al (1994) 'n of 1' trials comparing a non-steroidal anti-inflammatory drug with paracetamol in osteoarthritis. Br Med J 309: 1041–1046

'Single-patient' (n of 1) clinical trials showed that half the patients receiving NSAIDs for osteoarthritis did as well with paracetamol, thus confirming the conclusions of the foregoing citation.

14.5 Elliott MJ et al (1993) Treatment of rheumatoid arthritis with chimeric monoclonal antibodies to tumour necrosis factor alpha. Arthritis Rheum 36: 1681–1690

Important study suggesting that TNF-α plays a central role in the pathogenesis of RA.

14.6 Langman M et al (1994) Risks of bleeding peptic ulcer associated with individual non-steroidal anti-inflammatory drugs. Lancet 343: 1075–1078

Retrospective analysis of 1144 NSAID bleeders; odds ratio for bleeding was lowest for ibuprofen and diclofenac, highest for azapropazone and ketoprofen. Dose was also causally linked.

14.7 Carey TS et al (1995) The outcomes and costs of care for acute low back pain among patients seen by primary care practitioners, chiropractors, and orthopedic surgeons. N Engl J Med 333: 913–917

No difference in outcome, but primary carer was the cheapest.

Helewa A et al (1991) Effects of occupational therapy home service on patients with rheumatoid arthritis. Lancet 337: 1453–1456

Randomized study of 105 RA patients showing significantly improved joint function in the cohort receiving occupational therapy (did any of you ever suspect it didn't work?).

Meade TW et al (1995) Randomised comparison of chiropractic and hospital outpatient management for low back pain: results from extended follow up. Br Med J 311: 349–351

Patients treated by chiropractors derived more benefit.

14.8 Weinblatt ME et al (1994) Methotrexate in rheumatoid arthritis: a 5-year prospective multicenter study. Arthritis Rheum 37: 1492–1498

Two-thirds of the 123 RA patients started on MTX in this study were still taking it 5 years later, attesting to the drug's efficacy.

Porter DR et al (1994) Outcome of second line therapy in rheumatoid arthritis. Ann Rheum Dis 53: 812–815

Unlike the above, only one-third of patients treated with gold, penicillamine or sulfasalazine achieved prolonged disease control.

Kirwan JR et al (1995) The effect of glucocorticoids on joint destruction in rheumatoid arthritis. N Engl J Med 333: 142–146

Patients with early active RA had less X-ray progression if treated for 2 years with prednisolone 7.5 mg daily.

14.9 Szer IS et al (1991) The long-term course of lyme arthritis in children. N Engl J Med 325: 159–163

Failure of prompt initial diagnosis and treatment of Lyme disease may be associated with subsequent episodic arthritis, keratitis and (occasionally) encephalopathy.

14.10 Rashad S et al (1989) Effect of non-steroidal anti-inflammatory drugs on the course of osteoarthritis. Lancet ii: 460–462

Randomized study of 105 arthritic patients showing that aggressive NSAID therapy was in fact associated with more rapid joint destruction than was milder treatment, raising doubts as to the 'benign' nature of NSAID therapy.

CHAPTER 15

Skin disease

Physical examination protocol 15.1 You are asked to examine a patient who has recently developed a rash

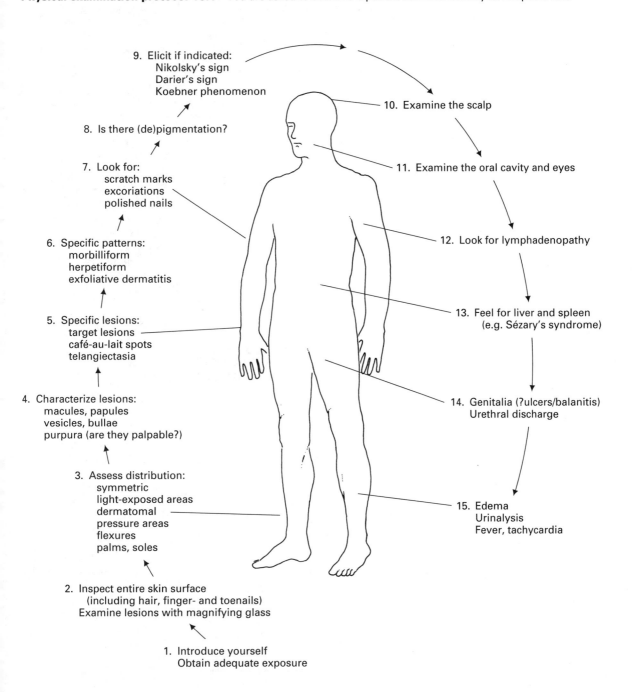

9. Elicit if indicated:
   Nikolsky's sign
   Darier's sign
   Koebner phenomenon

8. Is there (de)pigmentation?

7. Look for:
   scratch marks
   excoriations
   polished nails

6. Specific patterns:
   morbilliform
   herpetiform
   exfoliative dermatitis

5. Specific lesions:
   target lesions
   café-au-lait spots
   telangiectasia

4. Characterize lesions:
   macules, papules
   vesicles, bullae
   purpura (are they palpable?)

3. Assess distribution:
   symmetric
   light-exposed areas
   dermatomal
   pressure areas
   flexures
   palms, soles

2. Inspect entire skin surface
   (including hair, finger- and toenails)
   Examine lesions with magnifying glass

1. Introduce yourself
   Obtain adequate exposure

10. Examine the scalp

11. Examine the oral cavity and eyes

12. Look for lymphadenopathy

13. Feel for liver and spleen
    (e.g. Sézary's syndrome)

14. Genitalia (?ulcers/balanitis)
    Urethral discharge

15. Edema
    Urinalysis
    Fever, tachycardia

Diagnostic pathway 15.1   This patient has a spot diagnosis — what is it?

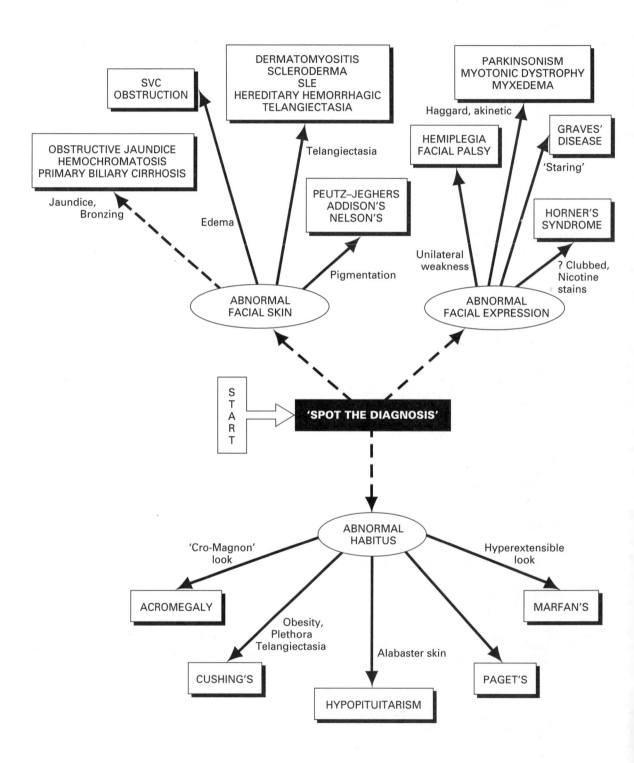

CLINICAL ASPECTS OF SKIN DISEASE

Commonest dermatologic short cases
1 Purpura
2 Psoriasis (± arthropathy)

Eponymous signs of skin disease
1 Nikolsky's sign →
   • Pemphigus (esp. foliaceous)
   • Porphyria (PCT, EP, VP)
   • Staph scalded skin syndrome
   — Denotes palpable shear-inducible separation of stratum corneum from underlying epidermis → blister formation
2 Darier's sign →
   • Urticaria pigmentosa
   — Denotes whealing of macule on rubbing
3 Koebner phenomenon →
   • Psoriasis
   • Still's disease
   • Lichen planus
   • Viral warts
   — Denotes skin lesions on areas of local trauma (e.g. scratches) due to papillary layer disruption

Skin rashes: diagnostic checklist for examinations
1 Purpuric
   — Vasculitis (is it palpable?)
   — Hematological (dependent distribution?)
2 Blistering
   — Vesicobullous
     • Pemphigus, bullous pemphigoid
     • Dermatitis herpetiformis (vesicular)
     • Porphyria cutanea tarda
   — Pustular
3 Exfoliative (scaly) or plaque-like
   — Psoriasis
   — Lymphoma (esp. T cell)
4 Suggesting systemic disease, e.g.
   — Herpes zoster
   — Eruptive xanthomata
   — Pretibial myxedema
   — Erythema nodosum
   — Acanthosis nigricans
5 Secondary syphilis (never hurts to mention)
6 Drug eruption (always mention)

Clinical patterns in skin disease
1 Asymmetric
   — Fungal
   — Contact dermatitis
   — Zoster (dermatomal)
2 Widespread symmetrical maculopapular
   — Drug eruption
   — Exanthem
3 Palms and soles
   — Erythema multiforme, Stevens–Johnson
   — Reiter's; pustular psoriasis
   — Secondary syphilis
   — Toxic shock; atopic eczema; 'pink disease'
4 Flexures
   — Psoriasis
   — Seborrheic dermatitis
   — Fungal, eczema, intertrigo
5 Limbs
   — Flexor aspects
     • Eczema
     • Lichen planus
     • Bullous pemphigoid
   — Extensor aspects
     • Psoriasis
     • Erythema multiforme
     • Dermatitis herpetiformis
6 Pruritic
   — Lichen planus
   — Dermatitis herpetiformis
   — Drug eruptions
   — Eczema, contact dermatitis, scabies

SKIN LESIONS OF GENERAL MEDICAL SIGNIFICANCE

Medical conditions associated with pruritus
1 Obstructive jaundice (e.g. PBC)
2 Chronic renal failure
3 Polycythemia rubra vera ('aquagenic')*
4 Hodgkin's disease; also CLL, lung cancer
5 Thyrotoxicosis; hypothyroidism
6 Estrogens: pregnancy, oral contraceptives
7 Parasitic infestations, esp. trichinosis
8 Drugs, esp. narcotic abuse

* NB: Exclude iron deficiency

Erythema nodosum: underlying conditions
1 **S**arcoidosis
2 **S**ulfonamides (and other drugs)
3 **S**treptococci (and TB, leprosy, toxoplasmosis)
4 Inflammatory bowel disease

Miscellaneous erythemas: diagnostic significance
1 Erythema induratum
   — Tuberculosis
2 Erythema ab igne
   — Myxedema, neuropathy
3 Erythema marginatum
   — Truncal rash in rheumatic fever
4 Erythema gyratum repens
   — Internal malignancy
5 Necrolytic migratory erythema
   — Glucagonoma

FACIAL RASHES

The central facial rash: diagnostic possibilities
1 SLE
2 Acne rosacea
3 Lupus pernio
4 Dermatomyositis
5 Porphyria cutanea tarda
6 Secondary syphilis

Differential diagnosis of facial telangiectases
1 Scleroderma
2 Hereditary hemorrhagic telangiectasia
3 Chronic liver disease (spider nevi)
4 Carcinoid syndrome
5 Ataxia telangiectasia (involve conjunctiva also)

Photosensitive skin rashes: predispositions
1 SLE
2 Porphyrias
  — Cutanea tarda
  — Erythropoietic
3 DNA repair deficiencies
  — Bloom's syndrome
  — Xeroderma pigmentosum, Cockayne's syndrome
4 Preexisting dermatosis
  — Rosacea; atopic dermatitis
  — Pellagra, Hartnup disease
  — Dermatomyositis, lupus
5 Drugs
  — Chlortetracycline
  — Chlorpropamide
  — Chlorpromazine

Differential diagnosis of sun-induced red weals
1 Polymorphic light eruption
2 Systemic lupus erythematosus
3 Erythropoietic protoporphyria
4 Solar urticaria

DISORDERS OF PIGMENTATION

Likely causes of diffuse hyperpigmentation in short cases
1 ACTH
  — Addison's disease
  — ACTH-secreting tumor
  — Nelson's syndrome
2 Chronic renal failure
3 Hemochromatosis
4 Primary biliary cirrhosis
5 Porphyria cutanea tarda
6 Drug-induced (e.g. busulfan)

Differential diagnosis of discrete hypopigmented areas
1 Vitiligo
2 Tinea versicolor
3 Tuberculoid leprosy
4 Ash-leaf macules of tuberose sclerosis
5 Morphea (localized patches of scleroderma)

SKIN APPENDAGES

Diagnostic features of the fingernails in systemic disease
1 Clubbing, nicotine stains
  — Lung cancer
2 Pitting
  — Psoriasis
3 Subungual splinters
  — Infective endocarditis

4 Telangiectasia, nailfold infarcts
  — Collagen diseases
5 'Half-and-half' (Lindsay's) nails
  — Renal failure
6 Leukonychia
  — Hypoalbuminemia (esp. liver disease)
7 Koilonychia (spoon nails)
  — Chronic iron deficiency
8 Onycholysis
  — Thyrotoxicosis
9 Yellow nails
  — Lymphatic hypoplasia (+ chylous effusions)
10 Blue lunules
  — Wilson's disease
11 Periungual fibromata
  — Tuberous sclerosis
12 Candida
  — Hypoparathyroidism

Etiological significance of splinter hemorrhages
1 Trauma
2 Infective endocarditis
3 Trichinosis (transverse splinters)

INVESTIGATING SKIN DISEASE

Immunologic aids to clinical dermatology
1 Pemphigus vulgaris
  — Serum antibodies to intercellular cement (70%)
  — Direct fluorescence
    • Epidermal staining with IgG, C_3
2 Pemphigoid (bullous or cicatricial), herpes gestationis
  — Serum antibodies to basement membrane (60%)
  — Direct fluorescence
    • Linear IgG and/or C_3 at dermoepidermal junction (i.e. subepidermal)
3 Dermatitis herpetiformis
  — ± Serum reticulin antibodies (25%)
  — Direct fluorescence
    • IgA in dermal papillae*
4 SLE
  — Direct fluorescence
    • Linear IgM, IgG or C_3 at dermoepidermal junction* (= 'lupus band')
  Discoid LE
  — Direct fluorescence
    • Negative in normal skin (cf. SLE)
5 Erythema multiforme
  — Direct immunofluorescence
    • Negative in affected skin

* In both normal and affected skin

Diagnostic procedures in dermatologic disease
1 Wood's lamp (black light)
  — Vitiligo
  — Ash-leaf macules of tuberous sclerosis
2 Dark-field examination
  — Syphilis
3 Tzanck preparation
  — Distinguishes herpes simplex from folliculitis
  — Distinguishes pemphigus from pemphigoid

4 20% potassium hydroxide (KOH) preparation
— Superficial fungal infections
5 Patch test
— Contact dermatitis
6 Skin scrapings
— Fungal infection, scabies
7 Punch biopsy
— Histopathologic corroboration (e.g. neoplasia)
— Culture (deep mycosis, bacteria, mycobacteria)
— Immunofluorescence (lupus, pemphigoid)

The bullous dermatoses: how to tell them apart
1 Pemphigus vulgaris
— Mucosal involvement typical, esp.
• Recurrent oral ulceration
• Conjunctivitis
• Genital, nasal, scalp or umbilical ulceration
— Age of onset 40–60
— Bullae are small, flaccid, fragile (rarely intact)
— Present as erosions and heal without scarring
— Histology → 'acantholytic' cells
— Autoimmune association
— Often requires *massive* steroid doses (120–240 mg prednisone/day)
— Rarely remits spontaneously; 'malignant' course
2 Bullous pemphigoid
— Mucosal involvement rare
— Mainly affects flexor aspects of extremities
— 80% patients > 70 years old
— Bullae are large, tense, non-fragile
— *No* acantholytic cells
— May respond to relatively low doses of steroid (e.g. 40 mg prednisone/day)
— May remit spontaneously; often self-limiting
3 Cicatricial (benign mucous membrane) pemphigoid
— Primarily affects conjunctivae, mouth, pharynx
— Classically afflicts middle-aged women
— Tense blisters → prominent atrophic scars
— May → entropion, symblepharon, dysphagia
— Requires long-term corticosteroid therapy
4 Dermatitis herpetiformis
— Typically manifests with (herpetiform) vesicles
— May affect scapulae, sacrum, scalp and extensor aspects of knees, elbows; buttocks
— Associated with pruritus, eosinophilia, intestinal villous atrophy and HLA B8/DRw3
— May respond to
• Dapsone (short-term)
• Gluten-free diet (long-term)
— May be aggravated by iodine ingestion
5 Porphyria cutanea tarda
— Atrophic scars on light-exposed regions
— Facial hypertrichosis; pigmentation
6 Acquired epidermolysis bullosa
— Atrophic scarring
— Associated with amyloidosis, malignancy
7 Pellagra
— Light-exposed regions → 'Casal's necklace'

DRUG ERUPTIONS

Immune mechanisms of drug-induced skin reactions
1 Type I reaction (urticaria)
Common causes
— Penicillin, sulfonamides
— Aspirin
— Sera, contrast media
2 Type II reaction (cytotoxic), e.g. ITP
Common causes
— Quinine
— Methyldopa
— Gold
3 Type III reaction (vasculitis), e.g. drug-induced lupus
Common causes
— Hydralazine, procainamide
— Sulfonamides
— Penicillin
4 Type IV reaction (contact dermatitis)
Common causes
— Topical antihistamines
— Topical neomycin

Clinical patterns of drug-induced skin reactions
1 Toxic epidermal necrolysis
— β-lactams, allopurinol
— Phenytoin, barbiturates, carbamazepine*
2 Erythema multiforme (± Stevens–Johnson; see below)
— Sulfonamides (sulfasalazine, co-trimoxazole)
— NSAIDs, esp. phenylbutazone*
3 Erythroderma
— Gold
4 Fixed drug eruption
— Barbiturates
— Phenolphthalein (in laxatives)
5 Serum sickness-like reactions (morbilliform, urticarial)
— β-lactams, β-blockers
— IV/IM proteins (serum, vaccines, streptokinase)
6 Small-vessel vasculitis (palpable purpura, esp. on legs)
— Penicillins, sulfonamides
— Allopurinol
— Thiazides, phenytoin, propylthiouracil

* and many others

Physical signs signifying severe drug eruptions
1 Fever, tachycardia, hypotension
2 Lymphadenopathy, arthritis
3 Glossitis, mucositis, facial involvement
4 Blistering, positive Nikolsky's sign (p. 363)
5 Confluent erythema ('red man')
6 Palpable purpura, skin necrosis

Clinical spectrum of drug-induced bullous disease
1 Erythema multiforme
— e.g. Co-trimoxazole

2 Photosensitization, e.g.
 — Psoralens
 — Demeclocycline
 — Nalidixic acid
3 Porphyria cutanea tarda, e.g.
 — Oral contraceptives
 — Stilbestrol (in prostate cancer)
4 Fixed drug eruption (→ hands, feet, penis), e.g.
 — Quinine: in tonic water
 — Phenolphthalein: in laxatives
5 Following coma → skin necrosis
 — e.g. Barbiturates
6 Pemphigus-like rash
 — Penicillamine
7 Pemphigoid-like rash
 — e.g. Frusemide
8 Pellagra-like rash
 — Isoniazid
9 Vasculitis → hemorrhagic bullae
 — e.g. Allopurinol*

* esp. in renal failure and/or concomitant diuretic therapy

Distinguishing features of Stevens–Johnson syndrome*
1 Systemic illness (fever, arthralgias)
2 Purulent or pseudomembranous conjunctivitis with corneal ulceration/perforation or symblepharon
3 Buccal ulcers, bullous stomatitis ± genital/anal ulcers Acute bloodstained crusting of swollen lips

* = erythema multiforme affecting mucous membranes

Drug eruptions: miscellaneous characteristics
1 Rashes due to drug sensitivity are classically
 — Symmetrical
 — Truncal
 — Pruritic
 — Associated with eosinophilia
2 Sensitization to drugs occurs
 — Most frequently with *topical* use
 — Least frequently with *oral* use
3 Drug rashes are distinctly *unlikely* with
 — Digoxin
 — Erythromycin
 — Benzodiazepines
 — Hormones, vitamins

Conditions predisposing to ampicillin rashes
1 Infectious mononucleosis (EBV)
2 CMV infection
3 Chronic lymphocytic leukemia
4 Concurrent allopurinol treatment

THERAPEUTIC APPROACHES TO SKIN DISEASE

Common measures in the management of drug eruptions
1 Withdraw suspected offending drug(s)
2 Emollients
3 Topical steroids
4 Oral antihistamines

Dermatoses responsive to topical steroids
1 Eczema

2 Psoriasis
3 Seborrheic dermatitis

Relative potency of topical steroids
1 High potency
 — Betamethasone dipropionate
2 Intermediate potency
 — Betamethasone valerate
 — Triamcinolone acetonide
3 Mild potency
 — Hydrocortisone valerate
 — Triamcinolone hexacetonide
4 Least potency
 — Hydrocortisone base (1%)

Treatment modalities in psoriasis
1 Tar baths
2 Steroids (topical)
3 Calcipotriol
4 Octreotide
5 PUVA
6 Cyclosporin A

Refractory fungal infection of nails?
1 Psoriasis
2 Contact irritants; trauma
3 Haven't treated for long enough (takes months)*

* Hence, always confirm diagnosis by nail analysis to ensure optimal drug therapy

Antineoplastic efficacy of synthetic retinoids
1 Regression of preneoplastic lesions
 — Oral leukoplakia
 — Senile keratoses (incl. transplant-associated)
2 ↓ Tumors in xeroderma pigmentosum patients
3 Mycosis fungoides (some responses)
4 Acute promyelocytic leukemia (p. 168)

UNDERSTANDING SKIN DISEASE

ULTRAVIOLET RADIATION

Medical consequences of ultraviolet radiation
1 UV-A (320–400 nm, long-wavelength UV, 'black light')
 — Low energy, high skin penetration
 — Responsible for tanning (*not* burning); used in tanning lamps
 — Present in solar radiation *all day*
 — Acute exposure implicated in pathogenesis of
  • Photosensitive drug eruptions
  • Porphyria rashes
 — Chronic exposure is implicated in
  • Skin aging
 — *High-dose* UV-A + psoralen sensitizers (PUVA: for psoriasis, mycosis fungoides) causes
  • Skin SCCs (incl. penis and scrotum)
 — *Not* absorbed by PABA
2 UV-B (290–320 nm, medium-wavelength UV)
 — High energy, high skin penetration
 — Attenuated by ozone layer

— Essential for endogenous vitamin D$_3$ production
— Absorbed by PABA-containing sunscreens
— Present in solar radiation mainly 10 a.m. – 3 p.m.
— Acute exposure causes
  • Sunburn (erythema)
  • Snow blindness (keratitis)
— Chronic exposure is implicated in
  • Skin cancers (SCCs, BCCs)*
  • Cataract
— May reduce immune surveillance and thus
  predispose to SCCs and skin infections
  • Leprosy, leishmaniasis
  • Reactivation of herpes simplex
3 UV-C (200–290 nm, short-wavelength UV)
— High energy, low skin penetration
— Used in sterilizing lamps
— May cause sunburn in climbers (↓ ozone; doesn't
  reach to sea level)
— May cause cataracts in experimental models

* Melanoma is associated with sunburn episodes, but relationship may be indirect; ocular melanoma has *no* relationship to UV

**Pathogenetic radiation types for various photo-
dermatoses**
1 Visible light
— Cutaneous porphyrias
2 UVA
— Polymorphic light eruption
— Drug-induced photosensitization
— Cutaneous porphyrias
3 UVB
— Lupus erythematosus
— Herpes labialis
— Vitiligo or albinism
— Xeroderma pigmentosum

THE SKIN AND CANCER

Classic cutaneous complications of cancer
1 Skin infiltration
— Metastases, e.g. breast cancer, melanoma
— Kaposi's sarcoma
— Histiocytosis X
2 Erythroderma
— Sézary's syndrome, mycosis fungoides
3 Excoriations (pruritus)
— Hodgkin's disease, polycythemia vera
4 Herpes zoster
— esp. Myeloma, lymphoma, CLL
5 Dermatomyositis* (esp. steroid-resistant variant)
— e.g. Ovarian/gastric/lung cancer
6 Radiotherapy effects
— Early: erythema, desquamation
— Late: atrophy, fibrosis, telangiectasia
7 Acanthosis nigricans (widespread, mucosal, pruritic)
— Gastrointestinal adenocarcinomas, esp. gastric
8 Thrombophlebitis migrans
— Mucin-secreting adenocarcinomas, esp. pancreas
9 Necrolytic migratory erythema
— Glucagonoma
10 Systemic nodular panniculitis (Weber–Christian)
— Pancreatic acinar-cell carcinoma

Acute febrile neutrophilic dermatosis (Sweet's)
— Acute myeloid leukemia
11 Xanthomatosis
— Multiple myeloma
12 Post-proctoscopic periorbital purpura; 'pinch'
purpura
— Myeloma with supervening amyloidosis
13 Erythema gyratum repens
Hypertrichosis lanuginosa ('malignant down')
Bullous pyoderma gangrenosum
— Not associated with any *specific* tumor type
14 Pemphigoid
Psoriatic exacerbations
Erythema multiforme
Bowen's disease
— Association with cancer *unproven*

* Associated with cancer in 15% cases; cf. polymyositis 9%

Inherited cancer syndromes with skin signs
1 Peutz–Jeghers syndrome (lip/buccal freckling)
— Gut polyps (mainly hamartomas)
2 Von Recklinghausen's disease
— Schwannomas, pheochromocytoma
3 Gardner's syndrome
— Osteomas, colorectal Ca
4 Cronkhite–Canada syndrome
— Gut hamartomas and carcinomas
5 Cowden's disease (multiple hamartomas)
— Thyroid and breast cancers
6 Muir–Torre syndrome (sebaceous tumors)
— Proximal colonic and genitourinary
  carcinomas
7 Tylosis (palmar-plantar hyperkeratosis)
— Esophageal cancer
8 Mucosal neuromatosis (MEN2b; p. 116)
— Intestinal ganglioneuromas, pheo-, Ca thyroid

URTICARIA

Urticarial problems in clinical practice
1 Ordinary urticaria
— May be IgE-mediated, e.g. reactions to insects
— May *also* be non-immunologically mediated
  • Histamine-containing foodstuffs (e.g. frozen
    tuna)
  • Arachidonic acid pathway inhibitors (e.g.
    aspirin)
  • Mast-cell degranulation (e.g. opiates)
— Topical therapy generally ineffective; oral
  antihistamines or exclusion diets may help
2 Chronic urticaria
— Defined as recurrent lesions for 3 months ±
  arthralgias, adenopathy, abdominal pain
— Mediated by histamine, *not* IgE; prick tests –
— Precipitating dietary factor identifiable in 25%
— Plasmapheresis or histamine antagonists may be
  useful; steroids contraindicated
3 Cholinergic urticaria
— Affects head/upper trunk, esp. young patients,
  after exercise or hot shower
— Painful pruritic lesions with 'blush'
— Rapid skin cooling may abort an attack

4 Cold urticaria: *familial*
  — Autosomal dominant; presents in infancy
  — Rash may appear *hours* after cold exposure
  — Associated fever, arthralgias, leukocytosis
5 Cold urticaria: *acquired*
  — Rash occurs within *minutes* of skin contact with cold water or ice (diagnostic test)
  — Syncope may ensue, may cause sudden death in young people (drowning)
6 Solar (U.V.) urticaria
  — Weal occurs within 1–3 min of sun exposure
  — Localized to sun-exposed areas
  — Differential diagnosis: SLE, drug reactions
7 Pressure urticaria
  — Affects pressure areas, e.g. feet, buttocks, back, palms, waist
  — Tender swelling 2–12 h after pressure injury
8 Scratch urticaria (delayed dermographism)
  — Redness, weals, itch occur hours after scratching
  — Distinct from *simple dermographism*, which affects 5% of people and is *not* pruritic
9 Vasculitic urticaria
  — Serious condition, may be life-threatening
  — Painful non-pruritic lesions lasting > 24 h
  — ± Fever, abdominal pain, arthritis, nephritis
  — Hypocomplementemia (C_3, C_4, THC), ↑ ESR
10 Angioneurotic edema
  — → Mucocutaneous junctions: lips, eyes, penis
  — Large tender swellings, often pruritic
  — Glottal edema may be a complication, esp. when angioedema occurs with anaphylaxis

NB: Urticaria does *not* occur in association with hereditary angioedema (C_1-INH deficiency; p. 188)

SKIN SYNDROMES

Sweet's syndrome: acute febrile neutrophilic dermatosis
1 Manifests with tender erythematous skin plaques (esp. head and neck, arms) plus fever and neutrophilia

2 Also → arthritis, conjunctivitis, mouth ulcers, proteinuria
3 20% of patients have a malignancy (e.g. acute leukemia); such patients have more severe skin lesions and cytopenias
4 Symptoms are generally steroid-responsive and may resolve within 2–3 months in patients without malignancy

The dysplastic nevus ('B-K mole') syndrome: features
1 Nevi typically 5–15 mm in diameter
2 Characterized by irregular borders and variegated color
3 Mainly affect trunk, but also sun-deprived areas
4 Often > 100 in number
5 Continue to appear after age 35
6 Histology
  — Melanocytic hyperplasia
  — Cytologic atypia
  — Spindle-shaped melanocyte 'nests'
  — Lymphocytic superficial dermal infiltrates
7 Autosomal dominant transmission
8 Risk of developing melanoma approaches 100% in DNS patients with positive family history of melanoma

Skin syndromes in HIV-infected patients
1 Kaposi's sarcoma
2 Opportunistic infections
  — Herpes zoster, varicella; CMV, HPV
  — Oral hairy leukoplakia (?EBV/*Candida*)
  — Norwegian (severe) scabies, fungal infections
  — (Myco)bacterial infections, incl. folliculitis
  — Bacillary angiomatosis*
  — Syphilis (primary or secondary)
3 Pathogen-non-specific skin presentations
  — Acute exanthem (at seroconversion; p. 186)
  — Xerosis (dry skin): itchy, lichenified
  — Seborrheic dermatitis (esp. scalp)
  — Psoriasiform rashes (± Reiter's syndrome)
  — Morbilliform rash with co-trimoxazole (in 70%)

* Responds to erythromycin; ? due to catscratch bacillus (p. 210)

REVIEWING THE LITERATURE: SKIN DISEASE

15.1 Kragballe K et al (1991) Double-blind, right/left comparison of calcipotriol and betamethasone valerate in treatment of psoriasis vulgaris. Lancet 337: 193–196

Randomized study of 345 Scandinavian patients, showing superior therapeutic activity for the vitamin D analog calcipotriol over the topical steroid betamethasone valerate.

15.2 Sheehan MP et al (1992) Efficacy of traditional Chinese herbal therapy in adult atopic dermatitis. Lancet 340: 13–17

Randomized study of 40 patients with refractory eczema. The group receiving 'traditional' herbs fared far better than did the 'placebo' herbs cohort.

15.3 Sowden JM et al (1991) Double-blind controlled crossover study of cyclosporin in adults with severe refractory atopic dermatitis. Lancet 338: 137–140

Study of 33 patients with refractory eczema, confirming the short-term efficacy of cyclosporin in such patients.

15.4 Ellis CN et al (1991) Cyclosporine for plaque-type psoriasis. N Engl J Med 324: 277–284

Double-blind placebo-controlled study of 85 patients with severe psoriasis; dose-dependent control of disease was achieved within 16 weeks, at an initial dose of 5 mg/kg/day.

15.5 Wilkinson SM et al (1991) Hydrocortisone: an important cutaneous allergen. Lancet 337: 761–762

Surprising study documenting a 5% incidence of contact allergy to hydrocortisone in a cohort receiving a related steroid in a nasal spray. Patch testing is usually false-negative in such cases, perhaps reflecting poor skin penetration by the drug.

15.6 Jonsson A et al (1991) Inhibition of burn pain by intravenous lignocaine infusion. Lancet 338: 151–152

Use of IV infusions of local anesthetic greatly reduced the need for opiate analgesia in this burns cohort of seven patients.

15.7 Kadunce DP et al (1991) Cigarette smoking: risk factor for premature facial wrinkling. Ann Int Med 114: 840–844

Cross-sectional study of 132 smokers and non-smokers, showing a 5-fold increased incidence of wrinkling in the smokers. In contrast, lifetime sun exposure of 50,000 hours only caused a 3-fold increased risk of wrinkles.

15.8 Brice SM et al (1989) Detection of herpes simplex virus DNA in cutaneous lesions of erythema multiforme. J Investig Dermatol 93: 183–187

Demonstration of HSV nucleic acid sequences in EM target lesions using polymerase chain reaction-derived DNA and in situ hybridization, suggesting a pathogenetic role for the virus.

15.9 LaGrenade L et al (1990) Infective dermatitis of Jamaican children: a marker for HTLV-1 infection. Lancet 336: 1345–1347

17/17 children with this syndrome of chronic Gram-positive skin sepsis were found to be HTLV-1-positive, whereas 11 of 11 without this condition were negative, strongly suggesting a pathogenetic relationship.

15.10 Kraemer KH et al (1988) Prevention of skin cancer in xeroderma pigmentosum with the use of oral isotretinoin. N Engl J Med 318: 1633–1637

63% reduction of tumor incidence during 2 years of treatment with 13-cis-retinoic acid, followed by a 9-fold increase on cessation.

Further Reading

1 BEST REVISION MATERIAL: **Your own notes**

These are always the most useful revision material since they are (or at least should be) custom-designed to cover your own weaknesses. Don't underestimate their value.

2 BEST CLINICAL TEXTBOOK: **Your patients' notes**

When it comes to learning clinical medicine, there's no substitute for getting out among the patients. Cajole, bribe or blackmail your seniors into demonstrating physical signs and the techniques for eliciting them; armed with this knowledge, find out where 'the cases' are, team up with a similarly motivated colleague and proceed to grill each other on your respective performances. Watch one, do one, teach one: that's how medicine's been for time immemorial and it's not about to change in your lifetime.

3 BEST GENERAL TEXTBOOK: Kelley's *Textbook of Internal Medicine*

Like expensive and weighty stethoscopes, expensive and weighty textbooks are not a prerequisite for passing medical exams. Owning one decent reference book can make life easier, however, and is probably worthwhile in the long run. Although largely a matter of taste – since almost all the big texts cover much the same content – for the time being this relative newcomer can be recommended for its conciseness, snappy editing and workmanlike index.

4 BEST MCQs: **MKSAP** (Medical knowledge self-assessment program; US)

For candidates who need a 'quiz-show' format to sustain their interest in the lead-up to an exam, this American Medical Association publication is good (it includes excellent state-of-the-art summaries of each subspecialty in addition to the self-assessment questions) – provided that your library can afford it. If not, look for other publications which feature detailed and authoritative answers: the (Australian) RACP self-assessment series, Lawrence & Hunter's *MCQs in General Medicine* and the *Pre-Test* series fall into this category.

5 BEST EDITORIALS: *The Lancet*

Up-to-date summaries of important (and fashionable) topics can be found here; an afternoon scanning the last 6–12 months' issues prior to your exam could be well spent. Although more abstruse than the *BMJ*'s efforts, the latter's editorials have of late drifted towards an emphasis on practice and politics rather than on medicine and disease.

6 BEST ORIGINAL ARTICLES: *New England Journal of Medicine*

The *NEJM* and the *Lancet* are the only two journals containing original articles worth perusing on a regular basis and the former has gained the edge since the last edition. So how do you get the most out of such articles when your time is limited? Try this: (i) skim through the Abstract – if the conclusions are earth-shattering, read the Introduction and Discussion; (ii) if (much more commonly) the Abstract sounds less than earth-shattering, just read the Introduction – in most cases it will provide a summary of a topical clinical problem as well as pointing out uncertainties in current knowledge (the latter being an important goal which traditional medical textbooks rarely achieve).

7 BEST REVIEW ARTICLES: *New England Journal of Medicine*

Review articles in any journal are worth a look. However, the *NEJM* articles often serve as a focus for exam questions and may thus be regarded in the same light as Original Articles from the candidate's perspective.

8 BEST SUBSPECIALTY TEXTS

The limitations of having to rely on library stock for your reading are obvious. The book you want may be unavailable, stolen, out-of-date, chained to the library shelf or so badly defaced that reading it becomes a cryptographer's exercise. Nonetheless, borrowing library books has two definite advantages: first, it's cheap and second, it provides some incentive to read the thing within a given time. The following recommendations are for those exam candidates who feel they need indepth or background information on a specific subject.

Cancer medicine
Short and readable:
UICC Manual of Clinical Oncology Springer-Verlag, Berlin
Reference:
De Vita VT et al (eds) *Cancer: Principles and Practice of Oncology* Lippincott, Philadelphia

Cardiology
Short and readable:
Schlamt RC, Hurst JW *Handbook of the Heart* McGraw-Hill, New York
Reference:
Braunwald E (ed) *Heart Disease* Saunders, Philadelphia

Endocrinology
Short and readable:
Watts NB, Keffer JH *Practical Endocrinology* Lea & Febiger, Philadelphia
Reference:
Wilson JD, Foster DW (eds) *Williams' Textbook of Endocrinology* Saunders, Philadelphia

Gastroenterology
Short and readable:
Christensen J *Bedside Logic in Diagnostic Gastroenterology* Churchill Livingstone, Edinburgh
Reference:
Sleisenger MH et al (eds) *Gastrointestinal Disease* Saunders, Philadelphia

Hematology
Short and readable:
Hoffbrand AV, Pettit JE *Essential Hematology* Blackwell Scientific, Oxford
Reference:
Lee RG et al *Wintrobe's Clinical Hematology* Lea & Febiger, Philadelphia

Immunology
Short and readable:
Male D *Immunology: An Illustrated Outline* Mosby, London
Reference:
Samter M (ed) *Immunologic Diseases* Little, Brown & Co, Boston

Infectious disease
Short and readable:
Grist NR et al *Diseases of Infection* OUP, Oxford
Reference:
Gorbach SL et al (eds) *Infectious Diseases* Saunders, Philadelphia

Metabolism, nutrition and genetics
Reference:
Stanbury JB et al (eds) *The Metabolic Basis of Inherited Disease* McGraw-Hill, New York

Neurology
Short and readable:
Wilkinson I *Essential Neurology* Blackwell Scientific, Oxford
Reference:
Swash M, Oxbury J *Clinical Neurology* Churchill Livingstone, Edinburgh

Pharmacology and toxicology
Reference:
Goodman LS, Gilman AG et al *The Pharmacological Basis of Therapeutics* Macmillan, New York

Psychiatry
Short and readable:
Burns AS et al *MCQs and Short Notes in Psychiatry* Wright, Bristol
Reference:
Kaplan HI, Sadock BS *Comprehensive Textbook of Psychiatry* Williams & Wilkins, Baltimore

Renal medicine
Short and readable:
Whitworth JA, Lawrence JR *Textbook of Renal Disease* Churchill Livingstone, Edinburgh

Respiratory medicine
Short and readable:
Flenley DC *Respiratory Medicine* Baillière Tindall, London
Reference:
Brewis R et al (eds) *Respiratory Medicine* Baillière Tindall, London

Rheumatology
Short and readable:
Moll JMH *Manual of Rheumatology* Churchill Livingstone, Edinburgh
Reference:
Katz WZ *Diagnosis and Management of Rheumatic Diseases* Lippincott, Philadelphia

Skin disease
Short and readable:
Fitzpatrick TB et al *Color Atlas and Synopsis of Clinical Dermatology* McGraw-Hill, New York
Reference:
Rook A et al (eds) *Textbook of Dermatology* Blackwell Scientific, Oxford

9   BEST BOOK FOR PASSING MEDICAL EXAMS:

.... I'm afraid I'll have to leave this one up to you.

Abbreviations

AA	Alcoholics Anonymous
ABPA	allergic bronchopulmonary aspergillosis
αFP/AFP	α fetoprotein
αHBD	α-hydroxybutyrate dehydrogenase
A_2	aortic component of second heart sound
A-a	alveolar-arterial (oxygen)
Ab	antibody
ACE	angiotensin-converting enzyme
AChRAb	acetylcholine receptor antibody
ACTH	adrenocorticotrophic hormone
AD	autosomal dominant
ADH	antidiuretic hormone (vasopressin)
ADP	adenosine diphosphate
AF	atrial fibrillation
AFB	acid-fast bacilli
Ag	antigen
AI	aortic incompetence
AIDS	acquired immunodeficiency syndrome
AIHA	autoimmune hemolytic anemia
a.k.a.	also known as
ALA	aminolevulinic acid
ALL	acute lymphoblastic leukemia
ALT	alanine aminotransferase (SGPT)
AMI	acute myocardial infarction
AMOL	acute myelomonocytic leukemia
ANA	antinuclear antibody
Ang	angiotensin
ANLL	acute non-lymphocytic leukemia
ANP	atrial natriuretic peptide
AP	anteroposterior
APC	adenomatous polyposis coli (gene, locus) or aspirin-phenacetin-caffeine or antigen-presenting cell
APCC	activated prothrombin complex concentrate
APML	acute promyelocytic leukemia
APSAC	anistreplase (thrombolytic drug)
APTT	activated partial thromboplastin time
APUD	amine precursor uptake and decarboxylation
AR	autosomal recessive, or
AR	androgen receptor
ara-C	cytosine arabinoside
ARDS	adult respiratory distress syndrome
ASD	atrial septal defect
ASO	antistreptolysin O (titer)
AST	aspartate aminotransferase (SGOT)
AT-III	antithrombin III
ATG	antithymocyte globulin
atm	atmospheres (pressure)
ATN	acute tubular necrosis
ATP	adenosine triphosphate
ATRA	all-*trans*-retinoic acid
AV	atrioventricular, arteriovenous
AVM	arteriovenous malformation
AZT	zidovudine (= azidothymidine)
BAL	dimercaprol, *or*
BAL	bronchoalveolar lavage
BAO	basal acid output
BCC	basal cell carcinoma
BCG	bacillus Calmette–Guérin
b.d.	twice-daily (dosage)
BJP	Bence-Jones protein
BP	blood pressure
BPH	benign prostatic hypertrophy
BSP	bromsulfthalein
BUDR	bromodeoxuridine
BUN	blood urea nitrogen
C1–7(8)	cervical vertebrae (nerve root)
$C_{3,4}$(etc.)	complement components
Ca	cancer
Ca^{2+}	calcium
CABG	coronary artery bypass graft
c-*abl*	cellular oncogene *abl*
CAH	chronic active hepatitis, *or*
CAH	congenital adrenal hyperplasia
cALLA	common ALL-antigen
cAMP	cyclic adenosine monophosphate
CAPD	chronic ambulatory peritoneal dialysis
CCF	congestive cardiac failure
CCK	cholecystokinin
CCl_4	carbon tetrachloride
CCU	coronary care unit
CD	cellular determinant
CDCA	chenodeoxycholic acid
CEA	carcinoembryonic antigen
cf.	confer (compare, contrast)
CFT	complement fixation test
CFTR	cystic fibrosis transmembrane conductance regulator
CGDC	chronic granulomatous disease of childhood
CH_{50}	total hemolytic complement
CHAD	cold hemagglutinin disease
CHOP	*c*yclophosphamide, *h*ydroxydaunorubicin (doxorubicin, Adriamycin), *O*ncovin (vincristine), *p*rednisone
C_1-INH	C_1-esterase inhibitor
CJD	Creutzfeldt–Jakob disease
Cl⁻	chloride ion
CLL	chronic lymphocytic leukemia
CMC	chronic mucocutaneous candidiasis
CML	chronic myeloid (granulocytic) leukemia
CMT	Charcot–Marie–Tooth disease
CMV	cytomegalovirus

c-*myc*	cellular oncogene *myc*
CN	cranial nerve(s) *or* cyanide
CNS	central nervous system
COAD	chronic obstructive airways disease
Con-A	Concanavalin A
c-*onc*	cellular oncogene
CPAP	continuous positive airways pressure
CPK	creatine phosphokinase
CPR	cardiopulmonary resuscitation
c.p.s.	cycles per second
CRA	central retinal artery
CREST	calcinosis, *R*aynaud's, *e*sophageal dysfunction, *s*clerodactyly and *t*elangiectasia (syndrome)
CRF	chronic renal failure
CRH	corticotrophin-releasing hormone
CRP	C-reactive protein
CRV	central retinal vein
CSA	cyclosporin (A)
CSF	cerebrospinal fluid, *or*
CSF	colony-stimulating factor
CSM	carotid sinus massage
CT	computed tomography
CTS	carpal tunnel syndrome
CVA	cerebrovascular accident
CVP	central venous pressure, *or*
CVP	chlorambucil, vincristine, prednisone
CXR	chest X-ray
2-D	two-dimensional (real-time)
D&C	dilatation and curettage
DAT	direct antiglobulin (Coombs') test
dDAVP	de-amino D-arginine vasopressin ('desmopressin')
DCA	dichloroacetate
DD$_x$	differential diagnosis
DES	diethylstilbestrol
DF-2	'dysgonic fermenter' 2 (*C. canimorsus*)
DFA	diffuse fibrosing alveolitis
DFO	desferrioxamine
DHCC	dihydroxycholecalciferol
DHEA	dehydroepiandrosterone
DHFR	dihydrofolate reductase
DIC	disseminated intravascular coagulation
DIP	distal interphalangeal joint
DISIDA	disopropyl iminodiacetic acid (cf. HIDA)
DL$_{CO}$	diffusing capacity to carbon monoxide (transfer factor)
DM	diabetes mellitus *or* dystrophia myotonica
DNA	deoxyribonucleic acid
DNS	dysplastic nevus syndrome
2,3-DPG	2,3-diphosphoglycerate
dsDNA	double-stranded deoxyribonucleic acid
DTs	delirium tremens
DTH	delayed-type hypersensitivity
DU	duodenal ulcer
DVT	deep venous thrombosis
D$_x$	diagnosis
EACA	epsilonaminocaproic acid
EB(V)	Epstein–Barr (virus)
ECG	electrocardiogram
ECHO	enteric cytopathic human orphan (virus)
ECOG	Eastern Cooperative Oncology Group (criteria)
EDTA	ethylenediamminetetraammonium
EEG	electroencephalogram
ELISA	enzyme-linked immunosorbent assay
EM	electron microscopy [erythema multiforme]
EMA	epithelial membrane antigen
EMG	electromyography
EN	erythema nodosum
ENT	ear, nose and throat
EP	erythropoietic protoporphyria
EPG	electrophoretogram
ER	estrogen receptor *or* endoplasmic reticulum *or* emergency room
ERCP	endoscopic retrograde cholangiopancreatogram
esp.	especially
ESR	erythrocyte sedimentation rate
EUA	examination under anesthesia
F VIII$_c$	coagulant moiety of factor eight
Fab	antibody fragments
FAB	French-American-British (classification)
5-FC	flucytosine
FDPs	fibrin degradation products
Fe	iron
FEV$_1$	forced expiratory volume in 1 second
FFP	fresh frozen plasma
FiO$_2$	concentration of inspired oxygen
FMF	familial Mediterranean fever
FNA	fine needle aspiration
FSH	follicle-stimulating hormone
FTA-ABS	fluorescent treponemal antibody absorption test
FTI	free thyroxine index
5-FU	5-fluorouracil
GABA	γ-aminobutyric acid
GBM	glomerular basement membrane
GBS	Guillain–Barré syndrome
GFR	glomerular filtration rate
GGT	γ-glutamyl transpeptidase
GH(RF)	growth hormone (releasing factor)
GHPS	gated heart pool scan
GIP	glucose-dependent insulinotrophic polypeptide ('gastric inhibitory peptide')
GI(T)	gastrointestinal (tract)
GN	glomerulonephritis
GnRH	gonadotrophin-releasing hormone
G6PD	glucose-6-phosphate dehydrogenase
GTT	glucose tolerance test
GU	gastric ulcer
GVHD	graft-versus-host disease
Gy	Gray (100 rad)
h	hour
HAV	hepatitis A virus
HB	heart block
Hb	hemoglobin
HbA$_{1c}$	glycosylated hemoglobin
HBcAg	hepatitis B core antigen
HBeAg	hepatitis B 'e' antigen
HbO$_2$	oxyhemoglobin
HBsAg	hepatitis B surface antigen
HbSC	sickle-C hemoglobin
HbSS	(homozygous) sickle-cell hemoglobin
HBV	hepatitis B virus
HCC	(25) hydroxycholecalciferol
(β)HCG	human chorionic gonadotrophin (beta-subunit)

HCL	hairy cell leukemia [HCl, hydrochloric acid]	L-DOPA	*levo-dihydroxyphenylalanine*
HCV	hepatitis C virus	LE	lupus erythematosus
HCO_3^-	bicarbonate	LES	lower esophageal sphincter
HD	Hodgkin's disease *or* Huntington's disease	Leu-1, 3a	monoclonal antibodies to T cell subpopulations
HDL	high-density lipoprotein	LFTs	liver function tests
HDV	hepatitis D virus (δ particle)	LGV	lymphogranuloma venereum
HEV	hepatitis E virus	LH	luteinizing hormone
HHV	human herpesvirus	LMN	lower motor neuron
HI	*Hemophilus influenzae*	LP	lumbar puncture
(5)-HIAA	hydroxyindoleacetic acid	LPHB	left posterior hemiblock
HIDA	hydroxyiminodiacetic acid (^{99m}Tc-labelled)	LRTI	lower respiratory tract infection
HIT	heparin-induced thrombocytopenia	LV(H)	left ventricle (hypertrophy)
HIV	human immunodeficiency virus	LVF	left ventricular failure
HLA	human leukocyte antigen	MALT	mucosa-associated lymphoid tissue
HOCM	hypertrophic (± obstructive) cardiomyopathy	MAO	maximum acid output
HPO	hypertrophic pulmonary osteoarthropathy	MAO(I)	monoamine oxidase (inhibitor)
HPT	hyperparathyroidism	MBC	minimal bactericidal concentration
HS	hereditary spherocytosis	MCHC	mean corpuscular hemoglobin concentration
HSP	Henoch–Schönlein purpura, *or*	MCP	metacarpophalangeal (joint)
HSP	heat-shock protein	MCQ	multiple choice question
HSV	herpes simplex virus [highly selective vagotomy]	MCT	medullary carcinoma of the thyroid
5-HT	5-hydroxytryptamine (serotonin)	MCTD	mixed connective tissue disease
HTLV	human T cell leukemia virus	MCV	mean corpuscular volume
H-V	His-ventricle	MDP	manic-depressive psychosis
H-X	histiocytosis X	M:E	myeloid:erythroid (ratio)
HZ	herpes zoster	MEN	multiple endocrine neoplasia
^{131}I	radioiodine	MESNA	sodium-2-mercaptoethanesulfonite
IAT	indirect antiglobulin (Coombs') test	MF	myelofibrosis [mycosis fungoides]
IBD	inflammatory bowel disease	MHC	major histocompatibility complex
IBS	irritable bowel syndrome	MI	myocardial infarction [mitral incompetence]
ICU	intensive care unit	MIBG	metaiodobenzylguanidine
IDDM	insulin-dependent diabetes mellitus	MIC	minimal inhibitory concentration
IDL	intermediate density lipoproteins	MIF	migration inhibitory factor
IEPG	immunoelectrophoretogram	min.	minutes
IF	immunofluorescence	MLC	mixed lymphocyte culture
IFA	indirect fluorescent antibody	MND	motor neuron disease
IFN	interferon	MOPP	*mustine* (nitrogen mustard), *Oncovin* (vincristine), *procarbazine, prednisone*
Ig	immunoglobulin		
IGF-1	insulin-like growth factor I (somatomedin C)	6-MP	6-mercaptopurine
IHC	idiopathic hemochromatosis	MR	mitral regurgitation
IHD	ischemic heart disease	MRC	Medical Research Council (UK)
IL-1	interleukin-1	MRI	magnetic resonance imaging
IM(I)	intramuscular (injection)	mRNA	messenger RNA
INH	isoniazid	MRSA	methicillin-resistant *Staph. aureus*
INR	international normalized (coagulation) ratio	MS	mitral stenosis [multiple sclerosis]
IP	interphalangeal (joint) [intraperitoneal]	MSU	midstream urine (specimen)
iPTH	immunoreactive parathyroid hormone	MTP	metatarsophalangeal (joint)
IQ	intelligence quotient	MVAC	methotrexate, vinblastine, doxorubicin, cisplatin
ITP	idiopathic thrombocytopenic purpura		
ITT	insulin tolerance test	MVP	mitral valve prolapse
IUD	intrauterine device	N	normal
IV(I)	intravenous (injection)	NADH	nicotinamide
IV	interventricular	Na$^+$	sodium
IVC	inferior vena cava	NAP	neutrophil alkaline phosphatase (score)
IVP	intravenous pyelogram	NB	note well
JCA	juvenile chronic arthritis	NBT	nitroblue tetrazolium
JVP	jugular venous pressure	NHL	non-Hodgkin's lymphoma
K$^+$	potassium	NMR	nuclear magnetic resonance
LAHB	left anterior hemiblock	NP59	^{131}I-6-β-iodomethyl-19-norcholesterol
LBBB	left bundle branch block	NSAIDs	non-steroidal antiinflammatory drugs
LCAT	lecithin-choline acetyltransferase	NSU	non-specific (-gonococcal) urethritis
LDL	low-density lipoprotein	OA	osteoarthritis

OC	oral contraceptive
OCG	oral cholecystogram
OPSI	overwhelming post-splenectomy infection
OX (2, 19)	Weil–Felix reactions
P_2	pulmonary component of second heart sound
PA	pernicious anemia
PA	posteroanterior
PABA	para-aminobenzoic acid
$PaCO_2$	arterial partial pressure of carbon dioxide
PAN	polyarteritis nodosa
PaO_2	arterial partial pressure of oxygen
PAO_2	alveolar partial pressure of oxygen
PAS	periodic acid-Schiff or p-aminosalicylic acid
PBC	primary biliary cirrhosis
PBG	porphobilinogen
PCK	polycystic kidneys
PCNA	proliferating cell nuclear antigen
PCP	phenycyclidine ('angel dust')
PCR	polymerase chain reaction
PCT	porphyria cutanea tarda
PCV	packed cell volume (hematocrit)
PCWP	pulmonary capillary wedge pressure
PDA	patent ductus arteriosus
PDGF	platelet-derived growth factor
PEEP	positive end-expiratory pressure (ventilation)
PEFR	peak expiratory flow rate
PERLA	pupils equal, react to light and accommodation
PGI_2	prostacyclin
Ph^1	Philadelphia (chromosome)
PHA	phytohemagglutinin
PI	prothrombin index (see INR)
PICA	posterior inferior cerebellar artery (lateral medullary) syndrome
PIP	proximal interphalangeal joint
PiZZ	phenotype for homozygous α_1AT deficiency
PMR	polymyalgia rheumatica
PNH	paroxysmal nocturnal hemoglobinuria
p.o.	orally
PR	per rectum [progesterone receptor]
p.r.n.	as necessary
PRV	polycythemia rubra vera
PS	pulmonary stenosis
PT	prothrombin time
PTC	percutaneous transhepatic cholangiogram
PTCA	percutaneous transluminal coronary angioplasty
PTH	parathyroid hormone
PTTK	partial thromboplastin time (with kaolin)
PTU	propylthiouracil
PUO	pyrexia (fever) of unknown origin
PUVA	psoralens/ultraviolet light (UV-A wavelength)
PVB	cis-platin, vinblastine, bleomycin
q (4 h)	every (4 hours)
q.i.d.	four times daily
$Q\text{-}T_c$	corrected Q-T interval
q.v.	which see (i.e. discussed elsewhere)
RA	rheumatoid arthritis or right atrium
RBBB	right bundle branch block
RBC	red blood cell
RBF	renal blood flow

RDW	red-cell distribution width (measure of anisocytosis)
REM	rapid eye movement
RF	rheumatoid factor
RIA	radioimmunoassay
RNA	ribonucleic acid
RNP	ribonucleoprotein
RPGN	rapidly progressive glomerulonephritis
RPR	rapid plasma reagin (syphilis test)
RSV	respiratory syncytial virus
RTA	renal tubular acidosis or road traffic accident
RV	right ventricle
R_x	treatment
SAP	serum alkaline phosphatase
SBE	subacute bacterial endocarditis
SC	subcutaneous
SCA	sickle-cell anemia
SCC	squamous cell carcinoma
SCID	severe combined immunodeficiency
SCLC	small-cell lung cancer
sec	seconds
SHBG	sex hormone binding globulin
SIADH	syndrome of inappropriate ADH secretion
SLE	systemic lupus erythematosus
Sm	Smith (antigen, antibody)
spp..	species
SRS-A	slow-reacting substance of anaphylaxis
ssDNA	single-stranded DNA
SSPE	subacute sclerosing panencephalitis
SSRI	selective serotonin uptake inhibitor
SVC	superior vena cava
SVT	supraventricular tachycardia
SXR	skull X-ray
$t^{1/2}$	half-life
T2–12	thoracic vertebrae nos 2–12
TB	tuberculosis
TBG	thyroid-binding globulin
Tc	technetium (^{99m}Tc = isotopic Tc)
TC	transcobalamin
TCC	transitional cell carcinoma
t.d.s.	thrice daily
TdT	terminal deoxytransferase
TF	transferrin
TFTs	thyroid function tests
TG	triglyceride
6-TG	6-thioguanine
TGB	thyroglobulin
T_H	helper T cell
THC	total hemolytic complement or tetrahydrocannabinol
TI	tricuspid incompetence
TIA	transient ischemic attack
TIBC	total iron-binding capacity
TLC	total lung capacity
TMJ	temporomandibular joint
TNF	tumor necrosis factor
TNM	tumor/nodes/metastases (staging system)
tPA	tissue plasminogen activator
TPHA	treponema pallidum hemagglutination
TPI	treponema pallidum immobilization (test)
TPN	total parenteral nutrition
TRH	thyrotrophin-releasing hormone
T_s	suppressor T cell
TSH	thyroid-stimulating hormone (thyrotrophin)

TSI	thyroid-stimulating immunoglobulin		VIP	vasoactive intestinal peptide
TT	thrombin time		VLDL	very low density lipoprotein
TTP	thrombotic thrombocytopenic purpura		VP	variegate porphyria
TURP	transurethral resection of the prostate		V/Q	ventilation perfusion
TXA$_2$	thromboxane A$_2$		VSD	ventricular septal defect
U2 (-6)	spliceosomal molecules		VT	ventricular tachycardia
UDP	uridine diphosphate		VWD	von Willebrand's disease
UMN	upper motor neuron		VWF	von Willebrand factor
URTI	upper respiratory tract infection		WAS	Wiskott–Aldrich syndrome
UTI	urinary tract infection		WBC	white blood cell
UV	ultraviolet		WCC	white cell count
VC	vital capacity		WDLL	well-differentiated lymphocytic lymphoma
V$_D$	volume of distribution			
VD	venereal disease		WPW	Wolff–Parkinson–White (syndrome)
VDRL	Venereal Disease Research Laboratory (test)		WR	Wassermann reagent (test)
VEB	ventricular ectopic (premature) beat		XD	X-linked dominant
VER	visual evoked response		XR	X-linked recessive
VF	ventricular fibrillation		ZES	Zollinger–Ellison syndrome